The Neuropsychology
of Attention

CRITICAL ISSUES IN NEUROPSYCHOLOGY

Series Editors

Antonio E. Puente
University of North Carolina, Wilmington

Cecil R. Reynolds
Texas A&M University

Current Volumes in this Series

AGING AND NEUROPSYCHOLOGICAL ASSESSMENT
Asenath La Rue

✗ BRAIN MECHANISMS IN PROBLEM SOLVING AND INTELLIGENCE:
A Lesion Survey of the Rat Brain
Robert Thompson, Francis M. Crinella, and Jen Yu

BRAIN ORGANIZATION OF LANGUAGE AND COGNITIVE PROCESSES
Edited by Alfredo Ardila and Feggy Ostrosky-Solis

HANDBOOK OF CLINICAL CHILD NEUROPSYCHOLOGY
Edited by Cecil R. Reynolds and Elaine Fletcher-Janzen

HANDBOOK OF HEAD TRAUMA: Acute Care to Recovery
Edited by Charles J. Long and Leslie K. Ross

HANDBOOK OF NEUROPSYCHOLOGICAL ASSESSMENT:
A Biopsychosocial Perspective
Edited by Antonio E. Puente and Robert J. McCaffrey

NEUROPSYCHOLOGICAL EVALUATION OF THE SPANISH SPEAKER
Alfredo Ardila, Monica Rosselli, and Antonio E. Puente

NEUROPSYCHOLOGICAL FUNCTION AND BRAIN IMAGING
Edited by Erin D. Bigler, Ronald A. Yeo, and Eric Turkheimer

✗ NEUROPSYCHOLOGY, NEUROPSYCHIATRY, AND BEHAVIORAL
NEUROLOGY
Rhawn Joseph

THE NEUROPSYCHOLOGY OF ATTENTION
Ronald A. Cohen

THE NEUROPSYCHOLOGY OF EPILEPSY
Edited by Thomas L. Bennett

RELIABILITY AND VALIDITY IN NEUROPSYCHOLOGICAL
ASSESSMENT
Michael D. Franzen

A Continuation Order Plan is available for this series. A continuation order will bring delivery
of each new volume immediately upon publication. Volumes are billed only upon actual ship-
ment. For further information please contact the publisher.

The Neuropsychology of Attention

Ronald A. Cohen
University of Massachusetts Medical School
Worcester, Massachusetts

In collaboration with
Yvonne A. Sparling-Cohen
Department of Youth Services
Boston, Massachusetts

and

Brian F. O'Donnell
Harvard Medical School
Boston, Massachusetts

Plenum Press • New York and London

Library of Congress Cataloging-in-Publication Data

Cohen, Ronald A., 1955-
    The neuropsychology of attention / Ronald A. Cohen.
        p.   cm. -- (Critical issues in neuropsychology)
    Includes bibliographical references and index.
    ISBN 0-306-43953-0
    1. Attention. 2. Neuropsychology.   I. Title. II. Series.
    [DNLM: 1. Attention--physiology. 2. Neuropsychology.   BF 321
C678n]
QP405.C715   1992
153.7'33--dc20
DNLM/DLC
for Library of Congress   92-49607
                                                               CIP

ISBN 0-306-43953-0

© 1993 Plenum Press, New York
A Division of Plenum Publishing Corporation
233 Spring Street, New York, N.Y. 10013

Printed in the United States of America

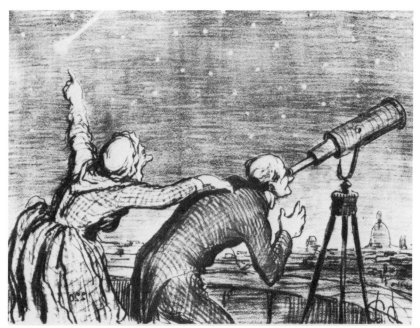

An unfortunate case of "hemispatial" inattention.

("*M. Babinet prévenu par sa portière de la visite de la comête.*" From *Le Charivari*, 1858, by Honoré Daumier. Babcock Bequest; Courtesy of Museum of Fine Arts, Boston, Massachusetts.)

Foreword

As you read this, you are probably unaware of how your left foot feels in your shoe. Although your brain was receiving sensory input from this foot, you were not aware of your foot because you were reading and not attending to it. However, this discussion led you to move your attention to your left foot and to become aware of it. When I was a medical student, I saw a patient who was unaware of both the left side of his body and the left side of his environment. Unlike people in normal health, who when instructed can become aware of the left side of the body, this patient could not be made aware of his left arm or the left side of his environment. The patient's defect was so profound that despite being hungry he was unaware of food on the left side of his tray and did not recognize that his left arm belonged to him. This left-sided body and spatial unawareness could not be accounted for by a primary sensory defect.

Although I knew that this man suffered from a large right-hemisphere stroke, I did not know the brain mechanisms that accounted for this profound example of unawareness. It was not until I had almost completed my neurology training in 1969 that I was able to return to this problem. At that time, most neuropsychological research was directed at understanding the language disorders associated with brain disease. There was almost no research on the neuropsychology of awareness and unawareness. Our early research reports on the neuroanatomical basis of neglect were met with open hostility. Not only did the proposal we submitted to the National Institutes of Health go unfunded, but the reviewer stated that if we ever discovered any new and interesting findings, it would certainly be serendipitous. Fortunately, about the same time that we started our research on attentional disorders, other laboratories were also initiating research in this area. For example, in 1970 Kinsbourne explained his hyperactive hemisphere bias hypothesis of neglect to the American Neurological Association.

Since that time, the number of excellent research articles dealing with neglect, awareness, and inattention has increased geometrically. Whereas in the 1960s there were only three groups conducting research on neglect and related disorders, today there are productive research groups throughout the United States. Almost every western European country has a research group performing research in this area and several countries such as England and Italy have multiple groups. In the past several years, investigators in Asian countries have also initiated research in this area and have published many excellent papers.

Currently, there are so many excellent research articles being published that, despite being an avid reader, I have difficulty keeping abreast of all of the advances related to the neuropsychology of attention. That is why I was so pleased that Dr. Cohen decided to write a book that summarized many of these advances. Dr. Cohen's book does more than summarize advances in the neuropsychology of attention. A summary would only describe the pieces of the puzzle; this book helps to put the puzzle together. Although the entire puzzle remains to be solved, only when the pieces are put together can one see what areas remain to be explored. Therefore, this book is more than a summary: it is a synthesis.

There are many methods by which one may study attention and attentional disorders. Physiologists have studied attention using single-cell recording, evoked potentials, and most recently neurophysiological imaging; cognitive psychologists have developed information processing models; and neuropsychologists and behavioral neurologists have attempted to fractionate behavior, test brain processing models, and discover the brain structures that support these modular functions. Cohen and his coauthors do a superb job of integrating the cognitive, physiological, and anatomical approaches to attention and attentional disorders.

The Neuropsychology of Attention is rather unique in its emphasis, as it is one of the few books in the field of neuropsychology that deals exclusively with the topic of attention. Not only does the book consider neuropsychological findings regarding the mechanisms underlying attention; it frames current knowledge regarding the neuropsychology of attention in the context of theoretical and empirical information regarding attention derived from other scientific disciplines. The book concludes with a consideration of neurobehavioral constraints on attention imposed by temporal and spatial dynamics, information processing speed, memory-attentional interactions, and the characteristics of neural systems. Cohen develops a unified theoretical framework and a comprehensive taxonomy for the neuropsychological analysis of attention that is a synthesis of this knowledge. This synthesis enables readers to obtain a better understanding of what has been accomplished in the field of attention and attentional disorders and allows readers to see what must be done in the future.

Kenneth H. Heilman

Gainesville, Florida

Preface

At the beginning of this project, I was struck by several paradoxes regarding the study of attentional phenomena within neuropsychology. On one hand, the concept of attention has been central to the historical development of psychology. Attention was considered a fundamental and inescapable aspect of human experience by Wilhelm Wundt, William James, and the other founders of modern psychology. On the other hand, for much of the 20th century, psychologists tried desperately to avoid acknowledging the need for an attentional construct. Because attention has an intangible quality and cannot be specified as a unitary process, many behavioral scientists considered the construct of attention theoretically incoherent. Some of their concerns regarding the nature of attentional phenomena were clearly justified. It is also apparent, however, that explanations of behavior and cognition that fail to account for attentional phenomena cannot fully capture human experience.

Recently, there has been a shift in zeitgeist, and attention has received more favorable treatment within the cognitive neurosciences. Humans cannot handle an infinite amount of simultaneous information. Therefore, cognitive processes must exist that direct our focus to information that is important, and that permit the selection of stimuli and responses from the large universe of alternatives. Regardless of whether one advocates the existence of a discrete attentional process, it is necessary to account for the occurrence of those phenomena that we normally label as aspects of attention. Consideration of the mechanisms underlying the selection of information and the control of stimulus and response processes is critical if we hope to understand human cognitive experience.

The necessity of studying the mechanisms underlying attentional phenomena is particularly evident within neuropsychology. Patients with brain disorders frequently do not perform at optimal levels, even when task variables are held constant. They may fail to detect an object in the environment, even though it can be demonstrated that they have adequate perceptual capability. Reference to performance deficits stemming from attentional dysfunction is common in clinical neuropsychology, though historically, few systematic approaches have been developed for assessing attention. Recently, this situation has begun to change, as greater effort has been expended in both developing methodologies for evaluating attention and understanding the brain mechanisms underlying attentional control and selection. Yet there continues to be a lack of coherence among concepts, models, and theories of attention, or the methodological approaches to the study of attentional phenomena.

This text attempts to provide a more systematic and integrated theoretical framework for the neuropsychology of attention. To accomplish this goal, it was first necessary to consider a large quantity of theoretical and empircal information regarding the phenomenology of attention for the many disciplines within psychology and the neurosciences. Because historically there has been relatively little exchange among these different disciplines, it was important to establish the features common to all approaches to the study of attention. Unless there is consistency in the constructs used to characteirze attention, a scientific analysis of attentional phenomena is impossible. With the establishment of a coherent conceptual framework, it is more feasible to consider the neural mechanisms underlying attentional processes. Information regarding the cognitive, behavioral, and neural bases of attention can then be more systematically applied to neuropsychological studies of brain dysfunction.

With these goals in mind, this text provides a synthesis of theories, concepts, and experimental findings regarding the neuropsychology of attention. The book is divided into three parts. Part I reviews the basic concepts necessary to neuropsychological considerations of attention. Several broad domains of theoretical and experimental information of relevance to the study of attention are addressed: (1) information-processing models; (2) alternative nonsensory models; (3) behavioral theories of attention; and (4) psychophysiological and neurophysiological evidence regarding the nature and mechanisms of attention. There has been little previous integration of attentional concepts developed from these different domains, although this is not altogether surprising when one considers the different scientific and philosophical perspectives that each represents. An attempt is made to present the strengths and weaknesses of each of these approaches, and to develop a more unified conceptual framework regarding the cognitive, behavioral, and neural mechanisms of attention. At the end of Part I, a theoretical framework of attention is presented that is applied to subsequent discussions of the neuropsychology of attention.

In Part II, this theoretical attentional framework is considered with regard to neuropsychological disturbances of attention. Consideration of the effect of brain damage on attention provides an important means of assessing the role of particular neural structures in mediating attention. The discussion here is not meant to be an exhaustive review of all neuropsychological data pertaining to attentional dysfunction in neurological and psychiatric disorders. Instead, the reader is introduced to several different neuropsychological perspectives on attention. In the first two chapters, the neuroanatomical systems involved in attentional control are discussed with consideration of the effect of localized lesions. Because there are extensive experimental data from studies of animal behavior, these chapters consider both human and laboratory animal studies of attention. The two subsequent chapters of Part II discuss how specific neurological diseases and psychiatric disorders affect attention. This discussion is followed by a consideration of the neuropsychological assessment of attention; covering both neuropsychological and more traditional psychological methods of evaluating attentional dysfunction. Experimental methods developed from information-processing approaches are also described. The final chapter of Part II describes several important neuropsychological models of attention. These models are distinguished from those described in Part I in that they are derived largely from studies of the effects of lesions on human attention. At the end of this chapter, a comprehensive neuropsychological taxonomy of attention is proposed.

Attention is determined by the interactive influence of multiple neural systems in response to incoming information from the environment. Characterization of the neurobehavioral bases of attention requries that the neural, behavioral, and physical parameters underlying attentional processes be specified. Part III departs from clinical neuropsychology to consider factors that must be examined if one hopes to specify the neuropsychological parameters underlying attention. These factors place constraints on human attention. We begin with a discussion of the relationship among consciousness, self-awareness, and attention. We then consider structural constraints on attention, including (1) processing speed; (2) memory–attention interactions; (3) the temporal dynamics of attention; (4) the spatial representation of attention; and (5) constraints imposed by the characteristics of neural systems. These five structural factors influence the capacity of humans to perform attentional operations. We also discuss computational methods and their application to the study of attention. This chapter is not meant to be an exhaustive review of current neural computational theories; rather, it is a consideration of the utility of this approach for neuropsychology. These computational models provide a formal theoretical system for the analysis of specific theories of attention and provide a test for the attentional processes within a neuropsychological framework. In the final chapter, a theoretical synthesis of the cognitive, behavioral, and neural mechanisms underlying the phenomena of attention is provided, and our neuropsychologial taxonomy of attention is reexamined in light of this synthesis.

In the past few years, we have witnessed explosive growth in the field of cognitive neuroscience, including an increased interest in the neural bases of attention. In fact, I have been impressed by the increased level of interest in the neuropsychology of attention, and by the efforts of many investigators to establish a clearer foundation for attentional research. In the future, we will undoubtedly see even greater cohesiveness of the concepts and methods used in the study of attention. I hope that this text will facilitate these efforts.

Ronald A. Cohen

Acknowledgments

This book would not have been possible without the support and efforts of Yvonne Sparling-Cohen, my wife, friend, and colleague. She made many suggestions, contributed to the writing of several chapters, and reviewed and edited the entire manuscript.

Several other people were instrumental in bringing this project to fruition. I am deeply indebted to them for their contribution and support. Many of the ideas in this book resulted from hours of discussion with my colleague, Brian O'Donnell. He contributed to and aided in the writing throughout the book and made major contributions to the chapters dealing with information processing theory, psychophysiology of attention, neuropsychological disorders of attention, and the assessment of attention.

Elliott Albers, whose friendship and approach to neuroscience helped to inspire this project, also reviewed early versions of the manuscript and provided useful input. Marc Fisher provided his support and neurological expertise throughout various stages of the project. Thanks also go to Richard Kaplan for our many hours of discussion, which helped to consolidate my ideas and provided a great source of enjoyment.

The writing of this book was facilitated by my collaboration with many friends, colleagues, and teachers. I am particularly grateful to Kenneth Heilman for his thoughtful review of the text, his valuable insights, and his inspiration to pursue the neuropsychological study of attention. Thanks also go to the other members of the neuropsychology faculty at the University of Florida, including Eileen Fennell, Edward Valenstein, Robert Watson, Russell Bauer, and Dawn Bowers; and to the neuropsychology faculty of the Neuropsychiatric Institute at UCLA Medical Center, including Asenath La Rue and Paul Satz. I am also grateful to Mieke Verfaellie and Howard Kessler for reviewing sections of the text. William Waters, who chaired my doctoral dissertation, was an important influence on my initial research of the psychophysiological correlates of attention. Chizuko Izawa, Seth Kunen, Arthur Rioppelle, and James May, my teachers during my early years of graduate study, provided me with a foundation in the cognitive sciences.

I also thank Michael Feuerstein who helped initiate this project and Eliot Werner who helped to make this book a reality. Special thanks go to Sue Woolford and the editorial staff at Plenum Publishing who brought the book to fruition.

Contents

I

Foundations of Attention

1

Introduction

Attention is a cognitive experience that is subjectively evident to each of us but is difficult to characterize. We are all aware of what attention is: the focusing of our inner resources and state of consciousness. The term *attention* is part of our everyday vocabulary. As children, we were instructed by our teachers to "pay attention." The television bombards us with information, soliciting our attention. In the military, a sergeant will order troops to "come to attention." The athlete who performs suboptimally may attribute the poor performance to lack of concentration. The construct of attention is used to account for a wide range of behavioral phenomena.

The use of the term *attention* to refer to a diverse set of behavioral phenomena led some behavioral scientists to conclude that attention is theoretically incoherent. Because attention describes many different behavioral and cognitive processes, it cannot be considered a unitary entity. Should attention then be considered a process at all? *Attention* may simply be a useful term that helps us to classify behavior, but that has little explanatory power. Is there, then, technical justification for the construct of attention? These types of questions regarding the scientific necessity of an attentional construct have some merit.

Attention is not a unitary process; rather, the term refers to a class of behavioral and cognitive processes that produce discernible effects. Just as conditioning is the by-product of other primary processes with more basic neurobiological mechanisms, so attention is comprised of smaller elements. Therefore, the multifactorial character of attention is not in its own right grounds for dismissing the construct of attention. Although attention cannot be reduced to a single neurobehavioral event, attentional processes account for an important aspect of behavior.

Attentional processes facilitate cognitive and behavioral performance in several ways. Attention serves to reduce the amount of information (the number of stimuli) to receive additional processing by the brain. At other times, attention enables a larger amount of information to receive additional processing. Humans are constantly flooded with an infinite number of signals from both outside and within. Attention frames this input with regard to the available capacity of the individual. Metaphorically, attention is like the aperture and lens system of a camera. By changing the depth of field and the focal point, attention enables humans to direct themselves to appropriate aspects of external environmental events and internal operations. Attention facilitates the selection of salient information and the allocation of cognitive processing appropriate to that information. Therefore, attention acts as a gate for information flow in the brain.

Attention directs behavior with reference to the spatial and temporal characteristics of the situation. As information quantity is reduced, the temporal-spatial frame of reference from which the information was selected is focused, and other temporal-spatial regions are deemphasized. Therefore, attention has often been thought of as a "spotlight" that illuminates certain areas, thereby enhancing performance in those areas. Because attention is the by-product of an array of processes, investigation of the neuropsychology of attention requires that we first consider the behavioral characteristics of attention. The behavioral and cognitive processes that constitute attention must be specified before we can hope to understand the neural bases of attention. A number of different types or conditions of attention have been described in the psychological literature over the years. These types include focused, selective, directed, divided, sustained, effortful, controlled, automatic, and voluntary attention. Other phenomena related to attention have also been described, such as concentration, vigilance, orientation, executive control, intention, and search. Experiential states associated with attentional processes have occasionally been labeled as *consciousness* and *awareness*. Ineffective attention is often associated with inattention, fatigue, distractibility, confusion, impersistence, neglect, or discontrol. Though the nomenclature associated with attention is sometimes unwieldy, it bespeaks the complexity and centrality of attention to behavioral experience.

MANIFESTATIONS OF ATTENTION

Perhaps the easiest way to characterize the varieties of attention that have been most commonly described is by describing situations in which they are evident. Attentional behaviors vary as a function of the task demands. Therefore, we will consider several behavioral situations that illustrate different attentional manifestations.

Focused Attention

The term *focused attention* refers to the essential aspect of attention that we described before: the amount of information selected at a given time relative to the temporal-spatial constraints of the situation. There are numerous examples of focused attention. When we attempt to solve a complex mathematical equation, we direct concentrated effort toward various solutions. A chess player's ability to come up with effective moves depends on an ability to focus in this way.

Selective Attention

The term *selective attention* refers to an aspect of attention that is highly related to focus. Selection is the process by which some informational elements are given priority over others. When we listen to the radio for a particular song, we exhibit selective attention. Selection always occurs relative to a temporal-spatial frame of reference. Even if we do not have an *a priori* basis for selection, our attention is directed by events in our environmental frame. If while driving we see a police car's flashing light in the distance, our attention is likely to be pulled to the spatial location of that stimulus.

Divided Attention

In reality, attention is always subject to division among a multitude of processes and potential stimuli. A teenager who does homework while watching television is engaging in divided attention. Signal detection research has devoted much effort to establishing the relationship between signals and noise, as well as among multiple sources of information. As we will discuss later, the debate has focused on whether attention to multiple sources at one time is possible. Divided attention is difficult because of *interference* created by the competing stimuli. Although evidence now suggests that people have some capacity for simultaneous divided attention, this capacity is fairly limited. As the number of simultaneous information sources increases, attentional performance declines markedly when the task requirements are demanding. The quality of performance on multiple simultaneous tasks depends on how automatic the tasks are. For instance, some typists are able to talk or carry on with other activities while they type. In such cases, typing ability has become very automatized. The distinction between *automatic* and *controlled* processes has been the subject of much research since the early 1980s.

Sustained Attention

The term *sustained attention* refers to the fact that attentional performance varies as a function of the temporal characteristics of the task. When a task requires attentional persistence over a relatively long time, it is said to demand *sustained attention*. The performance of a long-duration task places additional processing demands on the system. Sustained attention may tax an individual for very different reasons than short-duration tasks that require the detection of a stimulus among a multitude of distractors. Some types of sustained attention require high levels of *vigilance*, but few responses. For instance, a building guard may spend an entire night watching for intruders, although none may appear. Attention to such low-frequency events has different processing requirements from responses to high-frequency events in the short duration. The guard is confronted with a host of temporal factors such as sustained motivation level, *fatigue*, and boredom.

Effortful Attention

Some types of attention are much more effortful than others. Generally, tasks that require controlled processing require greater effort. Such tasks are also more apt to demand conscious awareness.

Furthermore, the effortful demands of tasks influence the capacity to perform multiple tasks. This is obvious even in cases of extreme physical exertion. It is not difficult to listen to a radio while engaging in moderate physical exercise like walking. However, it becomes increasingly difficult to maintain attentional focus when extreme physical exertion is required. At such times, people become increasingly aware of the signals being given out by the body (e.g., a pounding heart beat), so that giving continued attention to other information becomes impossible. Such interference effects due to effortful demands are evident in more subtle neuropsychological tasks that require motor performance along with a secondary activity (e.g., word generation).

Intention and Directed Attention

Attention is normally thought of as a process that prepares the individual for optimal sensory intake, analysis, and integration. Yet response-based factors play a significant role in governing the other attentional processes that we have discussed. Usually, attentional selection occurs relative to response demands. When confronted with numerous response alternatives, we direct our behavior to obtain information that will provide the best result. Although sensory selection may be elicited by the characteristics of the stimuli that are bombarding our senses, more often than not it is the product of a planned, goal-directed course of action. Volition has always been a controversial construct, so that there is usually reluctance to use concepts like *voluntary attention*. Yet it is clear that, in many situations, attentional behavior is generated as part of an *intention* to act.

Humans often generate a large number of covert response alternatives, which they test either overtly or through covert cognitive operations. These response intentions influence the value placed on certain stimuli and, in turn, affect the direction of attention. The act of *looking* is, in its own right, an intentional behavior. For instance, hunters who go into the woods looking for prey use a wide range of tracking behaviors that may increase the likelihood of finding an animal. The hunters' intentions guide their overt and covert responses and ultimately prime their level of vigilance to their target.

Some theorists may argue that we should not consider *intention* and behavior associated with response production attentional processes because to do so dilutes the construct of attention. If the goal is to specify one molecular process that we can call attention, it may be unwise to link *attention* and *intention*. However, if *attention* refers to a class of behavioral phenomena in accordance with our previous discussion, then both sensory attention and response intention should be considered aspects of attention. Certainly, both factors need to be accounted for in considerations of the mechanisms underlying attention.

CONSTRAINTS ON ATTENTION

Attentional performance is influenced either directly or indirectly by a number of factors that may not be considered aspects of attention in their own right, but that affect attentional capacity. Some of the factors that put constraint on the processes of attention are described below. Greater detail is given to these factors in Part III of this text.

Neural Constraints

The organization of the brain and the characteristics of neural activity clearly influence the properties of attention. On one level, this fact is obvious, though many cognitive theories completely ignore the nature of brain organization when considering mechanisms of attention. There is still much to be learned about how neural structure and function mediate attentional operations.

Processing Speed and Resources

The speed at which operations can be performed in the brain is a rate-limiting factor for some aspects of attentional performance. This fact has led to chronometric analyses of attention. Although the issues surrounding processing speed are complex, it is clear that there are some boundaries on attention that are created by the time required by certain cognitive events (e.g., the time required to move a finger after initial cortical activation). However, the exact parameters underlying processing speed, capacity limitations, and resources still require much investigation.

Memory and Attention

The characteristics of memory encoding, storage, and retrieval have great bearing on attention. Some investigators have viewed attention as being synonymous with short-term memory. Cognitive scientists have addressed this relationship, though the neural relationship of these two classes of processes requires much more research.

Spatial-Temporal Constraints

External reality is represented in our experience in a temporal and spatial organization. Therefore, the way time and space are organized in behavior, cognition, and brain is of great importance in considerations of attention. Attention is a process that is both temporally and spatially distributed. We attend against the backdrop of a temporal and spatial representation of our experience. We direct focus to certain spatial positions in order to make selections. Furthermore, time constrains our ability to select optimal targets consistently. Therefore, consideration of the temporal and spatial parameters should be essential to the study of attention.

Consciousness, Awareness, and Self-Directed Attention

The nature of consciousness and awareness has been central to the philosophies of many of the great thinkers of history. Yet, for the behavioral sciences, these constructs have generally been an enigma. With the reemergence of scientific interest in attention, there has been a need to consider these difficult concepts. Within many of the early cognitive theories, awareness was a necessary condition for attention. In fact, attention allowed for limited access to awareness. However, there is now evidence that not all attentional processes require awareness. The interrelationship of consciousness, awareness, and attention is only beginning to be considered by modern cognitive neuroscientists.

A UNIFIED NEUROPSYCHOLOGICAL MODEL OF ATTENTION

Given the convergence of information regarding the behavioral, cognitive, and neural bases of attention, it is now possible to generate a comprehensive model of attention. Obviously, such a model must be consistent with the available neuropsychological evidence regarding normal and abnormal states of brain functioning. In this text, we will build the case that attention depends on a minimum of four neurobehavioral factors: (1) sensory selection; (2) response selection and control; (3) factors that influence attentional capacity; and (4) factors that mediate sustained performance.

These four factors are not orthogonal, as they may share common neural mechanisms. However, they are distinct in that they are evident in different task situations, and also because each is most strongly influenced by particular sets of component processes. The component processes that contribute to each factor will be discussed in greater detail later. For now, we will simply list the most important component processes.

Sensory Selection

Attentional control initially occurs during relatively early stages of information processing, before the development of response intentions. Three related component processes appear to be involved in early sensory selection: *filtering*, *focusing*, and *automatic shifting*. The earliest form of selection occurs as a result of filtering mechanisms that are tuned to particular featural characteristics. Subsequently, attentional focusing is accomplished in higher order sensory systems that interact with motivational and response-mediational influences. The neural response of these sensory systems is either "enhanced" or "inhibited" by expectancies or information that primes attention. Automatic shifting of attention can occur as a result of focusing, in conjunction with the orienting response, which is controlled by habituation and sensitization.

Response Selection

Although early attentional selection is possible, attending is normally influenced by the response demands associated with a situation. Four component processes appear to be critical in selective response control: *response intention, initiation and inhibition, active switching, and executive supervisory control*. These component processes are interdependent and hierarchical. Intentionality, response initiation, and inhibition contribute to the capacity for active switching and executive control. These processes are largely under the influence of anterior brain systems located in the premotor and prefrontal cortex.

Active switching differs from automatic shifts of attention associated with the orienting response, as it involves an exploratory search of the environment. Looking and other observing behavior are the behavioral expression of active attentional switching.

Attentional Capacity

Humans have a limited attentional capacity. We cannot process an infinite amount of information simultaneously. Therefore, it is necessary to characterize those factors that limit attentional performance. In the course of this text, two kinds of general factors will be described that influence attentional capacity: *structural* and *energetic*.

The attentional constraints that we mentioned earlier are some of the structural factors that influence capacity. Structural capacity is limited by the constraints of memory, neural processing speed, the nature of temporal-spatial representation, and other neural system characteristics that influence how much information can be processed at one time. These factors combine to affect the global attentional *resources* of the individual.

In addition to these structural factors, there are energetic factors that reflect the short-term capacity of the system: *arousal* and *effort*. Although the concept of arousal has been troublesome for the behavioral sciences, it is clear that the brain contains activating systems that set a general energetic tone for the system. Though imprecise, the term *arousal* characterizes this energetic state. Effort is another energetic factor that reflects the momentary disposition of the individual toward a task. The level of effort is governed by multiple factors, including reinforcement-motivational influences.

Sustained Performance

An important aspect of attention is that it accounts for variability in performance over time. Sustained attention represents the end product of all of the other factors that we have mentioned. However, it should be considered a separate factor, as it characterizes the temporal distribution of these other factors. Sustained attention can be considered a function of *fatiguability* and conditions that support *vigilance*. Fatiguability may be a by-product of intrinsic biological constraints or the reinforcement contingencies associated with a situation. Vigilance is also affected by motivational factors, as well as the frequency of the targets to be detected. In addition, sustained attention is determined by the sensory selection, response selection, and capacity limitations that we have mentioned.

NEUROPSYCHOLOGICAL FOUNDATIONS

Attentional control is the by-product of processes associated with the four factors that we have described. There is now considerable information regarding the neural mechanisms underlying these factors. Neuropsychological studies of brain dysfunction indicate that the type of attention dysfunction varies as a function of the brain systems that are damaged. Lesions in anterior areas, including the prefrontal cortex, often cause disorders of planning, intentionality, and self-regulation. Unilateral lesions in sensory association areas produce problems in the sensory selection process. Lesions in the limbic system are likely to affect attentional capacity by changing memory registration, excitatory-inhibitory behavioral control processes, and the salience assigned to the signals that are processed. Damage to lower subcortical centers often disrupts the overall energetic tone and has attentional consequences.

Even though progress has been made toward an understanding of the processes of attention, the neuropsychology of attention is still in its infancy. The development of a unified neuropsychology of attention requires an integration of information regarding the cognitive, behavioral, and neural bases of attention. In this text, we begin with a consideration of basic scientific approaches to the study of these factors (Part I). We then consider clinical and experimental neuropsychological information regarding the neural mechanisms of attention (Part II). We conclude with a consideration of the neural and behavioral constraints on attention, hoping that this may provide structure and guide future neuroscientific efforts to understand attention.

Part I provides a basis for the neuropsychological model of attention that has been described. Early sensory selection is discussed from a historical perspective in the context of information-processing theories. Attentional capacity and resources, constructs that arose from these theories, are also reviewed. We then consider attentional models that emphasize the role of response selection and premotoric factors. Effort and fatigue are analyzed with regard to response control.

After this initial review of sensory and response-based models of attention, we consider how attention is accounted for within learning theory. Behavioral theories of learning tend to emphasize the influence of reinforcement contingencies in establishing discriminative learning and behavioral control. Reinforcement provides a means by which incoming information creates salience for the animal. Several phenomena first described in learning theories have special significance in the attention process. The orienting response and habituation are among the simplest forms of attentional behavior and therefore are discussed in some detail.

The concept of attentional capacity arose from information-processing considerations and then found support in studies of the arousal and physiological correlates of cognitive phenomena. Psychophysiological evidence regarding the manifestations and mechanisms of attention are discussed in some detail. This discussion is followed by a consideration of the neuroscientific evidence regarding the neural bases of attention.

The first part of the book lays a foundation for neuropsychological considerations of attention. The four-factor model of attention that we have introduced is then considered relative to the neuropsychological evidence regarding the brain systems involved in attentional control. The final sections of the book address factors that we must account for when considering attention. These factors should be incorporated in future parametric neuropsychological approaches to the study of attention.

Attention

A Component of Information Processing

BRIAN F. O'DONNELL and RONALD A. COHEN

EARLY PSYCHOLOGICAL THEORIES OF ATTENTION

Psychology emerged as a distinct discipline from philosophy and physiology in the last half of the 19th century. In the study of the mind, psychology was distinguished from philosophy by the introduction of experimental methods borrowed from scientific disciplines, especially physics; efforts to measure and quantify mental processes; and attempts to demonstrate empirically that a hypothesized mental process was common to many people, and not confined to a single author's introspection and inference. In terms of subject matter, psychology differed from philosophy in its emphasis on attention as a central concept within the domain of consciousness. In this section, we will review the concepts of attention advanced by psychologists in the 19th and early 20th centuries: Wilhelm Wundt, Edward Titchener, William James, and W. B. Pillsbury.

Wilhelm Wundt was a founder of experimental psychology, and attention was one of his major concerns: the first chapter of his introductory psychology textbook was devoted to attention and its relation to conscious experience (Wundt, 1973). The central place of attention was based on Wundt's definition of psychology as an investigation of the facts of which we are conscious, and of the laws that govern their relations and combinations. Wundt characterized consciousness as a large "apprehended" field of sensory and mentally derived content. Attention is focused on a small area of this apprehended field, and this small area makes up the "apperceived" element, or elements, of consciousness. The more focused attention is on a particular element, the less clear the apprehended background will be. What is the maximum size of this focal area? Wundt and other investigators soon found that the maximum number of perceptual or semantic elements that could be attended to concurrently was between three and seven. Wundt felt that this represented the maximum number of disparate elements that the mind could manipulate as a whole. The degree to which an impression was enhanced by attention was indicated by its "clearness" in consciousness. Wundt's conception of attention as a focal point in a wider field of consciousness would have pervasive influence in the further development of attentional models.

Edward Titchener was a student of Wundt's from the United States, and he returned to that country to continue his psychological research. In a review of the current literature on attention, Titchener (1908) argued that all models of attention involved the concept of the enhanced clearness of attended-to sensations and ideas. On the basis of this review, Titchener proposed a two-factor process of attention: increased clearness of attended-to sensations or ideas, coupled with inhibition of other impressions or memory images. Titchener, like his colleagues, wanted to put psychological models on an empirical or experimental basis, and he discussed the determinants of the clearness of sensory events. His list of the conditions of clearness anticipated entire categories of the experimental investigation of attention that subsequently emerged in the 20th century. For this reason, we will discuss them in detail.

Titchener discussed a range of stimulus properties that could increase attentional response (clearness): the intensity of a stimulus; the sudden onset of a stimulus, or a sudden change in its properties; stimulus movement; the cessation of a stimulus; and the novelty or strangeness of a stimulus, particularly when it had a quality that compelled attention, such as pain, or of stimuli that are "intimate, worrying, wicked things. The taste of bitter, the smell of musk, the sight of yellow belong, for me, to the same category; the least trace of them fascinates me" (Titchener, 1908, p. 190). (This last passage is one of the few in which these psychologists of consciousness touched on the influence of personality and unmentionable predilections on attention. Freud went virtually uncited in turn-of-the-century discussions of psychology.)

Titchener also discussed contextual influences on attention. Stimuli were likely to be attended to when a sensation was similar to the current contents of consciousness. He proposed a law of prior entry, suggesting that the stimulus to which we are predisposed takes less time than another stimulus to produce a conscious effect. He noted that the optimal interval between a preparatory signal and a stimulus was about 1.5 seconds. (The concept of prior entry resurfaced in this century in studies of stimulus priming). Attention allows fixation on a stimulus even when it is less salient than other ongoing events. For example, a person can attend to a speaker even when the speaker's voice diminishes in volume or when the noise level in the room is louder than the speaker's voice. Finally, Titchener observed that attention was labile, constantly shifting, and that this variation in attention was central in origin, rather than due to the fatigue of sensory organs.

William James was the most influential 19th-century psychologist working in the United States. The intellectual breadth of James's magnum opus, *Principles of Psychology* (1890), is quite remarkable, in part because of the breadth of the man himself: He held academic appointments in philosophy and physiology, in addition to his work in the field of psychology. James changed his view of attention in different works, and this discussion draws on his development of attention in *The Principles of Psychology*. James, like Titchener, felt that the empiricist philosophers had avoided discussions of attention because it contradicted a central premise of empiricism. The empiricists argued that experience shaped the mind, but attention implies that experience is chosen rather than given. James defined attention as "the taking possession by the mind, in clear and vivid form, of several simultaneously possible objects or trains of thought. . . . It implies withdrawal from some thing in order to deal effectively with others" (pp. 403–404). James clearly thought of attention as an active process, almost motoric in character, with both activating and inhibiting effects on conscious content. His view of attention also included a cognitive or motivational component, as he thought that the attention we focused on an object was a function of our interest in it.

James discussed attention in terms of several dimensions: the source of the attended-to content; the source of its interest; and its active or passive character. Attended-to objects could be either sensory or ideational in origin. Interest could be due to the immediate nature of the object or derived from the object's associations. James viewed attention as having two forms: passive and active. Passive attention was considered reflexive and effortless, whereas active attention was voluntary and effortful. James thought that volitional attention could not be sustained more than a few seconds without constant effort. Effort, then, was the result of conflict of interest in the mind, for example, when we have to focus attention on an uninteresting object for a remoter reward. If this effort resulted in the object's acquiring interest in itself, then the attention would be sustained passively. He argued that attention could not be maintained on an object that did not change, unless one intellectually considered different aspects of the object to maintain interest. James considered the possibility that our inward sense of effort in directing attention was the by-product of epiphenomena, that effort merely reflected external influences acting simultaneously on the mind. Although James appears to have rejected this position, his arguments anticipated the broad behaviorist agenda of making conscious phenomena an epiphenomenal function of environmental effects.

James suggested that attention had the general effect of improving performance, making us perceive, conceive, distinguish, and remember better than otherwise. In addition, it shortened reaction time, facilitating both sensory recognition and response selection. He stressed the importance of mental set in perception: "The only things which we commonly see are those which we preperceive, and the only things which we preperceive are those which have been labeled for us, and the labels stamped into our mind" (p. 444).

James also considered the phenomenon of inattention. He cited Helmholtz's argument that we leave impressions unnoticed that do not contribute to conscious discriminations (James, p. 456). For example, if I am kneading bread, I may not notice the individual sensations that combine to let me recognize the object that I am kneading as dough. Individual sensations such as the degree and orientation of pressure on each fingertip, and the temperature of the dough, its moistness, its elasticity, and its color—all merge into a unitary percept. We attend to the object itself and ignore its individual sensory properties. We lose awareness of a sensation, then, when it becomes integrated into a larger percept or concept.

Inattention may also be brought about by redundant stimuli. Predictable or repetitive stimuli also tend to fade from consciousness (Titchener, 1908; Wundt, 1973); Ebbinghaus (1973) also noted the role of practice in reducing the consciousness of complex sensory and motoric activities. The more practiced, and therefore the more habitual, an action, the less conscious effort it takes to perform it. Eventually, it becomes difficult for persons to describe exactly what they do to carry out a well-practiced, complex activity like reading or riding a bicycle. It is a truism in sports that great players seldom become great coaches, possibly because they have lost their awareness of the details of performance that preoccupy junior or weaker players.

W. B. Pillsbury, a professor of philosophy and director of the Psychological Laboratory at the University of Michigan, wrote a book on attention (1908) that summarizes the investigations and concepts advanced in the previous century. Pillsbury adopted the concept of attention as clearness put forward by Wundt, and he stressed the involvement of attention in other psychological processes like memory, as well as its biological basis.

Pillsbury, like contemporary psychologists, linked attention to what we would call working memory. Pillsbury believed that the number of separate objects that could be attended to at once was four or five for vision and five to eight for audition, and that the duration of a single act of attention was usually between 5 and 8 seconds.

His biological speculations regarding attention were surprisingly contemporary and must be regarded as inspired speculation, given the rudimentary understanding of neurophysiology and psychophysiology at that time. He concluded that the anatomical seat of attention lay in the frontal lobes, which were association centers mediating between sensory and motor areas of the cortex. He speculated that there were two physiological processes underlying attention: reinforcement, or facilitation, and inhibition. Reinforcement, or facilitation, was the increase in activity of one nerve cell due to the activity of another, and inhibition was the opposition of two cells in their activity. He ascribed fluctuations in attention and decay of attention over time to the effects of fatigue of cortical cells and the influence of rhythmic activity from the respiratory and vasomotor centers on cortical cells. He noted the association of attentional activity to motor phenomena, such as changes in sensory organs to focus on a stimulus, widespread contraction of the voluntary muscles, and alterations in respiratory and cardiac rhythms. He also appreciated the effects of neuropathology and psychiatric disorders on attention. He concluded that degenerations of the mind were usually accompanied by weakened or deranged attention. In psychiatric illness, mania was associated with instability of attention, and paranoia or obsessions ("fixed ideas") with distorted attention.

Summary

In the 19th century, psychology had emerged as a discipline distinct from philosophy. Its distinction lay both in its methods, which supplemented philosophical reasoning with experimental tests, and in its conceptual foci. Attention was intensely discussed and investigated by the foremost psychologists of the 19th century. Combining experimental techniques, psychophysiological speculation, and self-observation, these early psychologists made remarkable progress in the characterization of attentional phenomena. They described the structural and temporal properties of attention; its activation by top-down (mental) and bottom-up (environmental) events; and its biological correlates.

Attention was thought to be a focus within the larger field of consciousness, which could be directed to a very limited number of related concepts or percepts. The number of discrete objects that could be encompassed simultaneously was found to be between three and eight. Not only was the capacity of attention finite, but the focus of attention decayed rapidly in time and was subject to constant fluctuation. Attention both enhanced attended-to conscious content and inhibited the consciousness of nonattended-to content.

Attention could be passively elicited by events, or it could be volitionally deployed. Qualities of stimuli that passively elicited attention included intensity; stimulus onset and offset; changes in the properties of a stimulus; movement; and the novelty or strangeness of a stimulus. Stimuli could also elicit attention when they were anticipated or had interest to the observer. Active attention was effortful, volitional, and of short duration. Attention showed continual fluctuation over time, in both its content and its intensity.

In addition to the mental and temporal attributes of attention, early psychologists also theorized regarding its biological basis and peripheral effects. Reinforcing and inhibitory interactions between nerve cells were felt to mediate attention. The frontal lobes were thought to be a major anatomical structure involved in the elaboration of attention. Attentional activity was noted to influence voluntary musculature and cardiac and respiratory activity. It was observed that brain damage and psychiatric disorders frequently affected attentional performance.

After these pioneering investigations of attention, attention was to disappear from psychology in the United States with the domination of behaviorism. It is only in the latter part of the 20th century that attention has regained the degree of theoretical importance that these cartographers of the mind first assigned to it.

COMMUNICATION, CONTROL, AND INFORMATION PROCESSING

In 1949, Shannon and Weaver published a book, *The Mathematical Theory of Communication*, that was to have a profound influence on experimental psychology. The book proposed that communication could be analyzed mathematically in terms of information transmission and reception. Communication was defined as all procedures by which one mind may affect another or, even more generally, as the procedures by which one mechanism affects another mechanism. This concept provided a way for psychologists to begin to mathematically characterize the interaction of mental mechanisms, and to legitimize a psychology that once again would examine the activities in the black box between stimulus and response. The following description of communication systems is adapted from Weaver's introductory chapter in *The Mathematical Theory of Communication*.

Weaver categorized communication problems into three levels:

Level A: How accurately can the symbols of communication be transmitted? (The technical problem.)

Level B: How precisely do the transmitted symbols convey the desired meaning? (The semantic problem.)

Level C: How effectively does the received meaning affect conduct in the desired way? (The effectiveness problem.)

Communication theory, as originally developed, dealt only with Level A, the accuracy with which a sender could transfer a set of signals, patterns, or symbols to a receiver. Meaning and efficacy, although obviously dependent on the accuracy of the transmission of information, did not receive direct mathematical treatment in the original formulation of communication theory. These qualities would await (and resist) formal characterization by psychologists and computer scientists.

The Communication System

Shannon and Weaver discussed the communication system in terms of a general diagram, illustrated in Figure 2.1. The information source selects a desired message from a set of messages. A transmitter changes this message into a signal that can be transmitted over a communication channel. The receiver changes the signal back into a message and transmits this message to the destination.

A conversation consists of a series of communications. Each utterance takes place in a communication system. In spoken communication, the information source is the brain, the transmitter is the anatomy of the vocal system, and the signal is a series of pressure variations that are transmitted through the channel of air. The receiver is the ear and the eighth cranial nerve, and these systems convey the message to the brain of the listener, although in a radically different physical form.

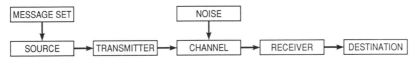

FIGURE 2.1. Shannon and Weaver's schematic of a communication system (1949), consisting of an information source, a transmitter, a communication channel, a receiver, and a destination. Adapted from Shannon & Weaver (1949).

The above describes a perfect transmission system, which, as Shannon and Weaver pointed out, is in reality always affected by noise. Noise consists of information or random distortions in the communication channel that are irrelevant to the message, and that may cause interference with accurate transmission. In the case of spoken messages, noise might consist of idiosyncratic aspects of the signal, such as an accent or a speech dysfluency, that make the message less understandable by the receiver; sources of noise in the environment, such as the noise of a construction site that two workers try to speak over; or noise introduced by defects in the receiver, such as that produced by hearing loss.

Although we have discussed a commonplace communication system that can be experienced behaviorally, communication systems may also be the information transactions within a nervous system or a mechanical system. For example, we could ask how effectively information was transmitted between different points in the brain, between working memory and long-term memory, or between the central processor of a computer and a video terminal.

Information

Information, in communication theory, is defined in a special way. Most important, information is not the same as meaning. In fact, Shannon and Weaver stressed that two messages, one meaningful and one nonsensical, can be equivalent in terms of information. Information is defined situationally by the number of messages that a sender can choose to transmit. It defines the relationship between what one does say and what one could have said. In the simplest situation, a response can be "yes" or "no." In this situation, the speaker is free to choose between two messages, and this freedom of choice is characterized by unity. In computer science or binary arithmetic, such a situation is said to contain one bit of information, which is encoded by an element that can take the values of zero and 1. The information of a situation can be mathematically expressed as the logarithm (base 2) of the number of messages that one can choose to transmit. If one can choose among 16 messages, then the information content is 2^4, and the situation is characterized by four bits of information. This mathematical description of information also defines entropy in a system, that is, the degree of randomness in a physical system. In this sense, the freedom of choice among messages is similar in its characteristics to the randomness of a physical system.

An extremely efficient message always has a maximum entropy or information value, so that the person has perfect freedom of choice in choosing the messages to transmit. In human communication by language, however, freedom of choice among the symbols of language is limited by previous choices. For example, if the first letter we choose for a word is q, it is extremely unlikely that our next choice will be anything but a u; if we choose *sh* as the first letters of a word, it is highly probable that the next letter will be a vowel; and if we choose the word *the* in a sentence, it is also probable that the next word will be a noun. This constraint of past choices on the nature of current choices is characterized as *redundancy* in communication theory. The ratio of actual entropy to maximum possible entropy in a message is called the *relative entropy* of the communication source. English has about 50% redundancy, as defined by communication theory.

Channels, Channel Capacity, and Coding

The channel by which a message is transmitted has a capacity, which limits the rate by which information can be transmitted. The channel capacity is therefore expressed as the amount of information that can be transmitted per second, and it uses bits per second as its unit.

The function of a transmitter is to encode a message, and the function of a receiver is to decode it. A central property of communication systems is that the transmission of information within a system can never exceed the capacity of the channel (C) divided by the information source output (H). Although this ratio (C/H) may be approached in communication systems, in practice optimal encoding results in longer and longer delays in the process of encoding, so that more efficient transmission of a signal extracts a cost in encoding time.

Noise and Redundancy

Redundancy may at first glance seem a negative quality: Who wants to be redundant? But in the natural world in which communication systems operate, redundancy in a message helps ensure that a message will be received accurately.

The receiver's uncertainty is a function of the information in a system: The greater the amount of information, the greater the receiver's uncertainty about which of many messages will be received. Another source of uncertainty exists, however, that degrades information content. This is the uncertainty introduced into a message by errors in transmission or by noise in the transmission channel. In order to receive a signal correctly, the receiver must subtract the spurious information added by noise from the information that is part of the original message. The effect of noise in a communication system is to increase the uncertainty of the receiver regarding the information in the message. This uncertainty due to noise is termed *equivocation*.

The relationship between these functional measures of communication can be expressed as:

$$H(x) - H_y(x) = H(y) - H_x(y)$$

where $H(x)$ is the information of the message source; $H(y)$ is the information of the received signals; $H_y(x)$ is the equivocation, or the uncertainty in the message source if the signal is known; and $H_x(y)$ the uncertainty in the received signals if the message sent is known, or the part of the received information that is due to noise. The right side of the equation is the useful information that is transmitted after the effects of noise are accounted for. The maximum rate of transmission of information (total uncertainty minus uncertainty due to noise) across a noisy channel is characterized by its capacity (C). The capacity of a channel sets the upper limit on the rate of information transmission in a system. Efficient coding may allow the actual rate to approach this limit, but it cannot be exceeded.

Because noise is a problem in natural world-communication systems, redundancy in language helps ensure accurate communication. It allows a message to be decoded even when it has been partially degraded by noise. For example, if I hear, with several sounds obscured, the sentence "I ate a —ice of can—lope," I am able by virtue of the redundancy of the English language, and my knowledge of what can be eaten, to reconstruct the original message. Therefore, in the noisy environment of natural communications, it is often advantageous to trade efficiency of communication for reliability through redundant coding.

Meaning

As Shannon and Weaver (1949) emphasized, communication theory has to do with the transmission of information from an engineering standpoint, and it generalizes across many forms of electrical and acoustical transmission systems. This model, however, does not characterize the meaning of a message, which is the realm of semantics. Weaver suggested that the general framework of the communication system could be extended to characterize semantic processing. For example, the first stage of decoding of the raw information content could be followed by another mechanism, the semantic receiver, which decodes the semantic characteristics of the message. The semantic receiver would be required to reconstruct the meaning of the original message, and somehow to resolve the ambiguities (uncertainty) inherent in any semantic communication.

Developments and Limitations

Communication theory influenced many researchers in psychology, who attempted to apply to the human mind its quantitative approach to characterizing information processing. After an initial period of optimism, it was found that information content and processing rates did not relate to human performance in a direct way (Posner, 1986). Consequently, although the models of mental processes developed from information-processing theory continued to be influential and resulted in a landmark volume by Broadbent (1958), the quantitative aspects of information processing found little place in the emergence of cognitive psychology. The failure of information content as characterized by communication theory to predict human performance can be related to Weaver and Shannon's observation that communication theory addressed only the technical problem of information transmission. The problem of how meaning is encoded and transmitted remains unsolved. The human information-processing system is probably equipped with innate structures that facilitate the processing of language and primitive visual attributes, which assists in the interpretation of information in the environment. Moreover, people continually develop new encoding and response systems, which allow the rapid processing of very complex activities, such as driving in rush hour or sight-reading music. Because of innate and acquired structures that facilitate the encoding and transmission of environmentally important information, the mathematically defined quantity of information in a stimulus has limited bearing on the speed at which it is processed, or on its demands on processing capacity in the nervous system.

PSYCHOLOGY AND INFORMATION PROCESSING

The development of communication theory in engineering had a profound impact on psychology. Since the 1920s, academic psychology in the United States had been dominated by a behavioral characterization of human and animal activity. Behavioral psychology places an emphasis on learning and observable behavior, typically associated with a reluctance to consider sensory or conceptual activities that cannot be easily related to environmental contingencies and simple motor behaviors. Communication theory, with its emphasis on the transmission of information, provided psychologists with a model that could enable investigators to theorize and test hypotheses regarding stages of information transmission within the nervous system.

Capacity, Channels, and Filters in the Human Nervous System

D. E. Broadbent's book *Perception and Communication*, first published in 1958, proved to have a seminal influence on the emerging field of the psychology of information processing and its successor, cognitive psychology. This book summarized experimental data from information-processing experiments and used them to describe mental activities and behavioral responses as components of an information-processing system. Broadbent used the communication system as a metaphor for relationships within the human nervous system: the relationship between a sensory receptor and the brain, or between the sensory system and memory, or between a perception and response generation. These relationships may all be considered communication systems. Each of these systems consists of an information source, a transmission channel or channels, and a receiver. The receiver, in turn, may function as a new transmission source. Each system may be conceptualized as a unit, and its properties may be studied by considering experimentally how different task demands affect outputs from the system, given a specific input.

The experimental data that Broadbent considered in the book are of fairly narrow range. Most of the information-processing experiments he described tested reception and response to oral speech under different conditions. The conclusions that he drew from these experiments, however, are quite sweeping.

Broadbent first noted that listening is usually a selective process, particularly listening to linguistic communications. In laboratory studies of selective listening, a subject typically heard two different messages over earphones or speakers and was required to listen to one of them and ignore (reject) the other. Choosing to listen to one message, particularly when some response is demanded, requires selection of the information source that is transmitting the relevant message, and filtering out extraneous messages. By filtering, Broadbent meant that some system in the nervous system excludes unwanted messages from further analysis, similarly to the way a radio tuner selects one channel (broadcast frequency) for amplification and excludes other broadcast frequencies.

Is this filtering of unwanted messages necessary? Can a person, with effort or learning, comprehend two messages at once? Broadbent concluded that two messages may be comprehended on simultaneous transmission if they carry little information. But as the information transmitted in these messages increases, only one can be wholly understood. After a point, increasing the amount of information transmitted does not increase the information received. This implied to Broadbent that the listener has limited *capacity*. As reviewed earlier, when the rate of information transmission exceeds the channel capacity of a system, the message will not be transmitted in its entirety. In fact, the messages involved will most likely be seriously degraded. If the information presented by the environment exceeds the capacity of the system, the system must select a limited amount of information to receive and must reject information outside this limited domain (channel). In humans, receptors provide vast amounts of information from moment to moment. Because we are unaware of much of this information in its raw form (e.g., the activity of individual pressure and heat receptors over the body), it must be filtered out completely or coded in a more succinct form before reaching awareness.

Where is this capacity limitation in the nervous system? Obviously, many sensations are received and processed in parallel by the nervous system and are transmitted across many thousands of nerve fibers. As these sensations are organized into perceptions, however, and these integrated percepts prompt responses, the capacity of the nervous system becomes more and more limited. With language, the central limit on processing is quite stringent, and typically only one extended message can be comprehended at a time. Moreover, although a person's capacity for response is limited, it does not appear that using different "channels" of response (e.g., speaking "yes" or "no" to questions asked in messages to the right ear, and writing "yes" or "no" to questions simultaneously posed to the left ear) increases the capacity to listen to more than one message at a time.

Because of this limit in capacity, the nervous system must exclude unwanted messages in order to attend to the message of interest. At the time Broadbent was writing, there was little physiological evidence of filtering. Investigators had shown that a variety of properties of speech sources could be used as cues or channels to allow a person to attend to a single speaker. These cues had to do with the physical properties of the voice, such as its gender, its spectral composition, or its position in space. Broadbent also considered evidence that semantic filters could be used by the nervous system. For example, a person's name elicits attention even if it is heard through an ignored channel. Broadbent cited results of experiments on "perceptual defense" that indicate that many people unconsciously reject or filter out words with sexual meaning.

Broadbent emphasized that the filtering of unwanted messages is not a complete rejection. A listener may notice the gender of the speaker in the rejected message; the fact that the message in the rejected channel is the same as the message in the attended channel (up to a 2- to 6-sec delay); or that the rejected message changes dramatically in spectral characteristics (e.g., from a voice message to a tone). The filtering system allows some information from an unattended-to channel to impinge on awareness, though only in a fragmentary way. Typically, these fragments are bits of the rejected message that were limited to a short duration (a few seconds). The narrative content of an extended message is always lost on the listener. Although Broadbent speculated that a person may be able to develop two higher order processing systems operating in parallel, there remains no evidence that this can be performed with auditory messages. When language reception or output occurs in different modalities, using memorized materials, or well-practiced responses, simultaneous processing can occur. James (1890) described 19th-century experiments requiring concurrent language operations, such as writing a poem while simultaneously reciting another poem. More recently, Hirst, Spelke, Reaves, Caharack, and Neisser (1980) reported that subjects can learn to read with good comprehension and simultaneously write sentences to dictation.

Immediate Memory

Can the limits on central capacity be expressed more exactly in terms of the amount of information that can be managed by a system, or the duration with which it can be held? Introspective psychologists had concluded before the turn of the century that a person could attend to only a few items at once (estimates generally ran from three to nine, depending on the type of item), and that, unless a reaction was highly practiced, only one coherent impression or thought could be considered at a time. These reports get at the heart of what has been labeled variously as *working*, *immediate*, or *short-term memory*. It is most clearly appreciated when we hear a telephone number that we need to remember until we can dial it on a phone. Most people report *rehearsing* the number mentally, repeating it over and over again, or visualizing the series of digits, until they can get to a phone and call the number. If interrupted during the rehearsal of a string of numbers by a question that requires a thoughtful response, a person often forgets the string of numbers, a finding indicating that it was stored in some impermanent form in a structure of limited capacity.

Broadbent synthesized experimental evidence that more exactly specified the characteristics of the short-term store, or working memory. He concluded that short-term memory is a distinct system from long-term memory. Information held in immediate memory is extremely limited in content, usually less than 10 items. The size of the items, in terms of information content, may vary greatly. Six or seven words contain much more information than a series of random digits, but both occupy similar amounts of space in short-term memory. Hence, the coding of information as meaningful units can greatly influence the raw amount of information held in short-term memory. Researchers came to refer to each item as a *chunk* of related information that could be coded as a meaningful unit. The limited storage capacity of short-term memory contrasts with the vast capacity of long-term memory, which is not filled in a lifetime of learning. Although our rate of learning appears to slow with advanced age, learning continues.

Not only is the capacity of the short-term store limited, but its contents decay rapidly. In fact, unless a conscious effort is made to retain specific information in short-term memory, it decays within a few seconds. Short-term memory ordinarily appears to hold information that represents the second-to-second results of sensory processing. It may, in fact, correspond to our introspective sense of conscious contents. (Although not discussed by Broadbent, the source of information stored in short-term memory may be supplied from long-term storage, such as images from the past or a plan of future action.) The transient nature of short-term memory contrasts with the permanence of long-term memory, which may hold memories from many years past.

Finally, the short-term memory store, as described by Broadbent, may hold information before filtering and may retain information after it has passed through central processing. If the short-term memory store occurs before complete filtering has occurred, then it is possible for information from a rejected channel of information to be briefly stored there and then processed after information from the attended-to channel has been analyzed. As long as the information from the processed channel can be analyzed before new information arrives, this strategy can be used by a perceiver. Long-term memory, on the other hand, stores only information that has passed the filter.

The Organism as an Information-Processing System

Broadbent summarized his conception of the information-processing system by using a diagram (Figure 2.2). This "information-flow diagram," as Broadbent referred to it, provided a simple framework for many further investigations and theories. The use of flow diagrams to illustrate theoretical relationships in the nervous system has itself become a ubiquitous tradition in the information or cognitive sciences. In its consideration of a "system for varying output until some input is secured" (p. 299), Broadbent incorporated the focus of operant and respondent psychology into this new framework.

Broadbent summarized the following principles as an initial set of conclusions about human information processing that the diagram renders in a kind of shorthand. He

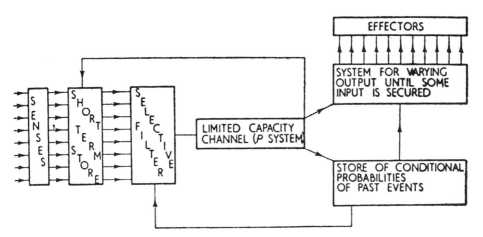

FIGURE 2.2. Broadbent's information-flow diagram (1958) for the organism. Information from the sensory systems is initially processed in parallel, enters a short-term buffer, and is filtered before entry to the limited-capacity channel (P system). Note the placement of the short-term store before, rather than after, the selective filter, as is typical in many subsequent adaptations of this model.

proposed that the nervous system acts to some extent as a single communication channel, so that it is meaningful to regard it as having a limited capacity. Because of the limited capacity of the central processing system (the P system), a selective operation is performed on the possible input into this channel by selecting information from all sensory events having some feature in common.

The probability of a class of events being selected for further processing is influenced by event properties (such as intensity or probability) and the state of the organism. The states of the organism that influence selection are commonly referred to as *drive states* in behavioral psychology, such as hunger, thirst, or sexual drive. One aspect of learning is the storage of the conditional probabilities of stimulus sequences that lead to reinforcement for that drive.

Incoming information may be held in a temporary store (immediate memory, or the short-term store) at a stage previous to the limited-capacity channel. The maximum time of storage is on the order of seconds, although information that has passed through the limited-capacity channel can be returned to the short-term store. This strategy, however, results in further reduction of the central, limited-capacity system for intake of new sensory information.

Finally, the amount of time taken to switch from one channel to another is appreciable, perhaps in the order of 1/6 second. Therefore, the ability of a person to monitor two channels of information deteriorates quickly when information in one of the channels requires sampling more than once per second.

Broadbent's Contribution

Broadbent was reserved regarding the contribution made by his model of human information processing, which was patched together from many sources. It has since come under attack on both theoretical and experimental grounds. Nevertheless, the influence of the information-processing model has been pervasive in the subsequent evolution of psychology. First of all, the overall model of information processing that Broadbent proposed remains influential. In part, this is true because he was careful not to overspecify the model and allowed for the possibility that people could change the relationship of systems within the model by adopting task-specific strategies. Researchers who subsequently debated the characteristics of filters often gave their models an all-or-nothing rigidity that Broadbent originally eschewed. Moreover, although seldom explicitly stated, a crucial change was made in the relationship between the short-term store and the filter system by later investigators. In Broadbent's model, the short-term store preceded the filter system and allowed the system to store input from secondary channels for later analysis. Consequently, multichannel monitoring of complex information could be carried out: in this model, there was no simple "bottleneck" that totally shut the door on unmonitored channels. In retrospect, Broadbent's conceptualization better describes the range of experimental data related to multichannel monitoring.

Even if Broadbent's model had been superseded by later developments and were of only historical interest, the impact of information-processing psychology would still be of great importance. Broadbent provided a compelling argument for the need to consider mentalistic (or computational) phenomena and summarized a variety of methods to experimentally test such models. These mental mechanisms were necessary to an understanding of the organism's responses to complex stimuli and environments; the importance of the size of the stimulus-and-response ensembles in the processing of demands; the impact of the demands placed on the capacity by meanings encoded in patterns and sequences; and the functional significance of the concept of short-term memory. Thus, Broadbent rehabilitated the work of the 19th-century psychologists who, largely through introspective techniques, had described many of these phenomena and had provided qualitative descriptions of constructs that were more formally developed in communication theory. Working memory and the limited-capacity system began to assume the characteristics of consciousness, a word banished from the annals of psychology for decades. Broadbent's mental flowchart, which was to have so many offspring over the years, captures something essential about the introspective and observed workings of the mind.

MODELS OF SELECTIVE ATTENTION

To be conscious of something in the physical or mental environment, a person ignores many other things. While you read this book, you are probably unconscious of the position of your body, the sounds of the heating system, the content of a conversation on the radio in the next room, or the typeface of the individual letters. Nevertheless, these diverse stimuli continually activate your sensory systems and may occasionally distract you. What sorts of systems allow a person to maintain attention on a text, bring it back after distractions, and block or filter out the many sensory impressions that continually activate the nervous system?

Selective Attention and Channels

Communication or information theory suggests that the nervous system, like electronic communication devices, can select to receive certain channels of information and can ignore or filter out the rest. Channel mechanisms are common in the electronic environment in which we live. A radio tuner selects one channel to amplify from the many that the antenna picks up in the environment, rather than receiving a incoherent composite of many programs simultaneously. Occasionally, two frequencies on the radio are too close to be resolved by the tuner. When this happens, the stations interfere with each other on the radio, and both stations are amplified. A listener or viewer can still make out the message of interest when two messages overlap, but it would obviously be difficult to understand a message when more than two were superimposed.

People are easily able to select channels of linguistic information. In a bar, there may be music playing and many other conversations being conducted, but a person is able to effectively single out and understand a particular speaker. If the background noise is very loud relative to the voice of the speaker of interest, however, this task becomes difficult, and reception of the message may break down entirely.

Information is continually being received from the environment by the senses. Because only a small amount of information can be consciously appreciated and generate responses, some sort of system exists to transmit one message to consciousness, and to filter out other messages. The concept of a filtering mechanism in the brain, as discussed previously, was developed by Broadbent (1958). The characteristics of this system, and its location in the stream of information processing, have produced a large body of investigation and a variety of models of selective attention.

Dichotic Listening

The ability of people to listen to one speaker, while ignoring another, has been widely used in an experimental procedure called *dichotic listening*. Its introduction to the field of attentional studies is generally credited to Cherry (1953). In a dichotic listening experiment, a person wears earphones through which two different messages are played simultaneously. The listener is usually asked to monitor one of the two messages, usually repeating it word for word as it is presented. This spoken repetition is called *shadowing the message*. If one message is presented to one ear, and a second message to the other ear, then it is easy for the listener to shadow the first message and ignore the other. If the rate of delivery of the messages is doubled, it is still possible to shadow effectively (Fairbanks, Guttman, & Miron, 1957). Because the rate of speech delivery does not have a marked effect on reception, sheer quantity of information content cannot be a primary limiting factor on performance. If the messages are presented from different perceived locations in space, selection remains efficient unless the sources are very close together. Giving selective attention to a spoken message is relatively easy when the sources of speech are separate in space, and more difficult when distinguished only by voice. Thus, it is much easier to attend to one speaker in a roomful of speakers than to one speaker on a conference telephone line, where the voices are not spatially distributed. This finding makes evolutionary sense, because it has been only recently that more than one speaker in a conversation can inhabit the same space. When the only difference between the messages is speech rate, performance becomes quite poor (Treisman, 1969).

Although subjects can attend to the information from one channel very effectively under quite adverse (noisy) situations, little information from other channels reaches consciousness. In a dichotic listening situation, in which different messages are presented to different ears, a subject may be aware that there is one or more other messages, and that the other message is given in a male or female voice, but may be unaware of whether the message is in English, or if the speech is played in reverse. When asked to listen for particular words in both the attended-to and the secondary channel, subjects typically detect most of the target words in the attended-to channel, and few in the secondary channel (see for reviews Kahneman, 1973; Moray, 1970; Neisser, 1967; Shiffrin & Schneider, 1977; Treisman, 1964).

The Search for the Bottleneck

These results led theorists to the concept of an attentional bottleneck in information processing. All information from the peripheral sensory system is initially processed in parallel for gross physical properties, and at some point in processing, one channel of information is selected from the various inputs. Channel selection is very effective when based on a sensory property such as spatial location and voice quality, although Broadbent did consider evidence that semantic or other particular features of a stimulus could be used for filtering. The selected information is allowed to continue through the system for further processing that is more serial in character, such as analysis of the meaning of a temporal sequence. Other information is filtered out from further analysis. This filtering may be due to active inhibition of the signal to prevent it from entering the domain of higher order processing, or due simply to the inability of the central processor to handle more than the gated channel. Because the most effective filtering appears to occur on the basis of simple sensory differences between the messages, it was suggested that the bottleneck (the switch from parallel to serial processing) occurs early in the information-processing sequence, immediately after sensory categorization of the messages into discrete bands. This early bottleneck model departed from Broadbent's original model of the filtering system, in which the filter was placed *after* the perceptual processing of multiple channels of information and the entry of information into short-term memory. In Broadbent's original description, therefore, information from unattended-to channels might be stored after perceptual processing in short-term memory, to receive more complete processing after a short delay. In fact, Broadbent reported experimental evidence that the flow of information into short-term memory and the limited-capacity system could change as a result of conscious task strategies.

This early bottleneck model did fit a broad range of experimental findings and agreed with our phenomenological experience of the consciousness of a seamless stream of unitary experiences. Nevertheless, several experimental findings were reported that showed that attentional processes were at work outside this model. Certain words, such as a subject's own name, were noticed (Moray, 1959). If the secondary message lagged behind the first message, this was often picked up by subjects (e.g., Cherry, 1953). And if the message on the attended-to channel switched over to the secondary channel, subjects would often follow it (Treisman, 1960).

These findings led to modifications of the all-or-none bottleneck model of selective attention, because the filter mechanism selected messages before semantic processing. If this was the case, how did words or phrases on the secondary channel receive semantic analysis of their content and meaning? Treisman (1964) proposed that secondary channels of information are not completely filtered, but attenuated. Attenuated information would be passed to higher levels of analysis only if it passed a threshold test. This test would identify words that had learned importance (e.g., one's name or a warning such as "Look out!"), or that were favored by contextual probabilities or recent use. Deutsch and Deutsch (1963) proposed that all incoming signals are analyzed for "importance," and that the most important message is selected for further processing, such as motor response or memory storage. This further processing is what enters awareness. Further processing of a given message may not occur at all, however, if a person's level of arousal is low, particularly when the message is not of great importance. (For example, when we are drowsy, we find it hard to follow the message in a mathematics text.) Although the system that assigns "importance" to a signal is not well described, the Deutsch and Deutsch model does imply that all signals receive extensive analysis, and that the most important signal is selected for further processing at a later stage. The model is vague regarding how much analysis is automatically allocated to all stimuli, where the late stage is located in the stream of information processing, and how experimenters can detect the processing of stimuli that usually do not enter consciousness and are not recalled. Treisman (1964) argued against the Deutsch and Deutsch model on economical grounds, in that such a model would make enormous demands on an information-processing system in order to rank all signals semantically by importance before selecting one signal for final, decision-related analysis.

The debate regarding whether an attentional bottleneck occurs early or late in the information-processing stream remains unresolved in the context of the dichotic listening paradigm. This lack of resolution may be due in part to limitations of the paradigm as it is typically used, and to limitations of the theory. In general, only two channels are used in such experiments, and pauses occur between words in the attended-to message, as well as between words, such as articles, that have very low information content (i.e., are highly redundant). Even if the bottleneck theory in its strongest form is correct (i.e., if only one channel can be processed at a given time), there is often time during pauses and redundant words or phrases to shift attention to another channel of information for the analysis of a word or phrase. There is evidence that words are automatically processed to a semantic level (Posner, 1980, 1986). Moray (1970) proposed that most ambiguities in the selective attention literature can be resolved by adopting a model in which, at any moment, a listener is sampling only one message, but the listener may switch between channels in the intervals between signals in the attended-to channel. This switch may be induced because of changes in the characteristics of the secondary channel (an orienting response) or because of task demands. This model has been around for a long time. William James (1890) cited his own experience and that of other investigators, which suggest that, during dual-task performance, attention oscillates from one task to the other. When these tasks require verbal performance—for example, reciting one poem while writing another—words sometimes slip from one poem to the other.

Broadbent's response to experimental findings that argued against an early, filter-based system was the development of a two-process model of attentional selection. Broadbent labeled these two processes *filtering* and *pigeonholing*. Filtering entails the selection of a stimulus for attention or further processing because it possesses a particular feature, usually a simple physical characteristic. In a selective listening situation, this feature might be the gender of the voice, its spatial location, or its loudness. Filtering occurs early in the time course of stimulus analysis, requires little controlled processing, and is most effective when based on the global attributes of incoming stimuli. Pigeonholing is the process that sorts stimuli that differ by multiple sensory attributes into response categories, or pigeonholes. If no category is appropriate, a stimulus is usually ignored. Because pigeonholing requires the detailed analysis of a stimulus on a number of dimensions, it occurs later in time, takes longer to complete, and requires more active processing than filtering. Human evoked-potential recordings suggest that filtering and pigeonholing are associated with responses that differ in their onset, scalp topography, and reactivity to stimulus information content (see Chapter 6).

In summary, as the filter model evolved, the selection process took on an unrealistic rigidity. Experimenters searched for a bottleneck because filtering was increasingly thought of as an all-or-none process. Some results favored an early bottleneck, some suggested a late bottleneck, and others suggested that more than one channel of information is processed at a time. These results led to the proposal by Broadbent that filtering on the basis of simple sensory features is an early, automatic, and global process that is complemented by a later, active, and slower selection process based on conjunctions of multiple stimulus features, and associated with large response sets. It should be noted that the filter model originally put forward by Broadbent allowed for the sampling of secondary or tertiary channels, although the degree to which these channels could be evaluated was limited by the demands of the primary channel, particularly by the rate of transmission in the primary channel. As will be discussed in a later section, a multiple-channel monitoring of transient signals does take place, and the strategies deployed for monitoring a range of channels by a person varies with the task demands.

Removing the Bottleneck

Ulric Neisser (1976) attempted to develop a theoretical position that eliminates the role of an attentional filter in perception. Neisser argued that, although it is correct in terms of information theory that many sensations are filtered out before reaching consciousness, or influencing behavior, this does not imply that there is a filtering system in the perceiver's brain. A perceiver picks up information that is consistent with current expectations, past experience, and plans. Other information is simply ignored. Neisser adopted Bartlett's term *schema* (1932) to describe the cognitive structure that directs perception. Neisser defined *schema* very broadly as "that portion of the entire perceptual cycle which is internal to the perceiver, modifiable by experience, and somehow specific to what is being perceived" (p. 54). Stimuli or thoughts that are inconsistent with the current schema do not intrude on consciousness, with a few exceptions. Innate schemata exist that are always active, such as a schema that directs attention to loud noises, pain, or sudden visual movements. Other such schemata are developmentally acquired. When one hears one's name called while reading, one's attention automatically shifts away from the text and to the speaker. These schemata are *preattentive processes*, which are always ready to be activated by appropriate stimulation but operate outside attention. Selective attention, for Neisser, is an active rather than a passive process. He likened it to motoric behavior: In order to pick an apple from a tree, one doesn't need to filter out all the other apples that one isn't going to pick.

Neisser's view dispenses with many of the problems of the filter model by emphasizing what it generally ignores: the importance of cognitive set, expectations, previous experiences, and goals in the direction and content of perception. What was formerly called attention now becomes a function of the current schema. Several difficulties arise, however, in defining attention as a function of active perception.

First, when a "top-down" model of perception is adopted, the ability of perceivers to make immediate sense of unexpected stimuli is poorly explained. When changing television channels, we are immediately able to perceive the content of the picture on the screen, even though it has no perceptual or semantic relationship to what has come before it.

Second, Neisser contended that systems do not exist within the nervous system to filter out a portion of the sensory input. He stated that such mechanisms have neither biological or psychological reality. The biological evidence suggests that both selection (or pick-up) and filtering (or inhibition) are elements of the neurophysiology of visual perception. The filtering and selection of stimuli constitutes a basic design principle within the visual system at a neuronal level (see Chapter 7). Stimuli or channels that are "selected" on the basis of task demands evoke very different physiological responses during the early stages of perception.

Schema models, as articulated by Neisser, emphasize the role of the perceiver in selecting information in the environment and define attentional focus as a function of schema. Much of Neisser's critique of filtering makes semantic rather than functional distinctions. Formally speaking, the schema model may also be described as requiring the filtering of unattended-to information, but Neisser argued against the need for an active process to inhibit the awareness of irrelevant information. In a certain sense, filter and schema models may describe complementary processes. Filter theory may describe the systems whose current operating characteristics are set by schemata. Although Neisser denied that such filter systems are necessary, physiological as well as psychophysical evidence has been accrued that points to their reality. In combination, these two theoretical currents give a more comprehensive view of the role of attention: Schemata determine why something is selected for attention, and filter theories describe how this happens and what constraints exist in comprehending the diversity of the signals that are presented by the environment.

Visual Selective Attention

On reviewing the selective attention literature, Moray (1970) concluded that different mechanisms are involved for different types of input. Visual signals, for example, are usually spatially extended but of short duration, whereas auditory signals, particularly speech, are extended over time and are presented sequentially. These different inputs probably require different processing strategies for optimal performance. Still, visual processing has properties that can be categorized as selective in nature.

Selective attention in the visual system usually occurs after extensive "preattentive" analysis of the visual field. The distinction between preattentive visual processing and attentional processing has been used by a number of investigators (e.g., Neisser, 1967; Treisman, 1964). The preattentive stage of vision includes processes that require little or no effort, that occur early in the temporal sequence of visual processing, and that operate across the entire visual field simultaneously. Automatic processes include such perceptual operations as the segregation of figure from ground, the maintenance of size constancy, and textural discriminations. Attentionally demanding visual operations, on the other hand, are usually carried out on circumscribed areas of the visual field and entail the serial scanning of large areas.

Gestalt psychologists (e.g., Kohler, 1947) have emphasized the organization of the visual field on the basis of such principles as stimulus similarity, proximity, and common fate. The automatic reorganization of the visual field that results in emergent properties and object discrimination is so effective that attentional processes play little role in Gestalt theory.

One problem with Gestalt principles is lack of an exact definition of concepts like *similarity* or *proximity*. In the case of similarity, there is no *a priori* basis for predicting which stimulus properties are perceptually similar, and which properties require cognitive effort to discriminate. More recent perceptual theorists have tried to distinguish properties that are automatically evaluated by the perceptual system and properties that require attention or effort to discriminate. Julesz (1981), for example, contrasted the automatic, preattentive segregation of the visual field on the basis of texture with the serial, focal attention used to search for specific objects within the visual field. Textural elements may be quite complex in appearance and may vary in orientation yet may still be automatically grouped together. Objects of focal attention may be physically dissimilar and distributed across the visual field but may nevertheless be grouped by category membership. Treisman (1960, 1964) argued that preattentive vision extracts a set of simple features, including color, size, contrast, orientation, curvature, line ends, and stereoscopic depth across the whole visual field. Objects that differ in a single simple feature are automatically discriminated (e.g., a green circle will perceptually "pop out" of a group of orange circles). Focal attention to a circumscribed location is required to identify an object on the basis of conjunctions of features, however. It takes effort, for example, to locate green squares amid a field of green circles and orange squares. The object, in this case, is defined by the conjunction of greenness and squareness. In order to examine a visual field for a conjunction of features, therefore, a viewer would need to search areas of the visual field sequentially. One appeal of Treisman's model is that simple features, perceptually defined, may be associated with specific populations of feature-sensitive neurons identified in the occipital cortex. An argument against this model is the observation that figures emerge from ground on the basis of conjunctions of many different features; yet this process is ordinarily very fast and effortless (i.e., preattentive).

Direction of the attention to different locations in the visual field has been likened to a spotlight that enhances the efficiency of the detection of events within the beam (Posner, 1980; Posner, Snyder, & Davidson, 1980). The direction in which the spotlight is directed is usually correlated with foveal position, but its effects can also be appreciated at more peripheral locations through experimental manipulations. This finding suggests that the spotlight is generated by analysis late in visual processing. Monkey experiments and lesion studies indicate that the parietal lobe and several subcortical centers are involved in the movement of the attentional spotlight across the visual field (Posner, Peterson, Fox, & Raichle, 1988).

Most studies of visual selective attention have used static visual displays. In a study by Neisser and Becklen (1975), subjects were asked to respond to significant events in one sports game that was superimposed over the image of a different sports game presented on the same viewing screen. The subjects were very effective in following and responding to the specified game, while ignoring the other game. Subjectively, the viewers were hardly aware of the ignored game. Neisser (1976) stressed that this study made it clear that selective looking cannot be attributed to differences between the attended-to and ignored games in their physical features or spatial origin, but must be attributed to expectancies and under-standing of the visual continuities of a sports game. In addition, the study illustrates that following visual events with temporal extension demands the same kind of exclusive attention that listening to continuous discourse requires.

In summary, selective attention in visual processing seems to occur late in the perceptual interpretation of a visual field. In fact, the integration of a visual scene may occur with little attentional selection. Visual selection takes place after extensive preattentive analysis and organization of the visual field, which occurs rapidly, automatically, and in parallel. Visual selection is required by tasks that involve the location of specific conjunctions of features or objects not isolated by preattentive processes. Visual selection over a static display entails scanning over sections of the visual field, a process that has been likened to the use of an attentional beam or spotlight. Spatial attention can be directed to specific sections of the visual field and can enhance later detection performance. Selective attention is also required for viewing a complex sequence of events over time, but the mechanisms that allow effective selection are unknown.

Attention and Signal Detection

The characteristics of the filtering system have also been evaluated by means of signal detection and recognition paradigms. Unlike dichotic listening experiments, these investigations have seldom used semantically complex material or messages that extended over long periods of time. Instead, these studies have used simple stimuli (tones, lights, and letters) in experimental settings where the information is just above the subject's threshold. These experiments have usually been designed to minimize the influence on the data of memory, response generation, or individual characteristics. In addition, such reduced paradigms have allowed the application of a mathematical characterization of filtering systems using signal detection theory to characterize the strategies and filtering characteristics of perception for a set of experimental conditions. Signal detection theory allows an experimenter to differentiate the detectability of the signal (d'), which varies as a function of noise within the nervous system, as well as of external noise, and an internal criterion for reporting the presence or absence of a signal.

Although signal detection experiments have addressed many of the issues posed by the dichotic listening experiments, there seems to be little interaction between these two experimental and theoretical currents. Swets (1984) provided a comprehensive review of findings from the signal detection literature. For the detection of auditory signals, several mechanisms were tested. Tanner and Norman (1954) proposed a dual mechanism for the selection of target tones. One mechanism is a single-channel (or single-band) receiver that can be placed anywhere over the hearing range, and that picks up one frequency or a narrow range of frequencies. This narrow-channel system corresponds to focal attention. It can be activated by telling a listener, "Raise your hand when you hear this tone (A flat over middle C)." The second system, which operates concurrently but is not limited by attention, receives information over the whole auditory spectrum and is activated by any sound. The narrow-channel system can pick up a specific frequency efficiently despite a low signal-to-noise ratio, as only the noise in the narrow channel of interest needs to be evaluated. The wide-channel system can pick up any signal, but because it is much less effective in dealing with the great amount of noise over the whole auditory range, it is far less sensitive than the narrow-channel model. A multichannel system has also been proposed, in which the listener can focus attention on more than one frequency channel at a time (Green, 1958).

Experimental evidence suggests that listeners can adopt either the single-channel or the multiple-channel approach when attending to auditory information. A single-channel approach is most effective when the listener knows that the information will arrive in a particular channel, and that the signal-to-noise ratio will be poor. A multiple-channel approach, although less sensitive to the signals in any given channel, is useful when the listener is not sure in which channel the information of interest will arrive (Swets, 1984).

Channel Selection over Time: Vigilance

Many tasks used in experimental psychology to investigate performance make stringent demands on processing capacity. Subjects are asked to view informative stimuli for a fraction of a second; to respond quickly; to recall information that has little meaning and no relevance to their everyday life; to respond rapidly to series of stimuli; or to perform more than one task at a time. Lapses of attention and errors of performance seem unavoidable under such conditions.

There is a class of tasks, however, that requires responses to events that occur only infrequently. Such tasks require *vigilance*, a state of readiness to respond despite long intervals of empty waiting. Such tasks are increasingly a part of modern occupations. Equipment operators monitor the consoles of automated factories, responding only to disturbances of function; radar and sonar operators wait for infrequent but perhaps very significant signals; an underling waits for an infrequent opening to interrupt a supervisor's monologue. Under such conditions, one's ability to sustain attention (as well as one's patience) is tried. And despite our best efforts, lapses of attention occur.

Broadbent (1958) suggested that lapses of attention consist of the tendency of observers to shift attention away from an information source after prolonged periods of observation, and to briefly sample information from another source. He considered several theories of lapses of attention in vigilance tasks. One possible explanation is a tendency toward the extinction of responses to a repetitive stimulus, due to a build-up of inhibition. However, the performance curve in a vigilance task is better characterized by oscillations in performance than by a progressive inhibition of response. Other mechanisms that appear to fit vigilance data are expectancy mechanisms, which relate performance level to signal probability. For low-probability signals, such as those in a vigilance experiment, processing requires more capacity, which may not always be available. In line with expectancy theory, highly probable events are processed more quickly than improbable events. Activation theories suggest that a person's arousal diminishes under conditions of impoverished sensory stimulation, as is typical in a vigilance task. Consistent with an activation model, manipulations that increase arousal—such as breaks from the task, environmental noise, feedback on performance, or the presence of another person—help maintain performance. Broadbent suggested another possible source of performance failure, based on the concept that the filter system is biased toward information sources that have not recently been active; that is, attention tends to wander between channels. This wandering would produce environmental scanning under conditions of low stimulation. Broadbent presented experimental data that suggest that the shift of attention from one channel to another and back again takes somewhere between 1 and 2 seconds. This oscillation between channels results in occasional lapses of attention from the monitored channel. One result is that prolonged signals are much less likely to be missed than brief signals. Broadbent concluded that vigilance decrements are probably best explained by occasional attentional shifts, which are more likely to occur under conditions of diminished activation and with low-probability stimuli.

Vigilance performance has received continued attention by researchers, probably because of its increasing importance in commercial and military activities. More recent reviews (Loeb & Alluisis, 1984; Parasuraman, 1984) have emphasized that vigilance performance and failures of attention do not represent a single process. Vigilance performance is influenced by both tonic and phasic factors, such as arousal, expectancy, and task demands.

In a comprehensive review of the vigilance literature, Parasuraman (1984) dissected vigilance into two aspects: the level of vigilance and the vigilance decrement. Overall performance in a vigilance task is described by the *level of vigilance*. The *vigilance decrement* describes the phenomenon of increasing error rates over the time course of a sustained-attention task. Performance can be described in terms of the sensitivity of the observer, quantified as signal detectability (d'), and by the observer's response criterion (beta). The overall level of vigilance is sensitive to the tonic level of arousal at the beginning of the task. If the arousal level is low, vigilance performance is usually poor throughout the task. Arousal can be altered by such factors as moderate heat, alcohol, and arousal's intrinsic rhythmicity (Parasuraman, 1984). Because diminished arousal lowers the sensitivity (d') of the observer to the signal, changes in response criteria do not improve performance. Physiological arousal tends to decline in any monotonous environment or under conditions of prolonged performance, although this decline in arousal is not always associated with declines in performance.

Phasic alertness (stimulus-specific, transient increases in arousal) tends to be associated with faster reaction time, a reduced criterion for making a response, and a higher error rate. This is true particularly in tasks in which the stimulus is present until a response is made.

The vigilance decrement is characterized as a gradual decline in the rate of detection of infrequent signals and an increase in response speed. This decrement appears to be due in part to changes in the observer's criterion to a more conservative one over the course of time. This change appears to be caused by an automatic readjustment of the criterion over time as modeled by expectancy theory. Observers adjust their criterion based on their estimate of signal probability. If an observer misses signals in a time interval, the observer's estimate of signal probability is always less than the true rate of occurrence. Consequently, the observer will adopt an increasingly stringent criterion for noting the occurrence of a signal as the time on task increases.

Factors that decrease sensitivity include increases in the time interval in which a signal can occur and the type of discrimination a task requires. Parasuraman (1984) divided discrimination tasks into two types: those requiring simultaneous or successive stimuli to make the discrimination. In *simultaneous-discrimination* tasks, all the information needed to make the discrimination is present simultaneously. As an example, a person might be asked to discriminate which of two objects is rectangular in shape. *Successive-discrimination* tasks require that a person detect a target that is specified as a change in some feature of a repetitive, standard feature. In terms of the preceding task, a person might instead be asked to discriminate rectangular objects from a series of objects presented one at a time. Successive discrimination requires that a person maintain some sort of representation in memory to perform the task. Parasuraman reviewed data that suggest that successive-discrimination tasks are associated with declines in sensitivity over time, whereas simultaneous-discrimination tasks are not. He interpreted these findings as indicating that the higher demands placed on the observer in successive-discrimination tasks require more resources, or effort.

Both Broadbent's and Parasuraman's considerations of vigilance performance suggest that multiple factors influence vigilance performance. Arousal affects overall performance level and observer sensitivity, while changes in criterion and task demands that influence sensitivity appear to be responsible for performance decrements over time.

Expectancy and Priming

Selective attention to a channel of information or a sequence of actions increases responsiveness to a specific group of stimuli over time. Vigilance also requires sustained attention to a channel or channels of information over time. Transient increases in responsiveness to a stimulus arrival comprise another attentional mechanism. These transient and often stimulus-specific states are experienced as expectancies and are usually studied experimentally with priming paradigms.

In general, people can react to an expected event more quickly than to an unexpected one. Experimentally, it was noted by early investigators that attention shortens reaction time. Titchener (1908) advanced a "law of prior entry," which stated that stimuli to which a perceiver is predisposed reach consciousness more quickly than a novel stimulus. The basis of the effect of attentional focus on processing time continues to be investigated. In Neisser's model of the perceptual cycle (1976), expectancy plays a major role in directing perception. Experiments and theories related to expectancies include studies of preparatory set, event probabilities, priming, and schemata.

Preparatory Set. If a person is simply warned that a stimulus demanding a response is about to appear, the response to the succeeding stimulus is facilitated. This effect is often ascribed to nonspecific arousal produced by the warning stimulus, because it is accompanied by physiological signs of arousal (Posner, 1986).

Event Probabilities. More probable events are responded to more quickly than less probable events. Even when global event probabilities are equivalent in a random sequence of two stimuli, short sequences of stimuli quickly generate an expectancy (K. Squires, Wickens, Squires, & Donchon, 1976). This effect corresponds to our commonplace experience that routine encounters require little thought in the generation of a response, but that novel or strange interactions generally demand conscious consideration before a response is selected.

Priming. The experimental paradigm most often used in the investigation of expectancy effects is calling *priming*. In a priming paradigm, a stimulus is presented to a subject that may provide information regarding the attributes of the succeeding stimulus. For example, if a person is required to press a key whenever a word appears on a screen, the word *color* primes the reaction time to the word *red*. If the word preceding *red* is unrelated to *red* (e.g., *wall*), then the reaction time to *red* is longer than when it is primed.

In the example above, the prime word provides the semantic category for the succeeding word (usually referred to as the *imperative stimulus* or *target*). Other priming words might be semantic associates (such as *blue* or *purple*); phonemic associates such as *bed* or *wed*, or the word itself. That is, if a word is presented twice, the reaction time to the word is shortened on the second presentation. Priming can facilitate decisions, such as whether a string of letters is a word or not (Schvanevelt & Meyer, 1973), or what the missing letters are in a word fragment (Tulving, 1983).

The basis of priming effects remains obscure. It is not clear to what extent they can be attributed to conscious as well as automatic facilitation of performance, and whether priming creates changes in the procedures used to access related memories, or in the structure of semantic memory itself. Priming effects are often modality-specific and are relatively unaffected by the type of cognitive processing that the priming word undergoes (Tulving, 1983). Posner (1986) suggested that primes activate isolable pathways or subsystems in the nervous system, and that priming phenomena can be used to show how such pathways undergo facilitation, inhibition, and decay of information transmission.

If the word preceding an imperative stimulus provides incorrect information about the stimulus (e.g., if *red* is preceded by the word *water*), the reaction time to the imperative stimulus is usually delayed. Possibly, the activation of the semantic network induced by the presentation of the first word must be inhibited before the activation of another semantic network can occur.

When the majority of priming words in a series are valid, the facilitation and inhibition of the reaction time to succeeding target words are maximal. If the majority of the priming words in a series are invalid, the facilitation of response occurs after a valid prime, but little or no inhibition occurs after an invalid prime (Posner, 1986). Posner (1986) suggested that these results indicate that reliable priming creates a greater degree of conscious activation, which is associated with greater facilitation when a prime is informative, and with greater inhibition when a prime is uninformative. Unreliable priming, however, does not result in as much conscious pathway activation. Posner interpreted these results as indicating that the conscious activation of a pathway or subsystem involves limited-capacity processes and possibly the inhibition of other pathways. Automatic activation, on the other hand, makes little demand on limited-capacity processes and does not result in the lateral inhibition of parallel pathways in the nervous system.

The priming effect decays over time, as the interval between the priming stimulus and the imperative stimulus increases. Priming effects are usually maximal for short inter-stimulus intervals (less than 2 seconds), but an effect can sometimes be detected after surprisingly long periods, up to several minutes (Kirsner & Smith, 1974) or days on a word-fragment-completion task. Whether the decay and persistence of the priming effect is related to automatic activation or conscious activation via rehearsal of the prime in short-term memory remains to be determined (Posner, 1986).

Schemata and Expectations. *Schema* is a usage coined by Bartlett (1932) to describe the mental structure that supports an integrated experience of the world, and that allows us to act appropriately within it. Schemata are generated in reaction to the current environment to represent our current understanding of it; to provide a basis for perceptual interpretations; and to allow the selection of appropriate responses, goals, and expectations.

Schemata play a central role in Neisser's concept (1976) of the perceptual cycle. In the perceptual cycle, a perceiver samples sensory information from the environment, that modifies the current schema. On the basis of the modified schema, the perceiver forms anticipations about the whole environment that guide further perceptual and motoric explorations. This cycle expresses perception as an active process and schemata as dynamic, rather than rigid, cognitive structures. Neisser defined the schema as the portion of the entire perceptual cycle that is internal to the perceiver, modifiable by experience, and somehow specific to what is being perceived.

Schemata represent such global structures that they do not represent a testable construct. Although Neisser suggests that schemata ultimately require biological explication, the scope of schemata precludes such a characterization with any current technique. Schemalike entities, such as scripts, however, have been useful in artificial intelligence research. The concept of schemata has drawn attention to the role of expectation, learning, and goals in perceptual activity. Perception does not work as an isolated system on neutral stimuli. It occurs in an information-processing system that has evolved to provide a functional representation of the environment. Perception is shaped by past experiences, is directed by future needs, and modifies the perceiver's worldview. Moreover, Neisser's argument that the entire schema must be considered in perceptual experiments, and that such experiments should be ecologically valid, brings into question the representativeness of the experimental techniques of mainstream cognitive psychology

Summary

The processes involved in selective attention to auditory messages have been studied since the 1950s. Several systems appear to operate in parallel to allow selective attention to task-relevant stimuli or messages, while allowing concurrent monitoring of the environment for meaningful but unanticipated or low-probability events. When one is shadowing continuous messages, little information can be gleaned from concurrent background messages that are more than a word or two in length. This finding suggests that semantic analysis can take place while one is monitoring a message, but only for transient periods. Such a mechanism may be associated with intermittent switching from the monitored to the secondary channel; with brief storage and a fragmentary analysis of unattended-to information in short-term memory; or with the parallel processing of aspects of the ignored message that reach consciousness only intermittently. In an elaboration of the filter model, Broadbent proposed that the early, fast, and automatic filter process is supplemented by a later, slower, and active pigeonholing process involved in the mapping of a repertoire of responses to a stimulus set. Broadbent suggested that pigeonholing is shaped by a perceiver's beliefs and expectations. Similarly, Neisser emphasized the top-down selection of stimuli for perception by schemata.

Auditory selective attention appears to entail a more exclusive focus on the information of interest than visual selective attention, but this finding may be due to differences in the paradigms between auditory and visual studies. Typically, auditory studies have used messages extended over time, whereas visual studies have used static, transient displays. Visual perception involves an automatic, rapid, and parallel analysis of the entire visual field, and it becomes selective only when this preattentive process fails to isolate particular task-relevant objects. Focal attention has been associated with a spatially limited spotlight that can sweep over the visual field. Selection can also be focused on temporally extended events, to the exclusion of other events.

Evidence from signal detection and recognition experiments using transient multiple signals suggests that listeners can elect to monitor single or multiple channels of information, depending on data quality and task demands. Similar conclusions can be reached from studies of the detection of transient auditory and visual stimuli. The selection of information for conscious attention therefore does not entirely inhibit the concurrent and automatic monitoring of major environmental events in either stimulus modality.

Vigilance requires sustained attention to a sensory channel or channels so that one responds to infrequent events. Vigilance deficits and decrements are due to multiple factors, including arousal, task demands, and unconscious criterion shifts in the performer. These factors affect both the sensitivity and the response criterion.

Expectancies decrease reaction time to events. Expectancy effects, unlike selective attention to a sensory channel, are quite transient. Expectancy effects decline rapidly after 1 or 2 seconds. A diversity of mechanisms underlie expectancy effects, which may be automatic or effortful in nature.

For almost two decades after the introduction of models of selective attention, little physiological evidence was available to support their biological reality. In recent years, neurophysiological (Chapter 7) and electrophysiological (Chapter 6) data have accumulated that suggest an association between these cognitive processes and local and distributed neural mechanisms.

AUTOMATIC AND CONTROLLED PROCESSING

The attentional demands of tasks, even very complex tasks such as reading or driving, often diminish with practice. Many perceptual judgments, such as depth perception or movement detection, seem to require little or no attentional effort at all. The characteristics of habitual or automatized performance were ignored for several decades in the development of information-processing models of the mental processes, which focused on how information is transmitted and transformed between static structures, usually as a function of intentional strategies.

In the 1970s, a number of researchers initiated lines of experimental and theoretical work that investigated the characteristics of mental processes that, although mediating complex sensory and motoric activities, proceeded with little effort, and often little awareness, on the part of an individual. Such processes, which are activated and proceed with minimal conscious effort, are usually termed *automatic processes*. These are contrasted with a second type of mental operations, which require intentional commitment and have been termed *conscious* (Posner & Snyder, 1975), *controlled* (Schneider & Shiffrin, 1977), or *effortful* (Hasher & Zacks, 1979; Kahneman, 1973). Controlled processes require mental capacity or resources; are greatly influenced by subject characteristics and conscious strategies; and are usually degraded when dual-task performance is required.

What Processes Are Automatic?

Because the bulk of the data in the literature of cognitive psychology was initially collected in the course of intentional activities, when the subjects were consciously using different strategies to modulate task performance, the first task of investigators arguing for a distinction between automatic and controlled processing was to define and demonstrate automatic processes. Posner and Synder (1975) proposed three criteria for an automatic process: the process occurs (1) without intention, (2) without giving rise to conscious awareness, and (3) without producing interference with other ongoing mental activity (i.e., automatic processes do not demand attentional resources). Posner and Synder used investigations of the Stroop effect to make the point that subjects cannot always avoid processing aspects of a stimulus that they desire to ignore. In the Stroop paradigm, subjects are asked to name the colors in which words are printed, when the words themselves spell the same color names (usually red, blue, and green). If the word spells a different name from the color that it is printed in, it is very difficult to avoid reading the words and simply to respond to the color of the type. Experiments on the Stroop effect suggest that color naming and word reading go on in parallel, regardless of the intentions of the perceiver, and that interference takes place in the generation of response output, when only one of these two automatic processes can be articulated. Because word reading has been shown to proceed faster than color naming, word reading interferes much more with color naming than the reverse. Posner and Snyder stressed the distinction between the automatic activation of information-processing pathways by stimulus characteristics, which do not require intention and which allow parallel processing within other pathways, and conscious attention to a given pathway, which requires capacity and results in the inhibition of other processing pathways (Posner, 1986).

Hasher and Zachs (1979) proposed that the codings of event frequency, location of objects in space, and temporal information about the order of events are all processed and encoded automatically by individuals, because they can recall this information without making any effort to learn it during an experiment. Hasher and Zachs (1984) then carried out a series of experiments describing the characteristics of the automatic processing of frequency of occurrence. Typically, two types of paradigms were used. Natural stimuli vary in frequency of occurrence in the environment, and subjects might be asked which occurs more frequently. For example, is *bacon* used more frequently than *pastrami* in English? People were surprisingly accurate in evaluating the relative frequency of such things as letters, pairs of letters, syllables, words, surnames, professions, and sources of morbidity and mortality, though they could not explain how they had acquired such knowledge, because such frequency information is seldom explicitly communicated. A second paradigm tested a person's ability to recall the frequency of occurrence of stimuli that were systematically varied. The protocols of Hasher and Zachs involved exposing a series of stimuli to a subject, which occurred from zero to six or seven times, and asking the subject to guess how many times each stimuli in a set had occurred. Again, the subjects were remarkably accurate in making such judgments, whether or not they had been instructed to keep track of the stimulus frequency. From such experiments, Hasher and Zachs concluded that frequency of occurrence meets six stringent criteria for automatic processing: (1) processing occurs without intention; (2) encoding is not improved by intentional strategies; (3) training and feedback do not improve encoding; (4) people vary little in their capacity to encode such information, regardless of their education or cultural background; (5) after the acquisition of an automatic process (if it is not innate), age does not influence performance; and (6) disruptions due to arousal, stress, or other processing demands have no effect on an automatic process. Experimental evidence, reviewed by Hasher and Zachs (1984), suggests that frequency of occurrence is processed automatically by all these criteria.

The six criteria proposed by Hasher and Zachs may be too rigid to describe the varieties of processing structures and strategies that people use. The same type of task (e.g., detecting a specific tone) may be automatic when the tone is very different from other sounds in the environment and may be effortful when the tone is more difficult to discriminate from other sounds. Evidence from studies of frequency of occurrence indicates that, under some conditions, frequency judgments are enhanced by instructions that affect intentional or incidental learning, and that frequency processing is degraded by concurrent task demands (Sanders, Gonzalez, Murphy, Liddle, & Vitina, 1987). Coding of spatial location is influenced by intention, competing-task-loads, practice, strategy, and individual differences (Naveh-Benjamin, 1987). These investigators concluded that the automatic and controlled processing distinction describes a continuum, rather than two distinct types of cognitive structures.

One problem with the models of automatic processing reviewed up to this point is the lack of elaboration of how these processes fit in with more general models of information processing and learning. The following theories of automatic and controlled processing, the first proposed by Broadbent in 1958, the second by Schneider and Shiffrin (1977) 20 years later, provide more comprehensive explanations of these processes.

Automatization and Capacity

Although Broadbent's *Perception and Communication* (1958) is usually cited as a key foundation of information-processing psychology, theories of mental automatization seldom consider the creative discussion of automatization in his chapter, "Verbal and Bodily Response." Broadbent's arguments can be related to the relationship between (1) the number of stimuli in a sequence that need to be considered to produce a response, and (2) demands on capacity. These relationships are illustrated in Figure 2.3, adapted from the original diagrams in Broadbent's book.

Figure 2.3a shows the relationship between stimuli and responses in a discrimination paradigm. This relationship requires that each stimulus be associated with a single response. Therefore, the ensemble of responses is equal in number to the ensemble of stimuli. Once a response has been made, the perceiver can forget the previous stimulus and move to the next one. This relationship describes the task demands posed when a person is required to repeat words immediately after hearing them. Stimulus–response associations, or response–consequence associations, make up the bulk of the experimental data obtained in behavioral learning experiments.

Figure 2.3b shows the relationship between stimuli and responses when responses are

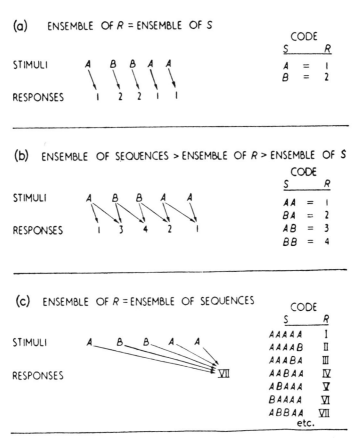

FIGURE 2.3. Automatic and controlled processing. The information demands posed by the relationship between stimulus and response ensembles. (a) A stimulus that invariably calls for the same response makes the least demands on an information-processing system. (b) A response that depends on a pattern of stimuli makes greater demands on system capacity. (c) A response that depends on mapping a response to each stimulus ensemble makes the greatest demands on system capacity. Example c is typical of linguistic communication, in which the usual unit of communication is a sentence or paragraph. Adapted from Broadbent (1958).

contingent on specific sequences of stimuli. In these situations, the perceiver must detect the spatial or temporal patterns of stimuli rather than react to the stimuli as independent events. Whereas the previously described stimulus– response relationship makes minimal demands on the storage capacity of the perceiver, pattern recognition requires the storage of representations in short-term memory until a pattern requiring a response accumulates. Pattern recognition requires greater capacity of the perceiver than the respondent or operant behavior modulated by individual stimuli.

Figure 2.3c shows the relationship between stimuli and responses when a novel sequence of stimuli must be assimilated before a response can be generated. This relationship is typical of speech comprehension, in which an entire sentence must be uttered before it can be fully comprehended and a response can be made to it. Although such sequential analyses are commonplace in humans, animals have great difficulty learning idiosyncratic sequences without cues. The analysis of sequences requires enormous computational capacity. Broadbent provided the following example: If a vocabulary of only 850 words is assumed, then comprehension of a sentence of a single word would require that the nervous system be able to represent 850 states. To comprehend a two-word sentence would require 850^2 states, or 732,500. A three-word sentence requires 850^3 (i.e., 60 million) states to represent all combinations. Broadbent argued that it is the capacity of a human's nervous system to deal with the information demands posed by sequentially coded messages that makes language possible. Whereas humans master sequential learning tasks readily, animals have great difficulty with them.

Schemata, Automatization, and Awareness

Broadbent related the classes of stimulus–response relationships described above to differing degrees of awareness. Responses based on single stimuli often proceed with minimal or no awareness. For example, a person may leave a room and shortly afterward not remember whether he turned off the light. Responses that are elicited by invariant patterns of stimuli may reach awareness, although people may not be able to describe the basis of the pattern. The perceptual organization of patterns is a major concern of Gestalt psychology. Bartlett (1932) referred to such informative patterns as *schemata*. Responses to unique, sequential stimuli in language are generally made with awareness: A person does not have to think how to put a shirt on, or what is road and what is sidewalk. But a person has to decide in some conscious way how to respond to a question. Broadbent noted that Bartlett (1932) distinguished between schematic memory and memory requiring consciousness. Memory for schemata (habitually encountered patterns of stimuli, or responses organized into a complex pattern) is often nonverbal and can be executed with little awareness. The components of a schema are frequently lost to awareness. Athletes are often mistaken about what they actually do when performing and are surprised by their motor behavior on videotapes. Bartlett argued that the recall of individual events in their temporal context, however, entails consciousness. For example, a woman recalls that she wrote a section of a book in the morning, went shopping in the early afternoon, and decided to prepare fettucini Alfredo for supper. This type of recall is now referred to as *episodic memory* (Tulving, 1983). Similarly, the performance of an action that requires the comprehension of a unique sequence of events requires consciousness. The performance and recall of behavior that requires the preservation of the sequential characteristics of events require more capacity than stimulus- or pattern-based behavior, and this is why they require, or at least enter, awareness.

Broadbent argued that *automatization* of a task occurs when performance can be reduced to an invariant stimulus–response relationship (Figure 2.3a), or to a schematic operation (Figure 2.3b). Typically, this process is highly practiced. As a task becomes more automatized, it requires less information from the environment in order to be carried out and places fewer demands on capacity within the nervous system. Consequently, it becomes less conscious and interferes less with the concurrent performance of other activities. If the stream of stimuli in the environment becomes unpredictable, however, the task will again demand capacity and require conscious performance.

As an example, while driving along a divided highway with little traffic in the daylight, you can easily listen to the radio, carry on a conversation, daydream, or make plans for future activities. As night falls, however, you enter an area of heavy construction. The road narrows, is bordered by concrete abutments, and makes sudden changes in direction. Traffic is congested, and cars move abruptly in and out around you, often without signaling, in the few places where there is room to maneuver. Despite these problems, you're late for a crucial appointment and want to make the best possible time, and therefore you try to take advantage of any opening in the traffic yourself. As you enter the construction zone, the predictability of freeway driving disappears, and much greater demands are placed on your nervous system. Consequently, your awareness of your decisions relating to driving increases, and your ability to think or listen to other things diminishes.

A Structural Model of Automatic and Controlled Processes

Broadbent and the experimenters he cited laid the groundwork for the investigation of automatic processes. It was not until 20 years later, however, that more detailed models of automatic processing were developed. Schneider and Shiffrin (1977; Shiffrin & Schneider, 1977) presented a comprehensive theory of human information processing that placed particular emphasis on the role of memory in modulating attentional processes. This theory was elaborated within the context of an exhaustive literature review, and several experiments were interpolated within the text. These authors were particularly concerned about the distinction between mental activities that require conscious control or capacity and those that seem to proceed automatically once they are initiated. Most important, their model and experiments explicitly dealt with the question of what sort of effortful processes can be automated with practice, and how performance changes as a result of automatization. Because of the scope of this model and its influence on subsequent theories, it will be described in detail.

The framework adopted by Schneider and Shiffrin is structuralist in its description of mental processing and associationist in its description of learning. *Memory* is described as a collection of *nodes* interrelated through learning. Each node consists of many information elements. When one element of a node is activated, all associated elements are activated as well, a principle called *unitized response*. The *long-term store* consists of inactive nodes. The *short-term store* consists of activated nodes, whose information is available for further processing. *Control processes* (decisions, rehearsal, coding, searching of stores) manipulate the input and output of information from the short-term store. A *control process* is a sequence of nodes activated by attention to accomplish a specific task. Such a process is flexible, temporary, and limited by the capacity of the short-term store. Because of this capacity limitation, controlled processes must be executed serially. *Automatic processes* are the learned, sequential activation of nodes in which (1) the same sequence is always activated by a particular input, and (2) the sequence is activated and run with little or no attention required. Once learned, an automatic sequence is difficult to suppress, ignore, or modify. Automatic processes, because they make minimal demands on the attention of the short-term store capacity, can run in parallel. Like Broadbent, Shiffrin and Schneider stressed the role of an invariant relationship between stimulus and response in enabling automatic processing.

The capacity limitations of the short-term store play a pivotal role in the theory. The short-term store serves two functions, providing (1) a storehouse for currently relevant information (sensory input and activated nodes) and (2) a work space for control processes. A large amount of information in the short-term store may be activated simultaneously, but only a small amount will persist for more than a few seconds. By incorporating a decay process within the short-term store, the model is able to explain how the system may occasionally react to sensory information that is outside the primary channel when its meaning can be extracted within a few seconds.

Schneider and Shiffrin tested this model in a series of target detection tasks. Subjects were required to search through a set of visual stimuli (letters and numbers) to detect the presence of targets corresponding to the items in a memory set. Schneider and Shiffrin predicted that when the memory set was distinct from the distractor set, a subject would be able to develop an automatic detection technique that would result in a gradual improvement in performance. Each stimulus was associated with a particular invariant response, a relationship that Schneider and Shiffrin referred to as *consistent mapping*. They predicted that automatic processing should be relatively unaffected by the number of items in the memory or stimulus set, because the sequence of nodes activated by a stimulus and leading to a response was always the same, and parallel processing could take place. In a *varied mapping* task, in which the stimulus and response relationships changed between trials, a controlled search process had to be used for each trial. The controlled search was serial, load-dependent, and exhaustive. In the varied mapping task, which required controlled, effortful, and serial processing for each task, the investigators predicted that little improvement would occur over trials.

These predictions were confirmed in a series of visual search and detection experiments. The investigators' paradigm can best be appreciated if we describe an experiment in detail. In one experiment, the factors of mapping (consistent vs. varied), stimulus set size, memory set size, stimulus duration, and presence of a target were varied. In the consistent mapping condition, elements in the memory set were never distractors and were distinguishable in category from the distractor sets (e.g., consonants vs. numbers). Therefore, the subject simply had to decide whether any character on a display was from a target category (e.g., a letter) or not. In the varied mapping condition, an element of the memory set on one presentation might be a distractor on another presentation, and the elements in the memory set were from the same category as elements from the distractor set (e.g., consonants). As predicted, in the consistent mapping condition, performance (correct detection) was little affected by load (set size) and was always superior to performance in the varied mapping conditions. In the varied mapping condition, performance decreased as a function of memory and stimulus set size, consistent with the notion that a controlled process is load-dependent. In both conditions, performance improved with increased stimulus duration.

Other experiments tested whether performance improved with practice on a consistent-mapping target-detection task. Two effects were found. First, performance levels slowly increased over many trials, while reaction time decreased, consistent with a change from controlled search to automatic detection. Second, when the items in the memory set and the distractor set were reversed after 1,500 trials, a negative transfer effect occurred. Performance on the task fell below, and remained below, initial performance for many trials. This finding was consistent with the idea that, after an automatic process is learned, it is difficult to modify or forget and may interfere with subsequent controlled processing in a similar domain.

This series of experiments and comments by Shiffrin and Schneider articulated the most integrated theoretical model for distinguishing automatic and controlled processes to date. The division of processing into controlled and automatic on the basis of the stimulus-and-response relationship made explicit a basic principle that could cut across many task situations. There is an unusual theoretical coherence in their model of automatic and controlled processing. This coherence is due in part to the development of Schneider and Shiffrin's theory within the existent, elaborated, and experimentally defined framework of structural information processing, and in part to its interweaving of attentional and memory processes. For example, although capacity is alluded to within the model, it is closely tied to the short-term store. The properties of the short-term store have been exhaustively investigated and therefore do not have to be experimentally defined again. In contrast, other investigators have defined capacity and processing resources much more broadly and have avoided identifying capacity with any particular phenomenological, information-processing, or neural system. Similarly, by describing the long-term store in associationist language, Schneider and Shiffrin (1977) placed automatic versus controlled processing within a richly elaborated model of memory. Finally, their theory predicts what classes of tasks can and cannot be automatized, a prediction that may give the model great generality.

The current limitation of the model is the lack of empirical data regarding the generality of their model across different experimental paradigms. Most studies of controlled and automatic processes use variations of visual target detection with similar task demands. Another limitation is the explicit exclusion of energetic factors, such as effort and arousal, from their model. Schneider, Dumais, and Shiffrin, 1984) attempted to integrate work in the area of controlled and automatic processing with the main currents of attentional theory and experimentation. Table 2.1 is adapted from Schneider *et al.* (1984) and specifies the relationship of these processes to a wide variety of attentional constructs.

CAPACITY, RESOURCE, AND SKILL

Frequently, we find that we can perform two tasks at the same time; for example, we can talk and simultaneously drive or walk; listen to music while eating dinner; plan our day's activities while putting on our clothes. Most of the examples of easily performed dual tasks combine quite different types of performance, usually well-practiced motor behaviors like driving or walking, along with equally well-practiced perceptual or cognitive activities. When we attempt to combine similar or difficult tasks, it may be difficult or impossible to perform them simultaneously. It is difficult to read and listen to a conversation at the same time, or to listen to music while playing a different piece of music, or to dress and eat at the same time without spilling something. Information-processing models discuss these problems in terms of the limited capacity of the nervous system and the relative automatization of concurrently performed tasks. A difficult problem that remains to be solved is the measurement of attentional capacity and the influence of such factors as effort or arousal on it.

Capacity plays a central role in explanations of how dual tasks are performed and how attention is divided among sensory, cognitive, and motoric tasks (Kahneman, 1973; Moray, 1967; Norman & Bobrow, 1975; Schneider & Shiffrin, 1977, Shiffrin & Schneider, 1977). Capacity represents the total number of processing resources available to an individual at a given time. Although limited, the resources that make up total capacity can be deployed on

Table 2.1.   Automatic and Control Processes[a]

Characteristic	Automatic process	Control process
Central capacity	Not required	Required
Control	Not complete	Complete
Integration	Holistic	Fragmented
Practice	Improves	Minimal effect
Modification	Difficult	Easy
Serial-parallel	Parallel	Serial
LTM storage	Little	Large amounts
Efficiency	High	Low
Awareness	Low	High
Attention	Not required	Required
Effort	Little	Much

[a]Adapted from Schneider, Dumais, and Shiffrin (1984).

more than one task, or on more than one stage of processing. However, when capacity is deployed on a secondary task, the primary-task performance frequently suffers because some upper limit of the available resources has been reached. In studies of human performance, the demand placed by a task on processing resources is called the task's *work load*. The greater the work load imposed by a task, the more the resources that are consumed, and the fewer the resources that are available for concurrent activities.

What are resources? Generally, theorists have avoided associating resources with particular mental or neuroanatomical systems; instead, they have described resources metaphorically. In a critique of resource models, Hirst noted that resources are described in at least two ways: as mental "fuel," such as effort, energy, or arousal, which is limited in quantity and drives cognitive processes; and as structural limitations, such as the content of short-term memory, which cannot be exceeded regardless of the amount of effort used in the task. Although resource theorists allude to both types of limitations, they tend to treat resources as a higher order entity, without bothering to differentiate its constituent mental elements. In the elaborate development of resource models by Navon and Gopher (1979), resources are described in economic terms. In the same way that economic output is constrained by the resources of a country, so are processing power and speed in the human information-processing system. Whereas economic resources are associated with concrete entities such as the labor pool, coal, or industrial capacity, processing resources in the human can be described only in terms of performance. Like most theories of attention, resource models posit systems that can never be directly observed or measured. Indeed, resources are not associated with any particular information-processing stages or neuro-anatomical systems but may be distributed among them in a flexible way. Given this degree of nonspecificity, the first step in developing resource theory was to conceptualize resources in such a way as to allow measurement of the resources that a task required, as well as how these demands changed as a function of task demands. In this discussion of resource models of attention, we shall follow Wickens's suggestion (1984) of using *capacity* to refer to the maximum amount of resources available for a task and *resources* to describe the actual amount of total capacity that is being used for a given performance.

One method of measuring the resources allocated to a task is to simply ask a person to vary the amount of effort put into a task. People are surprisingly effective in allocating resources to a task or tasks according to instructions (Wickens, 1984). In Figure 2.4, the increase in performance that occurs as greater effort is applied by a performer results in a gradual increase in performance. This curve is called a *performance–resource function* (Norman & Bobrow, 1975). When performance can be increased by devoting more resources to its execution, it is said to be resource-limited. However, trying too hard inevitably results in a degradation of skilled performance. Tasks based on the quality of sensory information may reach a performance limit that is determined by the quality of the information received, rather than the resources or processing strategies used by the perceiver. A listener can, with effort, detect particular sounds in a noisy environment. But if the sounds become too faint, or the environment too noisy, no amount of effort will increase performance. If the investment of additional resources no longer improves performance, the performance is said to be data-limited, rather than resource-limited. The curve in Figure 2.4 flattens as it enters the area of data limitation because increases in effort have no impact on the quality of performance.

The performance–resource function is a basic concept in resource theory, but by itself, it is a limited conceptual and analytical tool. Why worry about resources if the determinants of the curve can be expressed in such traditional terms as effort and skill? In addition, although resource theorists assume that increased effort translates into increased alloca-

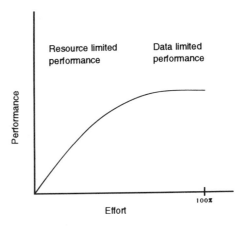

FIGURE 2.4. The performance level on a task is influenced by the level of effort only when task performance is dependent on the available resources. When task performance is limited by the quality of data, investing more effort will no longer improve performance.

tion of resources, it is not at all clear that this is what is occurring. As will be discussed in another section, effort has long been associated with the phenomenon of arousal. Arousal, unlike resources, is associated with specific physiological changes in the central and peripheral nervous system and, in this sense, is more directly measurable (although arousal has its own difficulties as an explanatory device). Moreover, advocates of resource models of attention rarely explain why processing resources should vary with effort rather than simply be available to whatever sensory or cognitive operations are currently being conducted.

Another method of quantifying the resources that a task requires is to have a person intermittently or continuously engage in a secondary task. The more resources required by the primary task, the fewer available for the secondary task. Consequently, a person's performance on a secondary task should become poorer when the primary task increases its demands on common resources. Analysis of dual-task performance has been the most common approach to measuring the relative demand on resources by a task. Dual-task analysis has several advantages. Tasks vary in the demands they place on the operator and are said to place varying work loads on an operator. Sometimes, this variation can be attributed to the computational aspects of a task: It is easier to square a number than to estimate its square root. More often, however, the source of the limitation is much harder to quantify: Is it harder to dress, drive a car, or listen to a conversation? If motivation and resources remain constant, however, the demands of different tasks on the resource pool may theoretically be compared by the amount they degrade the performance of a simultaneously performed task. Because motivation is assumed to be maximal throughout such experiments, it does not need to be considered as an experimental variable. Because the same pool of resources is available to all activities as needed, the source of the difficulty associated with a particular task need not be understood; only its experimentally defined demand on resources must be understood. Most important, if processing resources represent a single pool of "fuel" (Hirst, 1986), then if one knows the demands of two tasks on resources, it should be possible to *predict* dual-task performance. Such predictive power would be of great practical importance in the design of work settings when operators such as airplane pilots are required to monitor and respond to multiple sources of information.

Performance Operating Characteristics

Performance operating characteristics (POCs, also called *attention operating characteristics* or *AOCs*) are curves that describe the relationship between two tasks performed simultaneously at constant levels of effort (Kinchla, 1980; Navon & Gopher, 1979; Norman & Bobrow, 1975). Because the level of effort is assumed to be constant, the more the resources that are devoted to one task, the fewer that can be devoted to the second task. Figure 2.5 shows such a set of POC curves. The *y*-axis shows the level of performance on one task; the *x*-axis shows the level of performance on a second task; and the curves are idealized representations of how the performance on one task affects the performance level on a concurrent task. In a typical experiment, a subject learns how to perform two tasks. The performance of the subject on each task is then measured when the tasks are performed simultaneously. The subject is asked to devote varying amounts of attention to a primary task, and the concurrent performance on both the primary and the secondary tasks is measured. If secondary-task performance deteriorates when attention is directed to the primary task, the experimenter typically concludes that the two tasks share resources, and that the pool of available resources is not sufficient to allow both tasks to be concluded simultaneously at high performance levels. In Figure 2.5, this is illustrated by a curved POC. As the performance of one task improves, the performance of the second task deteriorates. If both tasks can be performed together at the same performance levels with which they can be performed separately, the tasks do not draw on the same resources, or they are data-limited rather than resource-limited. In this case, the POC for the two tasks is represented by lines at right angles (the solid and dotted line segments in Figure 2.5). Occasionally, the performance on one task can be facilitated by the concurrent performance of another task. For example, a musician may use a metronome to facilitate correct timing when performing a piece of music. This is called a case of *concurrence benefit*. Alternatively, simultaneous performance of a secondary task may always diminish the performance of the primary task, no matter how poorly the secondary task is performed. This relationship is called *concurrence cost*, and it is shown by the POC curve in Figure 2.5.

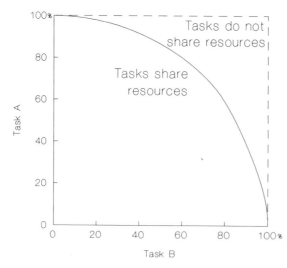

FIGURE 2.5. The performance (or attention) operating characteristics for dual-task performance. The shape of the curve depends on the degree to which Tasks A and B share cognitive resources. If the tasks do not share resources, then the dual-task performance levels remain the same as single-task performance levels (the lines at right angles). If the tasks do share resources, the performance on Task A will change as a function of the performance on Task B (the curved line).

Although learning effects are seldom investigated in studies of processing resources, dual-task performance may be improved in several different ways by practice (Navon & Gopher, 1979). The performance of individual tasks may be improved; the resources may be used more efficiently; tasks may be reorganized to reduce incompatibility; or the two tasks may be unified into a different task. The effect of practice is to increase performance (the POC curve gets higher), but the change in shape of the learning curve will vary somewhat depending on the type of improvement.

As the reader has probably already surmised, resource theory provides ample explanatory devices to account for a wide range of empirical findings. In this sense, it is a very difficult model to test, because it is difficult to conceptualize disconfirming cases. However, even with this great explanatory power, the assumption of a single resource pool shared by all concurrent tasks has not proved to be adequate to describe all experimental results. Most critically, it is usually not possible to predict dual-task performance reliably on the basis of the experimentally determined resource demands of individual tasks. The only way to determine dual-task performance remains to have an operator try to do both tasks at once, and to derive a POC curve empirically. Because of these difficulties, the concept of a single resource pool shared by all information-processing systems has been questioned. As an alternative, multiple-resource pools have been proposed, which are associated with different sensory or cognitive domains. Wickens (1984), for example, proposed that different resources may be associated with different modalities of input (visual vs. auditory), different stages of processing (encoding, central processing, or responding), types of encoding (spatial vs. verbal), and type of response (manual vs. vocal). Such distinctions, however, further complicate a model already overburdened with explanatory constructs, and they are extremely open-ended: Where does one stop drawing distinctions? If visual and auditory resources are to be distinguished, should not olfactory, tactile, kinesthetic, and gustatory resource pools be distinguished as well? The multiplication of interactions inherent in multiple-resource models precludes inclusive experimental design. If we consider all the possible combinations to be examined in Wickens's categorization of resource pools, for example, there are $2 \times 2 \times 3 \times 2 = 24$ conditions to be considered, presumably over a range of difficulty levels.

Critiques of Resource Models

Resource models address the broad question of why there are performance limitations, but they are very vague regarding what processes underlie resources and how they operate. And with the accumulation of experimental data, it appears that the single-resource model, which at least promised a mathematically and experimentally unitary model of resource–performance relationships, must be replaced by an impractically complex multiple-resource model. This combination of conceptual vagueness and rapidly escalating complexity has led to a mounting criticism of resource models, and to the development or resurrection of other models of multiple-task performance.

Interference Rather Than Competition

David Navon (1985), who coauthored a comprehensive theoretical paper on processing resources, argued that resource theory has been accepted for the lack of better alternatives that explain the splitting of attention among tasks. Navon argued that a model of multiple-task performance can be developed with the premise that resources are not required for task performance. He pointed out several methodological problems in resource models: POC curves, although closely identified with resource theory, are in reality theory-independent;

motivation effects are not readily explained by a constant resource model; and dual-task performance in typical experiments may be strongly shaped by experimenter demands. In such experiments, the instructions to the subject are usually phrased in such a way as to imply that dual-task performance must result in performance decrements, and the subject is usually given information about how much of a decrement to produce.

As an alternative, Navon proposed that tasks may be difficult to perform conjointly because they interfere with each other, not because they compete for resources. He went on to describe several types of interference effects. One familiar type is *cross-talk*. When two messages interfere with each other on a telephone line, it is not because they are competing for a central, limited resource. Rather, the co-occurrence of two messages produces interference. Similarly, processes in the brain may interfere with each other when they operate concurrently. Neuroanatomical evidence exists for this effect: Tasks interfere more when their processing centers are closer in cerebral space (Kinsbourne, 1970, 1982). Another source of interference may be *difficulty in making nonhabitual transitions*. When a given event invariably leads to the same response, all transitions within the nervous system are habitual. When, on the other hand, a given event forces a person to consider a number of possible responses, or to generate a new response, the transition from event to response requires nonhabitual transitions. The consideration of multiple interpretations of an event, and multiple responses, interferes with other processes that might be carried out in parallel. Habitual transitions are commonplace in our daily life. Driving home from work probably consists entirely of such responses. On the other hand, if a person is forced to detour from a well-known route to an unfamiliar section of the city, each intersection requires that a choice be made. The information processing at each intersection involves nonhabitual transitions between receiving the information obtained from the intersection, comparing it with a cognitive (or real) map of the city, and choosing whether to continue straight or to turn. While driving along the known route, the driver is able to mentally compose a memorandum; while negotiating the detour, the driver is not.

Skills

Neisser (1976) argued against the notion of limited capacity in the human nervous system. Neisser suggested, for example, that there is nothing about the structure of the brain to suggest whether and where channel limitations in information processing might occur. And although people tend to report conscious experience as something that is oriented around a single event or goal, this self-report may reflect only our cultural preconceptions and linguistic conventions rather than accurately describe the stream of consciousness in its totality. Neisser attributed dual-task difficulties, when they occur, to a variety of sources unrelated to capacity limitations. Skills are seldom learned in a way that facilitates their performance in conjunction. Skills can be combined during learning, or through reorganization, so that they allow effective dual-task performance. Musicians in ensembles commonly learn to play instruments and, at the same time, to listen and react to other instruments in the group. In support of this idea, Hirst, Spelke, Neisser and colleagues (Hirst *et al.*, 1980; Spelke, Hirst, & Neisser, 1976) performed a series of experiments in which the subjects learned to read prose while simultaneously writing words and short sentences from dictation. Initially, they were unable to do so, but after weeks of practice, they became quite efficient. There was even evidence from these experiments that the subjects processed and remembered semantic aspects of the dictated material. This intriguing study, unfortunately, has not prompted further investigations, and the strategy by which the subjects accomplished concurrent reading and writing is unknown. Unlike in the classical dichotic listening paradigms, the two messages were presented by means of different sensory modalities, and the subjects controlled the intake of one channel of information (the words that were read), so that they may have been able to use a variety of dual-task strategies.

Nevertheless, if dual-task performance at a semantic level is so malleable by learning, then a model positing fixed resources, which fix performance levels, becomes far less attractive (Hirst, 1986). On a theoretical level, although practice effects can be accommodated by resource theory (Navon & Gopher, 1980; Norman & Bobrow, 1975), they force the theory to deal with variations in individual skills and learning strategies in conjunction with individual variations in resources. Pragmatically, it indicates that POCs may radically change over comparatively short periods of time because of learning, so that they are, at most, transiently informative in predicting operator performance.

Hirst (1986) suggested that the concept of *skill* can replace the concept of *resource*. He admitted that *skill*, like *resources* is a vague concept. Unlike resources, however, skill does not carry a great theoretical burden with it. Instead of thinking about how a person's performance of multiple tasks reflects types of resources and demands on them, the experimenter thinks about how a person has developed or improved a skill. Skill emphasizes the observation that successful dual-task performance involves adaptations in the performer specific to those tasks that may not, and probably will not, generalize to other pairs of tasks. A skilled typist may be able to shadow (repeat) a message while typing (Shaffer, 1975), but this ability does not imply that the typist will find it easier than other subjects to read prose while writing from dictation.

Hirst summarized four techniques that can be used to facilitate dual-task performance: integration, automaticity, segregation, and time sharing.

Integration involves coordinating and combining two tasks in a single higher order task. An everyday example is dressing, which requires simultaneous movements of many body parts, as when putting on overalls. It takes a long time for a child to achieve this level of integration.

Automaticity involves practicing one task until it is automatic and then combining it with another task (e.g., driving and then talking while driving).

Segregation requires learning to keep tasks cognitively or neurally insulated from each other (reducing cross-talk).

Time sharing between tasks involves paying attention to one, then the other. Attention is not divided or shared in this situation but is switched from one message to another at junctions. Most students appear to learn to listen to a lecture while concurrently working on an assignment, with varying levels of efficacy.

It is perhaps notable that three of these strategies (integration, automaticity, and time sharing) were articulated and investigated by numerous authors in the 1800s (e.g., James, 1890) and were central concepts in Broadbent's model of information processing (1958).

Summary

Resource models ascribe the limitations in a person's ability to do more than one thing at a time to limits in processing resources that are shared by many mental systems. It appeals to our introspective feeling that our ability to attend is limited, and that the limit is quickly reached. Resource models, however, have had modest predictive success, are isolated from other currents of cognitive psychology and information-processing theory, and provide such a multiplicity of explanatory devices that virtually any pattern of performance can be retrospectively fit to the model. Capacity models suffer from a conceptual vagueness, primarily because of the reluctance of theorists (or their inability) to define the specific cognitive structures whose information-processing capacity is invariant between individuals and does not change as a function of practice. (One candidate for such a structure is working memory, which plays a central role in Schneider and Shiffrin's model of automatic and control processing.) If classical channel models were too restricted in scope to encompass exceptions to their general principles, it may be that resource models are too broad to provide useful conceptual tools.

Other explanations of multiple-task limitations, such as skill acquisition and interference effects, have been put forward to replace resource models in the analysis of multiple-task performance. These alternative models suffer at this time from a lack of conceptual detail, empirical investigation, and generality, which limits their attraction as a foundation for a cognitive model. In its strongest form, as articulated by Hirst (1986), skills do not generalize beyond a specific task domain, although the techniques of dual-task performance may be identifiable. This intrinsic lack of generality makes a skills approach unattractive to cognitive theorists seeking models with potentially strong predictive power.

Response Selection and the Executive Control of Attention

RONALD A. COHEN and YVONNE A. SPARLING-COHEN

Attention is considered by many cognitive theorists an extension of sensory processes. When we attend, some information is selected for further processing, and other information is ignored. Because attentional selection involves choosing one stimulus from a set of possible stimuli, it is easy to see why sensory selection has been emphasized in most theories of attention. However, attentional selection is also a "behavioral act," one that depends on motor activity, or at least on response execution and control. As we attend to stimuli in our environment, we direct our focus by looking, orienting our bodies, or preparing to respond either overtly or covertly. Furthermore, response preparation and selection are effortful and are subject to fatigue. In this chapter, we discuss how response selection influences attention, as well as the characteristics of attentional effort, vigilance, and fatigue.

RESPONSE SELECTION AND ATTENTION

Many of the information-processing models of attention discussed in previous chapters emphasized the role of "early" sensory selection processes. These models postulated a bottleneck through which incoming information is gated. A bottleneck reduces the number of information channels that are competing for address in the central processing system. Presumably, the bottleneck constrains the amount of information to be handled during serial processing. A bottleneck is necessary because humans have difficulty performing multiple simultaneous tasks, especially when the tasks are demanding. By reducing the amount of information to be responded to at each point in time, the system can avoid being overloaded. The sensory selection models (e.g., Treisman, 1964, 1969) place this bottleneck at a very early stage in the information-processing sequence during which little motor involvement would be possible.

Broadbent (1958) and Treisman (1960, 1964) have argued that the placement of a filter or a bottleneck soon after sensory registration is necessary to explain the transition from parallel to serial processing. Many of the early attentional theorists questioned whether attention can be handled by a set of processes in parallel because normally, humans can perform only a very limited number of activities simultaneously. Subsequent experiments have demonstrated that people can perform simultaneous tasks, as long as the demands of each task are not excessive. However, the capacity for attention to more than one task depends on many factors, such as the nature of the stimuli and the tasks, as well as the individual differences across people. Simultaneous stimuli processed by different perceptual analyzers can be dealt with in parallel (e.g., concurrent visual and auditory analysis), whereas simultaneous stimuli processed by a single analyzer must be handled serially.

These conclusions are based on two sets of observations: (1) people have difficulty dividing attention among multiple inputs, whereas they are able to easily direct attention to one stimulus, and (2) it is relatively easy to divide attention among the attributes of a single input, but it is difficult to focus on one attribute, while ignoring others. These findings supported the idea that a bottleneck is located at an early processing stage.

Late Selection Models

Motor and behavioral response-control processes have not been believed to be major determinants of attentional selection by most theorists working from an information-processing perspective. There have been several noteworthy exceptions. Deutsch and Deutsch (1963) proposed a model of attention that differs from that of the sensory selection theories. The model proposes that the attentional bottleneck occurs at a later stage of information processing. This late selection model of attention (or the Deutsch model) assumes that stimuli are perceptually processed regardless of whether they are attended to or not. All incoming information must activate at least those parts of the CNS involved in sensory registration. Deutsch and Deutsch proposed that the central processing system is capable of forming response biases determined by the preset weightings. These response biases are determined by either the momentary state of relevance or a more enduring response disposition. A momentary state may reflect a motivational or reinforcement effect. For instance, if the current state of the individual reflects hunger, then food names may have priority for attentional allocation. Dispositions are reflected in a tendency to respond to certain stimuli that have inherent organismic salience (e.g., a red stop light is universally important as a warning in our culture).

By emphasizing the importance of dispositions and momentary bias, Deutsch and Deutsch suggested that attention is determined by factors associated with response planning and response selection. Consequently, they placed the attentional bottleneck at a processing stage that is much closer to the point of response generation. Although their model does not go so far as to suggest that motoric action is the basis of attentional control, it does emphasize the importance of response-related factors in determining how attentional selection occurs.

The Deutsch model accounts for the capacity of subjects to perform some types of divided-attention tasks. However, it came under much attack because it does not account for attention in all types of tasks, particularly those in which it is not possible to preset a response bias. The model's weakness is most evident in connection with tasks of focused attention like the ones that Broadbent's filter theory (1958, 1963) was designed to address. Late selection models cannot easily account for the ability of subjects to preferentially select stimuli coming to a particular sensory modality (i.e., the left ear during dichotic listening), as it is not possible to create an a priori response tendency to favor words coming into a particular channel. Registration must first occur centrally, and then some sensory selection decision is made in favor of one ear over the other. For a late-stage attentional bottleneck to work in the dichotic listening task, it would be necessary that the incoming information activate central structures, then trigger response biases, which prompt a feedback arrangement for retrospective analysis of the ear in which the word has occurred. This sequence obviously involves a rather complex and rather lengthy process that would make attentional selection on the basis of stimulus features very difficult. Subsequent experimental analyses of this problem revealed that selection based on stimulus features is, in fact, much easier than selection based on response criteria.

The Deutsch model predicted that when attention is divided among concurrent stimuli, the detection of salient inputs should be relatively easy even if they are not the initial target of attention, because all incoming information receives perceptual analysis. Treisman and Geffen (1967) tested this hypothesis using a dichotic listening task with a shadowing paradigm. Subjects were required to shadow (repeat after a short delay) all words coming to one ear, with instructions to remain vigilant and to respond when they heard a particular stimulus word in either ear. The Deutsch late selection theory predicted that this task should not be difficult because if the response bias is preset to detect a particular word, it should not matter that one channel (ear) is always being attended to. Treisman and Geffen's findings did not support this conclusion, as the detection rates were very high for the attended-to channel (87%) and very low for the unattended-to channel (8%). These findings led many attentional theorists to conclude that the early-selection models are more accurate.

Not all theorists abandoned the idea of late-attention selection associated with response set. Norman (1968) expanded the Deutsch model to address the criticisms of it. Norman suggested that the human attentional system is capable of dealing differently with two types of information: sensory and pertinence. Sensory information may be gated at an earlier stage of processing, whereas information that increases the salience of the sensory input may be gated at a later stage, closer to the stage of response selection.

Norman's theory advanced the general attentional framework of Deutsch and Deutsch. It suggests that attention involves multiple processes, one of which is governed by response demands. Because the sensory information contained in a stimulus may cause early activation of the central processing system, the theory accounts for why attention to a stimulus set is not more difficult than attention to a response set. However, studies that tested the predictions of Norman's revised model (e.g., Kahneman, Beatty, & Pollack, 1967) found inconsistencies with some of the model's predictions, particularly the level of discriminability for unattended-to inputs.

Norman proposed that the activation of stimulus-processing units by response-relevant stimuli causes pertinence to increase, and that this increase has the effect of changing the attentional response criterion. In contrast, the early-selection theories of Treisman and Broadbent predict a change in the discriminability (d') of signal detection based on the relevance of the incoming information. Experimental studies that demonstrated a change in d' corresponding to the relevance of the information being processed again supported the early-selection argument. Selective attention seems to influence the discriminability of sensory attentional processing.

Neisser (1967, 1969) proposed an alternative account of attention that attempted to avoid the pitfalls that had led to the debate over the location of the attentional filter. He started with an assumption that perception is an active process of synthesizing incoming stimuli. Stimuli that are attended to differ from those not attended to, primarily because they are not acted on. Neisser argued that filtering is not necessary because selective attention is simply the act of selecting a stimulus for further processing. As an example, he described the selection of a sandwich from a tray containing a number of possible choices. In choosing a sandwich, the person does not filter or block the food that he or she does not select. Rather, the person selects a potential item and then gives it some further attention or examination, before eating it.

In this model, attention reflects the allocation of a limited processing capacity to stimuli chosen from various alternatives for further perceptual synthesis. Response preparation is incorporated as an important part of this process, as situational response requirements ultimately determine which stimuli are relevant and in need of focused attention. Accordingly, attention is the by-product of a selection process guided by response demands that choose certain stimuli for further processing. Perceptual synthesis was considered an effortful process. For Neisser, perceptual synthesis was related to factors associated with response production. He suggested that a separate passive, preattentive system may exist to perform the preliminary sorting of perceptual input before synthesis. However, he distinguished preattentive filtering from the active attentional processing that occurs during perceptual synthesis.

The debate over when the attentional bottleneck occurs (early sensory vs. late response stages) was bypassed by Neisser's model. Because he regarded responding and perceiving as intricately related, he avoided the question of whether attentional selection is driven by sensory or response-based factors. Neisser emphasized that attention is influenced by multiple processes. By equating perceptual synthesis with focal attention, this theory regards attention as a bridge between perception and the production of responses. Attention reflects the sensorimotor integration occurring during information processing. Neisser argued that the sensory and response components of attention are so intertwined that they often cannot be distinguished. Neisser made a point of distinguishing between focused attention and preattentive processing. He proposed that focused attention reflects awareness, whereas preattentive filtering occurs with little awareness.

Because behaviors requiring perceptual synthesis can be performed without much awareness (e.g., driving a car), some theorists questioned Neisser's linking of focal attention with awareness. Subsequently, models were proposed by other investigators (e.g., Hochberg, 1970) that addressed this point by separating perceptual synthesis from awareness. Still, it can be argued that Neisser had only redefined attention so as to create an arbitrary separation between attention and preattention, as the distinction made between perceptual synthesis and awareness is very similar to that made between the models of early- and late-stage selection which were described previously. Many of the predictions of Neisser's model are very similar to those proposed by Broadbent and Treisman.

The most noteworthy aspect of Neisser's model is that he replaced the concept of a filter with a component of active selection. This change enabled Neisser to incorporate both perceptual and response-based components into a unitary model. Therefore, the model differs from the sensory selection models primarily because of its emphasis that attention involves the active selection of stimuli with regard to potential responses.

Capacity Constraints and Response Demands

Kahneman's capacity model (1973) focuses on the factors that affect the ability of humans to perform at optimal levels, rather than the location of the attentional bottleneck (see Figure 3.1). The capacity model proposes that attention is controlled by both ease of sensory selection during early processing and a sensitivity, dependent on task demands, that rejects irrelevant information. The impact of task demands on the available capacity is manifested in the form of effort. When a task requires greater processing capacity, the task demand is reflected by the effort necessary to perform adequately. The need for greater effort ultimately increases the demands on the response system, making sustained performance more difficult.

This model proposes that capacity limitations are created by the energetic state of the individual. Kahneman related effort to the energetic state and linked the concept of generalized arousal to this limited capacity. The energetic state has implications for the

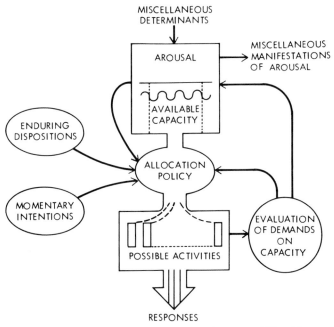

FIGURE 3.1. The attention capacity model. (From Kahneman, 1973, with permission.)

idea that attention is influenced by response demands, as energy expenditure is typically related to work load during behavioral responding.

The controversy over the location of the attentional bottleneck has subsided since the early 1970s, as evidence has suggested that attentional control emerges at several different stages of processing. Studies of selective attention to multiple inputs in parallel indicate that some types of attentional selection or filtering occur at early stages of sensory processing. Other studies have illustrated that response demands impose constraints on attention and serve to control the direction of attention. The characteristics of the attentional bottleneck that is observed depend on the experimental paradigm that is used.

This point has been illustrated by the studies of Schneider and Shiffrin (1977) and Hasher and Zacks (1979), which distinguished between automatic and controlled attention. Attentional effort was created by increases in memory load on tasks requiring the analysis of successive frames of spatial stimuli when the targets to be detected varied (variable memory set). The result was a significant slowing of reaction time as a function of memory set size. This slowing was also shown to be related to the informational content of the targets, as a determination of categorical information slows reaction times even more than simple word discriminations (Fisk & Schneider, 1984). These results suggest that attentional effort and control are strongly related to the demands of a task. Therefore, the need for attentional control may be induced by different types of experimental manipulations, some of which increase response demands, and others of which increase memory or cognitive processing demands.

With respect to the original question of whether response preparation, selection, or execution exerts control over attention, the answer must be yes. Whether this control is a function of motor, premotor, or higher order executive processes is less clear-cut. It is feasible that attention is determined by several different response-dependent factors, including (1) the demands of motor responding; (2) the positional orienting of the animal toward the available stimuli (looking); and (3) the covert organization and planning of the behavioral responses.

Motoric Influences on Attention

The idea that attention is related to response selection and production is not new. William James (1890) had proposed that the nature of the response occurring in a situation governs the associated mental experience. In his theory of emotions, emotional experience results from the labeling of overt motor responses. This model continues to be investigated by psychologists studying emotions, though James's original model, which considered the behavioral–motor response to be a precursor to the cognitive–emotional experience, is no longer viewed as favorably. Although there is some empirical support for the role of motor responding in governing or facilitating cognition (see Chapter 6), most cognitive investigators discount the idea that motor responding is the primary basis for cognitive phenomena like attention.

Theories advocating a motoric basis for cognition have largely been refuted, as experimental studies of animals and human subjects whose motor systems have been disrupted have failed to indicate cognitive impairment. When subjects were given curare, a drug that blocks the neuromuscular junctions of the peripheral musculature, they were still able to solve complex mental problems (Leuba, Birch, & Appleton, 1968). If the feedback from peripheral musculature were critical to attention or other cognitive operations, one would expect that these subjects would have lost their problem-solving ability. These findings led researchers to conclude that the motor system plays a minimal role in cognition.

Some investigators have criticized the curare studies on the grounds that the findings of decreased peripheral muscular activity, as recorded in these studies, may have been insufficient to rule out completely the role of the motor systems in cognition (McGuigan, 1978). Although peripheral neuromuscular response was blocked by curare, covert central motor activation may still have played a role in mediating cognitive performance. Some researchers even suggested that, although the muscular response was greatly reduced, small levels of muscular feedback may still have been influential.

Although there continues to be some support for the role of the motor system in cognition, the notion that motoric responding is the primary basis for cognitive processing appears untenable. There is overwhelming evidence to support the position that factors associated with central processing influence selective attention. Motor responding cannot be the central determinant of attentional control. Yet, the importance of motoric responding in attentional control should not be completely dismissed.

In the absence of normal sensory input, animals still attempt to select stimuli from the environment. For instance, an animal that is blind, deaf, and hungry moves about, exploring and searching for food, when placed in a novel environment. The animal's behavior is motorically directed, as it attempts to access the remaining cues regarding the location of food. The act of searching the environment is driven by an attempt to detect cues and ultimately to locate food. Therefore, motoric responding (i.e., searching) is initiated in an effort to select the appropriate stimulus.

Although the above is an extreme example, it illustrates that motoric responding is an important aspect of attentional behavior, one that is independent of sensory registration and selection. The motor act facilitates the development of dispositions and the orientation of an animal's behavior toward available cues. Although it can be argued that the intake of sensory cues normally precedes a motor response, this may not always be the case. Attention may be directed by the opposite sequence. In many cases, the animal may begin overtly searching the environment, looking for salient information that will trigger further attentional allocation. The catalyst for this type of search may be motivationally determined.

Even when overt motor responding is suppressed, one cannot rule out the possibility that systems related to motor responding are involved in attentional control. For instance, the use of curare to block motor responses proves that peripheral motor activity is not essential for thinking,but it does not discount the possibility that covert premotor activation and planning are responsible for problem solving. There may be many motorically based cognitive processes that do not produce visible overt responses. Certain types of brain damage produce neuropsychological impairments, known as *apraxias*, that are disorders of motor intention and planning, rather than disorders of overt movement. Motor-response planning and intention have obvious implications for the processes of attention. The fact that the motor system is hierarchically arranged makes the possibility of a premotor basis for attentional control feasible. This fact led Sperry (1952) to conclude, "The core of the perceptual process is not itself a motor pattern. It is more pre-motor or better pre-premotor in nature owing to the hierarchical plan of neural organization" (p. 309). Sperry concluded that "the entire output of our thinking has ultimately but one end, to aid in the regulation of motor coordination" (p. 299).

Motor Activation during Covert Processing

There are several lines of evidence suggesting that motor activation influences attention and the handling of incoming information. Subvocalization was once thought to be the behavioral basis for thought. Although most neuroscientists no longer give this idea much credence, there is evidence that covert verbal rehearsal produces motor activation. McGuigan and Rodier (1968) noted more motor activation (EMG) of the laryngeal speech apparatus in subjects who engaged in covert reading in the presence of auditory distraction (white noise) than in subjects who read in silence. This increase in motor activation presumably reflects efforts to overcome the division of attention between the relevant words and distracting noise.

Cohen and Waters (1985) found increased muscle activation associated with the covert processing of words during a level-of-processing task. The degree of EMG activation did not covary as a function of the level of processing (i.e., phonemic, low semantic, and high semantic), in contrast to heart rate and skin conductance measures, which did vary as a function of both the stage of covert processing and the level of processing. This finding provides a further indication that motor activation is associated with the covert act of attending to a word and to problem solving. However, the fact that EMG levels did not differentiate the levels of processing suggests that measures of gross motor activity may not be as sensitive to subtle variations in task demand as to other autonomic measures. Cacioppo and Petty (1981a,b) found a greater degree of EMG sensitivity to differences in task demand when labial monitoring was conducted. Therefore, certain muscle groups may reflect covert cognitive processes more than others.

Caution should be used when interpreting findings pertaining to the muscular correlates of covert cognitive processes. The motor activation noted in these experiments may simply have been a by-product of attention and problem-solving behavior, and not an important regulatory or facilitatory influence (see Chapter 6). The evidence regarding the impact of muscle activation on cognition is not conclusive. However, it is clear that the autonomic and muscular responses of the body are intricately linked to attentional processes.

Premotor Control of Attention

Disorders of Intention

Damage to cortical areas anterior to the motor strip frequently causes disorders of skilled movement (apraxia) and problems with response planning. Patients with apraxia can perform motor acts reflexively but can not intentionally generate simple motor repertoires on demand. For instance, they may catch a ball when it is thrown to them but may not be capable of demonstrating how to catch or throw a ball. An individual who cannot produce intentional responses is able to react to stimuli, but not to generate a sequence of planned responses. It has been suggested that a distinction should be made between the concepts of *attention* and of *intention* (Heilman, Watson, Valenstein, & Goldberg, 1988). The term *intention* refers to those processes involved in response planning and selection, and the term *attention* refers to the processes of sensory selection. This distinction is quite meaningful, though in practice, it is often difficult to dissociate these two components of behavioral control.

Looking and Attending

It goes without saying that where we look influences what we attend to. Of course, where we look may ultimately be determined by the stimuli in the environment that catch our attention. Looking and attending are functionally intertwined. There is also considerable evidence that these two functions are also physiologically interdependent. The complexity of the interactions between the sensory and the motor systems is apparent when one studies eye movements during attending. During visual search, saccadic eye movements are a fundamental component of attending. Although there are now experimental investigations that illustrate that visual selective attention is possible without eye movements, under normal conditions of attending in the natural environment saccadic activity plays a significant role.

Eye movements are under oculomotor control. They can be classified as either a *saccadic* or a *pursuit* motion. Saccadic eye movements are very rapid (3–5 sec) and occur without conscious or intentional control. Smooth pursuit eye movements are usually slower and correspond to an object of fixation that is moving in a field. Without these two types of eye movement, foveal vision is limited to approximately 2 degrees of the full visual field. Saccadic movements produce a shaping of the images that extend beyond this small range.

Through a combination of saccadic and pursuit eye movements, the individual is able to scan and search a dynamic environment that encompasses three spatial dimensions, and that often contains a multitude of stimulus elements. Most eye movements are saccadic, so that continuous motor planning and control are not required. Saccadic movements occur as a motor program that is based on a prior strategy, or they are elicited reflexively by changes in the stimulus set (i.e., the gaze is drawn to some potentially relevant feature in conjunction with the orienting response). It occurs as a rather automatic part of ongoing activity or tasks in which the individual is engaged.

Less frequently, looking involves an intentional tracking or search for objects in the environment (pursuit movements). These movements suggest a controlled attentional allocation that is voluntary. In both saccadic and pursuit movements, looking involves a response that is very precise and under the fine motor control of the oculomotor system (see Alpern, 1971, for a review).

Eye movement occurs in relationship to the presented stimuli and the task (see Figure 3.2). Studies of fixation patterns during the perception of pictures indicate that subjects tend to fixate repeatedly on major features of the picture (Yarbus, 1965). For instance, when one is viewing a face, fixation shifts between the eyes, the mouth, and other structural features. In

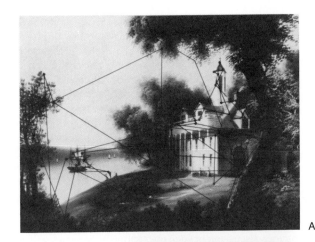

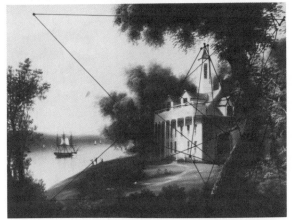

FIGURE 3.2. Effective visual search requires intact functioning of premotor systems such as the frontal lobe eye fields and other frontal lobe systems. (A) Normal subjects focus on the relevant features of pictorial stimuli. Consequently, they exhibit an organized pattern of eye scanning. (B) Patients with right posterior parietal lesions often exhibit a neglect of the left hemispace, though they may scan relevant features in their right hemispace. (C) In contrast, patients with severe frontal lobe dysfunction often exhibit ineffective exploratory search. While they may direct their visual attention to all spatial regions, they often fail to attend to relevant features, and their eye movements have a disorganized and random quality.

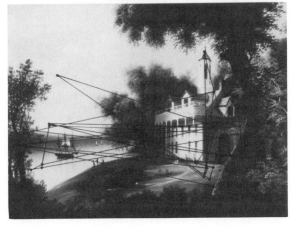

fact, analyses of the eye movement tracings during this task result in a picture that is an approximation of the original facial stimuli. Obviously, tracings of eye movements are based on motor output, rather than on actual sensory input. Yet, these movements seem to mirror the relevant visual features of the stimulus. Yarbus (1965) showed that changing the instructional set for this type of task influences the eye movements that occur, as the subject fixates to a greater extent on features relevant to the new task.

The eye movements of patients with frontal lobe lesions affecting the frontal eye fields show a great reduction in the quantity and precision of visual search movement. In contrast, damage to the primary visual cortex and associated areas in the parietal lobe does not result in such a disruption in eye movements (Luria, Karpov, & Yarbus, 1966). Patients with frontal lobe lesions also have a very different type of visual disturbance that involves an inattention to relevant details, as well as a failure to organize or integrate the details of the visual image into a meaningful whole. Therefore, frontal brain systems are critical to the active visual analysis of input and ultimately the process of *looking*. Without the involvement of this cortical system, perception of the entire visual field is possible, though the individual may fail to actively search the environment. The result of such ineffectual visual search is inattention. Because this line of evidence is important to an understanding of attention, further discussion of such inattention syndromes will be considered again later in this book.

Experimental Evidence of Premotor Attentional Control

Several recent investigations have explored the role of premotor systems in the control of attention. For the most part, these studies have used measures of eye movements, along with reaction time and performance data, to determine the speed and efficiency of attending across different regions of visual space.

Gawryszewski, Riggio, Rizzolatti, and Umilta (1987) conducted a series of experiments to examine how different attentional parameters affect reaction time. Their tasks required subjects to attend to a cue before the onset of the target stimuli. The subjects were required to respond differentially to the target stimuli and other distractor stimuli. The cue was in either a correct or an incorrect location with respect to the upcoming stimuli, thereby providing accurate or erroneous information about where the subject should look in space. The spatial position of the cues and targets across the vertical, horizontal, and depth dimensions was varied. Subjects could direct their attention along the dimension of spatial depth without eye movements. The first set of tasks involved a cue that gave spatial information that was incorrect with respect to the position of the upcoming target. When a particular point in space was attended to because of cuing, the subjects responded faster to targets occurring at less depth relative to the cued position than to target positions beyond the cued depth.

In a second set of experiments, subjects were again presented spatial cues that directed their attention to either correct or incorrect spatial positions. Their performance was compared to that on a task in which no prior cue was given. The subjects were much slower in responding to the unattended-to spatial positions than in a neutral condition during which no spatial information was cued. The investigators concluded that this second paradigm demonstrated that the neutral condition involved a state of diffuse, nondirected attention, as proposed by Jonides (1981). The time differences for responding under the three conditions (neutral, invalid cue, and valid cue) illustrated that incorrect fixation has an attentional cost. Gawryszewski, Riggio, Rizzolatti, and Umilta (1987) concluded that the increased time needed for incorrect fixation on a spatial position is most easily accounted for by the time required to substitute motor programs. This finding supports the notion that motor programs help to control spatial attention.

In a related study, Rizzolatti, Riggio, Dascola, and Umilta (1987) tested the hypothesis that reaction time differences that occur when one is attending to correct or incorrect positions are due to premotor factors. A paradigm similar to the one described in the previous experiment was used, except that the subjects were either cued to a specific position or instructed to attend to all of the possible spatial positions of the target stimulus. The subjects showed small but significant benefits from correct cuing to a specific location. More striking was the large increase in reaction times that occurred when the cue stimulus was presented at an incorrect location. The cost of incorrect cuing increased as a function of increased distance between the attended-to location and the position of the actual target. The costs were greatest when the subjects crossed horizontal and vertical midlines.

These effects could not be easily accounted for by a hemifield inhibition hypothesis (i.e., inhibition of one side of space by the other) because, within a particular hemifield, there was a cost of incorrect cuing. The hemifield inhibition hypothesis maintains that an all-or-nothing cost should occur across hemifields (Hughes & Zimba, 1987). The effect may be partially accounted for by the time required to either overtly or covertly orient across the two locations. However, the increased cost of orienting across the midline suggests that there is an additional factor influencing reaction time. Rizzolatti *et al.* (1987) concluded that this factor is the time needed to erase one oculomotor program and prepare another.

Neurophysiological support for the role of premotor factors in the control of spatial attention has been demonstrated in experiments involving laboratory animals, as well as brain-damaged human subjects. Rizzolatti (1983) described investigations by his group into the direction of attention in cats after lesions to midbrain structures, finding that attention was impaired in the vertical, but not the horizontal, dimension. Posner, Cohen, and Rafal (1982) demonstrated a similar disturbance in patients with supranuclear palsy secondary to basal ganglia damage.

Visual-Motor Integration during Attending

A complex relationship between the processes of visual selective attention and visual–motor integration has become apparent from neurophysiological investigations. For instance, Petersen, Robinson, and Morris (1987) reported that a thalamic nucleus, the pulvinar, has a capacity for spatial selectivity. The pulvinar is intricately interconnected with the association cortex, and also with neural systems involved in saccadic movements. Petersen, Robinson, and Keys (1985) demonstrated that the responses of cells in certain areas of the pulvinar correspond with saccadic movements in monkeys. Cells of this region also respond more to stimuli that are targets or cues for active responses, than to stimuli that are not linked to responding.

The influence of these cells on selective spatial attention was assessed by measuring the reaction times of monkeys to targets following valid or invalid cues, after a GABA agonist was administered (Peterson *et al.*, 1987). GABA (gamma aminobutyric acid) is a ubiquitous inhibitory neurotransmitter. After administration of the GABA agonists, reaction times were inhibited when the cue and the target were in opposing visual fields, but not when they were in the same field. A GABA antagonist increased reaction times under these same conditions. This effect was noted for both valid and invalid cues, though the magnitude was greatest for invalid cues. These studies suggest that movement is not the basis for the differences in reaction time. However, factors associated with the integration of feedback regarding saccadic movements and visual information may be the source of the reaction time differences. Therefore, attentional selectivity may truly depend on the integration of both sensory and motor information.

Goldberg and Segraves (1987) concluded that motor program selection and sensory enhancement should be considered separate attentional components. Sensory enhancement was demonstrated by recording superior colliculus and inferior parietal neuronal activation before saccadic eye movements (Bushnell, Goldberg, & Robinson, 1981; Goldberg & Wurtz, 1972; Wurtz, Goldberg, & Robinson, 1980). This response was interpreted as a neural substrate of visuospatial attention. A related response was noted in neurons of the frontal eye fields (Bruce and Goldberg, 1985; Goldberg & Bushnell, 1981; Goldberg & Bruce, 1986). Single-unit discharges from the frontal eye fields were noted before saccadic movements, a finding suggesting that the brain was choosing among competing motor programs. Approximately 60% of the cells of this region discharged before purposive saccadic movements. During a learning task, many of these cells (40%) responded only to visual stimuli, and not to movements.

The act of fixating attention modulates the response of frontal eye field neurons to electrical stimulation (Goldberg & Bushnell, 1981; Goldberg & Bruce, 1986; Goldberg & Seagraves, 1987). During attentive fixation, there is an increased threshold for evoking saccades, and a decreased amplitude and velocity of elicited movements. These responses also depended on the nature of the stimuli being attended to. Ambiguous stimuli produced premotoric activation, which may or may not actually trigger movement. The discharge of cells in the frontal eye fields and the superior colliculus depend on information derived not from sensory analysis, but only from a signal that triggers and targets a response in space. Premotor activation occurs in response to nonspecific information that a stimulus has occurred at a target position in space. Eye movements may then be directed without the need of detailed visual analysis.

An important characteristic of cells of these regions is their response to the disengagement of attention. Not only do they respond when a target stimulus appears, but they also respond to its offset. Fischer and Breitmeyer (1987) demonstrated that the engagement and disengagement of attention may involve processes that are somewhat independent of attentional fixation. The engagement of visual attention produces an inhibition of saccades, whereas disengagement produces a facilitation of these movements.

Attention as an Executive Function

Effective engagement and disengagement of attention requires that the prefrontal cortex be intact. Lesions of the prefrontal cortex create impairments of the suppression of reflexive glances. Patients with such damage have problems inhibiting extraneous saccadic movements to relevant targets and also encounter problems when trying to initiate goal-directed responses (Guitton, Buchtel, & Douglas, 1985). The prefrontal cortex seems to exert supervisory control over the attentional selection of motoric responses.

Within the field of neuropsychology, there has long been interest in how the brain exerts executive or supervisory control. The distinction that has been made in the cognitive sciences between automatic and controlled attention is at the heart of this renewed interest. Automatic attentional processes are executed with little motoric effort and typically involve sensory selection based on stimulus features. Attention becomes automatic when the response demands are minimal and the stimulus set is already a well-integrated part of long-term memory. The term *automaticity* refers to selections that can be performed without awareness or deliberate intention. Automaticity is also apparent when a stimulus pulls for attentional allocation, as in the case of the orienting response (OR) or classical conditioning. The capacity to perform multiple tasks simultaneously is a good indicator that automaticity has been involved.

In contrast, controlled attention is evident when a task requires effort. With effortful attention, it is difficult to process more than one stimulus at a time, a finding that leads to the conclusion that attention involves a channeling of serial processing. Effortful attention usually involves intention, deliberation, and awareness. The temporal characteristics of such tasks dictate that a series of actions be executed sequentially. Controlled attentional processes appear to be fundamentally different from the automatic processes of attention. Controlled attention is easy to demonstrate on tasks that require response production in conjunction with vigilance of some sensory attribute over long time periods. For instance, the performance of rotary pursuit (e.g., keeping a pen tracked on a rotating line) is an example of an attentional task that places strong demands on both the fine-motor and perceptual systems. Sustained performance on this task is difficult over a long time course. Tasks that are not well rehearsed, and that are therefore not part of "procedural" memory, are also likely to require a greater degree of controlled attention. Such a task cannot be performed automatically because the task is not fully encoded in memory.

Neuropsychological data arising from the study of brain-injured patients have added weight to the argument that premotor systems are important in controlling attention, through the regulation of response execution. The example of ideomotor apraxia illustrates the influence of premotor areas on the intent to act. Lesions of the prefrontal cortical regions also greatly affect the capacity to sustain attention (see Chapter 10).

Disruption of the prefrontal areas results in a loss of the ability to organize and execute responses that involve multiple steps. Although the ability to form and retrieve visual and auditory sensory and associative information may be unaffected, the capacity to handle such information consistently over time is usually impaired. The net result is that the individual with "frontal lobe" impairment can often respond correctly at a given instant but cannot do so on a regular basis. Furthermore, when a task requires that a sequence of associations be connected together in a stochastic manner to result in a course of action, there is often a breakdown in functioning.

What is the relationship of these brain regions and their associated functions to attention? With respect to our discussion of selective attention, it is obvious that damage to the frontal lobes does not necessarily impair the capacity for automatic attention. On an individual trial of a task, such patients can attend to specific stimulus features relatively well. However, when a task requires consistent attention to specific features over an extended set of trials, performance is typically impaired. Therefore, these response centers have an impact on controlled and sustained attention, with particular disruption of the ability to persist in tasks.

Summary

The findings of the early information-processing researchers generally supported the position that humans are capable of making attentional selections at very early stages of processing. However, it is unlikely that all attentional processes occur at these early stages. Attentional control also seems to be influenced by later response-based factors. Although motoric responding cannot by itself account for attentional control, an individual's disposition to respond and the outcome of that response dictate attentional allocation.

Response dispositions are generated by intrinsic "motivational" and state-dependent factors, which are typically modulated by extrinsic cues from the environment. The outcome of the dispositional state is the production of premotor activation, which shapes the "intentional" direction of future responding. The demands present in a particular situation influence the capacity to translate this intentionality into an accurate response. The tendency of animals to explore the environment sets the stage for attending. Attentional search generates the response alternatives from which the animal can select. Feedback from responding facilitates attending. Therefore, attentional control depends on sensorimotor integration, because response intentions must be coordinated with and directed toward relevant environmental targets. Models of attention that account for both sensory and response selection factors seem to have the greatest validity and utility.

Attention is mediated by factors associated with response production and control in several ways. Some motor responses seem to be associated primarily with directing attention to specific spatial positions. The act of looking is an example of overtly directed attention. Visual scanning through saccadic eye movements is a more covert process, but one that serves to focus the visual analyzing system on appropriate targets. These types of responses play critical roles in normal attention. Although there are recent studies that illustrate that spatial selective attention is possible without eye movements, saccadic movements are evident in normal conditions of attending. Recent evidence demonstrating that visual tracking may be initiated by subcortical mechanisms before cortical registration illustrates that these movements influence attentional preparations before sensory analysis. Though sensory spatial selection may occur without eye movements, visual scanning is normally intricately linked to the sensory enhancement associated with attentional processing.

In addition to eye movements, other overt responses facilitate attending. For instance, the positional orienting of an animal's body prepares it for further intake. We have also discussed several covert determinants of attention that are based on response demands. Premotor and prepremotor functions exist that influence the planning and execution of responses. These "executive" functions also modulate the allocation of attentional resources. Damage to the anterior cortical regions that are responsible for executive control results in clear-cut patterns of attentional disturbance. Although executive functions seem to be critical determinants of attentional control, they are much more difficult to study than overt sensory and motor responses. One of the challenges for future attentional research will be to specify the parameters of the influence of premotor and executive functions on attentional selection.

VIGILANCE, EFFORT, AND FATIGUE

The performance of any motor act requires effort. Within biological systems, effort can be defined in terms of the amount of work that a task requires and the energy requirements necessary to perform that work. In the simplest terms, effort can be determined by measuring metabolic expenditure. For instance, a runner who travels a distance of 1 mile burns a certain number of calories. The amount of energy consumption can be measured with relative ease and is quantifiable. Within this context, fatigue is also relatively easy to specify, as it reflects the decrement in neuromuscular capacity with repetitive activity. Neuromuscular fatigue occurs when a particular muscle is stimulated repeatedly in a short time period, without adequate compensation for the metabolic demands of the task.

Effort and fatigue are easily demonstrated in classical experiments in which electrical stimulation is repeatedly applied to a frog leg muscle. The amount of metabolic activity necessary to maintain the muscle contractions can be determined. This determination provides an indication of effort and work load. After repeated stimulations, the muscle begins to lose its normal operating characteristics. Eventually, a state of tetanus is reached, when the muscle can no longer respond. Under normal physiological conditions, this end point is never reached.

Unfortunately, this classic physiological interpretation does not account for many common behavioral experiences associated with effort and fatigue. For instance, effort is often reported by subjects performing behaviors that require little energy. Similarly, fatigue is noted as a function of sustained cognitive activity, even when there is no depletion of muscle capacity. The behavioral characteristics of effort and fatigue associated with normal task performance seem to bear little relation to the events occurring during extreme muscular exertion. The concepts of effort and fatigue that arise from the study of sustained cognitive operations seem to have a different basis from the processes described in traditional physiological studies.

Although neuromuscular effects do not seem to account for behavioral effort and fatigue, there is evidence that motor-response-production demands influence whether a task is seen as effortful and the likelihood that fatigue will result. Tasks that involve sensory analysis with minimal response requirements tend not to elicit these behavioral effects. Attentional tasks that have relatively easy sensory demands, but difficult response requirements, are likely to be described as effortful.

The terms *effort* and *fatigue* are often used to describe the individual's subjective experience. In such cases, the experience of effort and fatigue reflects the individual's self-awareness about declining task performance or an inability to persist. Self-awareness of fatigue may be an accurate appraisal of an actual behavioral effect. However, individuals may also report subjective experiences of effort and fatigue when there is no real decrement in performance. It is not clear whether sustained performance on tasks that are perceived as effortful always eventually results in the subjective experience of fatigue. Therefore, it is important to distinguish between effort and fatigue as physiological, behavioral, and subjective phenomena.

Vigilance and Sustained Attention

Behavioral fatigue was first analyzed in the context of experiments testing the "vigilance" of human subjects. The term *vigilance* refers to the ability of humans to keep watch for long periods of time. In terms of information processing, vigilance involves attending for long periods while anticipating a signal's occurrence. The signal rate may vary across studies. By definition, vigilance requires sustained attention. The goal is to determine what variables influence the subject's tendencies to stay on task or to become distracted. As described in Chapter 2, vigilance has often been studied within the context of information-processing theories that emphasize early sensory selection during information processing. Many of these studies were conducted with military applications in mind, such as determining the performance characteristics of radar operators.

The first important group of studies in this area was conducted by Mackworth (1950). The subjects in these experiments watched a simulated radar screen and responded when a double signal appeared. The signals were easy to see, so the task was not perceptually demanding. Yet, there were strong demands for sustained attention to a rather monotonous task. Mackworth found that subjects required to perform consistently over a 2-hour period showed rapid fatigue after approximately 30 minutes. Subjects who had rest periods between periods of vigilance tended to show no fatigue.

Although this initial finding seemed unambiguous, subsequent studies suggested that this effect was highly dependent on a host of factors. Broadbent (1950) illustrated that decreased vigilance did not always occur when no rest periods were given. The complexity of the task, the rate of stimulus presentation, and the rate of target occurrence influenced performance.

Colquhoun and Baddeley (1967) tested vigilance under four experimental conditions, in which the stimulus and target frequencies varied between a high and a low rate (see Figure 3.3). They found that accuracy was maintained for the longest durations when a high target and stimulus rate was used. The rate of decay was greatest when the stimulus rate was high,

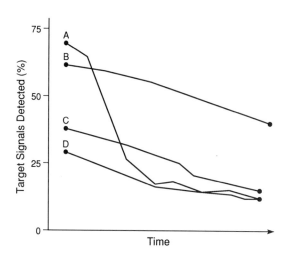

FIGURE 3.3. Sustained performance (vigilance) on long-duration signal-detection tasks similar to those described by Colquhoun and Baddeley (1967). Performance varied as a function of the proportion of the target signals relative to distractor items (noise) during both initial training and actual test periods. The greatest level of fatigue was noted when subjects were trained with a high rate of target signals but were then switched to a test task with a low proportion of targets (A). When the target rate remained high during both study and test phases, performance declined gradually (B). However, when the subjects were trained on tasks with low target rates, they performed poorly regardless of whether the test period had a low target rate (C) or a high target rate (D).

but the targets were infrequent. Under this condition, subjects initially performed well but then rapidly decayed so that after several test periods, their accuracy was worse than that of subjects exposed to a low rate of stimulus and target presentations. When the subjects were presented with a low rate of stimulus presentation, they showed poorer performance from the start but did not deteriorate much beyond their initial level. This finding led to the conclusion that expectancy and anticipatory factors played an important role.

Although these results held up for simple tasks involving the detection of a single target, contradictory findings were obtained by Jerison (1957, 1959). Subjects exhibited a decrement when monitoring one target but did not show a temporal decline when monitoring three targets simultaneously. This finding was rather surprising because attending to three simultaneous stimuli should be more effortful. Broadbent (1963) accounted for this effect by noting that the errors made in each type of task differed. When one signal source was used, the subjects made few false-alarm errors but tended to miss items over time. With three stimuli, the subjects initially made many more false-alarm errors. Therefore, these tasks produced different types of errors that reflected the degree of confidence that subjects had when making a response.

Broadbent and other investigators later refined their techniques by applying signal detection methods to the analysis of vigilance. Signal detection analysis provides an index of the stimulus discriminability and also the response criterion (β). Using these methods, Baddeley and Colquhoun (1969) found that varying the signal presentation rate influenced the way response tendencies (β) changed, but not stimulus discriminability. Other studies also supported these findings that d' does not change significantly over long task periods (e.g., Broadbent & Gregory, 1963, 1965; Colquhoun, 1961, 1966; Colquhoun & Baddeley, 1964, 1967). Only during special tasks involving sustained continuous visual attention were decrements in discriminability noted (Mackworth, 1965; Mackworth & Taylor, 1965). These results suggested that the task demands created by the rate of stimulus presentation influenced the way subjects were likely to respond. The reason was not clear, though the rate of presentation seemed to influence the subjects' expectancies and motivational state.

Vigilance has been analyzed for the role of variables such as motivational state and level of arousal (Corcoran & Houston, 1977; Corcoran, Mullin, Rainey, & Frith, 1977). Interestingly, when arousal (defined as the amount of irrelevant noise) was varied, the results were inconsistent with the predictions of expectancy theory. Greater noise levels facilitated performance (McGrath, 1963). As we will discuss later, some fundamental problems with the concept of arousal as used by early investigators have bearing with this finding. These results correctly indicated that the relationship between internal arousal state and performance is not a simple linear function. With respect to how arousal influences vigilance, it appears that this influence depends on how one defines arousal. The level of arousal and the task characteristics are both important. Arousal influences response tendencies, as reflected in the measure of response bias (β). Arousal's effect on discriminability is less clear-cut.

Several conclusions may be reached about the characteristics of vigilance or, more generally, sustained attention (Broadbent, 1971). When the information to be processed occurs at a high rate, there is likely to be an eventual decline in d' over a given time period. However, this decline can be prevented if the individual modifies her or his response criterion. In contrast, when signals occur at a low rate, d' does not change significantly. Instead, there is a tendency toward higher β levels, reflecting a change in the disposition to respond a particular way. Signals that have longer durations of onset do not show a decline in d' over time, but they may show a change in β, reflecting a change in the confidence of the operator. Therefore, it is primarily under conditions of high stimulus rate and low target rate that discrimination ability is reduced over time, a finding suggesting that, under this condition, an informational overload eventually occurs. Generally, the temporal effects of performing for long durations with low rates of stimulus processing seem to have more impact on the response characteristics of the individual than on perceptual discrimination capacity. Whether these tendencies are evident in the performance of individuals with impaired brain functioning is not yet well established.

Effort: An Attentional Component

Humans possess a limited attentional capacity that becomes evident when they are required to perform dual or multiple tasks. Attention can be directed to more than one activity, but at the cost of a reduction in the amount of allocation that can be directed to a particular task. Kahneman (1973) suggested that the level of momentary organismic arousal would set limits on attentional capacity. He considered effort synonymous with the momentary arousal.

A central assumption of Kahneman's model is that arousal and effort reflect the bioenergetics expended on task performance. In this sense, attentional effort is an analogue of neuromuscular effort as demonstrated in physiological studies. Kahneman used another analogy derived from the physics of electrical load to illustrate this concept. When a toaster is engaged, the result is a decrease in the available voltage for other electrical appliances. Furthermore, the capacity of the electrical system to handle all of the voltage necessary to operate household appliances depends on the nature of the system used to transmit the electricity (i.e., the wiring). Kahneman suggested that this analogy applies in principle to the process of attentional effort, although he acknowledged that a paradoxical situation exists. In the case of attentional performance, a moderate level of arousal produced by tasks of intermediate difficulty actually produces optimal performance.

Several fundamental differences exist between the electrical analogy and the attentional process. Electrical capacity can be exactly specified. On the other hand, arousal and effort are governed by task demands, organismic factors, and variables that are difficult to specify. Electrical usage always results in a certain amount of voltage utilization that depends on fixed and specific variables such as the resistance of the wiring and the amount of energy that is necessary to perform certain work, or other specific factors. In the biological system, the demand placed on arousal is determinable, but the organism may overshoot or under-shoot the optimal levels necessary for task performance.

Perhaps a more significant problem with this concept of effort arises from the ambiguity that is associated with the construct of arousal. Biological systems always show indications of arousal, even when there is no task to perform. Therefore, arousal is not singularly associated with the energy used for task performance, because it also reflects a basic characteristic of the physiological system. Of course, it could be argued that tonic physiological arousal is related to organismic maintenance, whereas momentary bursts of effort are reflected in phasic increases in arousal depending on the demands placed on the system. However, attentional effort and arousal may not refer to a single phenomenon.

The difficulties that have been encountered by researchers attempting to characterize arousal as a generalized phenomenon are described in Chapter 6. An eloquent neurophysiological argument against regarding effort, arousal, and activation as a unitary process was given by Pribram and McGuinness (1975). There seems to be strong evidence that the physiological responsivity associated with the various components of attention reflects different processes. Pribram and McGuinness used the term *effort* to describe the coordination of "arousal" occurring during sensory intake with the "activation" of sensorimotor readiness. According to their model, the coordination of arousal and activation is achieved through neurophysiological events reflecting cognitive processes such as the "chunking" of information in memory, which makes the system more efficient. Therefore, the relationship between effort and arousal is not straightforward.

Physiological Correlates of Effort

A wide range of physiological responses has been studied so that effort can be assessed as a function of task demand. For instance, Kahneman and Beatty (1966) measured the pupil dilation of subjects at rest and during the performance of effortful tasks. They found that the amount of pupil dilation that was detected correlated with the task's difficulty and the amount of effort required. It was also noted that the rhythmic activity of the pupil diminished during the performance of mental arithmetic. Porges (1972) found a similar relationship between heart rate variability and reaction times on tasks. The relationship between decreased physiological variability and effort has also been noted in other physiological systems (Kahneman, Tursky, Shapiro, & Crider, 1969; Thackray, 1969). Although effort is most easily demonstrated by the use of simple mental operations such as performing arithmetic problems, it should be noted that a relationship between effort and physiological activity has also been demonstrated on more complex tasks. For instance, several investigators have described relationships between autonomic measures such as heart rate and skin conductance and performance on cognitive tasks involving associative elaboration (Cacioppo & Petty, 1981a,b; Cohen & Waters, 1985; Jennings & Hall, 1980; Jennings, Lawrence, & Kasper, 1978). It is well known that time pressure increases the physiological responsivity associated with effortful tasks, as well as with the perception of effort that the subject has. Kahneman (1973) reported that pupillary response was not correlated as strongly with the familiarity of words that were being processed as with the pace and processing demands of the task.

Cohen and Waters (1985) demonstrated that incidental memory performance differences that occur as a function of the level of processing (semantic, phonemic) can be explained by the concept of attentional effort. They found that physiological activation was greatest during the processing of words that were later recalled, regardless of the level of processing. However, the semantic tasks tended to elicit greater physiological activation to more word-processing trials, and the subjects recalled more of the semantically processed words.

Unfortunately, it is difficult to attribute physiological changes solely to the effect of effort. For instance, anxiety, emotional state, and muscular demands can also cause changes in autonomic states that are very similar to the appearance of attentional effort. Although the demands for motor output tend to increase the amplitude of the response across different measures during the performance of effortful tasks, covert processing alone also produces sizable responses.

Task Difficulty and Effort

Another problem that commonly arises with use of the term *effort* is that *effort* can refer either to the demands of a task or to the intensity of the response production by the individual. It is often difficult to separate these two types of effort. Tasks that are very effortful require that the individual use high levels of attentional, cognitive, or behavioral resources to achieve adequate performance. On the other hand, a task may have minimal processing demands, and yet the individual may exert much attentional effort as a result of motivation to perform well. This is quite evident in students who are taking an important test of relatively well-rehearsed material, but who show considerable muscle tension as a result of anxiety and a desire to perform well.

Conversely, tasks that place effortful demands on the individual for optimal performance may actually elicit minimal effortful expenditures of cognitive resources. This effect is particularly evident if the reinforcement properties of the task do not elicit maximal attention. For example, for optimal performance (99% accuracy), a security guard may have to maintain heightened vigilance, which is very effortful. Yet, the guard may eventually learn that he can sleep through much of the night, and that the chances of an event's occurring is still very small. In this instance, the task demands great effort for optimal success but, in reality, can be performed with a minimal chance of failure with little effort.

These illustrations point to an important issue that has been addressed by investigators studying signal detection theory. An individual's biases that result from motivational factors, such as the payoff for adequate performance, influence response tendencies, as well as the types of errors that are likely to occur. When considering the nature of attentional effort, it is important to distinguish between the tendency of a task to require effort and the tendency of the individual to generate effort. Although the task may require "effort," the actual expenditure of effort by the individaul may be minimal. Information-processing approaches to the study of attention have often not taken these factors into account. In order to ensure parsimony, it was often assumed that an individual's expenditure of effort is directly proportional to the demands of the task at hand. However, this assumption reflects an ideal scenario. Life would be easier for researchers studying attention if individual differences in effortful exertion did not matter. However, in reality, they do matter, and attentional effort cannot be established without a consideration of both factors.

Hockey (1970a,b; 1978; 1979) addressed these issues when analyzing indicators of system states. He suggested that there are two types of variables that affect attentional performance: structural and strategic variables. Structural variables include such parameters as changes in capacity and processing speed that will be directly effected by task demands. Increasing noise in the environment would affect these structural variables. Presumably, physiological variations that are purely endogenous would also be considered a state variable. In contrast, strategic variables reflect the individual's strategy or approach to the situation. When assessing effort, it is important to consider the influence of both variable classes.

Haier, Siegel, Nuechterlein, and Hazlett (1988) reported interesting findings related to the role of effort in performance. They found that subjects who scored higher on intellectual measures actually showed less cortical activation while performing a given task than subjects who were less intelligent. This finding is noteworthy because it suggests that the need to generate greater activation may reflect the processing constraints that exist for a given individual. Although greater effort may produce better performance for a given individual, the need to generate greater effort, as reflected by cortical activation, may provide an index of the brain's processing powers. This finding may also fit the recent attentional work on the distinction between automatic and effortful processing. For the individual with stronger cognitive ability, more information can be handled through automatic attentional processes, and therefore, the degree of activation that is produced by effortful processing is less.

Intrinsic and Extrinsic Induction of Effort

Some tasks generate effort as a result of their demands but require that the individual have some external motivator to perpetuate this effort. For instance, performance on a paced serial-addition task may be very effortful, and in order to sustain performance, some type of external reinforcer may be necessary. The subject who performs this task is motivated by a desire to satisfy the examiner, or by a wish to perform well so as to demonstrate a high level of competence. In their own right, some tasks of this sort may not elicit much effort because they are rather boring. Therefore, the examiner's verbal praise and encouragement are necessary to boost motivation to the level that is necessary to sustain performance. Other tasks intrinsically elicit effort because they are salient, interesting, or inherently rewarding. For instance, a computer game that is pleasurable for a child is likely to maintain interest levels for reasonable periods of time, enabling sustained vigilance.

This type of effect accounts in part for the types of results seen when subjects perform different types of cognitive tasks. The levels-of-processing effect noted by Craik and Lockhart (1972) is an example. Using a levels-of-processing paradigm, Cohen and Waters (1985) found that subjects experienced greater attentional activation when performing semantic tasks than where performing phonemic tasks. Attentional activation was reflected both by subsequent incidental memory recall of material processed at different levels, and by the associated physiological reactivity. The attentional activation noted during the semantic tasks probably resulted because these tasks were inherently more interesting or meaningful to the individual.

An alternative explanation for these effects is that the semantic task required more attentional allocation than the phonemic task. Therefore, the increased attentional activation noted on semantic tasks may have been a function of the subjects' generating more effort to complete these tasks successfully. Although this is a reasonable possibility, the fact that attentional effort varied across processing levels within each subject suggested that the semantic task itself was drawing the subjects' attention. Furthermore, the subjects did not report that the semantic task was more difficult. Because the individuals' motivation and tendency to exert effort should have been consistent across all of the processing tasks, effort was probably generated by the nature of the task. This is not surprising because we would expect people to generate greater effort when a task is meaningful.

In everyday situations, it is not always easy to distinguish between effort generated as a result of extrinsic task demands and effort generated as a result of task salience. Yet, a formal analysis of the structure and characteristics of a particular task often yields this information. This distinction may also become obvious when subjects are asked to give subjective impressions of tasks, and these are compared with their performance. For instance, on the levels-of-processing task that we discussed, the subjects often indicated that the phonemic tasks seemed more difficult, even though they showed greater physiological reactivity on the semantic tasks. This reaction enabled a dissociation with regard to the type of effort that was generated (e.g., Cohen & Waters, 1985).

Neurobehavioral Characteristics of Fatigue

The term *fatigue* is traditionally used in physiological studies to refer to a neuromuscular event that occurs when a motor unit can no longer sustain its firing. Normally, when a muscle fiber is stimulated by a nerve impulse, there is a period ranging from several milliseconds to .2 seconds during which the fiber contracts and then relaxes. This response occurs when impulses of less than 50 Hz are sensed. However, with repeated stimulation at a rapid rate, there is a change in threshold, so that eventually the muscle ceases to respond. This phenomenon is characterized as neuromuscular fatigue. In humans, fatigue occurs first as a change in the state of the neuromuscular junction, which is followed by the decreased conduction capacity of contractile muscle tissue. Although the physiology of muscle fatigue is now understood in considerable detail, this type of fatigue does not seem to account for the experiences that are described by individuals who report cognitive or behavioral fatigue.

Whereas neuromuscular fatigue refers to a specific physiological phenomena, cognitive fatigue and behavioral fatigue are much more difficult to define, and the underlying mechanisms are not well understood. In fact, difficulties in defining fatigue led some researchers to question whether fatigue is a meaningful construct or an effect that can be measured (e.g., Broadbent, 1979). From the standpoint of behavioral analysis, *fatigue* refers to a decline or change in the quality of performance over time. Accordingly, fatigue is the overt manifestation of a reduced capacity of the individual to respond effectively. However, this definition does not take into account the endogenous characteristics of fatigue. The term *fatigue* is also used to refer to a subjective state of tiredness that may exist before attempts at performance.

Behavioral fatigue can be induced in several different ways. Forcing an individual to sustain attention to a task for excessive periods of time often results in reports of fatigue. Under conditions of sleep deprivation, patients often report fatigue. We also know that patients with certain neurological and psychiatric disorders report behavioral fatigue as a major symptom. For instance, fatigue is a frequent symptom of major depression, metabolic disorders, and multiple sclerosis. In these disorders, fatigue may be reported as indicative of the resting state of the individual, even when little behavioral effort is exerted.

Unfortunately, a problem exists in trying to characterize a single integrated form of fatigue, since the subjective experience of fatigue may or may not be correlated with actual performance changes. Should a concept of fatigue reflect the subjective experience of the individual or the neurobehavioral characteristics reflected in performance? This question troubled many early investigators and has led to many confounded findings. In fact, Broadbent (1957) and Bartley (1981) questioned whether fatigue was a meaningful concept in the behavioral sciences.

Significant problems are encountered in trying to predict the response characteristics of fatigue. Figure 3.4 illustrates four plots of hypothetical changes in response tendencies that may be expected during states of fatigue. The different patterns of fatigue reflect the fact that the characteristics of fatigue vary as a function of the behavioral task, the type of response that is measured, and the time frame of interest. Fatigue can usually be tested in experimental paradigms that provide temporally based vigilance measures. The reader is encouraged to consider Broadbent (1971) and Mackworth (1950) for excellent reviews of central issues related to the assessment of vigilance.

Line A in Figure 3.4 illustrates a gradual decrement in performance that may be

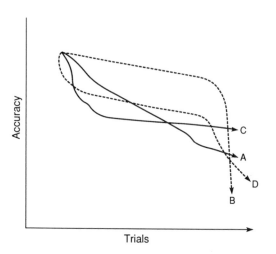

FIGURE 3.4. The temporal characteristics of fatigue are not always consistent across tasks or people. Four different fatigue patterns are illustrated. (A) Fatigue is often seen as involving a gradual decrement in performance over the entire task period (A). Howver, fatigue exhibits a more complex temporal function. For instance, after physical (neuromuscular) depletion, a very different pattern may be seen: A steep performance decline eventually occurs as the system's response capabilities are depleted (B). Up to that point, the level of performance may be relatively stable. Tasks with very intense attentional requirements may produce an initial rapid decrement from optimal levels of performance, until a sustainable performance level is reached (C). Fatigue of this type is associated with demands for attentional effort. Ultimately, fatigue may be best characterized by a combination of the functions illustrated in the first three curves. A rapid rate of initial performance decline is followed by a period of stabilization during which there is only a gradual performance decrement, with eventual severe performance decrement as a result of system failure (D).

predicted of a subject performing a sustained task of long duration. The response decrement expressed by this curve is characterized by a slow decline in performance throughout the entire period of the task.

Line B in Figure 3.4 illustrates a different pattern of fatigue characterized by a gradual decrement in performance over the initial period of the task. With longer durations, the rate of decline accelerates. This model would be predicted of a system that performs reasonably well until a state of depletion occurs that rapidly diminishes further response capability. This condition occurs with sustained neuromuscular responding.

Performance on tasks of shorter duration may result in the opposite fatigue pattern (Line C in Figure 3.4). Under conditions of intense vigilance, there may be a rapid decline in performance over the early phases of the task, with the subject reaching a more sustainable level of performance later during the task. This model fits with the findings of Mackworth (1950). A group of individuals who performed a vigilance task over a 2-hour period was compared with subjects in an experimental condition who performed the same task for half-hour intervals. Each subject in the experimental group alternated with another subject after each half-hour interval. Mackworth found a curve similar to that shown in Figure 3C for the subjects performing at a continual rate, whereas the subjects who alternated after a 30-minute period showed little decrement in performance.

It is likely that the pattern of fatigue observed in most individuals does not fit a simple curvilinear relationship such as those shown in the first three examples. The rate of decrement in performance is likely to vary as a function of the time frame of the task that one examines. Line D in Figure 3.4 is an example of a pattern of fatigue in which there is a rapid drop in performance during the early stages of a task, which then stabilizes to a slower rate. However, after a long period of performance, there is a rapid decline, as the individual becomes totally exhausted. This pattern may be typical of performance on monotonous tasks. Initially, the individual attempts to maintain an optimal rate of performance, which requires great effort and is not easily maintained. Over the early phase of the task, there is some success and optimal performance is maintained. Eventually, there is a decline to a more sustainable level of performance, at which stabilization occurs. During this period, there are only small declines in performance for a rather long duration. Eventually, even this level cannot be sustained as the individual reaches a state of total exhaustion. At that time, there is a rapid decline in the quality of performance. The point of this illustration is that the characterization of fatigue depends on the frame of reference that is chosen.

Fatigued subjects are often able to regain the capacity to perform for short periods of time, when a new response is required. This finding is interesting, but it also complicates most models of sustained attention and vigilance. This effect would not be predicted from models of neuromuscular fatigue, because a fatigued muscle does not show spontaneous recovery until some refractory period has passed. The patient who is behaviorally fatigued may perform near optimal levels in certain instances but may then perform suboptimally for a greater percentage of the time as the level of fatigue increases.

An adequate model of fatigue should account for the variability in performance noted during times of fatigue. This variability may result in an oscillatory function (Figure 3.5), so that the degree of variability, as reflected in the scatter of points around a regression line, increases over time. This type of occurrence has been noted in recent studies of the fatigue characteristics of patients suffering from multiple sclerosis (MS) (Cohen & Fisher, 1988; Krupp, Alvarez, LaRocca, & Scheinberg, 1988). Patients with MS often show the capacity to perform on various cognitive tasks as they become fatigued. However, they show an increased inconsistency in their responding over time.

The variable performance characteristics of the MS patients was evident in both their subjective reports and their task performance. Their performance on an adaptive-rate continuous-performance test became increasingly unstable over the time of the task. Their performance was characterized by a tendency both to miss target items and to exhibit slower reaction times. Additionally, they exhibited greater variability during later trials, which was reflected by greater variances in both accuracy and reaction time. Interestingly, the subjective reports of fatigue by these patients were much more variable than those of normal subjects. This variability followed a circadian pattern, suggesting that performance variability was mediated by an intrinsic rhythm.

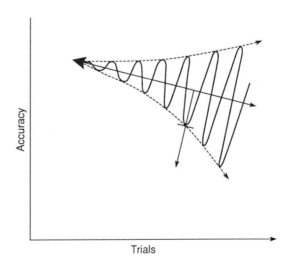

FIGURE 3.5. Sometimes the most striking characteristic of fatigue is an increased degree of performance inconsistency. Multiple sclerosis patients exhibit such a pattern of neuropsychological performance when tasks require effortful attention (Cohen & Fisher, 1989).

Accuracy

Trials

It is interesting that, in his early theoretical formulations, Clark Hull (1942) anticipated the need to account for response variability when he postulated an oscillatory function. This function was later criticized and deemphasized by other researchers exploring Hull's models of behavior. In postulating an oscillatory function that may be associated with fatigue, an obvious question arises. Is the increased variability that is noted over time a result of changes in some endogenous mechanism that regulates behavior, or is it determined by extrinsic stimulus factors that pull the individual away from the original task.

Tasks of very long duration are likely to be characterized by the presence of fatigue, as the individual's physiological system is no longer able to maintain adequate arousal. Endogenous factors affecting arousal probably play a critical role in cases of fatigue caused by factors such as sleep deprivation, certain neurological disorders, and physical strain. Under these conditions, fatigue reflects a steady state that may exist independently of the specific task demands that are placed on the individual. This state of fatigue creates a disposition that will affect further responding on a range of tasks.

The response decrements occurring during tasks of shorter duration are more difficult to account for by changes in the endogenous state of arousal. On short-duration tasks, the rate of fatigue normally corresponds with task demands at a given point in time; more demanding tasks should result in a faster rate of response decrement than less demanding tasks. Fatigue is a by-product of the task demands and the capacity to generate sufficient activation and effort.

Ordinarily, most people are able to override constraints placed on processing capacity rather well (Kahneman, 1973). Therefore, although high demands may elicit fatigue in the short run, it may become apparent only as an inconsistency in performance, as individuals can usually muster their resources to perform in a single instance. When subjects are sleep-deprived (Wilkinson, 1962), they may still show the capacity to perform adequately on short-duration tasks, but the cost is increased muscle tension. When negative consequences are associated with poor performance, subjects increase their effort and the result is increased sympathetic activation (Malmo & Surwillo, 1960). This finding suggests that people have reserved capacities that are not used except under extreme conditions.

Performance seems to be constrained by the information-processing capacity of the given individual. Although it is difficult to define information-processing capacity, or "resources" (as discussed in Chapter 2), there clearly are individual differences in performance and attentional capacity. Capacity may depend on a wide range of interacting variables, such as the type of information to be processed, the level of momentary activation that is possible, and the amount of noise in the environment. However, it is also determined by the intrinsic cognitive resources of the individual.

The fatigue that occurs on short-duration high-demand tasks seems to differ in fundamental ways from fatigue that occurs in less demanding long-duration tasks. Although attentional dysfunction may be the end product of both long- and short-duration fatigue, the performance characteristics may be quite different. One may question whether *fatigue* is a useful term if it refers to a number of different behavioral, subjective, and physiological phenomena. There is merit in this criticism, as more precise terminology would be useful to help distinguish among the different types of fatigue. However, in our view, it would be a mistake to discard fatigue as a useless concept. In our view, the concept of fatigue is necessary and useful. *Fatigue* refers to a response tendency, one in which an individual shows an inability to sustain continued performance.

Circadian Effects on Fatigue

Circadian factors greatly influence the induction of fatigue (Hockey & Colquhoun, 1972). Throughout the day, there are systematic variations in biological indices of the neuroendocrine and metabolic states. These variations follow a rhythm that is highly correlated with behavioral activity level in most species. Cognitive functions also vary in a circadian pattern. Folkard and his colleagues (Folkard, 1979a,b; Folkard & Greeman, 1974; Folkard & Monk, 1980) demonstrated that memory performance follows a circadian function, and that phase shifts in this rhythm disturb memory load capacity.

There is now evidence that the suprachiasmatic nucleus of the hypothalamus serves as a central clock regulating circadian rhythm. Lesions in this region disrupt neuroendocrine and appetitive rhythms (Lydic, Gander, & Moore-Ede, 1984). In a recent case study, Cohen and Albers (1991) demonstrated that damage to the suprachiasmatic region disrupted behavioral, cognitive, and sleep patterns in a woman with a craniopharyngioma. The primary feature of her disorder was a failure to maintain consistent levels of performance, as she showed wide fluctuations in behavioral state in short durations. This effect suggests that regulatory systems in the brain may control the consistency of behavioral state and may ensure against fatigue. The Cohen and Fisher (1989) study of fatigue associated with multiple sclerosis also demonstrated that this symptom follows a circadian pattern.

Summary

Effort is an important construct in considerations of attentional phenomena. Attentional effort reflects the allocation of cognitive and behavioral resources. Response demands create a pressure for attentional processing. However, effort is also associated with other task characteristics that are not necessarily associated with task complexity. Therefore, attentional effort is a function of demands for response preparation, of selection and production, and also of the limited capacity of the neural system.

Attentional capacity, effort, and fatigue are intricately related. Together, they influence vigilance, as well as the ability to sustain attention on complex tasks. Attentional capacity is determined by a range of factors: endogenous state, noise and stress, response biases produced by motivational factors, and the intrinsic resources of the individual. Therefore, the exertion of attentional effort and the tendency to fatigue are influenced by both intrinsic and extrinsic factors. Certain neurological diseases (e.g., MS) and psychiatric disorders (e.g., major depression) cause impairments of effort and fatigue. However, it is not yet clear whether the fatigue evident in these disorders has the same subjective, behavioral, or physiological characteristics. More research is necessary before the behavioral characteristics of effort and fatigue can be fully operationalized and applied systematically to clinical or work situations.

Contributions of Behavioral Psychology to the Study of Attention

RONALD A. COHEN and YVONNE A. SPARLING-COHEN

Behaviorism emerged in response to the early schools of psychology that had put a premium on the analysis of consciousness and subjective experience. With roots in the principles of associationism, objectivism, and logical positivism, behaviorism maintained that psychology should be an empirical science, its focus restricted to measurable behavior. This could be best accomplished by studying the characteristics of association formation between external events (stimuli) and the resulting responses. The term *conditioning* became synonymous with the process by which an associative linkage was established and learning occurred. By characterizing the relationship between the responses of the animal and the stimuli in its environment, learning theorists specified building blocks for more complex behaviors.

Today, it is possible to study attention from a cognitive information-processing perspective without ever addressing how behavioral learning theories accounted for attentional phenomena. A philosophical shift away from the tenets of behaviorism has occurred over the past decade. There were numerous reasons for this change of *Zeitgeist*. Many behavioral scientists reacted against the constraints that behaviorism placed on the study of human behavior, and its reluctance to regard many cognitive phenomena as being within the scope of scientific investigation. Also, the position of radical behaviorism that a consideration of physiological processes is irrelevant to an understanding of human behavior became untenable. Although the repudiation of behaviorism was justified in many respects, learning theory made important contributions to our current understanding of the behavioral processes, including the development of a scientific method for behavioral study that set a benchmark for other psychological sciences.

Behavior results from the interaction of an animal's long history of selection and the environmental stimuli of the moment. Although the present environment acts to direct behavior, how an animal responds to a particular stimulus depends on the result of previous encounters with it. For this reason, identical stimuli may elicit different responses within one animal at different times. Selection history provides one explanation of why different animals do not give the same response to a stimulus. The selection of stimuli and responses from larger sets of alternatives is a fundamental component of conditioning. Yet, most behaviorists accounted for behavioral selection without using a formal attentional construct.

Behavioral theories that sought to account for attentional effects usually used a bottom-up approach, as they argued that "selective attention" could be explained by means of basic behavioral concepts. Although their usual intent was to demonstrate that an attentional construct was not necessary, the result was a behavioral theory of attention.

Performance deficiencies are often attributed to inattention if there are adequate stimuli in the environment to direct a behavioral response but the individual fails to respond to these stimuli. Donohoe (in press) described situations in which "inattention" can easily be explained through basic behavioral concepts. He specified four behavioral conditions that are prerequisites for optimal attentional performance: (1) all stimuli necessary for a particular response must be present at the moment of the response; (2) the history of selection must be favorable for the desired response; (3) the environmental context must be stable; and (4) the target stimulus must not be affected by interfering stimuli. Attentional failures often occur when one or more of these conditions are not met. Heightened attention or hypervigilance may occur as the result of a transfer of previous learning to the new situation and contextual learning.

How behavioral models either incorporated or ignored attention is of both historical and conceptual relevance to our current discussion. With this in mind, a brief review of how learning theories incorporated and/or accounted for attentional processes is presented in this chapter. Because most readers of this book are already familiar with the basic tenets of the learning theories, we will restrict our focus to how behavioral approaches dealt with the construct of attention, in order to provide a somewhat different and useful perspective for students of attention.

EARLY LEARNING THEORY

Many of the concepts and methods derived from behaviorism are now so highly integrated into the behavioral and cognitive sciences that they are taken for granted. Even the most current models of cognition borrow heavily from constructs developed in the early learning theories. Examination of these theories reveals a remarkable consistency of conceptual themes.

Thorndike (1911; 1931) is credited with formalizing the first modern learning theory when he established a number of laws that he felt accounted for learning (see Table 4.1). These laws specify the conditions under which associative learning occurs. The *law of effect* is the most fundamental determinant of behavior, as pleasure or satisfaction determine what is learned. The law of effect was later expanded in the concept of reinforcement, which became a core of the operant theories of learning.

In addition to the law of effect Thorndike (1911) believed that learning is a function of other factors, including the individual's disposition. As Thorndike stated, "Not only is the situation important, but also the conditions of man" (p. 65). The influence of the predisposing state on learning is emphasized in the *laws of set, readiness, multiple responding, associative shifting,* and *assimilation.* The laws of readiness and set are directly concerned with the fact that an individual must be in a prepared state for learning to occur. The law of multiple responses posits that the activity of healthy animals results in the generation of a large number of responses. The amount of response production influences the association formation by affecting the number of stimulus–response (S–R) pairings that may occur. These three laws anticipated the need to account for organismic state when considering learning. Their emphasis on the preparatory state of the animal and its tendency to respond implies an attentional component.

TABLE 4.1.   Thorndike's Laws of Learning

Law of effect: Successful steps in learning are rewarded, and unsuccessful steps are omitted. Pleasure and satisfaction determine which responses are learned.

Law of readiness: the "conduction unit" must be in a state of readiness to form the association . If it is ready, the associative process results in pleasure, and if it is not, conduction results in "annoyance." Learning will occur only if the animal is prepared for learning.

Law of exercise: The use or disuse of an associative connection determines its durability. (This law was largely criticized and not well substantiated.)

Law of multiple resources: The ability to make a varied set of responses facilitates the process of learning. This and is related to the notion of trial-and-error learning.

Law of set: Previous experiences and disposition help to determine learning in the new situation. (The role of previous memory in determining the response to new situations is implicated.)

Law of associative shifting: The sensitivity of the animal to a particular type of stimulus will determine the ease of learning. (This was analogous to Pavlovian conditioning.)

Law of assimilation: The animal will act in a new situation in a manner that is consistent with the way it acted in similiar situations. (this law also suggests an important role for previous long-term memories in learning.

Law of prepotency of element: Stimulus elements in the environment produce different sensitivities in the animal, which influence the selection process. (Selection of stimuli does not occur at random but is based on prior weightings. This law has direct implications for current theories of attention.)

The law of associative shifting posits that an animal's flexibility in forming associations is a function of its sensitivity to input. Thorndike conjectured that animals normally exhibit great sensitivity and therefore rapid associative formation. The law of assimilation states that, once an association is formed, the organism responds in other situations in a manner similar to that learned in the initial situation, a predecessor of the stimulus generalization. Again, an attentional component seems to emerge. By emphasizing organismic sensitivity and the stability of behavior once it is learned, Thorndike proposed factors that would affect the direction of the behavioral response, as well as the conditions necessary for a response to new stimulus information.

The *law of prepotency of elements* has particular relevance to our discussion of attention. It specifies that individuals do not select stimuli at random but select stimuli based on their inherent informational or reward strength. The implications for selective attention are obvious. Environmental stimuli are seen as guiding the selection process.

Thorndike's laws posit broad parameters and rules governing learning and therefore are usually considered in the context of learning theory. Yet, these laws also provide a foundation for thinking about other behavioral control processes like attention. Although subsequent learning theories have provided greater specificity, the basic elements of Thorndike's laws are apparent in the major behavioral theories that followed: classical conditioning theory (Pavlov, 1927) and operant learning theory (Skinner, 1938).

CLASSICAL CONDITIONING

Pavlov approached the study of behavior from a biological perspective, as he searched for the physiological mechanisms underlying simple learning. He saw behavior as the by-product of the present environment acting on the organism. Pavlov's mentor Sechenov (1956) went so far as to conclude that even the most complex responses involved in thinking can be traced to the environmental stimuli of the moment. Pavlov observed that certain physiological reactions (e.g., salivation) always occur in response to the presentation of salient stimuli (e.g., food). He noted that this unconditioned response (UCR) occurs in a reflexive manner, except under conditions of satiation, when appetitive drive is reduced.

Normally, a salient stimulus such as food (unconditioned stimulus—UCS) elicits the UCR without the need for learning. Two qualities of the UCS are of relevance: (1) the UCS acts as a catalyst that guides behavior, and (2) the UCS is always biologically relevant. These qualities give the UCS the capacity to make other less salient stimuli into potential response catalysts through an associative process. This quality is important to our considerations, as it illustrates that this type of learning is propelled by biological pressures.

Pavlov (1927) considered conditioning a function of homeostatic mechanisms that ensure the maintenance of internal equilibrium relative to the external environment. The animal's behavior is dictated out of a need to conserve energy and resources. Accordingly, conditioning results in complete equilibrium of the animal's energy and physical state with the energy and physical state of the external environment. The presence of a strong appetitive or drive state (e.g., hunger) is necessary if learning is to occur. Although Pavlov did not direct formal study to the issue of "drives," steps were always taken to ensure the presence of a strong appetitive state before conditioning. Therefore, the presence of a UCR suggested the presence of biological drives.

The UCR would not have generated a great interest without Pavlov's discovery that animals could learn to respond to less salient stimuli through temporal association with the UCS. In natural environments, animals respond to a broad range of stimuli, many with little inherent biological value. Some of these stimuli are important only because they activate memories of previous situations of importance to the particular animal. Pavlov found that a normally inconsequential stimulus can be associated with a UCS to form a conditioned stimulus (CS), which will evoke a conditioned response (CR) with properties similar to those of the UCR.

Diagram of Simple Classical Conditioning

UCS → UCR	UCS → UCR	
CS → OR	CS → CR	CS → CR
(conditioning response)		
Preconditioning	Conditioning	Postconditioning

Following conditioning, a CS can serve to elicit the CR even when a UCS is not present. It acquires salience and a strength approaching that of the UCS. Higher order conditioning is possible because the CS serves to increase the informational value of other stimuli with which it is associated. By chaining a series of CSs, responding can be conditioned to stimuli far removed from the original UCS. Yet, higher order conditioning is still rooted in the initial organismic salience of a UCS.

Much of the conditioning research after Pavlov sought to establish the parameters governing the rate of learning and extinction and the pairing of the CS and the UCS. The time between the UCS and the CS was found to be critical to the strength of conditioning (contiguity). Although association formation is obviously a critical process in its own right, a number of secondary factors also influence conditioning. The animal's momentary energetic state is influential, as is the sensory-processing characteristics of the neural system. Before conditioning can occur, sensory registration must take place. Pavlov regarded the creation of temporary associations between the organism and the environment as only one of two major nervous system functions. The second major function is the analysis of external stimuli (i.e., perception and attention). This second function, which was largely ignored by subsequent behaviorists, is of obvious importance to our considerations of the role of attention in classical conditioning.

Expectancy and Anticipation

One of the strongest lines of evidence for an attentional component in classical conditioning is a demonstration of expectancy and anticipatory responses before the presentation of a CS. Rescorla (1967, 1969) demonstrated that the temporal relationship between the CS and the UCS has a bearing on whether expectancy and anticipatory responses occur in conjunction with the presentation of the CS. When the CS preceded the UCS by approximately .2 sec, the strength of conditioning was maximized. When the CS and UCS occurred simultaneously, or when the UCS preceded the CS, very weak conditioning occurred.

In an aversive conditioning paradigm, dogs were trained to avoid an unsignaled electric shock by jumping from one side of a shuttle box to the other. Once the dogs had acquired the response, a tone was introduced along with the shock. For one group of dogs, the tone occurred randomly, with no clear relation to the shock, and for a second group, the tone preceded the onset of the shock. Rescorla found that the dogs in the second group increased their jumping rates to the presence of the tone, and that the dogs in the first group did not, even though the number of actual pairings of UCS and CS were the same for the two groups. In other words, contiguity alone did not predict increased responding. The nonrandom pairing of the CS before the UCS was critical, presumably because it served as an anticipatory signal. These findings supported the idea that the CS is a temporal indicator of an impending UCS, which enhances the animal's attention by preparing it for the salient stimulus soon to appear. Some cognitive investigators have interpreted such expectancy as an indication of a cognitive expectancy of attentional process (Mandel & Bridger, 1973).

Generalization

Stimulus generalization provides a mechanism by which the conditioning of a response to one stimulus can spread to related stimuli. Although a CR will occur to stimuli sharing similar features with the original CS, the response magnitude decreases as a function of the psychophysical distance from the CS. For any class of stimuli, a response gradient can be demonstrated along a particular featural dimension (e.g., color).

The phenomenon of response generalization that has also been demonstrated during conditioning reflects an inverse property, that a CS conditioned to elicit a particular response may become effective in generating other related responses. For instance, a stimulus may initially be conditioned to produce a response of the animal escaping from an aversive stimuli. The animal may vocalize as it escapes, which is an associated response. Over time, the stimulus may serve to elicit vocalization.

The processes of stimulus and response generalization illustrate several additional features of conditioning theory that have a bearing on potential attentional mechanisms. In addition to a link between stimuli and responses, generalization implies the development of links between stimuli (S-S associations) and between responses (R-R associations).

Without generalization, the range of behavior is limited by the history of previous associative pairings among CS. If a stimulus has not been conditioned, it will not elicit a response. Generalization provides for greater behavioral diversity by accounting for the production of a CR to other approximations of the original CS. Similarly, response generalization enables variants of the original CR to occur secondary to the CS. In some regards, generalization reflects an error on the animal's part. With generalization, there is a loss of specificity of the S-R relationship. Yet, generalization also has adaptive value, as it decreases the likelihood that the animal will respond differentially to stimuli that are similar with respect to informational value.

Although stimulus generalization is not usually considered an attentional process in its own right, it may account for certain attentional effects. Because generalized stimuli do not have the same strength as a true CS, there is a diminished likelihood that they will elicit the appropriate CR. Therefore, attentional failures may actually reflect an attenuated response strength resulting from generalization.

THE ORIENTING RESPONSE

Perhaps no phenomenon was as essential to establishing an empirical basis for the concept of attention as the orienting response (OR). The occurrence of an OR marks the initial reaction of the animal to a new stimulus. This reaction occurs independently of the actual reinforcement properties of the stimulus and is largely based on the strength and the physical attributes of the signal. The orienting response consists of a large set of muscular skeletal, autonomic, and central nervous system responses that are triggered in a reflexive manner after registration of the stimulus. More than any other construct from conditioning theory, the orienting response provides a behavioral index of attention. The origins of the OR construct shed light on the intricate relationship between conditioning and attention. When choosing a stimulus to serve as a CS, it was evident to Pavlov that the stimulus should not already be a UCS. If a potential CS was strong enough to produce a UCR without conditioning, then that stimulus would compete with the original UCS rather than become associated with it. For a stimulus to be an adequate CS, it could not already be so salient that it already elicited a UCS. Yet, it had to be strong enough to result in sensory awareness. Pavlov was forced to isolate stimuli that met both conditions. The response generated by such stimuli was labeled as an OR, because it produced transient orientation of the animal to the signal. The orienting response construct was developed out of methodological necessity.

The OR marks the animal's registration of the CS, before pairing with the UCS-UCR. If an OR does not occur before conditioning, the CS is probably not gaining sensory or perceptual registration; therefore the likelihood that conditioning will occur is reduced. The inclusion of the OR in the model indicates the importance of the consideration of a sensory processing phenomenon before the event of conditioning. The fact that the OR exhibits a variable course over trials, and across different stimuli and contexts, implies that its role as an attentional index decreases in strength over time. The reduction in response strength is an indication that the potential CS is strong enough to elicit a brief attentional response, but not so strong as to maintain the behavior. This decline in strength of the OR is labeled *habituation*.

Habituation of the OR

An important characteristic of the OR is that it diminishes in intensity as a result of repeated exposures to neutral nonsalient and unreinforced stimuli. The OR and habituation are highly interdependent. Investigations of the OR have often focused on specifying the factors that influence the rate of habituation, as a way of delineating the processes underlying the OR and its maintenance. Habituation is of interest to students of attention, because it provides a process by which the animal can decrease its response to one stimulus, in lieu of another. Because attention depends on the ability to shift from one stimulus to another, the capacity to habituate is critical in allowing orientation to other stimuli to occur. Much research has focused on specifying the parameters underlying habituation in different experimental situations (for reviews, see Siddle, Stephenson, & Spinks, 1983; Waters & Wright, 1979).

The OR as an Attentional Index

Because the OR reflects the animal's reflexive response to occasional environmental stimuli, it has been called the "what is it" response. Through the OR, the animal is able to determine if a new stimulus deserves additional processing. The generation of the OR is highly dependent on the nature of the new stimulus that has occurred in the environment. Strong, salient, and particularly biologically relevant stimuli elicit UCRs, whereas stimuli of more moderate strength or salience are likely to result in a response that habituates. If a stimulus is too weak, it will not result in any response. Therefore, the OR is a response to moderately strong stimuli of potential relevance to the organism. This distinction is important, as it illustrates the relationship of the OR to the information contained in a stimulus. If a stimulus is so weak or nonsalient that it does not cause sensory registration, it will not result in an OR.

Many behavioral investigators following Pavlov focused their efforts on delineating the stimulus characteristics that influence the orienting response and habituation. Berlyne (1960) demonstrated that the capacity of a stimulus to elicit an OR depends on a variety of different featural and informational characteristics. To produce a response, a stimulus must be different from the general background environment. The distinction between stimulus and background may be based on a variety of characteristics ranging from simple psychophysical properties to complex qualities requiring semantic processing. For instance, incongruities in pictures (e.g., a camel with a lion's head) was shown by Berlyne to produce a large attentional response. A more detailed account of attentional influences of the OR is provided in Chapter 5.

OPERANT CONDITIONING

Operant conditioning theory had its roots in the principles espoused by Watson (1913) and in Thorndike's law of effect (1911), but it was formalized by Skinner (1938). Although operant theory emphasizes the formation of associations between stimuli and responses, it places special emphasis on the role of responding in governing the delivery of reinforcement. During classical conditioning, behavior is determined by a "respondent reflex" to the stimulus. Within an operant framework, conditioning does not originate from a reflex to environmental stimuli; instead, it results from the spontaneous behavioral repertoire of the animal. In classical conditioning, there is not a simple mechanism to account for how an animal produces completely new behaviors that are outside of its natural behavioral repertoire. The production of novel responses is not a problem for operant conditioning, as the animal's trial and error may result in a new response as it attempts to meet its goal of obtaining reinforcement.

An example of a response prompting a reinforcer is evident in a common human experience; the first utterings of an infant. The baby makes the sound *ma-ma*, which prompts the mother to pick the baby up and smile (+ reinforcer). This stimulus leads to further repetitions of the sound *ma-ma*, and eventually, an association is made. As in classical conditioning, increased responding occurs in operant situations as a function of both reward and aversive consequences.

Operant research led to the important observation that behavioral responding can be sustained by inconsistent reinforcement. During classical conditioning, without the presence of a CS, the CR will not occur. However, in natural situations, behaviors often occur when no external stimulus is present. For instance, an infant may cry in response to some internal distress, with variable reductions in crying based on the response of the parent. This partial reinforcement effect, which is an integral aspect of operant behavior, is not easily explained by classical conditioning. Operant research devoted much effort to characterizing how different schedules of reinforcement deliver influence responding. Behavioral selection is seen as a by-product of these schedules, and attentional phenomena are largely subsumed under this same set of principles.

An implicit assumption of operant theory is that animals have a natural disposition to respond. Once a behavior has occurred, the animal receives some consequence (reinforcer) from the environment that changes the probability of future responses. Although reinforcement guides the direction of behavior, responding is the catalyst for conditioning. This differs from the more passive nature of classical conditioning when learning is controlled by the influx of stimuli entering the animal. This distinction has significance for the role of attentional processes during conditioning. During operant conditioning, the animal must direct its behavior toward the available environmental alternatives in order to be reinforced. Although behaviorists minimize the role of covert processes like intention, they generally acknowledge that behavior is the outcome of the animal's history of "selection."

From a behavioral perspective, response selection does not imply selective attention or covert decision processes. The animal simply approximates the correct response in successive steps (often by chance) until it learns to respond in a manner that results in consistent reinforcement. These approximations are evident in operant techniques such as "shaping." The apparent haphazard nature of the animal's response approximations leads to the conclusion that the experimenter is generating the desired response through his or her reinforcement. Yet, shaping also illustrates that operant learning involves an active process: The animal gradually modifies its behavior to optimize the likelihood of a positive consequence.

Discrimination Learning

With repeated experience, we learn to discriminate between salient and nonsalient stimuli based on their utility as signals of consequential payoff. Operant researchers coined the term *discriminative learning* to refer to the process by which an animal learns that responses to one stimulus are reinforced, whereas responses to another stimulus either go unreinforced or result in punishment (see Figure 4.1).

Skinner (1938) demonstrated that pigeons could be trained to produce a desired response selectively and with much precision when presented with different stimuli. If a colored light was presented when the reinforcer was delivered, the animal eventually learned to respond to the colored light. The light had been made into a discriminative stimulus (S_d) upon which future responding could become contingent. Furthermore, the animal could learn to discriminate a particular color from others, thus producing specificity of learning and response selection. It is relatively easy to demonstrate how complex discriminations can be learned from simpler discriminations.

Although it was not the focus of operant investigations, it is apparent that discrimination learning depends on sensory and perceptual processes. The animal must be capable of detecting subtle differences among stimuli when making discriminations in complex environments. Furthermore, there is often a large number of stimuli with some reinforcement value. Therefore, selective response to a discriminative stimulus involves a complex and dynamic process. On any given learning trial, there may be competition among stimulus

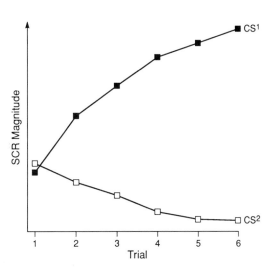

FIGURE 4.1. The acquisition of selective skin conductance response (SCR) to different visual cues during discrimination learning in a laboratory animal. Two conditioned stimuli (CS_1, CS_2) initally produce SCRs of the same magnitude. When CS_1 is paired with an aversive stimulus, and CS_2 is paired with a neutral stimulus, they rapidly differentiate in their salience. CS_1 produces an even greater SCR, and the response to CS_2 extinguishes. Conditioning of this type has been described as a basis for "attention" by behavioral learning theorists.

elements for further processing. The interaction of competing stimuli in a particular environmental context explains many "attentional effects" within the operant perspective. Therefore, when the animal is faced with multiple S_ds, responding will not occur in an all-or-nothing fashion. Instead, behavior is influenced by the interactive value of the multitude of cues, in conjunction with some memory of which S_d yielded the best outcome. This requires that the animal perform a series of operations that include the matching of the new stimuli with previous memories.

The dynamic nature of discrimination learning is illustrated in the work of Spence (1936) and subsequent neobehaviorists. Although Spence did not stress the need for an attentional concept in his early work, his example of successive discriminations provided a behavioral model of attention. Spence assumed that discrimination learning involves the following sequence in most learning paradigms: (1) the animal approaches a choice point on a task; (2) it then searches the environment for cues before it acts with a full response (e.g., running to one leg of a maze); and (3) it makes its response. At the choice point, probabilities can be attached to the likelihood that an animal will respond by making an approach response. These probabilities are determined by the weights derived from the previous reinforcement history. Spence was aware that, generally, an animal orients in different directions during acquisition learning. Therefore, there are multiple response probabilities associated with this "receptor-orienting" act for each trial. Even though conditioning may be interpreted as occurring on a given trial in an all-or-nothing manner, that trial actually involves multiple choice points. Each choice point requires a discrimination and then a reorientation. Because this orienting response is subject to rapid decrementing, the animal is capable of making multiple responses before responding with a full approach.

The ability to make increasingly complex discriminations is facilitated by previous learning of easier discriminations (Lawrence, 1949). A transfer of learning occurs that enables a progression toward more discriminations. Spence suggested that this transfer can be explained solely as a function of habit inhibition. However, the transfer phenomena can also be interpreted as an "attentional" process that is enhanced by learning (e.g., Zeaman & House, 1963).

Logan (1972) tested this possibility in a series of experiments and demonstrated that the ease of discrimination, the amount of training on the original discrimination, and the established criterion for moving to more difficult discriminations are all important dimensions that affect the transfer of discrimination learning. Using an easy criterion for successful performance on easier discriminations resulted in better discrimination learning performance than using very stringent criteria. This finding ran counter to expectations from theories of selective attention, which predict increased transfer when more stringent criteria are used. Logan concluded that, during discrimination learning, the generalization of response tendencies is more critical than the enhancement of stimulus selection ability. Logan chose to interpret his findings as nonattentional because they ran against the perspective of attention as a stimulus-driven process. However, as we discuss elsewhere, response selection may also be interpreted as an attentional process.

Observing Responses

Certain responses that have a primary function of enhancing the perception of stimuli are called *observing responses*. For instance, if you are at a crowded cocktail party and hear a potentially interesting conversation, you are apt to approach the speaker so that you can hear better. Observing responses are not a unique type of operant response; rather, they are the result of basic discriminative processes. Observing responses provide a behavioral explanation of paying attention.

Blocking

The term *blocking* refers to cases in which a discriminative stimulus fails to guide a response because another preceding stimulus has established a different response tendency. Blocking has been used to explain the phenomenon of base-rate neglect that occurs in some attentional paradigms. Bias for a more frequent stimulus accounts for the failure of subjects to respond to a target stimulus with a low rate of occurrence. Blocking provides a behavioral explanation for this bias.

EXTINCTION: A CONTROL MECHANISM OF ATTENTION

Extinction, the process by which an animal ceases to respond with a particular conditioned behavior, is a critical determinant of the selection and direction of responding. Extinction enables the individual to stop responding to a particular stimulus in lieu of another. This type of control is necessary if an animal is to switch its response and select new stimuli. Therefore, extinction is important in behavioral explanations of attentional selection.

During simple conditioning, extinction can be determined solely by measuring the rate of responding when a reinforcer or UCS is removed. For instance, if an animal is conditioned to salivate to a red light (CS) that is associated with food, and then the CS is repeatedly presented without the UCS, there will be an eventual decline in the strength of the CR over trials. Although extinction is a simple concept, the mechanisms underlying extinction are not well understood.

Several different mechanisms for extinction are possible: (1) associative trace decay; (2) inhibitory processes; (3) interference; and (4) response competition.

The associative-trace-decay hypothesis maintains that extinction occurs because of a physical degradation of a previously learned association. From an attentional standpoint, this hypothesis leads to the conclusion that shifts in selection are largely governed by the durability of the memory trace. Although there is now neurophysiological evidence accounting for this type of decay, it is difficult to explain most instances of extinction by using this hypothesis. Phenomena such as spontaneous recovery and recruitment indicate that the extinguished response is not totally removed from memory in many situations.

Neobehaviorists, following in the tradition of Hull and Spence, postulated that inhibitory processes are fundamental to extinction. Inhibition implies an organismic factor that suppresses the processing of the stimulus or the response. Inhibition is an important concept in our considerations of attention and will be addressed later in greater depth.

Interference and response competition (R_c) provide other mechanisms for extinction. With interference, the strength of the original behavior is not diminished, but its expression is blocked by competing stimuli or responses. Extinction does not occur in a vacuum; as a response decreases in intensity or frequency, other responses occur. Responses are essentially competing for behavioral expression. When one response fails, other responses occur. Evidence supporting the role of response competition comes from investigations of the nature of behavioral responding during extinction. Research has indicated that animals do not simply become passive during extinction. They engage in a variety of behaviors, including withdrawal and frustrative responding (Denny, 1946; Denny, Wells, & Maatsh, 1957). The notion that extinction actually involves an active process of generating alternative competitive responses characterizes the operant approach.

NEOBEHAVIORAL CONTRIBUTIONS

Behavioral Inhibition

The suppression or slowing of one behavioral response by another is referred to as *behavioral inhibition*. The presence of behavioral inhibition is often interpreted as a sign of neural inhibition, though as Konorski (1948, 1970, 1971) pointed out, behavioral inhibition may not always underlie neural mechanisms. Although behavioral inhibition may result from neural inhibition, there may be other causes for behavioral inhibition. Whereas neural inhibition is a tangible physiological event that involves the reduction of neural activity at a site by a secondary neural process, behavioral inhibition is more difficult to measure and is evident only in circumscribed paradigms. Therefore, the concept of behavioral inhibition has been the subject of considerable debate since it was first used. Yet, behavioral inhibition provides a useful concept for understanding how stimuli exert control over behavior and ultimately over attentional phenomena.

Numerous types of behavioral inhibition have been studied since Pavlov first described internal and external inhibition, including reciprocal, retroactive, proactive, conditioned, passive, latent, and inhibition of delay. According to Pavlov (1927), both extinction and habituation are associated with a decreased adaptation of neurons to a particular stimulus. Although this adaptation may occur passively, as a result of associative decay, Pavlov believed that inhibitory processes facilitate extinction. He considered behavioral inhibition an expression of some type of neural inhibition.

To test for inhibitory influences, Pavlov presented +CS with excitatory influences relative to the original CR with −CS having inhibitory influences. The order of the +CS and the −CS was varied across experiments. He found that when the +CS was presented first, the response to the subsequent −CS was diminished, whereas initial presentation of the −CS resulted in the opposite effect. These effects were labeled *positive* and *negative induction* and were used as illustrations of a behavioral inhibition. The occurrence of induction suggested that stimuli have excitatory and inhibitory influences on one another. Subsequently, the strength of induction was shown to depend on variables such as trial spacing, the interstimulus interval, the amount of overtraining, and the extent of exposure to aversive stimuli (Bernheim & Williams, 1967; Krane & Ison, 1971; Senf & Miller, 1967).

The occurrence of induction supports the position that inhibition plays a role in extinction. The suppression of a response to the second stimulus cannot be easily explained on the basis of a passive decay of the strength of the associative trace. Induction laid the groundwork for the concept of *conditioned inhibition*, thereby providing a basic behavioral mechanism to account for more complex stimulus interactions, such as compound stimuli.

Hull suggested alternative inhibitory processes in his theoretical system. He proposed that extinction was influenced by reactive inhibition (I_r). Hull proposed that I_r, which is a function of a negative drive state, results from sustained responding over time. I_r is regarded as independent of nonreward and is thought to naturally dissipate over time. Because of I_r, a competing response eventually develops that replaces the original response. Hull labeled this process *conditioned inhibition*. Conditioned inhibition represented a clear break from the assertions of most other behavioral theorists that inhibition is not a necessary construct (Skinner, 1938). Hull's inclusion of an inhibitory process suggested that organismic variables play a role in learning.

A second type of inhibition was noted by Spence (1956) and Denny (1946). They observed that frustration (FD) was encountered by animal subjects in certain situations of nonreward. Frustration is usually quite evident because the animal engages in active responses, with agitated movements and attempts to escape from the situation. This type of response appeared to be very different from the more passive effects of reactive inhibition. However, subsequent investigators attributed FD to the effects of response competition and schedule of reinforcement (Amsel, 1967).

Conditioned Inhibition

If separate discriminative cues are associated with the acquisition and extinction periods during conditioning, they have differential influences on the reemergence of the CR. Extinction is facilitated when there is a great distinction between the two cues. The presentation of the acquisition cue causes a slowing in the rate of extinction, whereas presentation of the extinction cue speeds extinction. Once a stimulus becomes a cue associated with either acquisition or extinction, it can be labeled as a conditioned inhibition (CI) or a conditioned excitation (CE). The presentations of a +CS or a −CS have reciprocal effects on one another, which are the basis of the process of "induction" that we discussed earlier. Therefore, conditioned inhibition and induction are related processes.

The application of CI or CE to other conditioning paradigms either enhances or suppresses the rate of extinction of other CRs. Whether a stimulus acts as a facilitator (+CS) or an inhibitor (−CS) depends on whether it elicits a CR that is compatible with or antagonistic to the response associated with the new task. Conditioned inhibition provides a mechanism for the mediation of both acquisition and extinction.

During CI, stimuli with inhibitory capacity reduce the strength of responses associated with the CS, whereas stimuli with excitatory capacity increase the response strength to the CS. Because the excitatory and inhibitory properties of the stimuli used to induce CI and CE are developed through previous trials of conditioning, the phenomenon of conditioned inhibition illustrates that stimuli can acquire excitatory and inhibitory characteristics. The interaction of stimuli with excitatory and inhibitory potentials can explain why behavior does not occur in an all-or-nothing fashion. The interactions of stimuli may produce a smooth response gradient that varies as a function of the addition or subtraction of CI and CE. Progressively stronger or weaker behaviors would result the further one moved along a particular dimension from the inhibitory or excitatory stimulus.

Konorski (1948, 1971) expanded the concept of conditioned inhibition to explain a general class of behavioral phenomena. Konorski's investigations suggested that the occurrence of CI is highly dependent on how the CS is reinforced. According to Konorski, reinforced CSs are very different from nonreinforced CSs. This was demonstrated in a series of elegant experiments that compared the rates of extinction and recovery of the CR when two CSs were simultaneously presented. One CS was reinforced with the presentation of a UCS, and the other CS was not reinforced. After a large number of trials, the response to the reinforced CS was extinguished. It was found that the strength and type of the CR that occurred in each condition was quite different. A stimulus that always signaled the arrival of reinforcement but then ceased to do so readily recovered its role as a signal. However, a stimulus that never signaled upcoming reinforcement during training could not easily be changed into a signal for reinforcement in future conditions.

These findings supported the existence of two forms of conditioned inhibition: (1) primary inhibition resulting under conditions of consistent nonreinforcement, in which a stimulus becomes resistant to serving as a signal, and (2) secondary inhibition resulting when a CS ceases to be reinforced after a period in which it was reinforced by a UCS. Secondary inhibition was regarded as producing a weaker inhibitory tendency. Konorski concluded that these findings indicated the presence of two antagonistic neural centers, one associated with excitation during reinforcement, and one associated with the inhibitory effects of nonreinforcement (a no-UCS center).

Measurement of Behavioral Inhibition

Much effort was directed toward finding ways of validating the presence of CI, and paradigms were developed to test for the strength of inhibitory and excitatory stimuli. These paradigms usually manipulated the type of stimulus presented during extinction. By showing differences in the CR when novel stimuli, habituated stimuli, or uncorrelated stimuli were used for CI, researchers were able to isolate the specific effects of conditioned inhibition. Seven paradigms have been used to determine that a stimulus has excitatory or inhibitory tendencies. All of these were based on the selective addition or subtraction of potential CI or CE during extinction. For instance, the combined cue approach required that the experimenter selectively introduce or remove stimuli from a stimulus complex (Kendler, 1971; Konorski, 1972; Rescorla, 1969). Stimulus termination procedures provide a good example of how these paradigms were used to measure CI. During stimulus termination training, the animal learns to respond in such a way that it can determine the duration of stimulus presentation. The introduction of CI or CE stimuli during these procedures differentially affects the animals' performance. For instance, Terrace (1963; 1968; 1971a,b) trained pigeons on an escape task to avoid aversive stimuli. The animals learned to discriminate a cue in order to make responses that would temporarily turn off the aversive stimulus (S−). The pigeons made a horizontal-vertical discrimination with the right foot. Later, when the S− was introduced, responses with the left foot resulted in the appearance of a white light and escape from the S−. Terrace noted that the pigeons produced responses to the S− that were antagonistic to the original S+ used in the discrimination task. These antagonistic responses were overt and were labeled as "active" inhibitory responses, as there was a competition established between the two incompatible responses to the S+ and the S−.

Terrace also observed other responses not directly related to the bar-press routine of the task. The pigeons groomed themselves and showed an increase in other activities that appeared to be means of avoiding the conflict and the resulting frustration. These responses were described as "passive inhibition." The most compelling evidence for inhibitory influences in this paradigm was the occurrence of aftereffects of exposure to the S−. Typically, the rate of responding to the S+ increased above baseline, and latency of response to the S+ decreased below baseline after exposure to the S−. This aftereffect suggested a compensatory mechanism in response to conditioned inhibitory influences (Terrace, 1963). Another stimulus termination method, the "advance procedure," has also been used to demonstrate CI within an instrumental framework (Honig, 1969, 1970). Animals were trained to respond in a manner that changed the future stimuli that were presented based on the performance of correct discrimination (i.e., to advance a slide carousel to the next frame). The amount of time that the stimulus was maintained and the number of responses that were made during the task represented the two variables of interest. A response gradient was demonstrated so that the S+ and the S− interacted in an inhibitory manner to affect the two variables of time and response rate. Furthermore, a peak shift was demonstrated based on a tendency for the point of maximum inhibitory strength to change as a function of training. This peak shift suggested that the stimulus value had changed as a function of inhibition.

Disinhibition

The recurrence of a CR with representation of the CS following extinction is known as *spontaneous recovery*. This response is usually short-lived because, without the presence of the UCS, the CR quickly extinguishes. Spontaneous recovery has been used as evidence of behavioral inhibition, as it seems to reflect a release from the inhibition that has occurred during extinction. If associative decay were the sole basis for extinction, spontaneous recovery would be unexpected, as there would be no remaining trace of the previous learning that could reemerge. The concept of disinhibition supported the theoretical position that extinction was induced by inhibitory processes. Some behaviorists who objected to the role of inhibition presented evidence that spontaneous recovery could be accounted for without inhibition. Yet, the concept of disinhibition had appeal because it suggested an active neural contribution.

Advocates of the role of inhibition in extinction argued that antagonistic relationships between two or more neural systems could account for resistance to extinction. It had been well documented that there is more resistance to extinction soon after initial learning, as the CR reappears in the presence of nonreinforcement. Over time, this resistance to extinction diminishes. Resistance to extinction could be explained by the interactive effects of two or more neural centers; as the influences of the two neural centers become more balanced, a more eradict response pattern would be expected, as a result of competition between the centers. Eventually, the neural response strength associated with the nonreinforcement becomes dominant; the result is a greater strength of extinction and a tendency for responding not to occur. This neurophysiological arrangement can be thought of as a dual-process model of inhibitory control.

In chapter 7, we discuss evidence that multiple subcortical neural structures are involved in different aspects of animal responses to reinforcement. As Konorski suggested, inhibitory activation may actually involve neural excitation in a particular neural system. This point is illustrated when one considers the effect of damage to the frontal cortex, which typically causes behavioral disinhibition. Even though neural activity in the frontal cortex is diminished, behavioral activity may be increased, an effect indicating that the excitatory neural activity of the frontal cortex exerts an inhibitory influence on behavior.

Amsel (1967) concluded that inhibition may have very different roles and characteristics in classical and operant conditioning. He went further to distinguish between the role of inhibition in classical conditioning with mediation and simple Pavlovian conditioning without mediation. Amsel argued that most of the operant behaviors that have been attributed to inhibitory effects can be explained on the basis of response competition (Rc). The weights assigned to different response possibilities during operant conditioning are determined by the relative reinforced strength of each response alternative. Operant response selection does not depend on inhibitory processes, because extinction is associated with the excitatory activation of a new response. He saw a role for inhibitory processes in classical conditioning.

Cue Dominance

The construct of attention was most directly addressed by neobehavioral theorists as they attempted to apply behavioral principles to complex situations. Some investigators incorporated the concept of selective attention into their behavioral models (Lovejoy, 1965; Mackintosh, 1965; Trabasso & Bower, 1968). Others argued against the need for an attention construct (Kendler, 1971; Logan, 1972). These behaviorists attempted to illustrate how more fundamental behavioral principles could account for attentional effects. Kendler's concept of cue dominance illustrates these efforts. The term *cue dominance* was used by Kendler and Kendler (1962) to describe the overshadowing of one stimulus by another. Stimuli are regarded as having different weights that affect the probability that they will elicit a response. When two stimuli are simultaneously presented, one is dominant and serves as the behavioral catalyst. This stimulus may also either facilitate or inhibit the strength of the second stimulus. This concept is an extension of the Pavlovian principle that stimuli in the environment trigger responding and guide behavior. Cue dominance occurs because of intrinsic or acquired qualities of the dominant stimulus.

Intrinsic cue dominance is derived from the inherent quality of the stimuli before learning (e.g., psychophysical dimensions). Intrinsic cue dominance occurs as a result of the influence on the organism of natural characteristics of the stimuli. For instance, certain animal species may have a preference for visual over auditory information. Kendler (1971) demonstrated an intrinsic dominance of color cues over shape cues in rats. Intrinsic dominance of brightness over orientation cues has also been shown for rats (Basden, 1969).

Although stimuli have inherent qualities that determine their potential cue dominance, this can be manipulated by varying the difficulty of discrimination in a particular psychophysical dimension. Furthermore, with repeated trials, animals may learn to perform discriminations more easily. Therefore, cue dominance results from the interaction of intrinsic stimulus qualities, the task's characteristics, and learning.

Acquired cue dominance was proposed to account for how stimuli with no inherent strength can gain cue dominance as a result of conditioning. Kendler and Kendler (1962) demonstrated acquired cue dominance in humans, by showing that certain cues prevail during reversal learning. During their studies of reversal learning, individuals were initially trained to make discriminations based on color and shape cues. Afterward, they were required to shift their responses to the opposite alternative and to ignore an irrelevant "extradimensional" cue. Following learning, the subjects exhibited dominance of the acquired reversal cue over the extradimensional cue with intrinsic cue dominance. Therefore, the strength of acquired cues may surpass that of intrinsic cues as the result of learning. Interestingly, humans show greater capacity for the development of acquired cue dominance than lower animals (Kendler & Kendler, 1962).

The learning of cue dominance was primarily attributed to the excitatory and inhibitory tendencies of the contextual stimuli that interact to produce an "effective excitory strength" (Kendler, 1971). With exposure to an ever-changing set of stimuli, the animal experiences variations in the effective excitatory strength as a result of conditioning. This, in turn, influences the selection of responses based on these cues. Because each stimulus in the field has both excitatory and inhibitory strength, the tendency to make particular stimulus selections can be mathematically specified by determining the interactive product of all stimuli in the set.

When multiple stimuli interact in normal environments, it is difficult to account for the selective influence of individual cues. Kendler (1971) suggested that, in such contexts, all of the elements exert simultaneous interactive influence through a process called *stimulus compounding*. The relative weights of all of the elements of the environmental set change when a new stimulus is introduced, which changes the overall stimulus value. A smooth gradient of excitatory and inhibitory weights results, which then strengthens as a function of the broad range of stimuli. Compounding enables multiple interacting stimuli to simultaneously provide cues that direct responding and influence behavioral selection.

During discriminative learning, animals either may use a number of individual stimuli that serve as independent cues or respond to some aggregate of cues (i.e., a stimulus compound). Some investigators have disagreed with the notion that, in complex environments, animals normally respond to a "compound stimulus." Wagner (1969) argued that the degree to which specific environmental cues exert influence over behavior during learning determines whether an attentional construct is necessary. If the animal's behavior is controlled solely by subtle variations in the environment, a separate attentional construct is not necessary, as attention is synonymous with stimulus compounding. Because discriminative learning often involves selective responding to successive individual cues, Wagner acknowledged that one might argue that an attentional construct is necessary. To avoid the need for an attentional construct, he sought to find a behavioral explanation for successive discriminations.

Wagner's modified continuity theory provided a conceptual solution to this problem. All sets of stimuli contain cues that are compounded over a succession of trials. At any given moment, the combination of elements in the stimulus set may or may not exert its maximal influence as a reinforcer. According to Wagner, the probability of a particular response selection is governed by the extent to which a set of stimulus components approaches maximal reinforcement potential with each successive discrimination. Wagner concluded that it is possible to account for attentional effects strictly on the basis of variations in the reinforcement values of a pattern of cues.

DRIVE AND MOTIVATION

Why do certain stimuli act as UCSs or have reinforcing qualities? Although reinforcement was a central component of early learning theories, the reason why stimuli are reinforcing was often overlooked. Pavlov (1927) assumed that appetitive drives exist that determine the strength of the UCS, but he did not explore the basis for these drives. Subsequently, the concepts of *drive* and *motivation* were used by psychologists who sought to account for the internal influences mediating stimuli and responses. *Motivational state* refers to internal conditions that control behavior. Specific motivational states have been labeled as *drives*.

Clark Hull (1943) was among the first behavioral theorists to consider drive a critical determinant of behavior. He postulated that drive increases habit strength (sHr), and that, during associative formation, drive exerts a multiplicative influence on the direction of behavioral responding. In his behavioral model, drive serves as a catalytic force producing an excitatory tendency (E). The organism acts in response to this drive state until satiation occurs, or until inhibition originating from other sources diminishes further responding.

Emphasis was placed on measuring how changes in level of drive influence the probability of responding.

Although Hull's concept of drive has much appeal because of its operational basis in mathematical formulism, it was plagued with problems. The use of deprivation time as a primary component of drive departs from the idea that drive is an internal energetic state that catalyzes action. Drive is most often thought of as a force or pressure that stimulates or prevents action. Hull's emphasis on deprivation time arose out of a hydraulic construct based on the idea that, over time, internal pressures build, so that there is a linear relationship between time and drive intensity. Unfortunately, this hydraulic principle does not work in all situations, as the correlation between deprivation time and intensity of appetitive behavior is not always strong. Under certain conditions, the behavior resulting from deprivation may be opposite what is predicted. Also, it was difficult to demonstrate drives for more complex behaviors, such as sex and curiosity.

Spence (1956) avoided some of these problems by distinguishing between motivation and drive. Spence proposed that reinforcement may effect motivational state, without directly reducing a drive. Hull had argued that all reinforcement acts through need reduction. For Spence, reward and nonreward were motivational incentives that might act independently of drive state. Using eyelid-conditioning experiments, Spence demonstrated that, by delaying reinforcement, one could actually inhibit responding. This finding was counter to the expectations of a drive reduction hypothesis, which predicted increased drive strength with delay. Therefore, drive and incentive could be dissociated. Spence proposed that a reaction threshold existed that mediated the animal's tendency to respond. The probability of responding was a function of the amount that the reaction potential exceeded this threshold.

Grice (1971) demonstrated that reaction threshold is not static. Using data from Taylor's work (1951) on eyelid conditioning and manifest anxiety, Grice was able to show that differences in the rate of conditioning between anxious and nonanxious subjects are a function of response threshold differences that vary between and also within subjects. This work suggested that the internal energetic state affects the rate of conditioning and suggested a role for arousal and attentional influences. Natural variations in drive and response threshold illustrate that the organismic pressures that catalyze behavior are not constant. Hull (1943) postulated an oscillatory function ($_sO_r$), which he felt accounted for natural fluctuations in reaction potential ($_sE_r$) of the animal. He linked behavioral oscillations to reinforcement, by suggesting that the rate of behavioral oscillation is a function of subthreshold reinforcements. The ever-changing set of external stimuli has an additive effect on the animal of producing an asynchronous pattern of behavioral oscillation. Grice (1971) proposed that behavioral oscillations are an intrinsic characteristic of animal systems that must be accounted for in considerations of behavioral performance. They would place an obvious constraint on attention, as variations in behavioral drive would influence the capacity for maximal responding at any moment.

SUMMARY

Behaviorists largely rejected the need for an attentional construct, as "attention" was considered theoretically incoherent. Yet, most behaviorists acknowledged the importance of accounting for the behavioral phenomena that are often grouped together under the label of *attention*. They made great efforts to account for attentional phenomena, without using formal attentional constructs.

In this chapter, we have discussed how processes derived from operant, classical, and neobehavioral learning theory have been used to provide behavioral explanations of attention and attentional failures.

We discussed three phenomena associated with classical conditioning of relevance to our attentional considerations: (1) the orienting response and habituation; (2) anticipatory responses; and (3) stimulus generalization.

The OR is an index of the animal's primary response to a new stimulus after sensory registration. It provides a distinction between salient and nonsalient information, as well as conditioned and novel stimuli. Because the OR habituates with repeated exposure, this response reflects transient attentional allocation.

Rescorla's demonstration that anticipatory responses occur in response to the CS illustrates that these stimuli have a greater role than simply mimicking the UCS. The CS provides information that enables a readiness for future responding. Anticipatory responses serve to prepare the animal for the upcoming stimulus, a role that has strong attentional overtones.

Stimulus generalization enables a spread of CRs to stimuli that are related in some manner to the original CS. It accounts for a more subtle form of attentional control, as the probability of a CR becomes a function of a range of stimuli with different weights. Therefore, the relationship between stimulus and response occurrences is inexact, as failures to respond to a stimulus may reflect the reduced probability associated with a generalized stimulus. The concept of *attention* is often used to account for the fact that, at times, environmental stimuli that are capable of guiding behavior fail to do so. Generalization provides one explanation for such failures.

Operant behavior is largely under the control of the schedule of reinforcement, and response selection is viewed as being governed by the animal's responses in attempts to be reinforced.

When a particular behavioral response fails to elicit the necessary outcome, alternative responses are produced. Therefore, extinction is not viewed as a passive associative decay, but rather as a process of active response competition, as the animal tries other response alternatives when its previous responses go unreinforced. It is easy to see how response competition could explain the capacity of animals to shift their responses in accordance with changes in environmental contingencies. Response competition provides an operant explanation for shifts in attention.

When an animal is conditioned to respond differentially to particular discriminative stimuli, it learns to select responses based on environmental cues. During complex operant tasks, the animal must make a response choice based on multiple cues. Often, response selection depends on the discrimination of very subtle cues. From an attentional perspective, the animal is using cues from its environment to make its best guess at the response that will result in the best outcome. Discrimination learning illustrates that the response to environmental cues is largely affected by reinforcement history and previous selections.

The neobehavioral approach was, in part, a reaction against the reluctance of traditional behaviorists to consider the organismic components of conditioning. Many neobehaviorists maintained that a consideration of internal mediational processes is necessary, and some even acknowledged the need for an attentional component. Behavioral inhibition and drive are the two concepts arising from neobehaviorism with the greatest relevance to attention.

Conditioned stimuli can be made to selectively facilitate or inhibit extinction. Conditioned inhibition provides a mechanism by which multiple stimuli can exert a combined influence on the direction of behavior. This idea was expanded by neobehavioral theorists who used the idea of conditioned inhibition to account for the development of compound stimuli. Compound stimuli are created by the sum of the interactions of all stimuli in the environmental context. This concept is central to many recent behavioral explanations of attention. Kendler's cue dominance theory and Wagner's modified continuity theory are examples of neobehavioral theories that seek to account for attention. In both theories, selective attention is viewed as the by-product of an ever-changing stimulus complex that exerts an influence on the responses that are generated. Variations in the stimulus set produce changes in the likelihood that particular response alternatives will be chosen. Behavioral inhibition is an expansion of the more basic principles of discriminative learning and generalization. However, by shaping the probabilities of particular responses in accordance with the interaction of multiple environmental cues, behavioral inhibition provides a neobehavioral explanation of how attention is directed. As we will discuss in Chapter 21, this concept has been integrated into the modern concept of an adaptive network.

Though many problems have been encountered by behavioral scientists when trying to operationalize drives and motivational state, these concepts continue to have utility. They are hypothetical physiological states that influence the direction of the animal's response. They reflect the fact that environmental stimuli are not the sole determinant of behavior. Natural variations in "drive" or, more specifically, internal neurophysiological states must be addressed if one hopes to account for behavioral control. The need to account for temporal variations in internal state is a consistent theme when one is considering constraints on attention. If animals operated continuously at their optimal state, their performance characteristics would be relatively constant. This obviously is not the case.

5

5

The Orienting Response
An Index of Attention

The orienting response (OR) is a fundamental component of classical conditioning. For Pavlov it provided a means of determining whether a stimulus could serve as a CR. The OR eventually became the focus of much interest in its own right, as it reflected the animal's initial overt reaction to a new, soon-to-be-conditioned stimulus. Because stimuli with little inherent salience elicit an OR before conditioning, Pavlov referred to the OR as a "what is it" reflex. The OR signals an observable attentional reaction before learning. For this reason, it has been of great interest to attentional researchers and is considered here in greater depth.

Stimulus Characteristics and the OR

The major determinant of the evocation of an OR is a change in stimulus characteristics (Lynn, 1966). The extent to which changes in stimulus parameters reflect the underlying biological importance of a stimulus determines the strength of a particular stimulus in producing an OR. Berlyne (1960) distinguished two types of stimulus properties that are likely to affect the production of the OR and thereby to influence attention. The first type of stimuli varies based on their physical properties, such as brightness, hue, and contour. The second type of stimuli varies based on higher order characteristics such as complexity, novelty, or significance. These characteristics are referred to as *collative properties*. Of course, these two stimulus classes represent a somewhat artificial dichotomy, as higher order stimulus characteristics, such as complexity, can ultimately be defined in terms of more basic psychophysical features (Spinks & Siddle, 1976, 1983).

Studies of the effects of simple psychophysical variations on the OR and on attentional response have indicated that human subjects are very responsive to small changes in visual stimuli. By changing the number or length of the sides on a complex shape, an attentional response may be elicited (Siddle, Stephenson, & Spinks, 1983). Similarly, small movements in a stimulus array usually result in an OR.

The response to movement seems to be inherent in even small infants (Gesell & Ilg,

95

1949). However, infants and adults both show a preference for responses to visual stimuli of greater complexity. This was demonstrated by Fantz (1958a,b, 1965, 1967) in studies that contrasted infants' response preferences to different stimulus characteristics such as patterns, contours, and dimensionality. Infants have been shown to have a response preference for patterned stimuli over homogeneous patches of color, random visual arrays over simple orderly arrays, curvilinear versus linear designs, and three dimensional versus two dimensional figures. There is a natural response tendency toward human facial features over other geometric shapes. In most cases, more complex stimuli elicit greater responsivity than simple stimuli. However, the response to human features suggests that complexity may be less critical than stimulus salience, human faces being perhaps the most significant naturally occurring stimulus.

Novelty and the OR

The novelty of a stimulus is important in predicting attentional response. In fact, Sokolov (1960, 1963, 1969) postulated that incongruity between the incoming stimulus and existing neuronal templates is the basis for the OR (The Neuronal Model). The neuronal template was considered by Sokolov to reflect memory created by previous stimuli. The incongruity that occurs when there is a mismatch between the new stimulus and prior stimuli is influenced by the novelty of the new stimulus. Novelty, in turn, reflects the distinctiveness of the new stimulus relative to the background environment and memories of previous stimuli.

Unfortunately, novelty is often difficult to determine outside controlled situations, in which an animal is reared with exposure to only a very limited stimulus array. In a natural environment, novelty must be inferred by the extent to which a stimulus is discrepant from the typical information surrounding an individual. Furthermore, if stimulus novelty is too great, it may lose its strength in eliciting an OR. With excessive novelty, the information conveyed by the stimulus becomes too difficult to extract. The result is that the stimulus takes on the characteristics of noise.

The problem of defining novelty is not trivial, as it points to a fundamental issue in the study of attention. Sensory processing occurs because of a need to extract information from the environment. Attention is the process by which information is selected. Yet, the quality of the stimuli in a given environment seemingly define the characteristics of the attentional response, as a stimulus that is either too similar to or discrepant from the environment will not produce a strong response.

Apparently, there is a window into which the information provided by stimuli must fit for it to be acted on. From a quantitative perspective, this window can be thought of as a mathematical function having an inverted U shape. Maximal response occurs when a stimulus is moderately complex. Excessive complexity takes on the characteristics of randomness.

The demonstration of an inverted U-shaped function relating attentional response to level of complexity does not resolve the problem of stimulus complexity. Complexity is easily dealt with when a single psychophysical dimension is considered. For instance, a stimulus array containing different geometric shapes is clearly more complex than one containing one shape. However, in natural environments, a multidimensional set of features is associated with a set of different stimuli. In such an environment, it is much more difficult to define complexity. In fact, complexity may be derived from the interaction of stimulus features, rather than from the nature of individual units. As we discussed in Chapter 4, stimulus generalization may play an important role in defining complexity in these conditions.

Information Content

Specification of the informational content of a given stimulus set should be critical to the determination of the effect of stimulus complexity on the OR. Spinks and Siddle (1976) quantified the level of information being presented in their stimuli (12, 26, and 60 bits) but did not find that the size of the skin conductance response (SCR) varied with information level. They did note that the number of ORs increased with stimulus complexity, as did the number of trials to habituation.

In other well-controlled studies, Verbaten, Woestenburg, and Sjouw (1979) found that more complex (60-bit) stimuli resulted in longer fixation times than less complex (12-bit) stimuli, though again, the size of the electrodermal response was not effected when no task instructions were given. In the second study, the subjects were told that a recognition task would follow the stimulus presentations. This time, the subjects showed no visual fixation differences but had greater skin conductance magnitudes, as well as a slower rate of habituation. In a later study, Verbaten and colleagues (1979) varied both informational level and task uncertainty and found that SCR and trials to habituation did not vary across conditions. However, fixation times were greater for the "uncertain" group.

These experiments indicate that the relationship of information level and stimulus complexity to the OR (as defined by the electrodermal response) is very subtle and task-dependent. When a task demand of future memory performance is given, greater autonomic responsivity occurs, with slower habituation. When no such demand is present, subjects attend to the complex stimuli longer, but do not show increased autonomic responsivity. In contrast, EEG desynchronization (as measured by alpha blocking) is unequivocally greater for complex visual stimuli (Berlyne & McDonnell, 1965; Gale, Dunkin, & Coles, 1969).

The dissociation of these different physiological systems, and the subtle influences of information complexity and task demand raise a number of interesting issues in the study of attention. The linking of task demand to electrodermal response suggests that expectancy may increase physiological activation because of the increased signal value of the complex stimuli. On the other hand, under conditions of no task expectancy, the complex stimuli do not cause autonomic activation but do result in greater visual fixation, presumably because of the greater interest evoked by complexity. The fact that autonomic response does not mirror "looking" under low-demand conditions indicates that this activation may be linked more to the salience generated by demanding tasks requiring future responding, than to the nature of the stimuli themselves. The stimulus characteristics affect the amount of visual gaze under low-demand conditions, but not necessarily the arousal that is produced. Central measures of brain activation correlate better with the process of visual fixation with low demand, as EEG reflects cognitive operations that may be more independent of the arousal generated by task demands, emotional salience, or other response-based factors.

Stimulus Uncertainty and Change

Thus far, we have dealt with stimulus complexity primarily from the standpoint of information level. However, stimulus complexity is also a product of the dynamic and temporal variations in stimuli. Most stimuli do not occur in isolation or in a fixed pattern. The effects of spatial uncertainty on visual fixation times was discussed in the last section. The uncertainty derived from the predictability of stimulus presentations produces a U-shaped relationship to the size of the SCR (Lovibond, 1969), as maximal response occurs when the probability of a stimulus occurring is 50%. Similar findings have also been noted in other physiological systems, including heart rate (HR) (Schwartz & Higgins, 1971). This finding suggests that information theory may help to delineate some of the characteristics of the OR associated with stimulus probability.

Stimulus variation is fundamental to the elicitation of the OR. Sokolov's original formulations (1960, 1963, 1969) dealt with the effects of subtle changes in stimulus parameters on the OR. Changes in stimuli are ultimately more important than the actual content of stimuli in determining the characteristics of the OR and habituation. When a series of stimuli is presented in one sensory modality (e.g., visual) and is then switched to another modality (e.g., sound), there is a large recovery of the OR (Furedy, 1968; Houck & Mefferd, 1969). Changes in tone, stimulus intensity, stimulus duration, stimulus omission, and word meaning have been shown to cause the reemergence of the OR (see Siddle *et al.*, 1983, for a review).

Changes in the pattern of stimuli appear to have a more subtle impact on the OR. When sequences of stimuli are presented in fixed orders, subjects show the greatest responses when there is a large discrepancy between the original sequence and the newly presented stimulus (Yaremko, Blair, & Leckhart, 1970; Yaremko, Glanville, & Leckhart, 1972). This finding is interesting because it indicates that the OR is sensitive to subtle aspects of the information in the stimuli. A habituated response quickly reemerges when subtle changes are made in the stimulus. This is a critical observation, as it suggests that, above all else, the OR is a signal of the organism interacting with a variable environment.

Stimulus Intensity and Duration

Relative to stimulus complexity, the effects of stimulus intensity are more clear-cut. A number of investigators have demonstrated a positive linear relationship between stimulus intensity and the size of the OR (e.g., Barry, 1977; Hovland & Riesen, 1940; Ray, 1979; Turpin & Siddle, 1979). As stimulus intensity increases, so does the size of the OR. With respect to habituation, most investigators have found that more intense stimuli require a greater number of trials for habituation. These findings seem to be fairly consistent across physiological modalities. In contrast, stimulus duration does not usually affect the amplitude of the OR (Raskin, Kotses, & Bever, 1969).

Interstimulus Interval

The interstimulus interval (ISI) has also been shown to affect both the OR and habituation. Very long ISIs tend to increase the size of the OR and to slow the rate of habituation (Gatchel & Lang, 1974; Geer, 1966). With ISIs greater than 120 to 240 sec, habituation may not occur (Schaub, 1965). With increasing ISIs, the stimulus is likely to retain its salience because it may appear as a new stimulus even though it has occurred before. During habituation, the amplitude of the OR has been shown to vary directly with the size of the ISI on the trial before (Winokur, Stewart, Stern, & Pfeiffer, 1962). This relationship indicates that the ISI duration not only affects the response to the immediate stimulus but also produces a spread of effect to subsequent trials. Long-term habituation effects have been found in many studies (Graham, 1973; Ohman, 1979; Stephenson, 1982; Wagner, 1976), suggesting that habituation may involve the formation of a longer term memory storage for the stimulus information.

The variability of the ISI also affects the OR and habituation, though the effects of variability are more dependent on methodological factors. Pendergrass and Kimmel (1968) compared variable and fixed ISIs on the skin conductance response and found that variable ISIs produced larger ORs when the subjects judged tone intensity. When a no-judgment condition was used, the results were opposite, with the fixed ISIs producing greater response. This dichotomous effect has been explained by a possible competing effect of "temporal conditioning" on simple habituation (Siddle *et al.*, 1983).

Characteristics of the OR

The most important criterion for labeling a response an OR is its tendency to habituate over repeated exposures to a particular stimulus. By definition, the OR is determined by its link with a given stimulus. With repeated presentations, an unimportant stimulus becomes less salient to the organism, and the result is a reduced response tendency. The link to a unique stimulus or set of stimuli is critical, as changes in the stimulus situation should result in the reappearance of a new OR. The appearance of the OR as an initial response to a stimulus that diminishes over repeated exposures reflects its relevance as an attentional measure. The OR marks the initial registration of a new stimulus at an organismic level, at a strength that is great enough to allow for further processing and conditioning.

Kahneman (1973) identified four components of the OR:

1. A phasic increase in physiological response to the stimulus that is alerting the individual.
2. The inhibition of other ongoing behavioral and physiological activity, including the heart rate deceleration that is often associated with the OR.
3. Orientation toward sources of future stimulation. The OR is in large part an expectancy response, priming the animal for further responding.
4. A subsequent generalized increase in physiological arousal, as seen through EEG desynchronization, cardiovascular responses, and increased muscle tension.

Although these properties determine whether a response fits the criteria of an OR, obvious questions remain: What are the physical properties of the OR, and what is the relationship of these properties to behavior? In other words, what is the functional significance of the OR. In the simplest terms, the OR may be composed of any physiological or behavioral response that occurs relative to a stimulus, and that habituates over presentations. Although the OR is distinguished from other responses by the criteria described above, the physical properties of the OR can vary across experimental situations, as different responses are measured.

Studies of the OR have examined a variety of responses, ranging from gross motor responses, such as a movement of the head in the direction of a sound, to molecular events occurring in the membrane responses of simple organisms (e.g., *Aplysia*). Interestingly, the characteristics of the OR and habituation are very similar across different organismic levels, even though specific physiological mechanisms may be very different (Kandel, 1978). The OR and habituation are very robust, as they are evident in most biological systems.

When the OR is examined at the level of systemic physiological response, a fairly specific pattern of response is observed. This response pattern has features that are dominated by autonomic sympathetic responses involving the multiple physiological systems. The OR involves increased skin conductivity (sweating), pupil dilation, vasoconstriction in limb musculature, central vasodilation, EEG desynchronization, and other associated changes in autonomic and musculoskeletal response. These responses have been well described by past investigators (see Kimmel, Van Olst, & Orlebeke, 1979, for a review).

Despite the diversity of the physiological responses associated with the OR, there are several components that have received the most consideration. The vasomotor and electro-dermal responses have been of greatest interest, for different reasons. The electrodermal response is usually studied through skin conductance, resistance, or potential measurement and indicates changes in the amount of sweat on the skin. These responses are very robust and also habituate in a dramatic fashion. The functional significance of the electrodermal response is not obvious. Yet, this response is a consistent correlate of the OR and is relatively easy to measure. Skin conductance and potential response increase with the greater activation accompanying the OR. These responses also reliably reflect habituation and are therefore particularly well suited to studies of this phenomenon. The electrodermal response is so well integrated with the OR that it has often been used as a primary criterion for identifying the OR.

The cardiovascular OR has also received considerable attention. Variations in cardiovascular responsivity are of obvious importance, as it reflects the behavioral and physiological demands placed on the animal. The OR can be differentiated from other associated responses (such as the startle and defensive reactions) as heart rate decelerates during the early stages of the OR. In contrast, heart rate typically accelerates during defensive and startle responses, and extreme vasoconstriction is noted across most somatic regions. The OR is similar to the startle and defensive responses in many other respects.

Although the direction of the HR and blood pressure responses provide the easiest way of separating defensive from orienting responses, there are several other bases for making this distinction. For instance, an OR may occur with either the onset or offset of stimuli, whereas the defensive response (DR) should occur only at the onset of a strong stimulus. Also, the OR should habituate more quickly, as was found by Jackson (1974). A major difference between the OR and the defensive response is the prediction of whether a recovery of the response will occur to subtle changes in the stimulus set that do not involve increased stimulus amplitude (i.e., dishabituation). The defensive response should occur only to high-amplitude stimuli and should therefore be unaffected by changes in information content at lower amplitudes. This distinction has been supported in studies of HR response (Graham, 1973).

The startle response has also been distinguished from the OR on the basis of a very rapid HR acceleration (Hatton, Berg, & Graham, 1970). The amplitude of the response is also great, and habituation is usually rapid (in contrast with the defensive response). This effect suggests that the startle is a different type of response that is less related to further information processing. The startle responses seems to be an extreme motor response to an extremely strong stimulus. The OR is certainly influenced more by the information-processing demands of a task, though there has been disagreement over whether the OR is associated with the sensory or the motor demands of a task (Graham, 1973; Obrist, Webb, & Sutterer, 1969).

As we will discuss in the next chapter, a differentiation in heart rate response is evident in cognitive tasks that normally fall outside the domain of the OR. The direction of the heart rate response depends on whether subjects are passively taking in information or the task requires a more active response (Lacey, 1959, 1967; Lacey & Lacey, 1957). The Laceys' studies suggested that the direction of heart rate response depends on whether informational intake and rejection are induced. Subsequent studies found that cardiac deceleration is often followed by a period acceleration of the HR, when an active response followed an initial period of sensory processing. This finding suggested an alternative conclusion, that cardiac deceleration is associated with sensory intake, and acceleration, with the preparation for a response. The directionality of the response may relate to attentional factors. Regardless of the reason for the bidirectionality of the HR, it is clear that the physiological response during stimulus processing is not a uniform phenomena.

HABITUATION OF THE OR

One of the most important features of the OR is that it habituates (see Figure 5.1). Over repeated trials, the size and frequency of the response diminishes rapidly. The variables that govern the rate of habituation are largely the same as those that govern the nature of the OR. The novelty, information content, complexity, intensity, and other stimulus factors determine the rate of habituation.

Habituation is a significant component of attention for many of the same reasons that extinction is relevant to understanding conditioning. Maximal response to new stimuli depends in part on habituation to previous stimuli. In a sense, habituation clears the registers for more salient stimuli. Therefore, it is useful to determine the effects of the introduction of new stimuli during habituation, or the re-presentation of a previously habituated stimulus.

The re-presentation of a habituated stimulus resembles the occurrence of spontaneous recovery after extinction. As in the case of extinction, several different hypotheses could account for the reemergence of the OR after habituation. One possibility is that habituation itself has little impact on the reemergence of the OR, and that spontaneous recovery is related solely to stimulus factors. Another possibility is that active processes serve as a gate to reject inconsequential stimuli and to enhance responses to consequential stimuli. This second hypothesis requires that inhibitory and excitatory processes influence habituation. One means of testing for these influences on habituation is through the paradigm of below-zero habituation training.

When a stimulus is presented beyond the point where it ceases to elicit an OR, one might predict that it would continue to affect the organism, producing an increase in the strength of habituation. Below-zero habituation should produce decreased spontaneous recovery of the OR when the stimulus is reintroduced. Contrary to this prediction, Waters

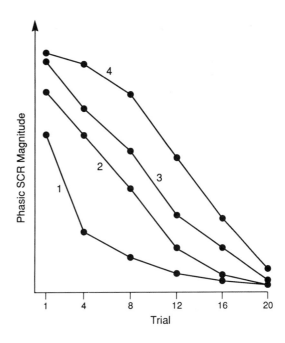

FIGURE 5.1. Habituation of the skin conductance orienting response as a function of repeated stimulus presentations of stimuli varying in featural complexity from 1 (least complex) to 4 (most complex).

and McDonald (1974, 1975, 1976) did not find evidence of below-zero habituation in a series of well-controlled experiments. In their first study, subjects received 55-dB tones until habituation was evident on two successive trials (i.e., zero response). One group of subjects then received no further stimulation until 3 minutes later, when a buzzer was presented followed by a re-presentation of the initial tone. The other group continued to receive 10 tones before the 3-minute delay. Waters and McDonald demonstrated no difference in spontaneous recovery between the groups. Their amplitudes of initial response during spontaneous recovery were similar, as were their rates of rehabituation. Interestingly, the subjects in the below-zero habituation group showed larger skin conductance responses to the buzzer than the subjects in the other group. This finding suggested that prolonged habituation below the point of zero response either is the equivalent of not being stimulated or is actually mildly aversive, thereby leading to sensitization.

In subsequent experiments in this series, Waters and McDonald (1975) demonstrated that prolonged below-zero presentations of the OR stimulus actually produced greater spontaneous recovery than during a control period. However, the amount of recovery was equal to the simple passage of time. In a later study (1976), four blocks of tone stimuli were presented, separated by 3-minute periods of time. This procedure enabled a spacing of habituation. Less spontaneous recovery was noted in this condition than in a time-matched control group. These findings suggested that activation-sensitization over time influenced spontaneous recovery and the rate of habituation. Whether the temporal variable alone influenced the below-zero effects was not clear.

In a final study, Waters, McDonald, and Koresko (1977) found that habituation plays a role in the ability to resist distraction. The introduction of distraction during habituation was found to increase the likelihood of a phasic OR.

These studies illustrate that events occurring during habituation have great bearing on the recovery of the OR, and that habituation is an attention-facilitation process.

Conditioning and the OR

Monotonous and inconsequential information provides a rate-setting factor for habituation. The less salient the stimulus, the faster the rate of habituation. Yet, the relationship between information type and habituation is not always easy to predict. Because all conditioning is preceded by an OR, habituation may interact with concurrent conditioning. Obviously, the introduction of a CS during habituation increases the likelihood of a larger OR to the inconsequential stimuli. The CS mediates the response to the nonsalient stimulus.

Two physiological responses have been associated with the transformation of OR-evoking stimulus; one process is very specific, and the other is nonspecific. When a stimulus initially serves as an OR, it tends to produce a nonspecific physiological response that is related to readiness and an expectancy of stimulus selection. During conditioning, the physiological response becomes more specific, with an increase in activation to the CS, but a decrease in the expectancy response (Ohman, 1983).

This distinction between the physiological responses associated with learning versus those that represent OR has been demonstrated in a variety of psychophysiological studies. For instance, Cohen and Waters (1985) demonstrated that the expectancy responses associated with a stimulus cue can be dissociated from the physiological responses generated during semantic learning during a levels-of-processing paradigm. The physiological response to the cue diminished over trials (habituation), whereas the response to the levels-of-processing task persisted across trials. Studies of this type illustrate that the OR can be differentiated from the physiological responses associated with other behavioral or cognitive processes. However, as a result of conditioning, these distinctions may become blurred.

INTENTIONALITY AND THE OR

The OR is normally viewed as an automatic involuntary response to environmental stimuli. If this is the case, then the OR and habituation must be governed by early processes associated with sensory intake. To what extent do response-related factors, including intention or volitional behaviors, influence the generation of OR. According to Maltzman (1979), a distinction must be made between voluntary and involuntary ORs. To illustrate this point, Maltzman analyzed the physiological responsivity accompanying the presentation of stimuli possessing different levels of semantic value. When subjects were given instructions to perform a cognitive operation on a particular word, they showed increased responsivity to all other words (i.e., semantic generalization). The semantic strength of the stimulus word was important in determining the size of an OR occurring to words. Task demand influenced the degree of semantic generalization and the semantic strength of a word. Maltzman concluded that this finding reflects a voluntary basis for the OR. Also, during problem solving, productive or goal-directed thinking results in greater physiological activation (e.g., Tikhomirov & Vinogradov, 1970). Physiological activation is often associated with increased emotional response, a finding suggesting that motivational factors may underlie the physiological response in these situations. Tikhomirov and Vinogradov (1970) found that, when subjects signaled their awareness of emotional excitement during problem solving (chess playing), they also showed a concomitant increase in galvanic skin response (GSR) over 1.5 sec after pressing a response key. Mandell (1968) postulated that two processes account for this relationship: one process that is cognitively (verbally) mediated and a second process that is the result of unmediated emotional conditioning. This dichotomy was demonstrated by showing different rates of extinction for each of these components, as the subjects continued to show unmediated emotional responsivity, even when they believed that they would no longer receive an aversive stimulus. Maltzman contended that this dichotomy does not necessarily indicate a dual process, as differential GSR responses can be explained solely on the basis of the semantic nature of the task.

NEURAL MECHANISMS OF THE OR AND HABITUATION

Sokolov (1960, 1963, 1969) proposed one of the first theories that accounted for the neural mechanisms involved in habituation of the OR (see Figure 5.2). According to this theory, habituation is determined by a stimulus comparator system that matches the newly presented stimulus to a neuronal model. Past exposures to related stimuli create expectancies of likely future stimuli. These expectancies influence the production of neuronal models, which serve as templates for the comparison of new input. The neuronal model is generated by a hypothetical model formation system, according to Sokolov. When afferent stimuli match the neuronal model, habituation occurs. A mismatch between the afferent stimuli and the existing neuronal model reflects the novelty of the new stimulus. Habituation is viewed as a function of the inhibitory influence of the model formation system in a second amplifying system. Without the influence of inhibition from the model formation system, the amplifying system would serve as a booster to amplify arousal. Reticular activation catalyzes the OR, but habituation occurs when the amplification process is inhibited. Reticular activation is inhibited when there is a similarity between the new stimulus and the neuronal model resulting from negative feedback along collateral pathways, which in turn inhibits the amplification of reticular activation.

Sokolov did not account for the neural mechanisms responsible for inhibition of the amplifying system in his original model but later proposed that the hippocampus may

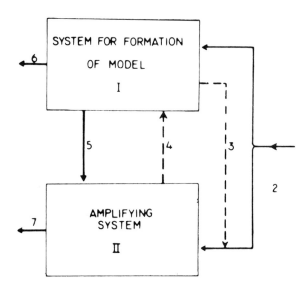

FIGURE 5.2. The neuronal model proposes that habituation results from neural systems that amplify and compare incoming stimuli with a neuronal model or template. A system that forms a model based on previous stimuli (I) and a system that amplifies the response to the stimulus (II) were proposed. Hypothetically, the two systems interact in a reciprocal relationship. The model formation system may also inhibit the input along sensory pathways prior to the amplification system. From Sokolov (1960, 1963), with permission.

play an important role in this process (1976). With repeated stimulation, the stimulus representation associated with past exposures modifies the response characteristics of the hippocampus. Neural cells of the hippocampus reduce their firing rate because of inhibition from collateral neurons that are potentiated by the repeated stimulus presentations. With decreased hippocampal firing to the stimulus, the neural network underlying the OR is uncoupled, as the reticular system is no longer stimulated. The collateral inhibitory stimulation may also potentiate inhibitory hippocampal cells, which in turn increase corticothalamic synchronization, further deceasing cortical activity in response to the new stimulus.

A test of Sokolov's model is its ability to account for a number of related phenomena, such as dishabituation and spontaneous recovery of the OR. The reemergence of the OR with representation of a stimulus after habituation is typically viewed as a form of disinhibition. The disruption of habituation to the original stimulus after a second stimulus is introduced (dishabituation) may reflect a release from inhibition. Sokolov proposed that this occurs because the characteristics of the stimulus are suddenly changed relative to the existing neuronal template. The incongruity of the new stimulus with the neuronal template essentially resets the organism's neuronal model, which then results in the reemergence of the OR.

Dual-Process Theory

Groves and Thompson (1970) described an alternative neural model to account for habituation and sensitization of the OR in their dual-process theory (see Figure 5.3). They suggested that the behavioral phenomenon of habituation is best explained as a function of two independent neural mechanisms in competition: habituation and sensitization. According to the dual-process theory, neural habituation occurs as a simple decremental function of Type H neurons along stimulus-response pathways (whose response tendencies shrink) with repeated stimulation. The decremental process of habituation results from iterated

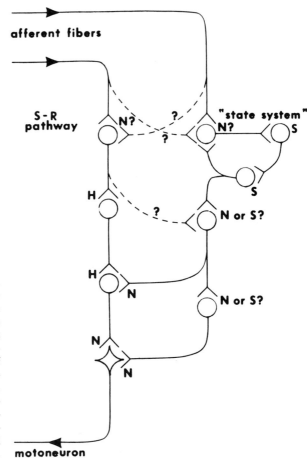

FIGURE 5.3. Schematic diagram of the dual-process model of sensitization and habituation. Two types of neuronal synapses (Types H and S) were postulated by Groves and Thompson to account for either attenuation or maintenance of the OR. H = habituation synapses, S = sensitizing synapses, N = nonplastic synapses, S–R indicates a stimulus–reponse pathway. The N synapses do not habituate or sensitize. From Groves and Thompson (1970), with permission.

stimulation. Habituation continues at an exponential rate until an asymptotic level is reached. The habituation rate is inversely related to interstimulus interval.

The second stage in the dual-process theory, sensitization, acts in opposition to neural habituation. Stimulation has a generalized effect of increasing the overall excitation level of the organism. With mild to moderate stimulation, there is an initial increase in sensitization along Type S neurons until a peak level is reached and then a decay in sensitization. Therefore, sensitization is a transient response, except under certain conditions. When a stimulus is very salient or intense, sensitization may be prolonged, and conditioning may even occur. The relationships between habituation, sensitization, and simple conditioning has been most clearly demonstrated in studies of simple organisms (Hawkins & Kandel, 1984). These mechanisms are discussed in greater detail in chapter 7 but can be summarized as involving differential presynaptic responses to stimulation.

The dual-process theory differs from Sokolov's stimulus comparator theory in several important ways. The dual-process theory specifies two independent processes for habituation and sensitization, whereas Sokolov did not separate these processes. This distinction has implications for the characteristics of habituation under different behavioral conditions. For example, the two theories differ with respect to predictions regarding the effect of dishabituation stimuli. By incorporating an independent, active process of sensitization in interaction with the process of habituation, the dual-process model has certain advantages. If habituation occurs solely as a function of an inhibitory influence, as Sokolov suggested, then dishabituation should follow principles that govern release from inhibition. When a stimulus is presented beyond the point that it ceases to elicit an OR (below-zero habituation), one might predict that it would continue to affect the organism, producing an increase in the strength of habituation. Below-zero training should then produce decreased spontaneous recovery of the OR when the stimulus is reintroduced. By increasing the strength of habituation with additional inhibitory exposures, the intensity of the response to a dishabituating stimulus should be reduced if habituation is primarily a function of inhibitory influences.

Alternatively, the dual-process theory maintains that dishabituation occurs due to a temporary masking of habituation by sensitization, without the requirement of increased inhibitory strength over repeated trials. Sensitization can override the effects of habituation and lead to potentiation of the OR by nonhabituated stimuli.

As Waters and McDonald (1974, 1975, 1976) demonstrated, below-zero habituation does not produce greater suppression of the OR. Spontaneous recovery of the OR was unaffected by below-zero training. While recovery from habituation is not influenced by below-zero training, Waters and McDonald (1974, 1975, 1976) found that the magnitude of the OR to sensitizing stimuli can be influenced by many different experimental manipulations.

Another strength of the dual-process theory is its parsimony. The stimulus comparator theory requires the complex interaction of multiple brain systems and therefore does not apply well to habituation in simple organisms or at lower neural levels. In contrast, the dual-process theory proposes neural mechanisms that operate across organisms and neural levels. Habituation and sensitization primarily reflect different presynaptic events rather than the interaction of entire neural systems.

The dual-process theory has been supported by many investigations of habituation in simple organisms, such as Aplysia (Kandel & Spencer, 1968; Kandel, 1978), and for a variety of reflexes across different levels of animal species. For instance, Thompson and Spencer (1966) demonstrated that the hindlimb reflex of the cat can be habituated and then dishabituates to other stimuli in a manner consistent with predictions of the dual-process theory. Human psychophysiological data support certain predictions of the dual-process theory (Waters & Wright, 1979).

While the dual-process theory has been validated for many types of habituation, some investigators have challenged the assumption that presynaptic processes account for all forms of behavioral habituation (Krasne 1976). The dual-process theory seems to be most clearly supported when considering habituation and sensitization in simple organisms and lower-level neural systems in more complex animals like primates. Pribram and McGuinness (1975) argued that simple presynaptic response decrementing processes, as proposed by the dual-process theory, are evident only up to subcortical thalamic and collicular levels.

ALTERNATIVE THEORIES OF HABITUATION

Other models have been proposed which account for the habituation of the OR and that expand on the dual-process or stimulus comparator theories. These models attempt to account for the type of habituation observed in humans and generally posit that in humans habituation and sensitization depend on the interaction of multiple neural systems.

Based on findings related to below-zero habituation training, Waters and Wright (1979) proposed a habituation-sensitization model (a modification of the dual-process theory) to account for factors that affect the maintenance of habituation (see Figure 5.4). Like the dual-process theory, the habituation-sensitization model proposes that habituation is solely a function of the decremental response of Type H neurons, along classical sensory pathways. However, Waters and Wright argue that sensitization cannot be accounted for solely as a function of Type S neurons, as sensitization by Type S neurons is very generalized and not stimulus-specific. In humans, sensitization is influenced by many stimulus-specific factors, such as the consequentiality of the sensitizing stimulus. Therefore, the habituation-sensitization model proposes that in humans, sensitization is a function of multiple neural interactions in the limbic-hypothalamic-frontal system.

The habituation-sensitization model proposes that within the hippocampus, Type A (activating) and Type I (inhibitory) neurons selectively facilitate or inhibit the response to stimuli along classical sensory pathways, depending on whether the stimuli are consequential or nonconsequential. Sensitization occurs independent of the decremental effects of habituation. While Type H neurons of the sensory attention system attenuate the OR based on continued representation of stimuli, other neural systems, including limbic, hypothalamic, and frontal cortical systems, selectively facilitate or inhibit further responding based on the degree of consequentiality. The habituation-sensitization model maintains many of the assumptions of the dual-process theory while placing more emphasis on the sensitization process.

Other investigators have proposed alternative theories which emphasize the importance of cognitive processes, such as short-term memory, in explaining habituation. Two of these models (Wagner, 1976, 1981; Ohman, 1979) posit that the OR is triggered by the "priming" of the stimulus in a limited-capacity short-term memory. Wagner's model is similar to Sokolov's neuronal model that emphasized the matching of incoming stimuli with existing internal representations. Wagner's model focuses on the relationship between short-term memory storage (STS) and the new stimulus. He suggests that there are two stages of priming which affect habituation. The new stimulus primes both its own representation in STS as well as the associative cues from retrieval of past memories of the stimulus. This model emphasizes the limited capacity of STS and therefore is very closely tied to information processing models. However, evidence for the presence of the priming suggested by this model is not very strong.

Ohman (1979) proposed an alternative information processing model that emphasizes the comparison of information held in long- and short-term storage. Short-term storage has a limited capacity. Therefore, there must be a constant interaction between new stimuli in STS and previously processed stored information. Ohman proposed that the OR springs from activation occurring when new stimuli are contrasted with the nonactive STS, which results in a heightened OR in the case of a mismatch. The OR is linked with a "call for central processing" rather than with actual cognitive processing. Ohman's model suggests that a dissociation can be made between activational components related to preparatory attention and subsequent cognitive processing.

The models of habituation proposed by Wagner and Ohman are interesting because they incorporate concepts derived from cognitive theories of attention to explain the OR and habituation. However, these models propose mechanisms for habituation that are complex, and the neural systems that might underlie these mechanisms are difficult to specify. As a result of this complexity, these models lack the parsimony of the dual-process theory, since a common mechanism for the OR and habituation across different neural systems cannot be assumed. Yet, habituation is observed in very simple organisms with nervous systems that have a minimal level of complexity (e.g., Aplysia).

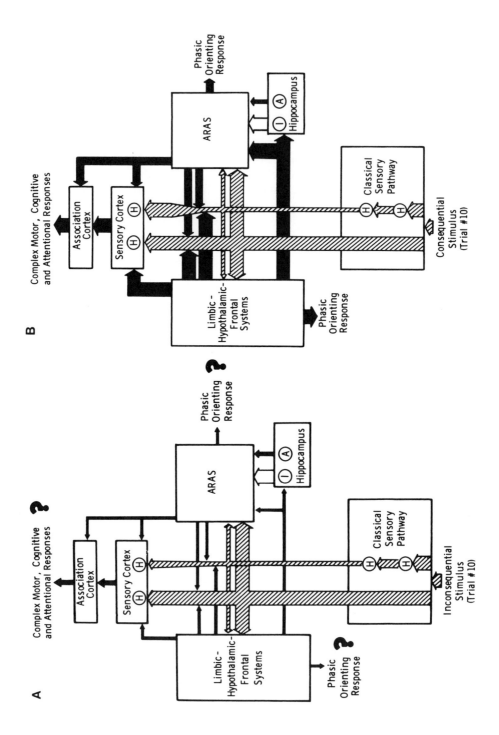

EVALUATION OF HABITUATION THEORIES

Past efforts to determine the validity of particular theories of habituation have often focused on the parametric characteristics of OR elicitation and habituation (see Stephenson & Siddle, 1983, for a detailed review of such efforts). The parameters that have been evaluated in these investigations include many of the variables discussed earlier in this chapter, including stimulus intensity, stimulus duration, stimulus information value, expectancy information, interstimulus interval, number of trials, stimulus change, and response to dishabituation. Unfortunately, no single theory has been fully supported by psychophysiological investigations of these parameters. Each theory makes certain predictions for which there is contradictory evidence. Consideration of tests of each of the parameters listed above is beyond the scope of this book. However, it is useful to consider some of the problems that arise when evaluation of theories of habituation is limited to only one parameter, stimulus intensity.

Each theory of habituation predicts different habituation characteristics as a function of stimulus intensity. For instance, Sokolov's stimulus comparator theory predicts a J-shaped function, with the habituation rate decreasing rapidly when stimulus intensity becomes intense. In contrast, the dual-process theory predicts that neural inhibition is unaffected by stimulus intensity. Sensitization is influenced by stimulus intensity, but in an indirect manner. Ohman's theory makes a completely different prediction: that increased stimulus intensity should result in increased processing allocation, which would actually speed the rate of habituation. Testing these predictions would seem to be a rather simple matter. Yet, experiments designed to evaluate the effect of stimulus intensity on habituation have not yielded conclusive results.

The relationship between habituation and stimulus intensity depends on many task characteristics. The distinction between short-term and long-term habituation appears to be of particular importance when accounting for this relationship. Short-term habituation refers to decremental effects that are relatively short-lived, whereas long-term habituation refers to an effect that is more durable. Short-term habituation probably occurs without the need for long-term storage of sensory representations. However, long-term habituation probably requires the involvement of a memory component for habituation to persist long after the afferent traces of the stimulus have decayed. For simple organisms, such as Aplysia, short-term and long-term habituation may share a common locus (Castellucci, Carew, & Kandel, 1978). However, in humans and other higher-order animals, the parameters associated with long- and short-term habituation may be quite different. A positive relationship exists between stimulus intensity and OR magnitude for short-term habituation, implying that habituation is likely to be slower with higher-magnitude stimuli. However, the initial level of the OR at the first stimulus presentation represents a confound when interpreting data regarding short-term habituation.

FIGURE 5.4. A habituation–sensitization model of selective attention (from Waters & Wright, 1979). (A) This flowchart illustrates the brain's response to the 10th trial of a consequential stimulus. The relative thickness of the lines reflects the relative strength of the inputs and outputs. A dark line indicates a modulating system, and a cross-hatched line indicates a sensory system; both are excitatory. Inhibitory impulses from the hippocampus are postulated (light line). The ascending reticular activating system (ARAS) produces arousal that is reponsible for production of the OR. (B) To a nonconsequential stimulus, the strength of the sensitization is reduced, and in turn, the likelihood of an OR decreases. In contrast to the neuronal and dual-process models, the model of Waters and Wright attempts to account for the roles of multiple brain systems.

Few investigations of long-term habituation in humans have been conducted. In one relevant study, Ray (1979) demonstrated that long-term habituation may not be consistent with short-term effects. Ray demonstrated that while subjects produced a greater initial OR as a function of stimulus intensity (i.e., decibel level of tones), there was no distinction in response as a function of initial intensity on a subsequent long-term test. While these results seem to provide some support for the theories of Ohman and Wagner, methodological factors limit the extent to which this finding generalizes to other conditions.

The phenomenon of dishabituation provides another illustration of the difficulties encountered when evaluating theories of habituation. The dual-process theory does not recognize a specific dishabituation process but instead maintains that a return of the OR after habituation training reflects the second, transient stage of sensitization. Studies of neural systems below the level of humans support the transient nature of dishabituation phenomena. However, in humans the dishabituation effect may be influenced by informational factors that may prolong the duration of dishabituation.

If one extends consideration to the other parameters of habituation that were mentioned earlier, an even more complicated picture emerges. Definitive conclusions regarding the validity of particular theories are difficult to reach solely on the basis of the current parametric data that exists from psychophysiological investigations of habituation. Data can be found that support each of the theoretical positions that we have discussed. Therefore, it may be that none of these theories fully accounts for the phenomenon of habituation.

An ideal model of the OR and habituation should provide for mechanisms with relative consistency across different levels of nervous system complexity. The dual-process theory accomplishes this consistency by maintaining that only two factors are necessary to account for behavioral habituation. The opposing actions of Type H and S neurons along classical sensory pathways account for both the decrement in the OR and the resistance to habituation. This theory explains many aspects of the OR without implicating specific neural systems.

While the dual-process theory has advantages because of its simplicity, it probably does not account for all forms of habituation. The demonstration by Waters and Wright (1979) that facilitation and inhibition of the phasic OR is both stimulus-specific and mediated by factors associated with stimulus consequentiality illustrates a problem in assuming a common habituation-sensitization mechanism for all forms of habituation. Since the dual-process theory postulates that sensitization is a nonspecific response, it should not be selectively influenced by stimulus characteristics. If stimulus consequentiality influences sensitization, then other neural systems must play a role in phasic activation-sensitization, as consequentiality implies a specificity of response not attributed to single neurons. While habituation and sensitization occur as the result of only two factors in simple neural systems, greater neural complexity may be necessary to modulate these responses in higher animal species and humans. Therefore, the dual-process theory of habituation and sensitization may help to explain subcortical responses of orienting and habituation but probably cannot account for all aspects of habituation in humans. The maintenance of habituation-sensitization in humans seems to depend on the interaction of reticular, hypothalamic, frontal-cortical, and limbic systems that produce both facilitatory and inhibitory influences. Sensitization may reflect the response of Type S neurons in sensory pathways and subcortical systems but also may be modulated by higher neural systems in humans.

Pribram and McGuinness (1975) stressed that the OR and habituation should be considered components of a broader attentional control system. They theorized that three separate neural systems control different aspects of attention through the interactive influence of three types of physiological responses, arousal, activation, and effort. The first system produces arousal that is reflected in sympathetic reactivity to sensory input. Pribram and McGuinness considered this arousal to be a function of the collative properties of the stimulus being processed. Activation is generated by a second neural system, which produces a state of tonic readiness. Pribram and McGuinness concluded that the basal ganglia and septal regions of the brain produce this type of activation in preparation for a potential response. Ultimately, arousal and activation compete as the animal orients to new stimuli while trying to maintain a state of motor readiness. Effort is considered to be the byproduct of the integration of arousal and activation in response to behavioral demands.

The effort required for the regulation and integration of arousal and activation is reflected by increased muscle activity elicited during cognitive operations. According to Pribram and McGuinness, a third neural system is responsible for the control of effort. They theorized that the hippocampus is the site of coordination of arousal and activation. The amygdala is also considered to be an important site in this process, as it influences sensory registration by assigning consequentiality to incoming stimuli.

The OR is comprised of both visceral and somatomotor components. Selective lesioning of different brain structures produces impairments of different components of the OR. For instance, lesions of the amygdala or frontal cortex destroyed the autonomic component but not the behavioral component of the OR (Bagshaw, Kimble, & Pribram, 1965; Kimble, Bagshaw, & Pribram, 1965; Douglas & Pribram, 1969). Therefore arousal, activation, and effort could be decoupled. Other investigators studying autonomic responsivity have demonstrated a similar dissociation between states of behavioral readiness, sensory intake, and effortful cognitive operations (e.g., Cohen & Waters, 1985).

Ultimately, it is necessary to evaluate theories of habituation from a neurobehavioral perspective. Since the goal of habituation theories is to account for underlying mechanisms, it is essential that these theories be evaluated with respect to the influence of specific brain systems. This is a relatively easy task when considering habituation in nonhuman species, and there is in fact a large body of neurophysiological evidence, much of which supports the dual-process theory. The task of studying the neural basis of habituation in humans is more difficult. Psychophysiological theories that propose neural mechanisms for habituation frequently infer the influence of particular neural systems without directly measuring the contribution of these systems. Psychophysiological methods frequently are only able to provide an indirect window into brain functions. Neuropsychological studies of the effects of ablation of specific brain structures provides a more direct means of evaluating these theories.

NEUROPSYCHOLOGICAL EVIDENCE

As we have described above, many neurophysiological investigations into habituation have supported the dual-process theory or modifications of this theory. Human psychophysiological studies have also provided partial support for the dual-process theory, though the evidence is equivocal. A fundamental test of the validity of the dual-process theory is whether habituation always occurs as a simple decremental process or whether, as Sokolov suggested, habituation is governed by inhibitory influences.

Ablation studies using laboratory animals have suggested that selective lesions of limbic and cortical brain structures alter different components of the physiological activity associated with the OR and attention (Pribram & McGuinness, 1975). Since ablation of the amygdala and the frontal cortex in primates disrupts the autonomic component of the OR, it is reasonable to assume that these neural systems also play a role in the human OR.

Not surprisingly, neuropsychological studies of the OR in human patients with brain damage have also indicated that the frontal brain systems play an important role in habituation. Following damage to the frontal lobes, patients frequently exhibit a dramatic failure to habituate (Luria & Khomskaya, 1966). Cohen (1991) demonstrated that following bilateral cingulate damage, patients exhibit abnormal habituation characteristics. Therefore, habituation appears to be modulated by multiple frontal systems.

In one of the largest neuropsychological studies of the OR to date, Oscar-Berman and Gade (1979) differentiated abnormalities in the OR and habituation on the basis of site of brain damage. Patients with aphasia due to posterior cortical damage did not exhibit abnormalities of either initial OR level or habituation when compared to normal control subjects. Patients with Parkinson's disease also did not exhibit abnormalities of these responses. In contrast, patients with Korsakoff's disease and Huntington's chorea exhibited marked abnormalities of the OR, as they had a reduced level of initial OR and also a reduced rate of habituation.

Some investigators have found differences in arousal response between patients with left and right hemispheric posterior brain damage (e.g., Heilman, Schwartz & Watson, 1978). However, these studies have not examined the OR under the same experimental conditions employed in traditional habituation paradigms. The hyperarousal response described by Heilman, Schwartz, & Watson (1978) in patients with right hemisphere brain damage may reflect abnormal activation relative to specific task demands.

In a recent well-controlled study, Meadows (1992) found that neither patients with left (n = 9) nor right (n = 11) hemispheric posterior brain damage exhibit abnormalities of either the OR or habituation to nonsalient auditory stimuli. However, a dissociation was found in autonomic response to emotional stimuli as a function of which hemisphere was damaged. This study illustrates the importance of distinguishing between the OR and other forms of arousal response.

Abnormalities of the OR have been described following subcortical lesions, particularly with limbic system involvement, in laboratory animals (Pribram & McGuinness, 1975). The impairment of the OR and habituation observed in patients with Korsakoff's disease and Huntington's chorea provides further evidence for the importance of these neural systems for normal habituation. Tranel and Damasio (1989) described a patient with intact electrodermal skin response following bilateral amygdala damage secondary to herpes encephalitis. This study raises questions as to whether the amygdala is essential to the human OR. However, in this study the patient's skin conductance response to repeated presentations of his name and familiar pictures was measured. Neither task qualifies as a true OR paradigm, since these stimuli are actually salient conditioned stimuli (CS) with obvious informational value. Therefore, while the amygdala may not be essential for an autonomic response to salient CS, it may be very important in modulating the OR to not-yet-conditioned stimuli.

In a recent, as yet unpublished, study, we examined the skin conductance OR in patients undergoing the WADA procedure as part of a presurgical evaluation in patients with partial complex epilepsy. Using angiographic procedures, sodium amytal was delivered by catheter at different times to the right and left posterior cerebral and right and left internal carotid arteries in three patients. The posterior cerebral injection affects visual processing systems unilaterally and also suppresses activity of the mesial temporal structures, including the hippocampus. The internal carotid artery injections do not affect posterior cortical activity and hippocampal activity is largely spared. Yet, activity of the anterior lateral temporal lobe and the amygdala is suppressed unilaterally, and frontal lobe functions appear to be affected bilaterally because of crossover of the drug. During the first minute of the assessment for each WADA procedure, a whistle with an amplitude of approximately 100 db was presented. Regardless of site of injection, patients exhibited intact skin conductance response (SCR) to the whistle and an increasing level of skin conductance level (SCL) following the posterior injection. In contrast, they exhibited a complete loss of the SCR and no tonic increase in SCL over the time of the drug's effect. This finding provides an illustration of how the skin conductance OR is strongly influenced by the actions of anterior brain systems, including the amygdala.

Despite evidence that implicates the limbic system, cingulate, and frontal lobes in habituation of the OR, there is relatively little neuropsychological data that directly show whether human habituation is best characterized by the dual-process theory or one of the other theories that we have discussed. However, my findings regarding the characteristics of habituation in patients with cingulate lesions sheds some light on this issue (Cohen, 1991). A dissociation was demonstrated between the slope of habituation and the trials and the criteria for complete habituation. Following cingulotomy, patients exhibited a rate of habituation between trials 1 and 2 that was actually more rapid than prior to the surgery. Yet, after surgery the patients failed to meet the criteria for complete habituation. They exhibited considerable variability in their SCR reactivity, with random fluctuations in response that suggested spontaneous recovery of the OR. These findings provide support for a modification of the dual-process theory, similar to that described by Waters and Wright (1979). Since the initial rate of habituation was essentially unaffected by the lesion, one can assume that this slope reflects the true rate of habituation. In fact, the slower rate of initial habituation prior to surgery may reflect the fact that under normal conditions the cingulate gyrus modulates the rate of habituation through selective excitation (sensitization) and inhibition. Following cingulate damage, the selectivity of this modulatory process breaks down and the true rate of habituation is unmasked. However, with the cingulate damage there is also a failure to regulate the sensitization process, resulting in random amplification of the OR response.

SUMMARY

The construct of the OR has been used to describe a range of phenomena. In a narrow definition, it refers to an automatic reaction to a new stimulus presentation. The OR has also been used in reference to a broader class of physiological and motoric reactions accompanying cognitive activity. This usage reflects one of the difficulties with this concept. It is probably a mistake to interpret the physiological correlates of attention and cognitive processes so broadly. On the other hand, it is impossible to characterize the OR as a single response. One solution to this problem is to restrict the use of the term *orienting response* to only those events accompanying the initial reaction to a new stimulus, but to accept that it is a response with multiple components. Therefore, for the purposes of future discussion, we use the term only to refer to the early attentional shifting associated with sensory selection.

Physiological Substrates of Attention

RONALD A. COHEN and BRIAN F. O'DONNELL

How the mind and body interact has been the focus of philosophical speculation since the time of Plato and Aristotle. The mind–body problem was central to the ideas of Descartes and many subsequent philosophers. Until the 19th century, it was commonly believed that "mental" experience was beyond the scope of physiological study. Cognition is still regarded by some scientists as a metaphysical entity without physical reality. This view was justifiable in light of the limitations of technology prior to the 20th century, and the great distance that seemed to exist between cognitive and physiological phenomena. As physiological investigations were often limited to the study of lower animals, it was extremely difficult to draw conclusions about the interactions of bodily state and cognition.

The advent of electrophysiology provided a nonintrusive means of studying the bioelectrical activity associated with behavior in humans. Early psychophysiological research was typically crude and plagued with methodological problems related to various technical limitations (e.g., Angell & Thompson, 1899). Nevertheless, a foundation was established for the investigation of the physiological manifestations of cognition. Although methodological complexities continue to present an interpretive problem in experiments, there is now abundant evidence that both central and peripheral bioelectrical activity reflect behavioral and cognitive processes. The observation of this physiological activity led to the concept of *arousal*, which became an important part of many theories of attention.

Modern investigations of the physiological correlates of cognitive processes have typically been motivated by two primary goals: (1) to discover the mechanisms underlying these processes and (2) to develop empirical indices that will mark the occurrence of a cognitive event, thereby providing a validation of that process. The value of specifying the physiological mechanisms underlying attention is self-evident. The need for an empirical physiological index of processes like attention is less obvious, but it can be understood in its historical context. The existence of attention and other cognitive processes has been the subject of much debate among behavioral scientists throughout this century. The demonstration of a physiological response associated with a particular process provides evidence of its existence.

Evidence of an attentional component has been provided by research in the fields of psychophysiology, neurophysiology, and, more recently, neuroscience. Attention has been shown to have both peripheral autonomic and central nervous system correlates. Early psychophysiological investigations demonstrated nonspecific relationships between the amount or intensity of cognitive processing and the autonomic response. In recent years, a dissociation of the components of cognitive processes has been possible with advances in these sciences. In this chapter, the psychophysiological evidence of an attentional component is presented. We then discuss how physiological reactivity provides an index of attentional allocation, as well as the physiological mechanisms underlying attention.

EMOTIONS, AROUSAL, AND PHYSIOLOGICAL RESPONSE

Emotional response provides one of the clearest examples of the relationship between cognitive experience and physiological response. We are all able to identify occasions in our lives when a sudden emotional experience resulted in a physiological response. For instance, a frightening event may produce changes in heart rate or rhythm and respiration, perspiration, and muscular tension. These visceral changes are autonomic responses associated with the fearful stimulus. The James–Lange theory of emotion (1884, 1922) provided a behavioral explanation of emotions, as it proposed that emotional experience is the by-product of the individual's labeling a behavioral response to a strong stimulus. James's (1884, 1922) well-known example illustrates this process: If a person encounters a wild bear while walking through the woods, he is likely to experience a series of physiological and behavioral responses as he flees from the situation. Retrospectively, he labels these responses as fear. Emotion can therefore be defined as the by-product of the labeling of physiological and cognitive responses, following a behavioral response to a stimulus. The James–Lange theory came under considerable criticism, largely because of objections to the sequence of behavior that it proposed for emotion.

Many investigators subsequently rejected the notion that emotions necessarily result from the interpretation of these bodily responses to a stimulus. Cannon (1929), the most influential early opponent of the James–Lang theory, argued that emotional stimuli elicit a CNS response that directly produces a broad set of behavioral, cognitive, and physiological responses. He classified these responses as a form of emotional "arousal," a generalized state of physiological energization that catalyzed behavior (Duffy, 1962; Schacter & Singer, 1962). Cannon considered arousal an undifferentiated physiological activation that accompanied different emotional and behavioral states. It provided a theoretical link between emotional response, physiological state, and the constructs of *motivation* and *drive*.

The concept of emotional arousal eventually came under scrutiny when some investigators noted that physiological activation is not undifferentiated. This finding argued against the idea of a generalized form of arousal. Ax (1953) studied the physiological response pattern accompanying various emotional states and concluded that the autonomic nervous system (ANS) response patterns associated with anger and fear differ. Ax proposed that physiological responses exhibit stimulus and response specificity and stereotypy. This means that some patterns of physiological response occur in certain situations regardless of the individual, whereas other responses are very specific to the individual regardless of the stimulus conditions. A generalized pattern of ANS activation may occur in most individuals with exposure to emotional stimuli (stereotypy), but certain situation may produce an enhancement of response in a particular physiological system (specificity). Differential physiological response patterns accompanying emotional states have been demonstrated by other researchers (Graham, 1973; May & Johnson, 1973; Schwartz, 1986; Weerts & Roberts, 1976). Later, we will discuss additional evidence against the concept of generalized arousal that has been provided by other studies that were not focused on emotional behavior.

Although the relationship between physiological response and emotional behavior is not as simple as was once assumed, it is clear that physiological reactivity is a strong correlate of emotions. The relationship between emotional and physiological response supports the position that behavioral and physiological responses are linked, and the physiological response is a fundamental part of emotional experience. Yet, the functional significance of these physiological responses is less obvious. Human cognitive and emotional experiences are derived from more primitive behavior. For instance, fear is often the by-product of previous experience with painful or aversive consequences. Therefore, emotions are influenced by organismic pressures. In an animal's struggle to survive, it seeks food, escapes from threatening situations, and rests to conserve energy. The visceral responses associated with these behaviors often serve adaptive roles by facilitating the desired response. When an animal is fearful, there is often a benefit in running away. The associated autonomic responses may enhance the animal's capacity for this response. Therefore, although visceral state may seem remote from human cognition, it is often indicative of the basic behavioral pressures or primitive drives that underlie more complex cognitive operations.

AROUSAL: AN ATTENTIONAL CATALYST

Physiological reactivity occurs not only during emotional behavior, but also in response to a wide range of behavioral events, including subtle forms of cognitive processing. Historically, these physiological responses were often attributed to a generalized arousal, and they were believed to reflect the underlying energetic state of the individual. The principle of bioenergetics maintains that, in any biological system, behavior is a reflection of the exchange of energy between the organism and the environment. The ways that energy is absorbed, stored, used, and lost by the biological organism are considered key determinants of the state of arousal and, ultimately, behavior. Bioenergetics had antecedents in the thermodynamic models of physics from the late 19th century and influenced Freud's psychoanalytic theory and many subsequent psychosomatic approaches. Behavior was seen largely as the result of the pressures created by a reserve of energy seeking release. This view of arousal was closely aligned to the construct of *drive*.

Many behaviorists rejected the notion of hydraulic pressures. They argued that this was a borrowed metaphor, with limited applicability to human behavior. They saw arousal as simply a nonspecific label for a specific type of response elicited by a stimulus. A central question emerged: Is physiological reactivity simply another type of response outcome, or does it reflect either specific or nonspecific factors that serve to catalyze behavior?

Arousal as a State Function

Behavior can be classified along a continuum of activity states. The conditions of coma and mania represent extremes at either end of this continuum, associated with states of behavioral hypoarousal and hyperarousal. During states of hypoarousal, decreased organismic reactivity is noted, whereas hyperarousal results in increased organismic reactivity. During states of hypoarousal, the EEG is slowed, and most autonomic reactivity is reduced. During states of hyperarousal, the EEG contains high-frequency asynchronous activity, and most autonomic measures are elevated.

Arousal has been used as an organizing concept that characterizes a "state function" for the animal. In theory, arousal reflects the energetic state of the animal. Arousal is governed by both the intrinsic properties of the biological system and the external environmental factors that modify the threshold for responding. Therefore, arousal is conceptually related to the construct of biological drive, which influences the direction of attentional response. Though the construct of arousal lacks theoretical coherence, in a broad sense "arousal" reflects the interaction of the physiological state, behavioral activity, and attentional allocation.

Arousal is often associated with attentional processes largely because of observations that attentional performance is impaired by extreme internal or external informational states. Conditions of organismic hyper- or hypoactivity tend to impair attentional performance. Similarly, extremes of emotion, information load, noise, and physiological activity often influence attentional performance.

Tonic and Phasic Physiological States

A distinction can be made between two types of physiological activity: tonic and phasic. Tonic activity is relatively stable, and it is nonspecific to any stimulus. Phasic activity is a transient response to some behavioral or physiological event. Both tonic and phasic physiological activity may vary over time. Presumably, phasic changes occur for brief periods, with a subsequent return to baseline, whereas tonic changes represent longer term shifts in baseline. It is not always easy to distinguish between tonic and phasic changes in physiological activity, as phasic changes may trigger tonic adjustments in level of activity.

In principle, tonic physiological activity reflects the state of the organism and sets the basal conditions that determine behavioral reactivity. Although tonic activity varies with the introduction of new stimuli, it is a less sensitive index of the momentary variations associated with a changing environment. In contrast, phasic activity reflects the temporal variations occurring in response to environmental or organismic changes occurring in the short term, typically in the range of 1–20 seconds.

The distinction between these two types of physiological activity depends on the time frame that one chooses to examine. It can be argued that tonic activity is the average of all the phasic responding that occurs in a given time period. From a practical perspective, however, certain physiological responses have a more tonic or steady-state character when viewed at a macroscopic level, whereas others are inescapably phasic in character. For instance, endocrine release may result in a phasic response, but the general nature of circulating hormones is usually thought to result in a tonic level that is slow to diminish (especially when compared to the fast responses of neurons). As we will discuss in Chapter 7, distinctions can be made between tonic and physiological responses for various levels of the nervous system, from autonomic responsivity to the activation of single neurons (Kotliar, 1983).

The tonic/phasic distinction is relevant to our current discussion of attention because the concept of arousal has been used as an explanation of both tonic and phasic physiological responses during behavioral and cognitive processes. Arousal in the form of tonic physiological reactivity has been considered a reflection of the animal's state of readiness, capacity, or threshold for responding. Phasic responses are often considered to be index of momentary behavioral and cognitive processes. The term *arousal* has been used to describe both types of responses, a usage that has unfortunately led to confusion and a weakening of the concept of arousal.

Tonic Arousal and Performance

The Yerkes–Dodson law (1908) described an inverted *U*-shaped relationship between arousal and performance. The law predicts that performance will be optimal at medium levels of arousal and will fall off at either high or low levels of arousal. This law arose out of experimental observations that the administration of aversive stimuli to animals improved learning performance when applied in moderate amounts. When too little or too much stimulation was provided to the animal during discrimination learning, performance was less optimal. This effect has been shown through paradigms in which behavioral and physiological "arousal" have been induced through pharmacological or environmental modifications. For instance, the administration of stimulants influences the quality of performance, presumably by altering the level of alertness. However, beyond a certain point, further stimulation reduces the quality of performance. Environmental and social pressures also influence performance in rough accordance with this function. For instance, the level of supervisory scrutiny in work situations produces a similar effect on performance. The manipulation of motivation and reward levels produces biases that also cause shifts in performance according to this function. The Yerkes–Dodson law holds up in a variety of behavioral contexts.

High and Low Arousal

The Yerkes–Dodson law predicts decreased performance under conditions of both very high and very low arousal (see Figure 6.1). The basis for reduced performance under conditions of low arousal is easier to explain than the effects of excessive arousal. Decreased arousal is associated with a decreased probability and intensity of response, whereas the opposite is true of increases in arousal level. Taken to an extreme, states of sleep or coma produce unresponsiveness and, of course, inattention because the organism is not sufficiently energized to respond.

The detrimental effect of very high levels of arousal on task performance is somewhat more difficult to explain. Easterbrook (1959) postulated that very high arousal restricts the range of stimuli that will be processed. Accordingly, with increased arousal, the individual's sensitivity increases, and this increase results in the rejection of irrelevant stimuli. (This process is similar to that described by Broadbent, 1958, in his filter theory of attention.) At

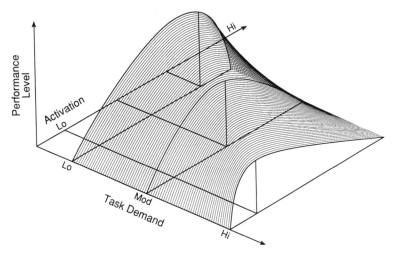

FIGURE 6.1. The Yerkes–Dodson principle. Performance varies as a function of task difficulty and level of arousal.

moderate arousal levels, this sensitivity has a positive outcome, because noise is filtered. However, with further increases in arousal, a point may be reached where there is too much sensitivity. With hyperarousal, Easterbrook postulated relevant stimuli may also be rejected, the result being decreased performance. According to this explanation, individuals who live in a state of continual hyperarousal will perform poorly on complex tasks because of a failure to be sensitive to all alternatives for solution of the task. It has been shown experimentally that increasing the level of arousal increases the probability of habitual responses.

Drugs such as amphetamine that increase arousal tend to restrict the processing of less relevant stimuli. The administration of drugs that decrease arousal (e.g., atropine) results in a less selective perceptual process. This occurs without any change in the functioning of the peripheral or central visual systems and therefore is most likely an attentional effect.

Environmental stimuli also produce similar effects. For instance, the introduction of noise during tasks may produce different results depending on the nature of the task (Broadbent, 1971). During sensory selection tasks, noise impedes performance. During response output tasks (e.g., writing as many digits as possible), noise may produce slight improvements in performance. In the first case, increasing arousal may be detrimental because it reduces sensory sensitivity, and in the second case, reduced sensory sensitivity may be helpful because it allows for the direction of attention to response output.

Although Easterbrook's explanation of the effects of hyperarousal is logical, there are many clinical instances in which this model does not work as well. For instance, the attentional deficits found in schizophrenics are believed by some researchers to result from an excessive activation of dopaminergic subcortical systems that causes an informational "gating failure" (see Chapter 12). Pharmacological increases of dopamine in these systems further diminish attentional capacity. This state of excessive dopaminergic activation can be thought of as involving excessive arousal, which ultimately makes the schizophrenic too sensitive to both relevant and nonrelevant stimuli. This example illustrates a problem in considering arousal a unitary process.

A distinction can be made between the effect of increased sensitivity with hyperarousal and other possible consequences of excessive arousal. Hyperarousal may also produce attentional lability or, alternatively, a narrowing of attentional focus. The hyperaroused subject may tend to be overly selective of certain information but may also show a tendency to be labile and to shift focus too easily when there is competing information. A metaphor for this phenomenon might be a laser beam. With increased energy, the beam may be more narrowly focused, thus having great specificity of direction. Yet, the increased energetics may also create a tendency for the laser beam to move too readily in its narrow focus from point to point. This effect would account for a simultaneous overselectivity and lability. Ultimately, attentional control is disrupted as a result of both effects.

Problems with Generalized Arousal

The Yerkes–Dodson law does not hold up in all situations. Predictions about arousal effects become much harder to make when several sources of arousal are interacting. The law holds up best when one considers the full range of behavioral energetic states (coma to agitated mania). Within this framework, arousal can be considered a unitary state that can be represented along a single dimension. The behavioral characteristics of arousal are easily identified and accepted by most people. If behavior is placed on a continuum, coma and lethargy fall on one end, and states of rage, mania, or agitation fall at the other.

One does not need to be a clinician to recognize the distinctions between these extreme states.

The concept of generalized physiological arousal was originally intended by early arousal theorists to be an analogue of behavioral state. Generalized arousal was thought by these theorists to directly correlate with both physiological and behavioral state. That behavioral state and physiological arousal should coexist along the same continuum seems intuitive. In fact, many of the early studies found evidence for such a relationship between physiological and behavioral states. However, the nature of physiological arousal has been problematic, as many exceptions to the predictions regarding generalized arousal exist. For instance, it is now well known that the stimulant Ritalin reduces activity level in hyperactive children. The original arousal theories would not have predicted this effect, as a stimulant should increase behavioral arousal. This paradoxical finding illustrates that there is not always a direct relationship between the direction of physiological responses and the direction of behavioral responses. The increased brain activation caused by Ritalin causes decreased behavioral arousal.

The analysis of sleep also reveals problems with the concept of a unitary general arousal. Sleep is usually associated with reduced arousal. Yet, not all areas of the brain have reduced activity during sleep. Therefore, generalized neural inactivity is not a characteristic of sleep.

Analysis of the electrical activity of the brain also reveals difficulties in the concept of arousal. The relationship between EEG and behavioral state is not always linear. For instance, although a fast low-frequency EEG usually indicates wakefulness, such activity has been noted during states of coma (Adams & Victor, 1981). The fact that certain drugs, like atropine, can cause cortical slowing without causing major behavioral effects is further evidence that EEG activity and behavioral arousal are not synonymous.

Most theories of generalized arousal (e.g., Duffy, 1962, 1972) predicted that measures of autonomic responses such as GSR, pupil dilation, or cardiovascular response would provide an index of the level of arousal. It is now evident that this prediction was also an oversimplification. Lacey and Lacey (1978) demonstrated that the cardiovascular response can be fractionated, as the occurrence of cardiac acceleration or deceleration depends on task conditions. The Laceys noted cardiac deceleration on passive attentional tasks that involved sensory intake. They noted acceleration when active directional attention was required for a task, a finding that they interpreted as reflecting the rejection of incoming stimuli. Evidently, a parasympathetic response causes cardiac deceleration when tasks require the passive perception of stimuli without a motor response. These findings suggest that arousal is not comprised of a unitary set of responses, and they led many of the original arousal theorists (e.g., Duffy, 1962; Lindsley, 1970) to recognize that both generalized and specific forms of arousal probably exist.

Alternatives to Generalized Arousal

It is now apparent that the original concept of generalized arousal lacked precision. The term arousal was used in an overinclusive manner to refer to all aspects of the internal state that mediate responses. As a result, many behavioral scientists have called for a rejection of the arousal construct. Others have suggested that the term arousal be used more selectively to refer to specific physiological effects.

Some of the problems associated with a concept of arousal can be resolved by reconsidering the nature of the tonic physiological activity associated with different behavioral states. Kahneman (1973) suggested that three conditions of high arousal can be delineated: (1) a generalized pattern of sympathetic nervous system dominance; (2) a pattern of increased motor inhibition, with associated alertness; and (3) a pattern of relaxed perceptual intake. These types of arousal vary with respect to the amount of motor activation that is involved. The pattern of arousal associated with generalized sympathetic activation is similar to the arousal described by the Yerkes–Dodson law. When a situation requires motor involvement, effort, or strain, there is usually an associated generalized sympathetic response. Also, when a situation has very aversive characteristics, it tends to produce a tonic state of sympathetic activation that is associated with an emotional interpretation.

In contrast, the state of readiness that is produced by a warning signal in an otherwise neutral situation is more closely associated with the classical interpretation of the orienting response (OR). Under these conditions, motor inhibition occurs to allow the animal to prepare for future responding. If the animal did not inhibit motor responding, a motor response might be produced that was antagonistic to the response necessary in a new situation. The autonomic responsivity associated with this state of alertness is different from the sympathetically dominated type of arousal. Central nervous system activation is associated with both types of arousal, though presumably different cortical areas are involved in each case.

Kahneman (1973) argued that transient changes in "arousal" are critical to an understanding of attentional processes because it reflects the momentary allocation of effort to the processing and analysis of a new stimulus, as well as the anticipatory state that enhances future attentional allocation by affecting the "capacity" of the channels that are available. Kahneman used the term *arousal* to describe the activation produced by different cognitive processes. Complete characterization of attentional activity may require a consideration of the nature of arousal, the orienting response, and the relationship of bodily responses to information processing.

Pribram and McGuinness (1975) proposed that a distinction be made among the physiological reactivity associated with sensory intake (arousal), the responses resulting from sensory and response anticipation and readiness (activation), and the responses resulting from the interaction of arousal and activation (effort). They proposed that different neural systems control these three aspects of attention. This model has some similarities to Kahneman's notion of arousal. Activation is the equivalent of Kahneman's second type of arousal. However, Pribram and McGuinness's description of effort differs from that of Kahneman.

The physiological equivalents of arousal, activation, and effort are very intertwined and are often difficult to dissociate. Yet, it is possible to create tasks capable of making these dissociations. For instance, arousal precedes activation during categorization. Reasoning may produce a different temporal order, as activation precedes arousal. The basis for this serial characteristic is the very nature of the task. Categorization depends first on sensory intake, and then a readiness for future stimuli. The sequence of these processes requires that arousal precedes activation. During reasoning, sensory analysis is less critical, so that sensorimotor readiness may be a more dominant response. Psychophysiological investigations of the physiological activity associated with arousal, activation, and effort during verbal processing have indicated that different forms of physiological reactivity are associated with the stages of cognitive operations required for a task (Cohen & Waters, 1985).

Ohman (1979) proposed a model to account for the relationship between arousal and attention that characterizes arousal in much the same way as Pribram and McGuinness characterized it. However, Ohman emphasized that memory serves as a control mechanism that directs attention, as the salience of previously presented information stored in memory governs what is attended to. His model suggests that the relationship between long- and short-term memory allows a distinction between the controlled effortful and automatic attentional processes that we discussed in Chapter 2. The inclusion of memory in this physiological explanation of attention adds further complexity to the construct of arousal.

As our understanding of the complex matrix of mechanisms underlying attentional control increases, an ever-growing number of responses are likely to be considered determinants or variants of "arousal." Therefore, it is reasonable to question whether the construct of arousal should be rejected.

One of the main criticisms of the arousal construct has been its lack of specificity. The term *arousal* has been used to describe a wide range of states of bodily activation. *Arousal* has been used to describe not only physiological state, but also the subjective state of excitation that may exist in certain situations. Arousal is said to result from neurochemical effects, stress, noise, emotional state, social pressures, and a host of other conditions encompassing almost the entire range of human experience. The construct of arousal is often used rather loosely, as a descriptive term. There is frequently little concern for how arousal is operationally defined, or for how the construct is used to explain many different psychological phenomena. Terms such as *arousal, activation*, and *effort* have often been used interchangeably to account for the physiological manifestations of an "energized" behavioral state.

Although the construct of arousal lacks theoretical definition, it maintains remarkably resilience, perhaps because of the descriptive value of the term. Almost everyone can identify with the sudden changes in physiological response accompanying certain emotional states. Although these responses may actually be made up of a multitude of different physiological reactions, the association of this activation with a behavioral or subjective event leads to the interpretation of generalized arousal. If the concept of arousal is rejected, we will need another concept that will capture this relationship between bodily response and behavior. Rather than doing away with the concept of arousal, many psychophysiologists have tried to provide a more careful definition. Others have suggested that the term *arousal* be reserved for the description of certain phenomena, and that other constructs be used to refer to more specific forms of physiological reactivity.

Although there are problems with the concept of arousal as originally proposed, it would be a mistake to reject the concept. The term *arousal* serves to describe a number of physiological changes that occur during states of behavioral activation. It also reflects the energetics accompanying different behavioral states. Although arousal may not exist as a single uniform phenomenon, the term retains descriptive utility. Whether we call the physiological activity accompanying attentional performance *arousal* or choose to use some other label may make little difference.

PHYSIOLOGICAL CORRELATES OF ATTENDING

Demonstration of galvanic skin response activation during problem solving by Pillsbury (1908) provided one of the first pieces of evidence that peripheral physiological response may reflect cognition. Woodworth (1938) extended these findings to other physiological systems. Eventually more complex cognitive tasks were used, and a relationship between cognitive demands and physiological response was found (Maltzman, 1955).

Arousal and the OR

The phasic changes in central and peripheral physiological activity that accompany cognitive processing were originally interpreted as manifestations of the orienting response. The OR concept explained how complex cognitive processes could be derived from more molecular behavioral events. For instance, Maltzman (1955, 1968, 1979) used the OR concept to illustrate how semantic generalization could result from the interrelationship between the OR and classical conditioning. This work was a noble effort to bridge concepts coming from several theoretical frameworks, including learning theory, psychophysiology, and cognitive psychology. Natural links seemed to exist among phasic arousal, the OR, and the behavioral processes underlying cognition.

Some investigators were uncomfortable with models that used the OR to account for the physiological responses that accompany a very diverse set of cognitive processes. The tasks used to elicit physiological activation were much more complex than the standard paradigms of classical conditioning on which the OR construct was based. When the OR was equated with all of the physiological responses associated with behavior, the OR concept became overly inclusive and diluted, and was reduced in its operational utility. The OR concept had been extended well beyond its original intent. In reaction to this issue, some investigators departed from a strict OR interpretation. They concluded either that the peripheral physiological reactivity accompanying cognitive processes reflected a nonspecific, generalized arousal, or that specific responses reflected particular underlying processes. Therefore, some physiological reactivity was considered different from the activation accompanying the OR.

Autonomic Attentional Indices

Thus far, we have discussed evidence that there is a relationship between physiological activity and cognitive processes like attention. Given this relationship, does physiological reactivity provide an index of attentional processing? This question has been addressed through investigations that examined the pattern of physiological response associated with tasks varying in the type and intensity of attentional demand.

There is considerable evidence that autonomic nervous system activity correlates with changes in attention. The earliest studies that addressed this relationship arose out of the investigations of the OR and habituation. Studies of the OR typically relied on the monitoring of behavioral or physiological activity during repeated exposures of an animal or a human subject to a stimulus. Habituation was reflected by decreased responding over trials and was thought to reflect decreased attention to a nonsalient stimulus. The OR and habituation effects are robust and are easily demonstrated in experimental situations. The OR seems to indicate passive attention. It was originally proposed to be a reflex, but later evidence seemed to suggest that the OR is centrally mediated by the brain.

Cardiac Deceleration Reflects Attentional Intake

The presence of heart rate deceleration during sensory processing was detected in early psychophysiological studies (Darrow, 1929; Freeman, 1948). This finding was later elaborated in studies that found (Lacey, 1959, 1967; Lacey & Lacey, 1978) that the direction of cardiac response depended on the task. When a subject was asked to perform a perceptual task without response requirements, deceleration was noted. However, when a task required problem solving or other more active responses, cardiac acceleration was noted. This was an exciting finding because it suggested a specificity of bodily response under different information-processing requirements. The Laceys proposed an intake–rejection hypothesis that suggests that the intake of information is associated with cardiac deceleration. According to the Laceys, active processing requires the rejection of incoming information, which is accompanied by cardiac acceleration.

The directional nature of the heart rate response makes sense from the standpoint of the OR theories, which predict a deceleration to unexpected stimuli (Graham & Clifton, 1966). The major difference between the standard OR methodology and Laceys' paradigm is whether the stimulus eliciting the response is expected or unexpected. The fact that cardiac deceleration occurs for a few seconds either before an anticipated stimulus or after an unanticipated stimulus suggests that the autonomic correlate of attention is similar in both cases.

The characteristics of a task that will produce deceleration are similar to those discussed for the OR. The stimulus event must be salient to the individual. The size of the cardiac response depends on stimulus intensity, onset, and the placement of the anticipatory stimulus relative to a primary task. Temporal factors appear to be important in determining the characteristics of the deceleration. Other factors, such as the perceptual difficulty of the task, the rate of stimulus offset, and the performance level of the subject, also influence the degree of deceleration that is noted (Jennings, 1986a,b).

Several explanations have been given for the cardiac deceleration accompanying sensory intake. The Laceys' intake–rejection hypothesis suggests that cardiac slowing facilitates the processing of incoming information as the animal reaches a state of readiness. A slower heart rate indicates a higher degree of readiness and receptivity according to this hypothesis, perhaps because of a quieting of the system. Jennings *et al.* (1978) suggested that cardiac deceleration results from the clearing of the system of previously processed information, or from the maintaining of processing capacity.

Graham (1979) proposed that cardiac deceleration is associated with the stimulus characteristics of the situation. Distinctions among the startle, orienting, and defensive responses may account for whether cardiac acceleration or deceleration will occur. Graham argued that the degree of perceptual clarity or discriminability accounts for the directionality of the response. She postulated the cardiac response to be the result of a reflex inhibition.

An alternative position to account for cardiac deceleration was offered by Obrist (1981), who argued for the importance of motoric activity in the control of cardiac function. Because passive attention is usually associated with a generalized reduction in motor activity, cardiac deceleration may result from motoric factors. Obrist suggested that this may result either from a direct effect of motoric changes on heart rate, or from a direct reduction of arousal that causes a quieting of both motoric and cardiac activity.

The biological bases for cardiac deceleration during anticipatory attending are unclear. Obrist's argument has intuitive biological relevance. If cardiac deceleration is associated with a generalized quieting of motoric activity during passive attending, then it is relatively easy to account for the linkage between the cognitive process of attending and the physiological response. However, if the Laceys' or Graham's hypotheses are correct, there must be another biological reason for the deceleration. Perhaps the fact that passive attending does not require the same metabolic demands as active motor responses accounts for cardiac fractionation. Cardiac deceleration would be associated with a quieting of the system and a conservation of energy. If motoric quieting is not the mechanism underlying this response, some type of sensorimotor readiness that is generated by the brain must also produce this physiological response. Graham's hypothesis of reflex inhibition depends on a brain stem mechanism responsible for triggering the reflex.

Cardiac Acceleration During Directed Attention

Psychophysiologists have focused more on the phenomenon of cardiac deceleration than on cardiac acceleration, probably because the finding of deceleration is counter to the expectations of theories of generalized arousal, as generalized arousal would accelerate heart rate. Cardiac deceleration during anticipation and passive attending is a good example of the specificity of the autonomic response that may accompany attentional processes. However, as we have previously indicated, attention may also involve an active direction of resources to some task. When a subject engages in a problem-solving task, attention is directed to the problem at hand. The character of this type of attention is quite different from the examples of sensory intake described previously, and this type of attention is usually accompanied by cardiac acceleration.

Increased physiological activity during problem solving has been reported in numerous studies since the early 1960s. Physiological activation has been attributed to a range of responses, including increased heart rate, respiration, muscle activity, skin conductance, and pupillary response (see Duffy, 1962). Of these responses, the acceleration of the heart rate that is noted during effortful processing seems to be a particularly reliable index. Lacey, Kagan, Lacey, and Moss (1963) demonstrated that cold pressor stimuli, mental arithmetic, and problem solving on anagram tasks produced cardiac acceleration, whereas listening to a white noise produced deceleration. Skin conductance increased during all of these tasks, a finding suggesting that it is a less specific measure of cognitive activity.

The degree of cardiac acceleration that occurs in a situation has been shown to be a function of task difficulty, stress, and conditions that increase the effortfulness of a task. It has also been shown to vary as a function of the level of developmental maturation. Jennings (1971) demonstrated that more mature children have greater heart rate acceleration than less mature children on Piagetian tasks. Therefore, cardiac acceleration seems to reflect factors related to both the traits and the state of the individual.

Several studies have been conducted to determine the aspects of information processing that accompany cardiac acceleration. For example, Kahneman, Tursky, Shapiro, and Crider (1969) asked subjects to add numbers on a serial addition task. The subjects had to perform a transformation by adding either 0, 1, or 3 to four integers. They found that the condition in which the transformation required adding 3 to the integers produced the greatest amount of acceleration.

In another study, Tursky, Schwartz, and Crider (1970) dissociated two components of the information processing required for mental arithmetic: memory load and mental transformation. In this study, the subjects were given instructions to transform integers through addition after the stimuli were presented. The physiological response to stimulus intake could be dissociated from responses associated with mental transformation. Cardiac deceleration was noted during the stimulus intake phase, and acceleration was noted during the transformation operation.

In order to determine which aspects of information processing accounted for these physiological responses, Jennings and his colleagues (Jennings, Lawrence, & Kasper, 1978; Jennings, Averill, Opton, & Lazarus, 1980; Jennings, 1986a,b) conducted a study in which memory load was varied, while subjects performed transformation tasks. The subjects in this experiment performed tasks that were serially arranged so that information input was followed by a period of memorization, which was followed, in turn, by a period during which the subjects were asked to add the integers. Unlike in the study by Tursky *et al.* (1970), cardiac acceleration was noted when the subjects added numbers that were visually presented, and when they added numbers in memory. Deceleration was noted on a silent reading task, and during a rule determination task. These findings indicate that the directed attention of adding numbers can produce acceleration that overrides any deceleration associated with stimulus intake. Jennings proposed that this finding might indicate that acceleration is associated with memory processing, motivated inattention, or the energy requirements of the task.

Jennings and Hall (1980) tested the relationship of several factors to the acceleration of heart rate during mental arithmetic. Memory load was varied (5 or 10 items), and the subjects provided self-reports about the energy requirements of the task. After an encoding period, the subjects were assessed on retention and recognition tasks. Surprisingly, the amount of acceleration occurring during these tasks did not relate to memory load. Also, acceleration did not vary as a function of the ratings of task difficulty. These results suggest that the direction of attention during the mental transformation operation influences the physiological response.

A question is raised by these experiments: To what extent does memory play a role in generating cardiac acceleration? The findings of Jennings and Hall led to a conclusion that acceleration is related to attentional direction rather than memory processes. This interpretation is consistent with the findings of other investigators studying a range of cognitive phenomena such as problem solving, logical reasoning, decision making, imaging, and memorization (Coles & Duncan-Johnson, 1975; Schwartz & Higgins, 1971; Silverstein & Berg, 1977). Although acceleration occurs during all of these cognitive operations, it was consistently attributed by these authors to attentional direction.

In an attempt to dissociate the attentional and memory components of stages of processing, Cohen and Waters (1985) used the levels-of-processing paradigm. Encoding was a function of the type of task that their subjects engaged in while processing a set of words. The subjects were initially presented with an anticipatory signal on each word trial, which appeared 5 seconds before the word onset. The word was then visually presented, and the subjects were instructed to perform one of three types of tasks (phonemic, low semantic level, and high semantic level) using the word. The processing was initially covert, as the subjects were instructed not to respond except by generating a solution in their own minds until after the word disappeared from the screen. They then made an overt verbal response based on their processing of the word at one of the three levels. Several physiological responses, including heart rate, skin conductance, EMG, and skin temperature, were recorded during the three stages of the task for words processed at all three cognitive levels (see Figure 6.2).

Cohen and Waters found that their subjects showed greater heart rate acceleration and skin conductance responses as a function of the level of processing used in processing the words. Those words processed at the high and low semantic levels had greater cardiac acceleration and skin conductance response than words processed at the phonemic level during both the covert and the overt verbalization phases of the task. The two semantic levels differed in heart rate and skin conductance response only during overt verbalization. The acceleration of heart rate was greatest during the verbalization phase, though during the phonemic task, acceleration was no greater during verbalization than during covert processing. These findings suggest that the cardiac and skin conductance responses noted during these tasks varied as a function of the demands associated with the level of processing, and not as a function of the requirement of producing a verbal response. Interestingly, the subjective ratings of the subjects indicated that they found the phonemic task most effortful and difficult, even though their physiological response was greatest during the semantic tasks.

Memory performance was also greatest for words processed at the high semantic level, followed by words at the low semantic level. Phonemically processed words were recalled less well. The correspondence that was noted between physiological activation and memory performance indicated that the levels effect may have been associated with the increased attentional activation required for or elicited by the semantic tasks. The physiological activation associated with recalled and nonrecalled words was compared for the various stages of processing. Regardless of the level of processing, the words that were later recalled

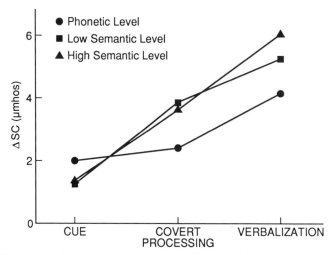

FIGURE 6.2. Heart rate and skin conductance vary as a function of the stage of processing and also of the cognitive operations required for task performance. Physiological response induced during incidental memory encoding reflected effortful attentional allocation (Cohen and Water, 1985).

had greater associated cardiac acceleration and skin conductance than the nonrecalled words during the word-processing periods. This was an important finding because it indicated that, irrespective of the level-of-processing effect, when greater amounts of activation were elicited on a particular trial the word was more likely to be recalled. In general, the semantic tasks elicited greater attentional direction and physiological activation, which were associated with better memory performance. However, words that were not processed semantically still had more likelihood of being recalled if the activation was greater during processing.

These studies illustrate several points relative to the question of how physiological activation relates to attention and other cognitive processes. It is apparent that cardiac acceleration is associated with the direction of attention to demanding tasks. Although various types of cognitive tasks may elicit this response, it appears that acceleration represents an activation that reflects the intensity of processing allocated to task completion. Greater activation is often associated with enhanced memory performance, though this effect seems less related to memory load or other factors associated with memory itself. Instead, physiological activation may reflect attentional resources. Memory encoding appears to be very dependent on attentional processes (e.g., Cohen & Waters, 1985). In fact, memory encoding and attentional allocation are very difficult to disentangle, particularly from a psychophysiological standpoint.

Pupillary Responses and Memory Load

Cardiovascular activation is sensitive to factors associated with attention. Does this mean that all autonomic responses are primarily indicators of attentional allocation? Although the jury is still out on this question, there is evidence that other peripheral physiological responses reflect other cognitive operations. The most obvious example is the demonstration that pupil dilation is related to memory load (Kahneman & Beatty, 1966). In this initial study, the extent of pupil dilation was shown to vary as a function of the number of digits to be encoded in memory (see Figure 6.3). It was found that dilations occurred approximately 300–500 msec following the onset of processing, a finding suggesting that memory load induced greater mental effort (Kahneman, 1973). This finding was of particular interest because pupillary response would be expected to be more closely linked to cognitive

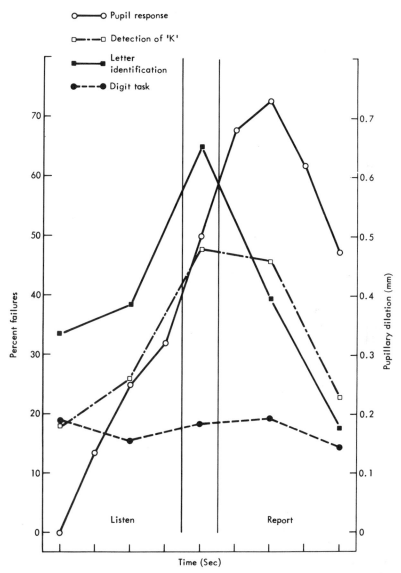

FIGURE 6.3. Pupillary response varies over the time period of a task as a function of attentional demands. Kahneman (1973, with permission) illustrated how this response is influenced by demands for passive and active attention.

processing than some of the other visceral responses we have discussed, as pupillary response is directly associated with the sensation of visual input.

Subsequent studies by Beatty (1979, 1982) have confirmed that pupil dilation is influenced by many different cognitive tasks. On language tasks, letter matching produced smaller dilation than grammatical reasoning tasks. On calculation tasks, the difficulty of multiplication has been shown to relate to the degree of dilation. Difficult visual-perceptual discrimination judgments produce greater dilation than easy perceptual tasks. Therefore, pupil dilation reflects not only the information load placed on memory, but in a broader sense, on overall attentional effort.

MOTOR ACTIVATION DURING ATTENTION

Muscular activation has also been shown to reflect attention and other cognitive processes. This is not surprising if we recognize that attention often involves the redirection of the body toward a new stimulus. Accordingly, motoric activity during covert cognitive processing would signal the preparation for attentional or behavioral redirection. The idea that motoric activation may be associated with covert thought processes is not new. Watson's radical behavioral position (1913) proposed that covert verbalizations serve as the basis for those behaviors that we label as thinking. Attempts to relate motor responding to thinking and other psychological experiences are found in the early psychological works of James, the structuralists, and other theorists who laid the foundation of psychological theory. Of course, some of these theorists viewed motoric activity as an indicator of the content of thinking, and others viewed this activation as the basis of the thought process itself.

Muscular activation during cognitive processing was demonstrated by Jacobsen (1938) and more recently by McGuigan (1978), Cacioppo and Petty (1981a,b), and others. The early investigations indicated that, during thinking, generalized muscular tension throughout the body increases. Although Jacobsen demonstrated that motor activity is an index of cognitive events, he did not go so far as to implicate a role for covert motor activity in thinking, nor did he prove that this activity is necessary for cognition. Findings that cognitive functioning is unimpaired after the introduction of curare provided evidence that motor behavior is not critical to thinking. Feedback from muscles is also not critical to motor control or cognitive performance (Taub, Williams, Barro, & Steiner, 1978). Despite these findings, which seem to reduce the significance of motor activity in cognition, there is some evidence that motor functioning may facilitate or organize cognitive processes.

Locke and Fehr (1970) demonstrated that the EMG activity associated with the memorization of words depends on whether the words are labial or nonlabial phonemes. Labial phonemes that were covertly rehearsed produced EMG activation. Therefore, muscular activation may reflect a specific form of motoric readiness associated with producing certain sounds. EMG activation may reflect the generation of an articulatory representation of information that has been processed. Glassman (1972) found that, when EMG was suppressed, subjects showed fewer errors of acoustic confusion. However, a subsequent study found the opposite effect, as suppression of EMG weakened acoustic discrimination performance and did not have an effect on memory. These conflicting results raised the possibility that the effect of muscle activation on performance depends on a number of task-related variables, such as the level of difficulty.

The relationship between task-processing requirements and muscular tension has been shown in several recent investigations. Cacioppo and Petty (1981a,b) demonstrated that the level of EMG activity recorded from a lip site was related to the level of processing required of the subject during covert performance. Because their task required a yes-no button response, this activation could not have been directly related to a need to respond verbally.

They did not find a differentiation from a forearm site, a result suggesting again that any muscle activity that occurs during covert processing is likely to be related to subvocal speech mechanisms. Cohen and Waters (1984) did not find a levels-of-processing differentiation of EMG activity in either frontal or laryngeal sites. They did note a progressive increase in muscular tension across the three stages of their task (anticipation, covert processing, and verbalization).

DO BODILY RESPONSES FACILITATE ATTENTION?

There is clear evidence that autonomic responsivity reflects attentional allocation. However, do these peripheral physiological responses facilitate or help to regulate attention? To what extent do the visceral and muscular responses accompanying information processing actually influence attentional performance?

General arousal theory predicted a functional relationship between physiological state and cognitive performance, as arousal was viewed as the energetic catalyst for performance. Kahneman's capacity model (1973) proposed that arousal regulates the size of the channel through which information can pass. Many psychophysiologists who have rejected the concept of arousal are still interested in the effects of autonomic reactivity on performance.

Studies showing increased physiological responsivity for items later processed into memory (e.g., Cohen & Waters, 1985; Jennings & Hall, 1980) have demonstrated that phasic physiological response is associated with performance. However, these studies do not indicate the functional significance or behavioral impact of these responses. They illustrate only that physiological responsivity accompanies and gives an index of attentional allocation.

The primary means of determining the impact of autonomic physiological response on performance is to induce physiological reactivity through the introduction of some external stimulus, and then to examine performance. Several early investigations sought to induce differing states of physiological arousal, in order to test effects on learning. Kleinsmith and Kaplan (1963) used a paired-associates learning task with words that had either high or low affective quality. The highly affective words (e.g., *rape*) produced greater skin conductance responses during initial presentation, and greater recall after 45 minutes. This result was interpreted as reflecting a facilitatory effect of arousal on the formation of long-term memory (LTM).

Kleinsmith and Kaplan's findings were replicated in other memory paradigms (e.g., free recall). Dissociations between the effects of induced arousal on short term memory (STM) and LTM have been found, as a negative effect of arousal (physiological activity level) on immediate recall has been noted, in contrast to a positive effect on long-term storage.

Although these general findings held up in other studies of skin conductance, the interpretation of the results came under scrutiny (Craik & Blankstein, 1975). The major objection among cognitive researchers was to the inference that arousal affects memory consolidation. Because there was little support for an effect of arousal on memory consolidation, these authors favored other explanations for the relationship of arousal and memory performance, including the possibility that induced arousal influences the subject's orientation to learning.

Induced Arousal

Kleinsmith and Kaplan's learning effects were tested with many other forms of induced arousal in studies by other researchers. Several approaches have been used, including the modification of informational content from the environment. Several studies have borrowed from Broadbent's work (1957, 1963, 1971) on the effects of noise on performance, which demonstrated that moderate levels of noise enhance performance. Unfortunately, the findings regarding the effects of noise on performance are somewhat complicated and difficult to interpret. One group of investigators demonstrated that noise improves short-term retention on serial learning tasks, but not on nonserial tasks (Hamilton,Hockey, & Quinn, 1972). Other studies have suggested that noise weakens the ability to form associative clusters (e.g., Smith, Jones, & Broadbent, 1981). Therefore, the effects of arousal produced by noise may depend on what aspects of memory processing one examines, as well as the paradigm that is used.

The effect of noise on autonomic state raises some interesting issues about the nature of arousal. Although continuous and intermittent noise typically produce changes in autonomic response, these changes are transient. Autonomic indices usually recover after several minutes. If this is the case, one must question how noise influences attention from the standpoint of arousal. Poulton (1979) argued that noise may have a catalytic effect by influencing an interaction of neuroendocrine functions with behavioral reinforcement contingencies operating in the particular situation.

In other studies, Hockey (1970a,b) demonstrated that noise enhances attention to highly salient stimuli that have priority and leads to reduced attention to other signals. A number of other effects have been found that demonstrate that noise facilitates performance on various tasks. The activation of attention was viewed as the basis for these effects. Hockey argued that arousal is induced by noise that creates a selection bias for high-certainty responses. This argument suggests that noise creates a narrowing of the attentional channel.

Induced Physiological State

Studies that manipulate environmental information do not directly control for physiological state. Arousal is inferred from notions of a generalized arousal, and many of the problems discussed with regard to the concept of generalized arousal emerge. It is not clear that noise or informational intensity equates with physiological arousal.

Physiological state has been artificially aroused through the introduction of drugs in a number of studies. For instance, Revelle, Humphreys, Simon, and Gilliland (1980) gave subjects a stimulant drug at different times of the day and examined their performance on achievement testing. These authors also compared subjects who were judged to be introverted or extroverted on personality measures. The investigators predicted that the effects of induced arousal from the stimulant would depend on personality type and time of day. Unfortunately, the results of this series of experiments was not straightforward, as impulsivity-based personality measures related to temporal pattern rather than level of arousal. A number of conceptual problems have been addressed in reviews of this study. However, this study does illustrate that alterations in physiological state do not produce a simple change in performance. A number of factors, such as personality type, time of day, physiological state, and perhaps other unaccounted-for variables, interact to influence performance.

It is wrong to assume that pharmacological manipulation produces a uniform bodily response or consistent predictable effects on performance. Stimulants like amphetamines and caffeine produce sympathetic nervous system activation, which is expected to produce increased "arousal." However, these drugs also have direct CNS effects, some of which may produce responses other than stimulation. For instance, stimulants produce reticular activation and also cause greater activity in other neural systems. Increased frontal lobe activation may actually cause greater behavioral inhibition. Therefore, it is simplistic to assume a unitary relationship between physiological activation and behavior.

Attempts have been made to induce physiological activation in specific systems in order to study its effect on performance. For instance, Cacioppo & Petty (1979) produced cardiac acceleration in his subjects by stimulation with a cardiac pacemaker. He found that performance on complex cognitive tasks was enhanced in subjects whose heart rates were paced at 88 beats per minute (bpm) rather than 72 bpm. However, these results have not been replicated. Several other investigators have failed to find consistent relationships between induced heart rate and performance in college students, or on reaction time tasks. Folkard (1979a,b) found that induced muscular tension improved the ability of subjects to reject distracting stimuli on sorting and interference tasks. Induced muscle tension also reduced memory performance. Folkard suggested that muscular tension blocks subvocal speech, which is necessary for memorization. Although there are findings that suggest that autonomic response facilitates attentional processing, additional research is necessary on the effects of the physiological activation of specific systems on performance.

CNS EVOKED-POTENTIAL CORRELATES OF ATTENTION

Peripheral physiological reactivity provides a useful, but indirect, index of attentional processing. Analysis of the mechanisms underlying attention can be inferred from the way autonomic responses vary across cognitive tasks. However, these responses do not directly reflect neural activity of the brain. Therefore, there are advantages in the use of central physiological measures in analyses of the mechanisms of attention.

The electroencephalogram (EEG) shows changes in frequency as part of the orienting response, indicating that attentional processing can evoke gross changes in CNS bioelectrical activity. The analysis of EEG activity, however, has serious limitations. First, changes in EEG frequency take place over a relatively long time course and cannot provide a good temporal resolution of neural processing. Second, the neural generators of EEG frequency changes are poorly understood. Finally, over any given time period, much of the EEG activity issues from neural activity that has nothing to do with the experimental manipulation. If the signal of interest is small in amplitude, it will be obscured by background noise.

Averaged evoked potentials provide a means of measuring sensory EEG responses that improves the signal-to-noise ratio and resolution in the time domain, and that enhances the possibility of isolating sources of the EEG activity in the brain. This technique involves averaging the EEG response to repeated stimulation of the nervous system. The resulting waveform is called the *averaged evoked potential*. Because evoked potentials provide a unique window for observing the interplay between sensory and attentional processing in the human CNS, we will consider this technology in detail.

Sensory Evoked Potentials

When sensory receptors are stimulated, a series of negative and positive deflections time-locked to stimulus onset may be subsequently evoked in the EEG. Because these potentials are evoked by sensory stimulation, they are called *sensory evoked potentials* (EPs). Because of the small magnitude of the EP in relation to ongoing background noise, many stimulus trials must be averaged to yield a stable EP.

EP waveforms are quantitatively characterized in terms of components. Unfortunately, there is no consensus in the field about the formal definition of a component (Sutton & Ruchkin, 1984). For the paradigms discussed in this chapter, components are identified with specific positive and negative deflections in the averaged EP. The deflections are labeled by their polarity and their order of appearance. The polarity of a deflection is either positive or negative, denoted by the prefixes P or N. N1, for example, would be the first major negative deflection observed after the presentation of an auditory stimulus. N1 generally occurs about 100 milliseconds (msec) after stimulus onset and is, for this reason, sometimes labeled N_{100}. Labeling components by their polarity and latency after stimulus onset (e.g., N100, P300) is another frequently used convention in the EP literature.

EP components are functionally categorized into two types: exogenous and endogenous. *Exogenous* components of the EP are responsive primarily to properties of the stimulus, such as duration, intensity, and frequency. Typically, exogenous components have short latencies (less than 100 msec after stimulus onset). They usually originate from the primary sensory pathways and projection areas. The morphology and scalp distribution of exogenous components vary greatly between stimulus modalities and are relatively little affected by task demands.

Endogenous components of the EP vary with psychological factors such as task relevance, expectancies, and stimulus probability. EPs associated with endogenous components are frequently referred to as *event-related potentials* (ERPs). Several ERP components occurring between 60 and 600 msec after stimulus onset are highly reactive to attentional processes. The study of these components has provided a rare opportunity to relate neurophysiological responses in humans to mental processes inferred from experiments in cognitive psychology.

The Negative-Difference Response and Auditory Selective Attention

In 1973, Hillyard, Hink, Schwent, and Picton (1973) reported an ERP produced by selective attention. The subjects in their experiment heard streams of tones rapidly presented in both ears. The tones were made up of frequent, low-pitched stimuli, interrupted by an infrequent high-pitched stimulus. The subjects were instructed to listen in one ear or the other, and to detect the infrequent tones presented to that ear. When the EPs to the tones were evaluated, it was found that stimuli to the attended-to ear were associated with a prolonged negativity beginning at 60–80 msec after stimulus onset. This negativity was present to both target and nontarget tones in the attended-to ear. This processing negativity appears to be an electrophysiological index of sensory channel selection. Hillyard and Hansen (1986) referred to this negativity associated with selective attention as the negative difference (Nd) response, as it can be best visualized by subtracting the EP generated by the ignored stimuli from the EP generated by the attended-to stimuli (see Figure 6.4).

Hillyard and Hansen (1986) reviewed work from the previous decade studying the Nd response. The properties of the Nd component are characteristic of a sensory filter as described by Broadbent (1958) and discussed in section 2.2. The Nd component appears to stimuli that can be distinguished on the basis of a single stimulus attribute, including pitch, location, intensity, or speech as opposed to nonspeech (Hillyard & Hansen, 1986; Naatanen, 1982). If a complex stimulus attribute is used to define the channel, the Nd component appears but is greatly delayed in latency. The short onset time of the Nd component suggests that it represents a tonic set that selects material before full cognitive analysis. Finally, the Nd response occurs to all stimuli that belong to the attended-to channel, regardless of their task relevance or probability. Hillyard and Hanen argued that this evidence suggests that Nd reflects the facilitated processing of stimuli as a result of early sensory selection on the basis of a physical attribute or "channel cue."

These findings support the hypothesis that there is a physiological system associated with auditory selective attention. The existence of such a system does not, of course, rule

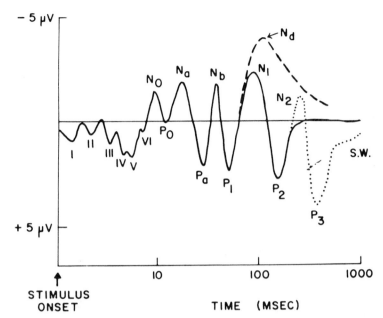

FIGURE 6.4. Event-related potentials generated by auditory stimuli in a variety of experimental conditions. Exogenous deflections or components are indicated by solid lines, and endogenous components are indicated by dashed or dotted lines. Deflections I through VI are exogenous potentials generated primarily by brain stem structures. Waves N1 and P2 are exogenous late auditory potentials. The dashed line (Nd) represents a negative deflection produced by the auditory stimuli within an attended-to channel. The dotted lines represnt the components of the P3 complex, typically evoked by rare, task-related auditory stimuli. In this illustration, responses with negative voltage are represented by upward deflections. From S. E. Hillyard (1985), with permission.

out the existence of a different selection system that operates after stimuli have been more fully analyzed, such as the selection system suggested by Deutsch and Deutsch (1963).

ERPs and Visual Selective Attention

Posner, Snyder, and Davidson (1980) proposed that selective attention to a region of the visual field acts like a spotlight, which enhances responses to stimuli within its beam. The perimeter of the beam metaphor is sharply demarcated, approximating an all-or-none boundary. Other investigators (e.g., Downing & Pinker, 1985) have suggested that the enhancing effect of the attentional focus gradually diminishes from a central location.

Mangun and Hillyard (1987, 1988) used ERP techniques to test whether spatial attention enhances responses to stimuli within a sharply demarcated "beam," or area of the visual field, or if the effects of focused attention decrease along a gradient. Subjects fixated on a midline point and were asked to focus their attention on a midline, a right, or a left location and to respond to targets in that area. They were asked not to move their eyes from the midline even when they attended to lateral locations, and trials that were associated with lateral eye movements were discarded.

In addition to the primary task, the subjects in one Mangun and Hillyard study (1988) were asked to respond to targets occurring in nonattended-to positions on the video display if they happened to notice them. ERPs were recorded for a 800-msec period after stimulus onset. Mangun and Hillyard found that the occipitally maximal P135 (msec) positive deflection decreased in a graded fashion as the target became more distant from an attended-to location. This effect was mirrored by a graded decrease in target detection. A late negative deflection at about 250–275 msec, on the other hand, was present only to target flashes in the attended-to sector. These results supported a spatial gradient of attention.

Spatial attention affects neural response at an early point in the stream of visual processing (at about 135 msec) and may be associated with a gating or filter system in the striate or prestriate cortex. Because the amplitude of ERP components increases with spatial attention, whereas the ERP morphology remains constant, the filter mechanism may operate by changing the sensory gain of the affected neurons. An all-or-none response occurs later in time, possibly reflecting a greater degree of stimulus specificity with the progression of cognitive processing.

ERP evidence also suggests that selection by color is subserved by mechanisms different from those used in selection by spatial location. Although spatial attention enhances the existing components in an ERP, color selection generates new ERP components (Hillyard & Munte, 1984). Color-form selection may be associated with greater activity over the left hemisphere (Harter, Aine, & Schroeder, 1982). Spatial selection occurs earlier than color selection (Harter *et al.*, 1982; Hillyard & Munte, 1984). When a stimulus is in a nonattended-to sector of the visual field, color has no effect on the ERP. The filtering of specific spatial and color attributes occurs earlier in the ERP than components reflective of conjunctions of color and spatial attributes. These findings support the hypotheses that separate feature analyzers exist for color and spatial discriminations, that the timing of these discriminations differ, and the stimulus features are extracted before conjunctions of features, that is, that the processing of features proceeds in parallel before an object is identified and placed in space.

In summary, ERP findings have provided insights into the time course and components of visual attentional processes. Attention to a spatial sector influences electrophysiological response between 70 and 150 msec after stimulus onset. Spatial attention occurs over a gradient within the visual field and appears to represent a filtering mechanism that operates by influencing sensory gain. The mechanisms subserving spatial selective attention appear to be temporally and electrophysiologically distinct from those subserving color selection. In general, these data support an early sensory selection process that passes relevant information for further processing and filters irrelevant information.

THE P3 COMPLEX AND ATTENTION

The P3, or P300, component has received continued experimental attention since it was first reported by Sutton, Braren, Zubin, and John (1965). The P3 is a long-latency endogenous component of the evoked potential that can be elicited by auditory, visual, or somatosensory stimuli. In a typical paradigm, the P3 is evoked when a subject attends to rare target tones among a train of more frequently presented nontarget tones. P3 usually appears at a latency between 250 and 800 msec after stimulus onset. It is generally preceded by a negative deflection (N2) and followed by a deflection whose polarity varies with scalp topography, the "slow wave" (Squires, Squires, & Hillyard, 1975). These endogenous components are shown in Figure 6.5.

Although N2 and P3 usually appear sequentially, they are dissociable. The topography

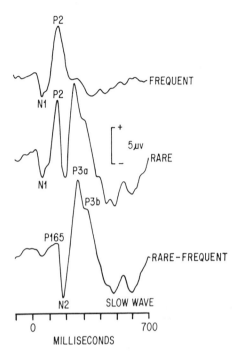

FIGURE 6.5. Event-related potentials averaged from frequent 1000-Hz tones and rare, target-2000 Hz tones (probability = .10). Frequent tones elicit the N1–P2 components and rare tones elicit the endogenous N2–P3 components. Subtraction of the waveforms generated by rare tones from frequent-tone waveforms isolates the endogenous components (P165, N2, P3a, P3b, and slow wave). In this illustration, scalp positivity is represented by upward deflections.

of N2 is modality-specific; that is, its peak amplitude appears at different locations on the scalp depending on the modality of the stimulation (Simson, Vaughan, & Ritter, 1976, 1977). P3 shows a modality-nonspecific scalp topography, with peak amplitude over the parietal area of the scalp. These findings suggest that the neural generators of the N2 response vary with the modality of stimulus presentation, and that the generators of the P3 response are invariant. N2 appears to a stimulus mismatch whether or not the stimulus is task-relevant, whereas the P3 response is attenuated or absent under these conditions (Näätänen, 1982).

The neural generators of P3 are not known with great specificity. Evidence from depth electrode recordings and correlations with magnetic fields suggests that medial temporal lobe and frontal lobe structures may be involved (Okada, Kaufman, & Williamson, 1983; Squires et al., 1983). Medial temporal lobe lesions in humans and, monkeys have little effect on the scalp-recorded P3 responses, however, a finding suggesting that other structures in the brain contribute to the P3 complex (Halgren, Stapleton, Smith, & Altafullah, 1986; Paller, Zola-Morgan, Squire, & Hillyard, 1988; Stapleton, Halgren, & Moreno, 1987).

Characteristics of the P3 response in humans provide strong evidence for the existence of a modality-independent physiological system in the brain that is activated in the course of attentional processing. In the remainder of this chapter, the responsivity of the N2 and P3 components of the EP (the N2–P3 complex) to environmental and cognitive factors modulating human performance is considered. The first section reviews experimental factors that influence the amplitude and latency of the P3 response, as well as hypotheses regarding the functional significance of P3. The second section summarizes the effects of brain dysfunction on the N2–P3 complex. The final section provides an interpretation of the N2–P3 complex derived from 19th-century models of attention.

Probability and Task Relevance

Variations in stimulus probability are associated with changes in N2–P3 amplitude (Sutton *et al.*, 1965). The effect of probability on P3 amplitude is enhanced when the stimuli are task-relevant (Duncan-Johnson & Donchin, 1977). When a stimulus is ignored, the P3 deflection that occurs (P3a) may represent a different component from the P3 deflection to a task-relevant stimulus (P3b) (Squires *et al.*, 1975). A large P3 response can be elicited by very discrepant or novel infrequent stimuli (Courchesne, Hillyard, & Galambos, 1975). Task-relevant stimuli are usually associated with N2–P3 activity even when the stimuli are equiprobable in relation to the irrelevant stimuli (Sutton *et al.*, 1965). N2 amplitude is less sensitive to task demands, a finding suggesting that it may represent an automatic match–mismatch detection process (Naatanen, 1982). At short interstimulus intervals (1–2 sec), the amplitude of P3 is inversely related to stimulus probability, approximating its information content as defined by classical information theory ($-\log 2p$) (Campbell, Courchesne, Picton, & Squires, 1979). P3 amplitude to a feedback signal regarding a previous judgment on a target detection task is related to the joint probability of the initial stimulus and the subject's response, termed *outcome probability* (Friedman, Hakerem, Sutton, & Fleiss, 1973) or contingent probability (Campell *et al.*, 1979). The N2 and P3 responses diverge from the classical orientation response in their resistance to habituation, even over prolonged periods of time (Rohrbaugh, 1984).

Sequential stimulus structure also contributes to N2–P3 amplitude. The first stimulus of a series elicits a N2–P3 complex. A tone preceded by one or more of the same tones shows diminished N2–P3 amplitude, and one preceded by a series of differing tones shows larger amplitude responses. Squires, Wickens, Squires, and Donchin (1987) used a linear additive model defining expectancy as a combination of decaying memory for events, structure sequence, and global probability for different stimulus sequences. The model accounted for 78% of the variance of N2–P3 amplitude. Duncan-Johnson and Donchin (1977) also found that global probability and sequential structure have independent effects on the P3 complex. At long interstimulus intervals, P3 responses can be evoked by stimuli regardless of probability.

In summary, global stimulus probability and stimulus sequence are important determinants of the amplitude of the N2–P3 complex. These effects interact with the task relevance of the stimulus. Extremely discrepant or novel stimuli can produce a P3 response in the absence of task demands, a finding suggesting that the attentional response represented by P3 may be codetermined by bottom-up and top-down processes within the nervous system.

Stimulus Evaluation

Both the amplitude and the latency of the P3 response are related to stimulus discrimination and evaluation. Stimulus intensity is inversely related to P3 latency (Papanicolaou, Loring, Raz, & Eisenberg, 1985). Increased difficulty of discrimination is associated with increased N2 and P3 latency (McCarthy & Donchin, 1981; Ritter, Simson, & Vaughan, 1972; Squires, Donchin, & Squires, 1977; Walton, Halliday, Naylor, & Callaway, 1986). Task demands that increase the complexity of stimulus evaluation increase P3 latency and reaction time (RT), whereas task demands that increase the difficulty of response selection increase RT latency without affecting P3 latency (McCarthy & Donchin, 1981). For example, the Stroop interference effect prolongs RT without affecting P3 latency, a finding suggesting that the delay in processing in this task is due to response interference rather than perceptual interference (Warren & Marsh, 1979). Variations in visual stimulus intensity, contrast, and complexity have additive effects on P3 latency (Walton *et al.*, 1986). These results have led several investigators to propose that either N2 or P3 latency provides an index of stimulus discrimination in the nervous system (Kutas, McCarthy, & Donchin, 1977; Ritter, Vaughn, & Friedman, 1979; Squires *et al.*, 1977). The N2 and P3 components, however, occur too late after stimulus onset to be a direct marker of stimulus discrimination (Goodin & Aminoff, 1984). Because RT is not temporally contingent on P3, it appears more likely that P3 latency represents the further processing of a stimulus contingent on initial discrimination, and parallel to response selection.

Guessing and Betting

The amplitude of the P3 response increases if a person correctly guesses the character of the next stimulus. Interestingly, if there is a payoff for correct guessing, the amplitude is greater even when the subject is told the correct choice beforehand and the actual appearance of the stimulus provides no further information (Sutton & Ruchkin, 1984).

Mental Load and Cognitive Resources

The finding that the amplitude of P3 is modulated by task relevance and attentional focus, and by its latency to stimulus evaluation, led investigators to link P3 amplitude to the conscious deployment of limited-capacity processing resources (Posner, 1975; Wickens, Kramer, Vanasse, & Donchin, 1983). Several lines of research are consistent with this formulation and suggest that P3 is sensitive to the mental load presented by a task.

Dual-task performance diminishes P3 amplitude on the primary task when the secondary task makes demands on perceptual resources, though not when further demands are made in the elaboration of a response. RT is responsive to both types of demands (Israel, Chesney, Wickens, & Donchin, 1980; Israel, Wickens, Chesney, & Donchin, 1980). Wickens *et al.* (1983) hypothesized that if the processing resources allocated to a primary and secondary task are reciprocal, this relationship should be reflected in variations in P3 amplitude to stimuli in both tasks. Using visual tracking as the primary task and an auditory oddball sequence as the secondary task, they compared P3 amplitude to stimuli within each task. As the resource demands of the primary task were increased, the P3 amplitude evoked by primary-task events increased, whereas those elicited by the auditory stimuli used in the secondary task decreased.

Automatic and controlled processing in visual search tasks (Schneider & Shiffrin, 1977) have also been investigated in EP and RT paradigms. These initial studies suggest that P3 amplitude reflects the mental demands on limited-capacity perceptual resources. In two studies using a mapping task (comparing a stimulus to a set of items in memory) N2–P3 amplitude was comparable whether the task required automatic or controlled processing, and both P3 and RT latencies were shortened in the automatic- compared to the controlled-processing task (Hoffman, Simons, & Houck, 1983; Kramer, Schneider, Fisk, & Donchin, 1986). Memory set size also had an effect on amplitudes: N2 amplitude was smaller, and P3 amplitude larger, with increased memory set size (Kramer *et al.*, 1986). The persistence of an N2–P3 response in the automatic condition suggests that practicing a controlled mapping task may reduce the slope of stimulus evaluation and reaction time on memory set size to zero and may reduce reaction time, but that the task still requires perceptual resources for performance.

THE N2–P3 COMPLEX AND BRAIN DYSFUNCTION

The N2–P3 complex has been studied in relation to normal aging, in psychopathology, and in neurological brain disorders. The most intensively studied clinical populations include patients with dementing disorders, schizophrenia, and depression. Variations of oddball paradigms, with or without RT measures, have been the most frequently used EP tests used on clinical populations. In an oddball paradigm, infrequent, task-relevant stimuli are used to elicit a P3 response. The P3 component has been the most generally measured EP component in these disorders, although some studies have also reported characteristics of other components.

Aging

After adolescence, N2 and P3 latency show a continuous increase in latency. The rate of prolongation is about 1–2 msec per year. A decrease in P3 amplitude has also been reported (Pffeferbaum, Ford, Roth, & Koppell, 1980; Squires, Sanders, & Wanser, 1986; Syndulko, Hansch, Cohen, Pearce, Goldberg, Montan, Tourtellotte, & Potvin, 1982).

Dementia

Dementing disorders such as Alzheimer's disease, multi-infarct dementia, and Parkinson's disease are usually accompanied by prolongation of N2 and P3 (Goodin, Squires, & Starr, 1978; Hansch, Syndulko, Cohen, Goldberg, Potvin, & Tourtellotte, 1982; O'Donnell, Squires, Martz, Chen, & Phay, 1987; Syndulko et al., 1982).

Psychiatric Disorders

Both N2 and P3 amplitudes have been consistently reported to be reduced in amplitude in schizophrenia (Levit, Sutton, & Zubin, 1973; Roth, Horvath, Pfefferbaum, & Kopell, 1980) and depression (Pfefferbaum, Wenegrat, Ford, Roth, & Kopell, 1984; Levit et al., 1973). N2 and P3 latency are usually reported to be within normal limits in these disorders, although there have been reports of slowing in schizophrenic patients (Baribeau-Braun, Picton, & Gosselin, 1983; Brecher, Porjesz, & Begleiter, 1987; Pfefferbaum et al., 1984). Because N2 and P3 latency are usually within normal range in schizophrenia, whereas RT is slowed, this particular type of psychopathology may reflect disturbances of response selection and execution more than stimulus evaluation (Duncan-Johnson Roth, & Koppell, 1984).

N2–P3 and Neuropsychological Measures

Few EP studies provide behavioral or intellectual descriptions of patient groups beyond diagnosis. In the case of dementia, the groups under study have often been heterogeneous in diagnosis as well as in severity. Specific intellectual or psychiatric disturbances relevant to such constructs as attention, learning, or degree of depression have seldom been measured or correlated with specific EP changes.

Several studies, however, have investigated the neuropsychological correlates of P3 latency changes in normal aging, dementia, and Parkinson's disease. In normal aging, P3 latency correlates with digit span performance (Polich, Howard, & Starr, 1983). Among older adults, P3 latency is negatively correlated with tests of verbal and spatial intellectual performance (Kraiuhin, Gordon, Meares, & Howson, 1986; O'Donnell, Friedman, Squires, Maloon, Drachman, & Swearer, 1990). In dementia and Parkinson's disease, P3 latency is also negatively correlated with intellectual performance (Hansch et al., 1982; O'Donnell et al., 1987, 1990; Polich, Howard, & Starr, 1983).

In summary, the N2–P3 complex is delayed over the course of normal aging and is further delayed in dementing disorders associated with diffuse brain damage. In aging, dementia, and Parkinson's disease, P3 latency is negatively correlated with psychometric measures of intellectual and memory function and appears to index changes that have a diffuse impact on mental function. Psychiatric disorders are consistently associated with reduction in N2–P3 amplitude, with component latencies within normal limits or mildly delayed. This pattern of results may indicate that N2–P3 latency prolongation is a marker for the clinically significant slowing of mental processes or diminished overall capacity, whereas diminished amplitude is associated with disorders affecting motivation or arousal.

SIGNIFICANCE OF THE N2–P3 COMPLEX IN ATTENTION

The P3 component has been described as indexing uncertainty (Sutton *et al.*, 1965), affective value (Sutton & Ruchkin, 1984), orienting (Ritter, Vaughn, & Costa, 1968), expectancy (Squires *et al.*, 1976), equivocation (Ruchkin & Sutton, 1978), stimulus evaluation (Kutas *et al.*, 1977; Squires *et al.*, 1977), context or schema updating (Donchin, 1981), and short-term memory reset (Grossberg, 1988). This multiplicity of hypotheses regarding the functional significance of P3 reflects the diverse range of the experimental manipulations that can affect P3 amplitude, or latency, or both measures. As is evident from the preceding review, the N2 component is reactive to many of the same factors as P3, although it may represent a more automatic phase of stimulus evaluation. Donchin (1981) suggested that the P3 component represents the CNS equivalent of a subroutine, which is invoked in a variety of cognitive operations. Alternatively, because the P3 may not consist of a single component but may instead be the sum of a number of components overlapping in time (Sutton & Ruchkin, 1984), the characteristics of the P3 complex may index more than a single CNS function.

Information-processing theory provides a vehicle for understanding the relation of the P3 response to stimulus detection, event probabilities, and attentional capacity. Information-processing constructs apply to aspects of the P3 response but do not provide a superordinate category that encompasses the embarrassing diversity of conditions that elicit the response. In a given paradigm, a subset of stimuli elicits a P3 response, which varies in amplitude and latency. What common mental process is associated with this subset of stimuli?

Factors that influence the generation of the P3 response include the intensity of a stimulus (Papanicoloaou *et al.*, 1985); the sudden appearance of or change in a stimulus (Sutton & Ruchkin, 1984); novelty (e.g., Sutton *et al.*, 1965); priming; and stimulus cessation (Simson *et al.*, 1976). The P3 is usually generated in experimental situations that require some sort of active discrimination by the subject (e.g., counting or key presses). These experimental characteristics correspond to the properties of active and passive attention as described by Wundt, Titchener, James, and other 19th-century psychologists (see Chapter 1).

As we have discussed previously, attention may be elicited actively or passively: to bottom-up stimulation or to top-down selection. Are there P3 paradigms that illustrate this dichotomy? A number of investigators have reported that novel or extremely disparate stimuli can evoke a P3 response in the absence of task demands, though these responses often vary in scalp topography from the task-related P3 response (e.g., Courchesne *et al.*, 1975). N. K. Squires, Ollo, and Sanders (1986) developed a series of conditions that show that similar P3 responses can be either passively or actively elicited. If two tones are sufficiently disparate in their characteristics (e.g., interpolating a rare, high-pitched, loud tone with a frequent, low-pitched, soft tone), the rare tone will evoke a P3 complex regardless of whether the subject is actively processing the tones. If two tones are very similar, the P3 complex will appear only if the subject performs a conscious discrimination to pick out the rare tones in a sequence. P3 responses evoked by both conditions are shown in Figure 6.6.

The passively evoked P3 complex is earlier in latency than the actively evoked P3 complex and habituates more rapidly, but their scalp topography and relationship to individual differences such as aging are similar. Using short tone sequences containing a discrepant tone, Polich (1989) also produced a passive P3 response with similar amplitude and topography to actively evoked P3 responses. These findings suggest that the P3 response represents a shift of attention to a novel stimulus which may be due to automatic (orienting) or control (effortful) processes. These results provide a physiological demonstration of the dichotomy between passive and active attention that was phenomenologically described by William James (1890).

SUMMARY

In this chapter, we have reviewed evidence supporting a relationship of the physiological activity of the visceral, musculoskeletal, and central nervous systems to the processes of

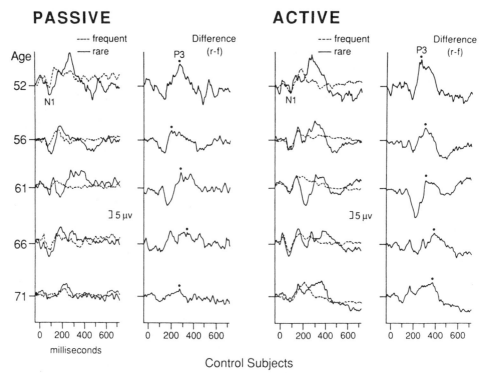

FIGURE 6.6. Passive and active P3 responses in five control subjects. Passive P3 responses were recorded to disparate tones in the absence of task demands, and active P3 responses were recorded to target tones that were counted by the subject. *Passive condition*: ERPs recorded to rare 3000-Hz tones (85-dB, probability = .10) and frequent 250-Hz (70-dB) tones without task demands. Note the positive deflection in the subtraction ERP after 200 msec. *Active condition*: ERPs recorded to rare 1500-Hz tones (probability = .10) and frequent 1000-Hz tones, both at 85 dB. In this illustration, scalp positivity is represented by upward deflections. From O'Donnell *et al.* (1990).

attention. Three goals underlie efforts to characterize the physiological correlates of attention: (1) physiological validation of the presence of an attentional process; (2) indexing of the strength and parameters of attentional allocation; and (3) a delineation of the mechanisms underlying attentional control. The first two goals have been accomplished in electrophysiological studies of peripheral and CNS response characteristics. The goal of characterizing underlying neural mechanisms has been more elusive, though psychophysiological data provide information about the likelihood of certain mechanisms.

Generalized arousal was originally proposed as the determinant of an organism's functional "state" and was felt to be an energetic catalyst for behavior. Models of attention have often included an arousal component in order to account for this catalytic process. Recent evidence has indicated that the construct of a uniform, generalized arousal oversimplifies the physiological underpinnings of behavior. Neuro- and psychophysiological studies have demonstrated that the autonomic and CNS activity associated with particular behavioral states is not uniform or generalized. It can be dissociated into multiple components, often resulting in paradoxical relationships between physiological and behavioral response. Furthermore, certain responses (e.g., heart rate) fractionate under different task conditions, a finding indicating that the physiological correlates of attention are also not uniform, as would be expected with a generalized arousal. Nonetheless, the concept of *arousal* provides a useful, though theoretically incoherent, construct for characterizing a nonspecific relationship between behavioral and physiological activational level and performance. Although the interacting neurophysiological mechanisms underlying arousal do not covary in a linear manner, there is a general relationship between behavioral state and attentional performance, and to some extent, peripheral and central physiological activity correlates with these states. Arousal is one determinant of the organismic "state" function.

The term *arousal* has also been used to account for phasic physiological responses accompanying cognitive processes. However, this overextends the concept of arousal. As Pribram and McGuinness (1975) suggested, it is probably best to consider these phasic responses independent "activational" states. The phasic physiological reactivity associated with attentional demands has also been considered a manifestation of the OR. Although these responses are associated with the OR when a new stimulus is introduced, the OR and habituation concepts by themselves do not adequately account for all of the physiological effects noted during attending. For instance, the autonomic activation associated with effortful processing suggests a process that is independent of the elicitation of the OR.

As physiological activity can be shown to reflect cognitive processes, and particularly attention, can we conclude that these responses provide an index of attentional allocation? The answer appears to be yes. We have discussed evidence demonstrating that autonomic response varies relative to the extent of attentional allocation, demand, and effort. Autonomic and musculoskeletal response patterns can be dissociated, depending on the type of attentional operation required. Pupil dilation, increased skin conductance, and muscle tension usually occur when attentional demands increase. Heart rate is a particularly sensitive index of attentional allocation. The cardiac response varies as a function of whether passive sensory intake or active-effort processing is usually present.

Although autonomic variables provide an index of cognitive events, including attentional processing, the extent to which changes in visceral states actually influence attention is less clear. Many peripheral physiological responses produced potential functional advantages for animals that help to explain their relationship to attention. For instance, cardiac deceleration is often part of a general quieting of the body in preparation for new information that may indicate the need for a rapid response, such as flight from a predator. Yet, the extent to which alterations in the peripheral autonomic state actually facilitate or inhibit attention is not yet well established. There is some evidence that induced changes in autonomic state affect attentional performance, though the jury is still out on this issue.

Peripheral physiological responding has yielded information regarding the potential mechanisms underlying attentional control. In particular, findings pertaining to the OR, habituation, and the dissociation of the components of attentional processing have been fruitful. However, visceral responding provides an indirect measure of underlying neural processes. Electrophysiological recordings of CNS activity enable more direct measurement and inferences about the neural mechanisms of attention.

Event-related-potential measures provide physiological evidence for several key mechanisms and relationships during information processing. ERPs are particularly useful in defining the time course of different stages of processing. Studies of auditory and visual selective attention suggest that the sensory selection of specific channels of information takes place on the basis of common stimulus properties. This selection process is physiologically manifest as early as 60–100 msec after stimulus onset and appears to support the hypothesis of an early sensory filter. Studies of the P3 complex suggest that stimulus probability or novelty has a profound impact on neural information processing and is associated with the activation of several distinct physiological responses. An early, modality-specific response, exemplified by mismatch negativity (N2), automatically registers the appearance of a stimulus disparity in a stream of events. It is similar to Sokolov's definition (1960) of a passive orienting response and can be observed at latencies as early as 150–200 msec. The P3 response, whose latency is influenced by stimulus evaluation time and whose amplitude is influenced by event and response probability, is also associated with discrepant stimuli. It can be observed to task-relevant stimuli at low levels of detectability and can be related to the pigeonholing, or categorization, phase of attentional selection. Although it is commonly elicited in the context of task demands, the P3 response can also be observed to very discrepant or novel stimuli in the absence of task demands. The P3 response is modality-nonspecific and may represent a common attentional process that can be activated by both bottom-up and top-down pathways.

In addition to providing physiological support for classical information-processing constructs such as sensory filtering, pigeonholing, and information content, ERP findings parallel descriptions of attentional factors described by 19th-century psychologists. In particular, the conditions that elicit attention and a shift an attentional focus through consciousness bear a striking resemblance to experimental factors that provoke and influence the P3 response.

Neural Mechanisms of Attention

Much of our knowledge of the neural substrates of attention has been derived from investigations of sensory and motor system neurophysiology. Studies of the neural bases of conditioning have provided a second important source of information. Only recently have direct neurophysiological investigations of attention been attempted, generally by extending findings obtained from sensory, motor, or conditioning paradigms. In this chapter, we discuss some of the experimental evidence regarding the neural basis of attention, derived from four areas of investigation: (1) sensory physiology; (2) conditioning; (3) inhibitory control processes; and (4) the orienting response (OR) and habituation.

The relevance of each of these topics to attention should be apparent by this point. Because attention is often considered a sensory selection process, the mechanisms of sensory registration and integration are the building blocks of attentional processes. Sensory physiology has developed to the point where investigators are now considering how information is processed after initial sensory registration.

Because attention is also a process of response selection and preparation for eventual action, the neural bases of motor and premotor control are also relevant to attention. In the past, neurophysiological investigations of sensory and motor functioning stopped short of considering sensorimotor integration, largely because it was extremely difficult to localize integrative processes at either a systems level or with respect to single neurons and circuits. However, advances in neuroscience have enabled researchers to go beyond the primary sensory and motor cortex to study the functional and neural properties of secondary and tertiary cortical areas. These cortical regions seem to be involved in the multimodal integration of information and have been implicated in attentional control. It now appears likely that attention is not under the control of a unitary brain system. Interactions of cortical and subcortical systems seem to play a role in producing attentional behavior, which complicates the issue of studying the neural basis of attention.

The mechanisms underlying conditioning are also relevant to considerations of attention. As we discussed in Chapter 4, behaviorist scientists have often considered attention a component of conditioning. Therefore, it is not surprising that information regarding attention should arise from studies of conditioning. The primary focus of most neuroscientists who study conditioning has been the identification of mechanisms for associative learning and memory formation. Although conditioning depends on the formation of relatively long-term changes in the neurobiological character of the neural system following stimulation, attention is reflected in the more transient relationship of the stimulus and response at a particular moment. Investigations of the neural bases of longer term associative changes have led to information about shorter term phenomena such as habituation and sensitization.

The processes of habituation and sensitization are also cornerstones of current models of the OR. Because the OR is a fundamental component of attention, it is easy to see why researchers interested in attention have devoted much effort to discovering the neural mechanisms underlying the OR, sensitization, and habituation. These processes are also essential components of conditioning and therefore serve to bridge attention and memory. This topic is given specific consideration in Chapter 5.

Within both the behavioral sciences and the neurosciences, "inhibition" is considered a primary control process that enables the modulation of competing response tendencies. Inhibitory processes have been proposed in neural models of a wide range of behavioral phenomena, such as extinction, habituation, spontaneous recovery, generalization, discriminative learning, the development of compound stimuli, and cue dominance. Because inhibitory processes seem to play a significant role in attentional control, neural mechanisms may account for the inhibitory control on attention.

The goal of this chapter is to provide a broad overview of four domains with relevance to the neuroscience of attention. This is not meant to be a comprehensive review of each of these domains, but a historical perspective that will illustrate the emergence of attention in the neurosciences. More detailed descriptions of neural models for specific attentional operations are provided in subsequent chapters of this text, along with evidence for attentional mechanisms derived from studies of brain dysfunction.

ATTENTION AS A COMPONENT OF CONDITIONING

Attention and memory are generally considered separate but interdependent processes. Both attention and associative formation are fundamental components of learning. Attention and memory formation are different stages of information processing during conditioning. Attention reflects the variation in responding based on an ever-changing external environment and internal psychobiological state. Although these variations are influenced by current conditioning and previous memory, they are also influenced by a variety of other factors, such as perceptual, motor, and physiological demands. The attentional construct is necessary to account for the fact that our responses constantly vary in a shifting universe of stimuli. Attention establishes the interface in a delicate relationship between salient memory of past information and the active excitatory and inhibitory influences of new information arriving in the form of a continuous flow of new stimuli.

Memory can be viewed as the end product of attention. When information processing is directed to a particular stimulus, this stimulus may produce a permanent change in memory. Conditioning has two components: an attentional component that consists of those neuronal processes involved in sensory and response selection, and a memory component that pertains to the formation of long-term changes in some neuronal substrate. From a neurophysiological standpoint, these two components of conditioning can be distinguished based on whether the changes in neuronal activity are relatively long- or short-term. The formation of memory depends on the registration of information from the environment. Attention increases the likelihood that processed information will result in memory. Conversely, the way in which information is encoded, stored, and retrieved from memory influences attentional demands. This point has been well documented by studies of controlled and automatic attention.

The strong interrelationship of attention and memory dictates that neural mechanisms governing associative formation also influence attention. Both attention and memory formation depend on the plasticity of certain neural systems. *Plasticity* refers to the ability of a neuronal unit to undergo either transient or permanent change in its neurochemical, physiological, or morphological character as a result of some external or internal stimulus. From the standpoint of conditioning, attention and memory formation represent different stages of a behavioral process through which the organism modifies its response characteristics as a function of environmental information. A common substrate of memory formation and attention is their dependence on the plasticity of certain neural systems.

Conditioning results in the production of a relatively stable behavioral response. The stability of the response indicates that the behavioral association has been encoded into memory. Some behavioral responses are less durable and are driven by more transient characteristics of the stimuli in the immediate environmental context. These behavioral responses usually reflect a short-term attentional state that does not necessarily develop into a permanent memory change. In an attempt to understand the nature of memory formation and storage, some neuroscientists have devoted considerable effort to determining the neural bases of these short- and long-term changes in state. The term *neural plasticity* has been used to characterize the capacity of certain neuronal structures to exhibit durable modifications in their neurobiological properties as a result of stimulation and conditioning.

Memory formation depends on the capacity of particular neural structures to exhibit plasticity in response to changes in incoming stimuli during conditioning. The demonstration of neuronal plasticity is also critical to understanding the neural mechanisms of attentional control. Although attention does not require long-term modifications in neural response, it does depend on shorter term modifications in neuronal activity with at least some durability. For a neural response to be classified as a component of attention, it must be shown to be separate from the direct activation of sensory system neurons occurring in response to sensory registration. Attention may occur without sensory activation from any new inputs when the animal is preparing to make a future selection of stimuli. The short-term neuronal activation or plasticity associated with attention must be different from both phasic short sensory activation and the more permanent changes associated with memory. Attention depends on an intermediate level of associative durability.

Bioelectrical Indices of Conditioning and Attention

The earliest techniques for studying the neural mechanisms of behavior involved the assessment of behavioral performance before and after lesions were made to particular structures. An alternative to the use of lesioning techniques is the analysis of bioelectrical activity from specific neural sites during conditioning. Recordings of neuronal bioelectrical activity using microelectrode techniques have provided evidence of the formation of temporary associative connections.

Changes in the neural activity of various brain structures to stimulation have been demonstrated in many neurophysiological investigations. The measurement of bioelectrical changes in a primary method of neurophysiology, which is often accomplished through single-unit recordings. Whereas the neuronal bioelectric response to sensory and motor processing has been analyzed extensively, the study of attention and memory has been much more difficult. To account for the phenomena of attention and memory, it is necessary to show that patterns of activation persist even after stimulation ceases, or in anticipation of stimulation. The elicitation of a specific pattern of activation to a cue preceding a conditioned stimulus (CS) can be interpreted as an indication of an attentional response. If the pattern of physiological activity changes as a function of the presentation of previously processed stimuli, there is indication that the stimuli have formed a memory that is reactivated (Kamikawa, McIlwain, & Adey, 1964; Kotliar & Yroshenko, 1971; Morrel, 1967). These changes in neurophysiological response are now described by many investigators as examples of neuronal plasticity.

Kotliar (1983) provided a useful taxonomy of the forms of neural response (plasticity) occurring during conditioning. The major differentiations include the distinctions made among (1) associative and nonassociative neural responses, and (2) tonic and phasic responses. The associative-nonassociative distinction was made to reflect the fact that not all types of neuronal activation during conditioning result in the formation of permanent association or memory trace. Kotliar concluded that the neural response to stimuli that have already been conditioned is different from the neural response to those that are not part of the associative system. Furthermore, distinctions can be made in the response to stimuli that are weak or neutral and those that are strong or novel. Nonassociative neural responses occur based on variations in stimulus characteristics or possibly response demands. Kotliar related nonassociative responses to the *neuronal model* proposed by Sokolov (1963) to account for the OR. The neural response occurs as by-product of the degree of mismatch between new stimuli and existing associative stimulus templates.

Distinctions between the tonic and the phasic forms of bioelectrical reactivity during conditioning illustrate the different component processes. Within classical conditioning, phasic modifications in neural activity reflect a temporary response to a CS, and tonic responsivity indicates more permanent changes in the dynamics of activity in a certain cell following conditioning. Both tonic and phasic activity changes have been described by researchers, though phasic changes are generally easier to demonstrate because they require only the reorganization of neural responsivity in the presence of or in anticipation of the CS. Although it is possible to account for many attentional effects on the basis of phasic modifications in activity, contrasting tonic and phasic modifications in bioelectrical activity helps to distinguish attentional effects from the formation of new memory.

Long- and Short-Term Neural Modifications

The demonstration of differences between long- and short-term modifications in neuronal bioelectrical activity is necessary if one hopes to distinguish between the processes of attention and memory formation. Historically, long-term changes have often been referred to as *tonic modifications*, and short-term changes have been referred to as *phasic modifications*. Tonic modifications in the activity of single neurons indicate the formation of a relatively permanent memory trace. Kotliar (1971, 1983) demonstrated tonic modifications in the neural activity of neurons in the sensorimotor cortex of laboratory animals. There was a change in the firing rates of single neurons following conditioning to pain. This modified neural responsivity persisted between trials of stimulus presentation, a finding indicating that the response was not simply activation produced by the aversion stimulus. Ramus, Schwartz, and John (1976) also described a distinction between stable and plastic neural discharge patterns during behavioral generalization.

Long-term changes (i.e., tonic modifications) in neuronal activation following conditioning have now been demonstrated by a number of other investigators (see Thompson, Clark, Donegan, Donegan, Lavond, Madden, Mamounas, Mauk, & McCormick, 1984; Woody, 1967, 1970). Although these modifications in neural response often involve either an increased rate of activity or a change in the pattern of activity following conditioning, it is also possible to produce tonic decreases in the rate of activity of neurons as a result of conditioning. Such decreases have been noted in the responses of neurons from midbrain regions. This reduction in neural activity may reflect conditioned inhibition. Therefore, conditioning may produce very different neural responses across the different centers of the brain.

It is much easier to demonstrate short-term response changes of individual neurons during behavioral performance. For instance, recordings from neurons of the visual cortex provide clear indications of neural activation during stimulus intake. Similarly, phasic activation of neural cells of the motor and premotor areas is evident before the production of a response. Although sensory and motor activation can be directly correlated with the demands of a particular task, it is also possible to produce transient activation of cells not directly connected to sensory intake or response production. Short-term modifications may also correlate with other behavioral processes, such as the attentional orienting of the animal and associative formation.

An analysis of transient bioelectrical activity during conditioning suggested that many brain regions demonstrate plasticity that seems to relate to the formation of temporary associative connections (Jasper, Ricci, & Doane, 1962; Kimble & Ost, 1961; O'Brien & Fox, 1969). These studies differentiated among sensitization, habituation, and conditioning events based on the characteristics of the single-unit activity of neural cells. Early studies had suggested that it might be difficult to distinguish whether the electrophysiological response to the CS was related to sensitization or conditioning (Grant & Norris, 1947). However, studies by Woody (1970) indicated that sensitization and conditioning can be differentiated based on when the single-unit activity is elicited. Sensitization and habituation represent temporary changes in behavioral state, as compared to the relatively durable modification occurring during conditioning.

Although the goal of most studies of conditioning has been to delineate the substrates of memory formation, findings of transient changes associated with sensitization and habituation have relevance to the study of attention. The neuronal responses associated with sensitization and habituation have a direct bearing on the mechanisms underlying the orienting response (OR). This response has been considered an important component of attention. For some time, it has been known that these behavioral responses have physiological analogues, although this link has usually been assumed based on an analysis of autonomic indices that at best provide indirect measurement of neuronal events. The demonstration of sensitization and habituation through single-unit recording has indicated that these processes are fundamental cellular responses. Therefore, some components of attention may be represented at even the simplest organismic levels.

CONDITIONING IN SIMPLE NEURAL SYSTEMS

Attempts to understand the neural mechanisms underlying different forms of learning has led investigators to search for model systems capable of providing unambiguous demonstrations of the essential components of conditioning. With this goal in mind, investigators have searched for evidence of memory trace formation in very simple organisms, in which the basic neural mechanisms can be more easily defined.

Kandel and Spencer (1968) suggested that two event markers can be used to classify whether neuronal activity in simple organisms is associated with conditioning: (1) if there is characteristic change in neuronal response to stimuli that meets the criteria for a CS, and (2) if there is specificity of the response to particular stimuli in the environment. The first marker determines whether a neural response is in fact associated with a special class of stimuli modified by learning, or whether the response is a component of a previously learned response. It also establishes a distinction between conditioning and sensory registration. The second marker, response specificity, helps to establish the type of conditioning that has occurred. Kandel and Spencer distinguished between two types of conditioning (classical and alpha). By delineating the neural response specificity, the investigator can determine whether a stimulus had activated a specific memory or procedural response, or whether it is eliciting a more generalized emotional response. By means of this framework, cellular responses can be classified as having either associative or nonassociative characteristics. The fact that not all conditioning events involve associative memory processes is worth noting, as nonassociative conditioning has many of characteristics of an attentional process.

There has been considerable progress in defining the changes in neuronal response occurring during conditioning in simple organisms (Castellucci, Pinsker, Kupfermann, & Kandel, 1970; Crow & Alkon, 1980; Hawkins, Abrams, Carew, & Kandel, 1983; Kandel & Scwartz, 1982; Spencer, Thompson, & Nielson, 1966). These and other studies have demonstrated a specificity of conditioning based on the change in membrane properties and the synaptic responsivity of certain neural structures. For the most part, these neuronal changes have not involved the formation of new synapses; rather, they have resulted from changes in the response characteristics of existing connections. Neurochemical factors have been shown to play an important role in modulating the strength of specific neural connections.

Studies of *Aplysia* by Kandel and his colleagues (Kandel & Spencer, 1968; Kandel, 1978; Kandel & Schwartz, 1982, 1983) indicated different neural mechanisms for habituation, sensitization, and associative formation (see Figure 7.1). All three mechanisms are contained in the *Aplysia*'s neuronal and synaptic system. These investigators viewed the processes of habituation and sensitization as nonassociative forms of conditioning, whereas they saw classical conditioning as involving associative formation. Kandel considered habituation the simplest form of learning, as it reflects a decrease in response to nonrelevant stimuli. Habituation has been shown to involve a depression of neurotransmitter release at synapses between sensory and motor neurons in *Aplysia* (Castellucci *et al.*, 1970). The phenomena of habituation in *Aplysia* has been tied to changes in Ca^{2+} influx at the synapse.

Sensitization was considered a more complex form of conditioning, by which the animal strengthens its response to a variety of neutral stimuli after exposure to an aversive or potentially threatening stimulus. This complexity is also evident in the mechanisms that have been demonstrated to account for this type of learning. Sensitization was shown to involve presynaptic facilitation of responding through activation of cyclical (AMP). Again, a host of neurotransmitters influences this process, as does the opening of K^+ channels. Sensitization is also a more elaborate process than habituation, as the activation of one pathway may increase responsivity in other pathways (Hawkins & Kandel, 1984).

Within simple organisms like *Aplysia*, conditioning represents the highest level of learning. It differs from sensitization because there is a specific response produced by pairings of an unconditioned stimulus (UCS) and a CS. Kandel and his colleagues conditioned *Aplysia* by the pairing of a strong electric shock to the tail (UCS) and a weak CS to the siphon of the organism. The withdrawal response (conditioned response—CR) occurring during classical conditioning has been shown to be an enhanced form of sensitization (Hawkins *et al.*, 1983). This finding suggests that the enhanced activation occurring at presynaptic levels facilitates the temporal association of the UCS and the CS.

Hawkins and Kandel (1984) proposed a model to account for the habituation, sensitization, and classical conditioning of the gill withdrawal reflex in a simple invertebrate organism (*Aplysia*). In Figure 7.1A, neural mechanisms for stimulus specificity and generalization of classical conditioning in *Aplysia* are illustrated. The first conditioned stimulus (CS_1) excites two sensory neurons ($S.N._1$, $S.N._2$), while the second stimulus (CS_2) excites $S.N._2$ and a third neuron ($S.N._3$). Since both conditioned stimuli excite $S.N._2$, generalization occurs. Only when a CS is presented to the tail S.N. prior to a UCS, does presynaptic facilitation occur through the facilitator interneuron (FAC. INT.), enabling conditioning.

In this model, habituation, sensitization, and classical conditioning depend on subtle biochemical events. Figure 7.1B illustrates the underlying neural mechanisms that have been identified in *Aplysia*. With repeated stimulation of the siphon sensory neuron, prolonged

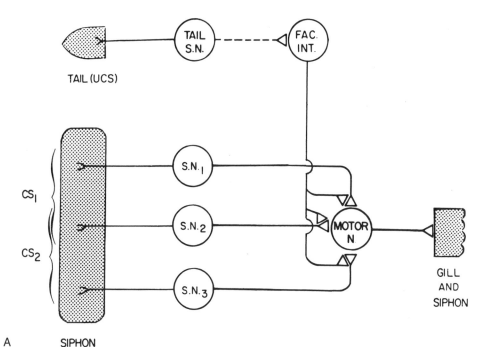

A   SIPHON

FIGURE 7.1. A model proposed by Hawkins and Kandel (1984, with permission) to account for the habituation, sensitization and classical conditioning of the gill withdrawal reflex in a simple invertebrate organism (*Aplysia*). (A) The first schematic diagram illustrates the mechanism propsed by Hawkins and Kandel for stimulus specificity and generalization of classical conditionings. CS_1 and CS_2 are conditioned stimuli, UCS is unconditioned stimuli, $S.N._1$ and $S.N._2$ are sensory neurons, and FAC. INT. is facilitator interneuron. (B) The second schematic diagram illustrates the neural–biochemical mechanisms for habituation, sensitization, and classical conditioning that have been identified in *Aplysia*. CA^{2+} is calcium, $s\text{-}K^+$ is potassium involved in sensitization, cAMP is cyclic adenosine monophosphate. Details regarding both figures are described in the text.

inactivation of calcium channels (Ca^{2+}) in the presynaptic neuron occurs. This inactivation leads to decreased Ca^{2+} release with each action potential and decreased neurotransmitter release. The behavioral outcome is habituation. Sensitization occurs due to prolonged inactivation of potassium channels ($s\text{-}K^+$) in the siphon sensory neurons, when there has been stimulation to the tail and presynaptic activation of facilitator neurons. A sequence of neurochemical steps results, with activation of adenylate cyclase in the sensory neuron terminals and increased levels of free cyclic adenosine monophosphate (cAMP). Next, activation of a second enzyme, cAMP-dependent kinase, causes protein phosphorylation, which closes a particular K^+ channel. This effectively decreases the total number of K^+ channels open during the action potential, and enhances subsequent action potentials, Ca^{2+} influx, and ultimately neurotransmitter release. Classical conditioning is similar to sensitization, except that a specific activation of the defensive response to conditioned stimuli (CS) that are temporarily paired with unconditioned stimuli (UCS). The selective enhancement of responding to the CS may result from an interaction of Ca^{2+} influx with serotonin-sensitive adenylate cyclase in the sensory neuron terminal.

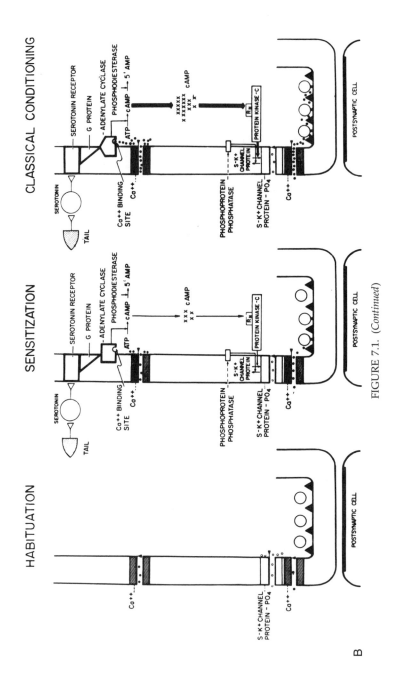

FIGURE 7.1. (*Continued*)

Hawkins and Kandel (1984) argued that the specificity of the associative response to the CS produced during classical conditioning is due to activation generated by its pairing with the UCS. Generalization of learning may occur because of the spread of the activation of sensory neurons and interneurons that share a connection with the primary target neurons that are excited during associative learning. As a result of sensitization, responding becomes more nonspecific during generalization. Other behavioral processes, such as extinction, second-order conditioning, and blocking, have also been illustrated by the use of simple organisms like *Aplysia* as model systems.

The eloquent demonstrations of mechanisms responsible for conditioning in simple organisms was a major advance in the field of neuroscience, as it demonstrated for the first time some of the neurochemical mechanisms of conditioning. Unfortunately, as one moves from *Aplysia* to more complex animals, the parsimony of this model system is harder to maintain. It is not clear whether the same fundamental principles of neural responsivity that account for conditioning of *Aplysia* hold true in the more complex neural systems of higher animals like humans. The degree to which there is consistency across the vast number of neural structures of the mammalian brain has not yet been established. Therefore, it is difficult to determine whether the neuronal responses associated with habituation, sensitization, and classical conditioning described by Kandel and his associates will be shown to be similar to the neuronal events occurring during more complex forms of behavior, including attentional processes.

Cellular Modifications During Conditioning

The recent explosion of studies of the neural basis of conditioning in simple organisms (e.g., *Aplysia*) has led to an understanding of the important biochemical changes occurring at a synaptic level. That learning involves a change in synaptic responsivity is now widely accepted. Furthermore, many neuroscientists now believe that these synaptic changes reflect relatively stable morphological changes in cellular structures during conditioning. Modification in the molecular characteristics of the neuron and its membranes is thought by many to be the basis for these synaptic changes.

The observation of change in synaptic characteristics during conditioning requires the correlation of biochemical events with specific events occurring during learning, which is not an easy task. Some investigators using this strategy have demonstrated the biochemical mediators of conditioning as described earlier in the work of Kandel's laboratory. Others have looked for long-term bioelectrical changes that occur during conditioning. This approach is analogous to that described by Kotliar (1983) as the tonic reorganization of neural activity. Two types of neural responses seem to exist at the synaptic level: (1) postsynaptic potentials (PSPs) and (2) contingent synaptic action. The PSP is shorter lived, lasting for minutes to hours, whereas the contingent synaptic action is more permanent (Libet, 1984). Contingent synaptic action is more difficult to measure, as it is expressed through the potentiation of neural activity produced by other neurotransmitters, rather than through direct activation of the synapse. In fact, the PSP may be viewed as the by-product of the contingent synaptic actions in the case of the reactivation of previously conditioned stimuli.

Differences in the speed of the PSP vary depending on the specific neurotransmitter and postsynaptic receptor that are involved (Ashe & Libet, 1981; Libet, 1970). For instance, the PSP produced by Acetylcholine (ACh) at nicotinic sites is very fast (0.05–0.1 sec), whereas that occurring at the muscarinic receptor is much slower (0.1–0.3 sec). There is an indication that dopamine may modulate the slow muscarinic PSP to make it even slower (1–4 hr). These responses have been demonstrated in sympathetic neurons and appear to be characteristic of higher level neurons. Slow PSPs differ from fast PSPs in a number of ways, including (1) the nature of the bioelectrical input (i.e., the volley frequency necessary to elicit response); (2) the tendency of slow PSPs to respond to a varied (heterogeneous) set of neural inputs; and (3) the electrical membrane characteristics associated with the slow PSP.

The characteristic slow response of the same PSPs make them good candidates for the formation of the more long-term contingent synaptic action. However, if such a long-term change is to occur, there must be a mediator that serves to enhance the strength of the neural activation and to make it more permanent. The interaction of PSPs produced by ACh with the prior effects of dopamine seems to provide for such mediation (Libet & Owman, 1974; Libet & Tosaka, 1970). Cyclic AMP produces an action similar to that of dopamine and ACh by enhancing long-term effects. In contrast, cyclic Guanosine Monophosphate (GMP), which acts as a mediator of slow muscarinic PSPs, produces a paradoxical interference within the formation of contingent synaptic action. The antagonistic effect of cyclic GMP is not permanent, as the receptor is not destroyed. This biochemical antagonist is very specific, as it acts only when dopamine or cyclic AMP is also present.

The existence of slow PSPs points to a mechanism to facilitate associative formation through the establishment of longer term potentiation. Faster potentials are less likely than slow PSPs to result in memory formation. Furthermore, these potentials have specific modulation through different neurochemicals in temporal relationship with incoming sensory inputs.

The development of long-term potentiation (LTM) appears to be the best explanation to date of the formation of memory. Long-term potentiation describes a neurophysiological process by which an association is formed. Although slow PSPs provide a bioelectrical basis for LTM, presumably there are also molecular changes that are the basis for this effect.

Baudry and Lynch (1979, 1984) have suggested that glutamate may be an important transmitter involved in memory formation in the hippocampus. Glutamate has a strong excitatory tendency and shows release after the electrical stimulation of hippocampal regions. Antagonists of glutamate inhibit this activity. An interaction between glutamate and calcium ions has been demonstrated, in which calcium stimulates glutamate binding to neural membranes.

Lynch and Baudry (1984) proposed a model for the transient morphological changes that may be associated with memory formation. These changes are produced by "proteases," which are enzymes that activate calcium and that cause changes in the configuration of the synaptic membrane. The change in membrane configuration was proposed to be a function of biochemical changes in neurofilaments and several other proteins that are termed *cytoskeleton-associated proteins*. This label reflects the characteristics of these proteins in defining the structure of the membrane in response to biochemical changes. In the context of memory formation, synaptic stimulation appears to result in changes in receptor structure and number.

Plasticity in the Mammalian Nervous System

Although Pavolvian conditioning appears to be the most complex form of conditioning in *Aplysia*, it is considered a rather low level of learning in mammals. The fact that specific-adaptive conditioning (e.g., the eyelid CR) can be learned without the presence of any brain tissue above the level of the thalamus illustrates this point (Norman, Buchwald, & Villablanca, 1977). This type of finding led some researchers to conclude that procedural tasks can often be learned with minimal levels of cortical involvement, with major involvements of the brain stem, the midbrain, and the cerebellum.

Motor System

Thompson and his colleagues (Thompson, Berger, Berry, Clark, Kettner, Lavond, Mauk, McCormick, Solomon, & Weisz, 1982; Thompson *et al.*, 1984), after localizing specific-adaptive learning to deep cerebellar nuclei (dentate and interpositus), demonstrated a mechanism underlying motor learning to aversive stimuli. Lesions in these regions abolished memory of previously learned procedural responses, and injection of certain neurochemical blockers caused selective, but reversible, change in both the behavioral and the bioelectrical responses of nuclei in this region.

Studies of other subcortical structures also reveal an important role in memory formation, particularly for motor tasks associated with classical conditioning. The red nucleus has been shown to be capable of forming new synapses (sprouting). Tsukahara and his co-workers demonstrated that sprouting occurs following classical conditioning (Tsukahara, 1981, 1984; Tsukahara, Oda, & Notsu, 1981). The neural activity of the red nucleus increases following conditioning trials. Although the relationship between the development of a functional synapse during conditioning and the anatomical characteristics of this synapse is still not entirely clear, the plasticity of cells in the red nucleus suggests a basis for associative formation. The involvement of both the red nucleus and the cerebellum in classical conditioning reflects the role of motor systems in the associative process.

Sensory Systems

There is also evidence of plasticity in the neuronal responses of sensory systems that seems to have implications for the processes of attention. Sensory attentional selection requires a mechanism by which neural cells in sensory regions can change their sensitivity when environmental biases shift. Recent studies of sensory plasticity suggests that such a mechanism is more than a remote possibility. For instance, Alkon (1982) conducted work on the classical conditioning of a simple organism, using light as a CS. His findings indicated changes in the photoreceptivity of the sensory system in the invertebrate *Hermissenda*. This organism rotates its orientation in response to the direction of light input. However, vertebrates do not exhibit such a close relationship between associative formation and sensory receptors.

Plasticity of neural activity in the auditory cortex has been demonstrated by means of both multiple- and single-unit recordings. Different patterns of neural discharge were shown to develop to a reinforced stimulus (CS+) and a nonreinforced stimulus (CS−) (Oleson, Ashe, & Weinberger, 1975). The pattern of activity reversed when the reinforcement was switched one week following initial training (i.e., the CS+ became the CS−). Recordings from the ventral cochlear nucleus also showed similar effects, although the pattern of neural discharge in this area developed after that in the auditory cortex. Also, responses in the cochlear nucleus extinguished after one week, a finding indicating that this is not a site of more permanent association.

Detailed analysis of regions of the auditory cortex indicated that only one of three regions showed plasticity during the discriminative learning of responses to different CSs (Ryugo & Weinberger, 1976). Studies of other types of learning, including instrumental conditioning, have yielded similar results (Gabriel, Miller, & Saltwick, 1976). Single-unit recordings of cells in this region of the auditory cortex have supported the finding of plasticity and again indicate some differentiation in the responsivity of cells to conditioning (Diamond & Weinberger, 1984). Furthermore, neural cells in the auditory cortex appeared capable of developing tuning functions, so that they become more sensitive to tones of a certain frequency. This finding suggests an obvious basis for discrimination learning.

Neural plasticity is found to varying degrees in many other sensory systems. Kotliar (1983) described experiments in which neural responsivity of the somatosensory cortex to tactile stimuli was assessed. No change in cortical activation was noted under conditions of repeated pairings of a CS with a UCS. However, cells in this region appear to be very sensitive to different forms of stimulation and are particularly responsive to pain. Therefore, Kotliar concluded that associative formation may depend on the presence of stronger stimuli. Under conditions of strong tactile stimuli, including pain, there appeared to be selective neurons that demonstrate plasticity to associative processes. Furthermore, when multimodal stimuli were used (e.g., sound and tactile stimulation), the greatest degree of change in neural response occurred. When painful stimuli were used, the percentage of cells showing modification in activity was greatest (90%). These findings point to two important factors affecting the associative formation in this sensory system: (1) the more salient the stimulus (i.e., in reinforcement strength), the greater the degree of neural modification that is possible, and (2) increasing the modalities of stimulation seems to enhance the neural response.

The existence of sensory system plasticity is important to our consideration of attention for several reasons. If modifications in sensory associative networks are possible, the idea that the visual system contains an invariant "hard-wired" organization can be negated. Furthermore, this finding suggests that modifications in sensory discrimination or filtering may be influenced by state-dependent attentional factors.

Some investigators have argued that physiological plasticity in sensory systems is related primarily to establishing a linkage of responses to specific stimuli (Birt & Olds, 1981). This argument is supported by the fact that activity of the auditory cortex does not contribute directly to motor responding or control. Plasticity in this region is unlikely to be the basis of processes associated with response production, as the neural reactivity of this region is poorly correlated with avoidance responses (Gabriel *et al.*, 1976).

Weinberger, Hopkins, and Diamond (1984) provided an alternative hypothesis, that the plasticity of neural activity in sensory systems may be related to the establishment of stimulus significance. If this is the case, the neural response of sensory regions like the auditory cortex would occur as a function of associative processes, through which a "tuning" of sensory signals occurs. Such a process would obviously be critical to discrimination learning, and ultimately to selective attention, because it would account for an increased selection bias for certain acoustical frequencies that have been enhanced.

The demonstration of sensory conditioning may account for how a stimulus set is established. In Chapter 4, we discussed the concept of stimulus compounding. Modified continuity theory and the concept of cue dominance predict that excitatory and inhibitory interactions among stimulus elements from the environment give a behavioral explanation of attention (Kandel, 1978; Wagner, 1979). This explanation of attentional effects depends on the demonstration of stimulus interactions that result in modified sensory association networks. Findings that indicate that modifications of sensory neurons during conditioning are possible provide some support for these behavioral theories.

Bioelectrical Activity in Humans

There have been relatively few studies of the neural response of single or multiple units in humans. An obvious difficulty in such research arises from the invasive nature of implanting depth electrodes. The study of seizure disorders has provided one avenue for this type of research, as depth electrode recording is often used for diagnostic purposes. Penfield and his colleagues stimulated a number of cortical regions and found that stimulation of the temporal lobes elicited memories in 7.7% of patients (Penfield, 1958; Penfield &

Rasmussen, 1950; Penfield & Roberts, 1959). He interpreted this finding as an indication of a veridical memory trace for past events. There are some theoretical and methodological problems that raise questions about the validity of this conclusion. Yet, these demonstrations provide important information about the nature of memory representation.

Subsequent neurophysiological investigations have provided a more systematic analysis of the neural activity of limbic and temporal structures (e.g., Halgren, Squires, Rohrbaugh, Babb, & Randall, 1980; Halgren, Squires, Wilson, Rohrbaugh, Babb, & Crandall, 1989). These studies resulted in findings that were similar to Penfield's. However, repeated stimulation of the cortex at a single site produced a variety of unrelated memories. These centers seemed to be important to the evocation of memory, though not necessarily to the specific content of those memories. These findings suggested that memory encoding and activation may be focally determined by events occurring in temporal-limbic structures, whereas representation is more widely distributed.

There have been few data from depth-electrode or single-unit recording directly focused on attentional control, though studies of primates have recently emerged that have used these methodologies. A larger number of data pertaining to the nature of electrophysiological response during attention are available from the study of event-related potentials (see Chapter 6). However, it is difficult to localize function by using surface recordings of this type.

Sites of Neuronal Plasticity in Humans

The well-known attempts by Lashley (1929) to identify the local brain regions responsible for memory storage resulted in failure. Lashley was unable to localize the missing "engram." He concluded that all parts of the brain participate, with "equipotential," in the performance of habits. Lashley's findings had a tremendous impact on the brain sciences for years, as memory and learning were assumed by many behavioral scientists to be nonlocalized.

Lashley reached his conclusions because of his inability to isolate a specific center of memory storage. However, these conclusions seem to have been premature, as subsequent investigations indicated that several brain structures are critical in normal learning. For instance, damage to the prefrontal cortex was shown to impair monkeys' learning ability (Jacobsen & Nissen, 1937). The critical regions of the prefrontal cortex responsible for learning were later specified with more precision (Butters & Pandya, 1969). In other studies, Scoville and Milner (1957) discovered that bilateral damage to the medial temporal areas of patients who had undergone surgical resections resulted in a severe amnesia. The patient H.M.'s amnesia proved to be pervasive and long-lasting, though it turned out that his lesion was also very large, involving the amygdala, the uncus, and much of the hippocampus and associated gyrus. Debate ensued about which structures were actually responsible for the amnesia (see Squire, 1987, for a review). Since the discovery of H.M., several other patients have been identified with more specific lesions of the hippocampus and related structures. These cases showed varying degrees of amnesia. The finding of severe amnestic disorders in patients with other diseases affecting diencephalic structures (e.g., Korsakoff syndrome) provided additional evidence pertaining to the anatomical locus of memory formation (Isseroff, Rosvold, Galkin, & Goldman-Rakic, 1982; Zola-Morgan & Squire, 1985a,b).

As more than one cortical area has been implicated in memory operations, some psychologists have taken the position that memory is not localized but is distributed throughout the cortex in a statistical fashion (e.g., John, 1972). There is in fact growing support for the concept of a distributed associative memory in neural networks of cortical areas related to particular sensory modalities (e.g., Mishkin, 1982; Mishkin, Ungerleider, &

Macko, 1983; Ungerleider & Mishkin, 1982). Interest in the distribution of associative memory in neural networks has led to major developments in the cognitive neurosciences.

It now appears that there are both localized centers for conditioning and memory formation, such as the limbic and paralimbic structures, and a nonlocalized distributed network of stored memory. Whether memory formation depends on a functional circuit such as that described by Papez (1937) or on the activity of specific structures by themselves is not entirely clear. However, the fact that certain brain structures (e.g., the hippocampus) exhibit a remarkable degree of plasticity has now been established.

The role of the limbic system, in particular the hippocampus, in the formation of associative memory is now well established. Limbic structures also seem to mediate the relationship between the UCS and the CS during classical conditioning. Inhibitory signals from these structures may have a particular impact on the extinction of previously conditioned responses. The limbic system appears to have great plasticity and is particularly rich in its neuronal reorganization capacity (Kotliar, 1969; Morrell, 1967; Olds & Hirano, 1969).

Segal (1973a) recorded the activity of 473 cells in various limbic areas and found that the CA3 fields of the hippocampus had the shortest latency of response to stimuli that had been previously conditioned. During extinction of the response, cells of the dentate region of the hippocampus showed the most rapid change in activity, and that cells of the CA3 region of the hippocampus followed. Subsequently, the cellular activity of the CA1 region and the central hippocampus changed. Cells of the cingulate gyrus and the septum did not respond differentially to extinction. Based on these findings, Segal concluded that the CA3 field of the hippocampus served to integrate conditioned responses through the facilitation of the conditioned signals in the dentate region.

The tremendous level of interest in the nature of limbic system functioning is largely due to its apparent importance to semantic memory. However, this is not the only brain region that exhibits plasticity, nor are all forms of conditioning localized in this system. Conditioning deficits can be created by lesioning other subcortical structures. For instance, defects of classical conditioning have been associated with lesions below the level of the limbic system, including the cerebellum, the red nucleus, and the septum. Oakley and Russell (1972) found that decorticate rabbits could still learn through classical conditioning. Lesions of the cerebellum (Thompson, Berger, Berry, Clark, Kettner, Lavond, Mauk, McCormick, Solomon, & Weiss, 1982; Thompson, Clark, Donegan, Lavond, Madden, Mamounas, Mauk, & McCormick, 1984) abolished a specific CR (eye blink).

The work of Olds and his laboratory (Olds & Milner, 1954; Olds & Hirano, 1969; Olds, Mink, & Best, 1969; Olds et al., 1972; Phillips & Olds, 1962, 1969) provided much of the early evidence for differential conditioning effects across brain systems. In one study, changes in neural activity were monitored across numerous sites during the generalization of classical conditioning to tones (1–10 Hz). Neural activity that correlated with the conditioning process was noted at all brain levels: reticular formation, posterior and lateral groups of the thalamus, a field of the hippocampus, and several cortical areas. However, there was a lack of activity in reticular areas of the midbrain, in other thalamic regions, and in several fields of the hippocampus.

Interestingly, the posterior thalamus appeared to be the region with the greatest amount of neuronal activity during conditioning. Olds (1973) felt that this activity was nonspecific, as the nature of activity did not vary with learning conditions (e.g., discriminative stimuli). Kotliar (1983) argued that, although there is a lack of relationship between thalamic activity and conditioning, this actually reflects the independence of thalamic cells during conditioning. The posterior thalamus appears to be sensitive to conditioning but manifests itself through changes in background activity that ultimately influence the gating of information flow into the cortex. By acting as a relay center, the thalamus plays a large role in attention, as it influences the way information is selected, as well as the level of cortical activation. These information-processing effects are separate from the process of associative memory formation.

The reticular formation of the brain stem also exhibits neural activity that correlates with conditioning. Kornblith and Olds (1973) demonstrated that a reorganization of activity of this region precedes behavioral change during classical conditioning. Over repeated trials, cells of the reticular formation showed a tendency to stabilize at the initiation of new presentations of the CS. This stabilization correlated with the orientation response (OR) elicited by the CS.

Because conditioning can be observed in neural systems at various levels of the nervous system, some neuroscientists have tried to establish which structures are required for particular types of conditioning. Studies by Woody (1967, 1970) and Thompson and his colleagues (1982, 1984) have indicated that the dentate nucleus of the cerebellum must be intact for the occurrence of a normal CR, whereas other forms of learning (e.g., declarative memory) depend on the presence of an intact hippocampal or limbic system. Thompson argued that there is a hierarchical arrangement of learning and memory; simple forms of classical conditioning require a lower level of neural organization (e.g., cerebellar), whereas symbolic learning requires a greater level of neural organization with limbic and cortical involvement. Such a distinction is the basis for the view that there are multiple traces of memory. Simple Pavlovian conditioning occurs with only the requirement of subcortical systems like the cerebellum, whereas declarative memory requires cortical and limbic involvement. Hierarchical arrangements would have implications for how attention and memory interact.

Because conditioning can be observed in neural systems at various levels of the nervous system, some neuroscientists have tried to establish which structures are required for particular types of conditioning. Studies by a number of investigators (e.g., Woody, 1967, 1970; Thompson et al., 1982, 1984) now indicate that no cortical involvement is necessary for the CR to occur, as decorticate animals continue to show eyelid conditioning. These authors concluded that brain stem systems in the regions surrounding the fourth ventricle (e.g., the red nucleus) are necessary for "nonspecific" conditioning, whereas the dentate nucleus of the cerebellum must be intact for the conditioning of "specific-adaptive" motor responses (e.g., eyelid conditioning). Other forms of learning require that higher levels of brain organization be intact. For instance, damage to the hippocampus and other limbic and cortical areas is likely to disrupt declarative learning. This finding suggests a hierarchical arrangement in the neural systems underlying learning and memory. Simple classical conditioning requires a lower level of neural organization (e.g., cerebellar), but not neces- sarily higher cortical involvement. Complex forms of learning depend on neural involvement at all levels.

Thompson and his colleagues (Thompson et al., 1982, 1984) argued that type of find- ing is neurophysiological evidence for multiple systems of "memory trace" that account for at least three different forms of learning: nonspecific learning, specific learning, and cognitive memory. The simplest conditioning involves nonspecific traces associated with conditioned emotional states such as those seen during classical conditioning. Specific adaptive memory traces reflect a higher level of neural organization, as they involve the learning of a specific motor or autonomic response of deal with particular stimuli. The highest level of cognitive learning is now often described as declarative memory and is capable to dealing with symbolic associative information extracted from sensory stimuli. There is now considerable neuropsychological support for multiple forms of memory (Moscovitch, 1982; Cermak, 1984; Schacter, 1985; Squire, 1987).

The existence of a hierarchical multitrace arrangement of this type has important implications for the study of attention. Different attentional processes are likely to be associated with each type of conditioning. Nonspecific learning is likely to elicit a non-specific expectancy or orienting response that directs the animal's attention. Specific, adaptive learning is likely to involve attentional processes that may facilitate the registration of cues to control behavioral response. Declarative learning would require a much more complicated form of attention involving the integration of sensory intake, response activation, and effort relative to the particular task.

INHIBITORY CONTROL PROCESSES FOR ATTENTION

Inhibitory processes have long intrigued behavioral and neuroscientists because of their potential role as behavioral and neural control mechanisms. Inhibition provides an explanation of how an animal may terminate one behavior in lieu of another. Unfortunately, the concept of behavioral inhibition has been very problematic (see Chapter 4). Because the concept of inhibition has been used to explain the mechanisms for both behavioral and neural processes, one must be careful when referring to inhibitory processes. Occasionally, ambiguity is associated with the use of the term *inhibition*. Demonstrations of behavioral inhibition are sometimes misinterpreted as indications of neural events, when there may not always be a natural relationship between these types of inhibition. Neurophysiological inhibition may not reflect behavioral inhibitory events. Therefore, it is important that investigators specify the type of inhibition that they are concerned with, so as to not confuse behavioral and physiological effects.

In contrast to behavioral inhibition, clear evidence of neural inhibition has existed since the earliest developments in neurophysiology. Brunton (1883) defined inhibition as the process by which one neural structure causes the cessation of activity in another structure. Sherrington (1947) demonstrated inhibition in his classical studies of muscle activity. He illustrated that muscular contractions are normally accompanied by a suppression of activity in other muscles. Studies of the feedback control of muscles and the sharpening of sensory inputs (Eccles, 1964) have illustrated the role of neural inhibition in both sensory and motor systems. Advances in the field of neurophysiology since the early 1980s have provided a more exact definition of the forms of neural inhibition (Sheperd, 1979).

Konorski (1948, 1970, 1972) provided one of the first comprehensive taxonomies of inhibition based on both neurophysiological and behavior considerations. Four classes of inhibition were postulated: (1) reciprocal inhibition; (2) antagonistic inhibition; (3) unidirectional inhibition; and (4) lateral inhibition. These types of inhibition differ with regard to the neurophysiological level at which they are noted. These forms of inhibition are also observable by means of neurophysiological recording techniques and therefore are more than theoretical conjectures.

Reciprocal inhibition occurs when different neural centers arranged in some structural organization exert an antagonistic influence on each other (see Figure 7.2). Excitation of one area suppresses the excitation of another area. The interaction is reciprocal, lending to the name of this form of interaction. Reciprocal interaction has been demonstrated at different levels of the nervous system ranging from spinal reflexes (Sherrington, 1947) to single-unit recordings (Eccles, 1964). Reciprocal inhibition can even be applied to behavioral and physiological responses that are incompatible (e.g., wakefulness and sleep).

Antagonistic inhibition differs from reciprocal inhibition in that the centers of inhibition are not paired and do not necessarily have a completely reciprocal relationship. Examples of this type include behaviors that are controlled by different neural structures, in which excitement at one structure tends to lead to decreased excitement in the second structure.

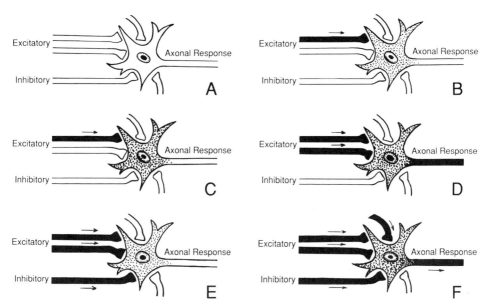

FIGURE 7.2. This series of diagrams illustrates the interaction of excitation and inhibition resulting in temporal and spatial summation for for a single simple neuron: (A) the neuron at rest; (B) partial depolarization following summation to below firing threshold; (C) temporal summation may be followed by suprethreshold polization after multiple impulses are summed; (D) spatial excitatory summation produces depolarization when together they reach the firing threshold; (E) when excitatory impulses spatially summate with inhibitory impulses, depolarization may be prevented; (F) if the neuron receives more excitatory impulses, causing further excitation, the inhibitory influence can be overridden and depolarization will occur.

Antagonistic inhibition has a less reflexive quality, and the antagonism may occur partly because of the functional inconsistency of certain behaviors (e.g., fear and sexual responses). In this case, the two responses are controlled by different neural systems that interact in such a way that fear and sexual responses are incompatible.

Unidirectional inhibition occurs when one brain system exerts influence on another, usually through direct pathways. The most striking example of this form of inhibition is the relationship between the cortex and the subcortical systems, including the hypothalamus. The destruction of cortical areas often results in disinhibition, with a failure of the animal to suppress arousal and excitatory behaviors such as rage or sexuality. Unidirectional inhibition is critical to a systemic control of the behavior and therefore is of particular interest to neuropsychologists. This type of inhibition will receive much more attention in latter chapters of this text.

Lateral inhibition is probably the most molecular form of neuronal response mediation. It occurs when adjacent neurons exert influence on each other; the result is usually a modulated and delicate response. Lateral inhibition occurs at various levels of the nervous system and is probably intricately related to associative processes in the cortex. It is also evident in the motor system, as adjustments in fine movements are made. However, the most classic form of lateral inhibition is seen in the visual system in the interaction of visual cortex nerve cells. Complex interactions of adjacent neural areas has been shown to be critical in generating visual contrast effects (Hubel & Wiesel, 1963, 1968; Pollen & Ronner, 1975).

Neural Mechanisms of Inhibition

Inhibition has been demonstrated through paradigms in which stimulation was presented at one site, followed by stimulation to a second site. The effects of previous stimulation on the second center were recorded through electrophysiological monitoring. If the frequency, amplitude, and general characteristics of the electrophysiological response varied, the presence of inhibition was demonstrated. In fact, inhibitory effects have been shown by means of a variety of techniques based on this fundamental paradigm. Investigations of single-unit activity have provided evidence of inhibition in the interactions of individual neurons (Eccles, 1964).

Inhibition has been demonstrated at various levels of the nervous system. Studies of the spinal reflex (Lloyd, 1941, 1946) and of the influence of cortical activity on brain stem activity (Nakamura, Goldberg, & Clemente, 1967) have attempted to illustrate inhibitory neural relationships. Sechonov (1956) noted that stimulation of the brain stem produces an inhibition of lower reflex activity, which was termed *general inhibition* and is analogous to the unidirectional inhibition described earlier. Within the field of neurology, a release of inhibition has often been observed following injury to a patient's brain. J. Hughlings Jackson (1958) gave detailed accounts of this phenomenon and suggested that a brain structure has inhibitory control over behavior if, when that structure is lesioned, there is a "release" of that behavior. This suggestion led to a number of studies in which lesions were produced in various animal neural structures so that investigators could observe behavioral release. Although the conclusions derived from this type of methodology have been criticized because it is difficult to prove that inhibitory effects are due to a specific lesion, much information about the systemic nature of inhibition was derived.

Recent neuroscience methods have used neurochemical means of blocking neural pathways or structures, as a way of producing greater specificity of effect. Furthermore, following the introduction of a chemical that blocks a particular pathway, it is possible to provide an agonist that will stop the chemical's effect. This technique helps to illustrate that the inhibition is actually related to the effects of a given structure and not to generalized effects of the injury. The reversal of effects produced by the agonist serves as a good experimental control. This technique is now used by many neuroscientists studying neuronal function. For instance, an inhibition of flank-marking behavior in hamsters can be produced with the introduction of a vasopressin antagonist to the medial preoptic area of the hypothalamic region. (Ferris & Albers, 1984; Ferris, Singer, Meenan, & Albers, 1988). When vasopressin was reintroduced into this region, the behavioral response was reversed as flank-marking behavior increased.

Limbic Influences on Inhibitory Control

The hippocampus, fornix, and amygdala, and aspects of the medial temporal lobe, the cingulate region, and forebrain pathways, are often collectively referred to as the *limbic system*. The hypothalamus is also often included as part of the limbic system, perhaps because of the high level of integration of the hypothalamus with other limbic structures, as well as its role in emotional behavior and "drives." Yet, there are many other functional differences between the hypothalamus and other limbic structures, so we consider the hypothalamus separately. Information about the behavioral role of the limbic system has come in large part from studies of laboratory animals. Neuropsychological studies of brain-injured humans have provided a less well-controlled, but important, second source of data. Damage to the limbic system is widely known to impair the ability of humans to learn. Acquisition rates decline with damage to this area, and memory performance becomes disrupted. The limbic system also seems to play a critical role in the regulation of appetitive state and drives, particularly in relationship to hypothalamic influences. Hess (1957, 1969) proposed that the limbic system influences behavior through opposing excitatory and inhibitory mechanisms. Because the general impact of limbic system damage on attentional control will be discussed in Part II, for now we will limit our focus on how this region exerts inhibitory control over behavior and, specifically, attention. The studies that are cited are not meant to provide a comprehensive review of the inhibitory functions of the limbic system; instead, they provide a historical background. The inhibitory processes that are described have particular relevance to attentional control.

Hypothalamic Influences

Investigations of the effects of stimulation to the hypothalamus have been conducted to determine whether the repetitive presentations of conditioned stimuli have excitatory or inhibitory influences. Thomas (1972) implanted electrodes in the lateral and posterior hypothalamus of cats. The electrodes generated electrical stimulation that elicited specific responses of fear or rage in these animals. Postmortem analysis of the site of electrode placement revealed that the lateral hypothalamic placement was associated with the lateral hypothalamus that was dorsal to the fornix. The posterior site near the mammillary bodies was associated with fear.

In one study, Thomas presented two tones of different frequency and a light as the CS, which preceded the presentation of the electrical stimulation (UCS). Responses were measured by the amount of strain produced as the animal's chest moved (CR). Thomas found that the CR occurring to unreinforced conditioned stimuli (CS−) generalized early in conditioning. This finding suggested that the hypothalamic response was subject to inhibitory effects. Interestingly, it was also noted that the CR (chest movement) was different from the normal UCR to the stimulation.

In subsequent studies, Thomas used a similar technique, but measured autonomic response (blood volume). This time, a dissociation in response occurred to the CS− and the CS+. The amount of vasoconstriction increased when the CS+ was presented along with the UCS. However, when a CS− was presented with the UCS, there was less constriction compared to when the UCS was presented alone. In the case of both the CS− and the CS+ presentations, there was a rebound phenomenon, with vasodilation occurring following the test trial. When the UCS was presented alone, this rebound did not occur. Therefore, a link between facilitatory and excitatory effects of CSs on hypothalamic activity was indicated.

The role of the hypothalamus in generating many behaviors associated with emotional response and drive state is well established. The studies that have just been reviewed suggest that hypothalamic responses can be conditioned, and also that these responses are subject to inhibition and facilitation by external stimuli. There is also evidence that the hypothalamus may exert inhibitory influences on other responses. Ultimately, there appears to be a reciprocal relationship between the hypothalamus and other neural systems, including the cortex. For instance, when certain hypothalamic nuclei are stimulated, appetitive responses may occur that cause functional suppression of responses mediated by the cortex. Conversely, cortical activation may inhibit hypothalamic impulses.

Stimulation of the upper brain stem results in different patterns of motor response, which are accompanied by an inhibitory rebound response. Grastyan, Szabo, Molnar, and Kolta (1968) implanted electrodes in hypothalamic, mesencephalic, and hippocampal regions of cats. A three-stage experiment was conducted in which stimulation to these areas was provided selectively, and the movement of the cats in a circular cage was recorded. During the first stage, the movement of the cat during stimulation was found to be circular. In Stage 2, the cats could press a switch that switched off stimulation, whereas in Stage 3, the cats were placed in a smaller cage during Stage 3, in which contact with a switch caused stimulation (a reversal of training).

The motor responses that occurred under different stimulation conditions were shown to vary as a function of whether the stimulation occurred with a negative or a positive motivational state. Also, the direction of movement depended on side of the brain that was stimulated. Movement to the same side as the brain hemisphere that was stimulated (ipsiversive) occurred when positive reinforcing stimuli were present. This finding suggested an approach response to this positive motivational condition. On the other hand, movement to the side opposite that of the hemisphere of stimulation (contraversive) occurred under negative motivation conditions, an effect suggesting an avoidance response. Often, this movement effect occurred following stimulation (rebound). The presence of this rebound with opposite vectors suggests an inhibitory/facilitory process acting relative to the automatic and strong response elicited by stimulation.

The nature of stimulation was found to have an important bearing on the nature of responding. Stimulation of the lateral hypothalamus and the mesencephalic areas tended to produce initial contraversive movement, followed by increased variability in the direction of movement with prolonged and more intense stimulation at one locus. The stimulation produced ipsiversive movement at lower stimulation levels, and contraversive movements with more intensity in a second group when another locus was stimulated. Again, variability increased with longer durations of stimulation. In a third group, stimulation always produced ipsiversive responding. The intensity of the stimulation was an obvious variable of importance in this study, as it determined the quality of experience and ultimately whether the animal would approach or avoid.

Interestingly, in other studies, Grastyan, Szabo, Molnar, and Kolta (1968) demonstrated that ipsiversive stimulation not only was correlated with avoidant behavior but also tended to induce sleep in cats. This paradoxical effect suggests that the movement did not cause the motivational state; rather, the stimulation elicited a broad excitatory state with both activating (motor) and inhibitory (sleep) components.

Hippocampal Influences

The approach to food under conditions in which cats are restrained has also been shown to produce inhibitory neural responses of the hippocampus. Molnar and Grastyan (1972) trained cats to lever-press in order to have food delivered. Later, the cats were restrained behind a Plexiglas door, through which they could observe the feeding device. In this experiment, restraint was not aversive, except that it prevented feeding. Hippocampal activity was measured during restraint and then following release. Activity during restraint was desynchronized, whereas immediately following release, there was synchronization with an increase of theta activity. However, this synchronization was not associated with approach to the food, as initially after release, the cats explored the restraint area. Therefore, the change in hippocampal activity seemed to be associated with vigilance or "hyperorientation" to the environment. Desynchronization occurred again as the animal eventually approached the food. An interesting finding of this study was that approach to the stimulus did not occur immediately after release. The intermediate period of hypervigilance seems to be associated with an inhibitory effect generated by the restraint.

Clark and Isaacson (1965) found that hippocampal destruction resulted in a failure to inhibit responding under conditions of punishment. This finding suggests that the hippo-campus normally inhibits responding following punishment. After lesioning of the hippo-campus, the animal lost this inhibitory control and initiated responses. Schmaltz and Isaacson (1966) noted that change from continuous to intermittent schedules of reinforce-ment tended to augment the amount of disinhibition, presumably because the initial contin-uous reinforcement schedule produced increased excitatory influences from the hypothalamus.

Isaacson (1972) conducted experiments to contrast the effects of lesions and epileptiform activity of the hippocampus. Epileptic activity was induced by the infusion of penicillin into the hippocampus. Isaacson found that animals with induced seizure activity in the hippo-campus failed to learn a task within 400 trials, whereas animals with lesions were able to master an active avoidance task in a time consistent with that used by normal control animals. This finding suggests that the hippocampus and other limbic structures have different responses based on the type of required task. Isaacson (1982b) maintained that the hippocampus plays an important role in attentional control.

Investigations of habituation of the OR have suggested that the hippocampus exerts both activational and inhibitory influences on dishabituation. Vinogradova (1970) demon-strated that hippocampal neurons both increment and decrement to repetitions of stimula-tion. The type of response depends on the particular task's characteristics.

Amygdaloid Influences

The amygdala's response to hypothalamic excitation differs from that of the hippo-campus. Animals with lesions to the amygdala show great problems in initiating respond-ing (Kemble & Beckman, 1970). Pribram (1969) postulated that removal of the amygdala causes a hyperstability by disrupting the temporal organization which has developed by habituation to recurring events such as those from visceral activity (p. 00). This conclusion was supported by studies of habituation in monkeys following removal of the amygdala (Bagshaw & Pribram, 1968; Bagshaw, Kimble, & Pribram, 1965; Bagshaw, Mackworth, & Pribram, 1970). Monkeys in these cases showed a general reduction of arousal as measured by galvanic skin response (GSR), as well as changes in the rate of habituation.

As was the case with the hippocampus, the exact effects associated with the amygdala depend on the nature of the task and the neurophysiological intervention. However, across all recent studies, it is evident that both the hippocampus and the amgydala are critical to memory formation. Mishkin (1978, 1982) and Murray and Mishkin (1985, 1986) provided strong evidence that the amgydala is important to normal memory functioning. When the amygdala and hippocampus were selectively lesioned, different effects were found, depending on the combination of the lesions used. Lesions to medial temporal structures created inability to perform visual object-recognition tasks, and lesions to the amygdala affected the ability of monkeys to associate visual stimuli with reinforcement (Spiegler & Mishkin, 1981). This finding indicated that the amygdala is involved in stimulus–reward association. Ultimately, the extent of global memory dysfunction seems to relate to the amount of combined damage to all limbic structures: amygdalothalamic and hippocam-pal (Mishkin 1978, 1982).

Some researchers have argued that the amygdala serves as a gate between cortical association areas and the reinforcement centers of the hypothalamus (Mishkin, Malamut, & Bachevalier, 1984). Although the memory functions attributed to the limbic system are well established, the role of these structures in gating information flow between the cortex and the hypothalamus is usually less emphasized. This role as a gate reflects the inhibitory influences of the limbic system. It is this role that has particular relevance to the study of attention. Although the structures of the limbic system are critical to the formation of memory, this role is most relevant to the processes of conditioning: the production, consolidation, and elaboration of associations. On the other hand, these structures also seem to have other roles, as the limbic system has an active part in the processing of information.

An obvious question arises: Does the limbic system's inhibitory influences and role in information processing (attention) result solely from the capacity of structures in this region to form memory, or do these structures have different roles that interact? The interrelationship between memory formation and attentional processes must be recognized and will be discussed in greater depth in Chapter 10. Despite this relationship, it appears useful to consider the information-processing role of the limbic system separately from its capacity to form memory. The limbic system appears to be important to the balance between reinforcement-driven excitation produced by the hypothalamus and inhibition produced by the cortical systems. This balance may be central to defining a mechanism for attention and may also be separate from memory formation.

Septal Influences

The septal region also exerts inhibitory influences on behavior, particularly under conditions of nonreward. Damage to the septal region has been shown to cause a failure of extinction to positive reinforcement (Dickinson, 1972; Raphaelson, Isaacson, & Douglas, 1966; Schwartzbaum, Kellicut, Spieth, & Thompson, 1964). However, the effects of this damage are somewhat selective, as there is generally little change in responding when conditions of nonreward are not involved. In other words, the septum seems to be involved in the mediation of behavior under conditions of frustration associated with non-reinforcement. This effect is characterized by hyperemotionality and rage reactions to frustration.

Dickinson (1972) trained rats in a go–no-go paradigm in which the rats were to respond when a certain stimulus occurred and not to respond to a second stimulus. Rats with septal damage had much difficulty inhibiting responses to the no-go stimulus. In a second experiment, rats were not given the no-go condition but instead had an active response alternative for the second condition. Therefore, the second experiment did not require a reduction in responding. This time, the rats with septal damage did not show problems in their performance when compared to normal control rats. This finding indicated that the act of not responding was critical to the problems encountered and illustrated the inhibitory role of the septum in normal behavior. Interestingly, enhanced performance on alternation and go–no-go tasks have been described in several experiments (e.g., Carlson & Cole, 1970; Carlson & Norman, 1971; Carlson & Vallante, 1974), suggesting that the relationship between attentional performance and septal damage is complex and task-dependent.

Damage to the septum creates several different dysfunctions that depend on which discrete areas are lesioned (Grossman, 1976). Attempts to dissociate the deficits associated with septal damage in rats have suggested that, although prolonged extinction and problems with nonreward occur in all cases of septal damage, there is a dissociation in other response characteristics depending on the discrete septal region of involvement. For instance, lesions to the stria medullaris have the greatest effects on passive-avoidance tasks (Van Hoesen, MacDouglass, & Mitchell, 1969), and damage to regions innervating the fornix have the greatest effects on certain instrumental tasks involving schedules of reinforcement that require waiting before responding (MacDougall, Van Hoesen, & Mitchell, 1969). This dissociation suggests that, although there is a critical common component in all forms of septal lesion, the specific nature of the deficits may depend on which septal nuclei are damaged, as well as on the projections from the septum to other neural structures (Grossman, 1976).

When an animal with septal damage persists despite nonreinforcement, one might assume that there is a reduction in the aversiveness that the animal experiences as a result of the lesion, which in turn should facilitate responding. However, Dickinson (1972) found that animals with septal damage actually experience increased aversiveness and continue responding nonetheless. Also, persistence effects with septal damage did not appear to be related to an increase in drive state. One explanation of the persistence may be that the tendency to respond increases as a result of increased drive or an energizing effect of increased frustration. However, Dickinson found that there was no difference between the impaired and the normal rats on this variable. The effects of septal damage seemed to be primarily disinhibitory, and to be associated with reduced extinction of reward expectancies.

The interaction of different neural regions for modulation of inhibitory effects was illustrated by Gray (1970), who argued that the effects of frustrative nonreward are mediated by septohippocampal system, with the septum affecting hippocampal theta rhythms. Gray used stimulation techniques to show the opposite phenomenon from those described previously: the blocking of frustrative nonreward.

The processes of neural and behavioral inhibition play an important role in modern theories of neurobehavioral control. Although neural and behavioral inhibition are often related and interdependent, they must be thought of as separate processes. One cannot assume that all forms of behavioral inhibition are produced by neural inhibition. Nor are all neural inhibitory events reflected in overt forms of behavioral inhibition. Yet, both are relevant to our understanding of behavioral and cognitive processes, including the control of attention.

Neural inhibition is apparent at many levels of the nervous system. There are also several forms of neural inhibition, which are likely to influence attention in different ways. In this chapter, we have focused primarily on inhibitory influences occurring across systems. The interactions of hypothalamic impulses with limbic modulation seem to provide an important basis for the regulation of appetitive, affective, and emotional state. The excitatory and inhibitory interactions across structures of the limbic system establish the values attached to stimuli that are processed. After receiving incoming stimuli, we typically experience an orienting reaction. Afterward, our tendency to continue attending to the stimulus depends on the salience of the stimulus. This salience is determined by the fit that occurs between the new stimulus, memories of similar events, and the motivational or affective weighting that is associated with that memory. The value that is associated with the stimulus influences future behavior through its excitatory and inhibitory influence. Inhibitory processes are of particular relevance to the control of attention, as they account for a possible mechanism by which the individual stops responding to a previous input and shifts to a new input or internal signal.

We have not focused on the types of inhibition found between neural cells in a particular region. The processes of lateral and temporal inhibition noted in studies of sensory perception illustrate how the interactions of neurons in a particular system account for complex effects. These interactions may account for nonlinearities in the way information accumulates in the system. Within modern computational theories that postulate parallel attentional processing, these types of inhibition may account for how a neural network changes its attentional disposition. Both neural and behavioral inhibition are likely to have important places in future attempts to understand the neurobehavioral bases of attention.

NEURAL MECHANISMS OF SENSORY SELECTIVE ATTENTION

Thus far we have considered neural mechanisms for attention which involve multiple interacting systems. While short- and long-term potentiation can be demonstrated in single neurons of simple organisms, the way that these events combine in human cognition is still relatively unknown, except at a systemic level. Is there evidence of processes like attention, selection, and filtering in the activity of single neurons?

Visual Mechanisms of Attention

The influence of stimulus properties and attentional factors on neuronal activity has been most clearly demonstrated in the visual system. From these investigations, overwhelming evidence has accumulated that the visual territory of the brain can be functionally divided into local subsystems that are responsive to specific types of visual properties. As Zeki and Shipp (1988) noted, the organization of the visual cortex, with its many functional divisions, bears little resemblance to the subjective experience of the visual environment, which is perceived as a unified whole. Introspective experience, therefore, provides only intermittent glimpses of the mosaic of the parallel, localized operations that underlie visual perception.

Selective neuronal responses to properties of the visual field are generated by several means. A neuron may be biologically reactive to specific types of visual properties. For example, one class of cone cells in the retina is chemically most responsive to only one portion of the visible light spectrum. The activity of one neuron may be influenced by other local neuronal activity. For example, the activity of a neuron responsive to movement in one direction may inhibit the rate of firing of a neighboring neuron that responds to movement in a different direction and vise versa. Neuronal activity may be increased or inhibited by task demands. This top-down modulation may be due to a general change of arousal, which influences the activity of neurons on a global basis, or to selective modulation of a particular neuronal ensemble to detect a specific visual event. In the following sections, we review the neuroanatomy of the visual system and the evidence for the modulation of neuronal response by intrinsic, local, and global mechanisms.

In this literature, the response properties of a neuron are usually described in relationship to a visual receptive field: the area of the retina that, if stimulated, will increase or decrease the firing rate of the neuron. In the retina, receptive fields were first described by Kuffler (1953), who found that ganglion cells in the retina are frequently associated with center–surround antagonism. He described two types of cells with this property. In the first type (on-center, off-periphery cells), the cell increases its firing rate when its field is stimulated centrally and decreases its firing rate when illumination is peripheral to the center of the field. In the second type (off-center, on-periphery cells), the cell has the opposite response pattern: Central illumination causes the cell to reduce its firing rate, and peripheral illumination increases it. Work by Hubel and Wiesel (1977) demonstrated that neurons in the primary sensory cortex demonstrate receptive fields that show remarkable selectivity, responding only to stimuli with a specific orientation, position, or width. Other investigators have found that cells are tuned to properties such as spatial frequency, phase, motion, and direction of motion.

The Neuroanatomy of the Visual System

The visual system encompasses a vast and functionally heterogeneous territory within the brain. When photons fall on the retina, they stimulate rod and cone cells within the retina. The rod and cone cells, in turn, stimulate several layers of interconnected cells, terminating in a layer of ganglion cells. The axons of the ganglion cells project backward from the eye in a bundle that forms the optic nerve. The optic nerves cross at the optic chiasm. After the chiasm, the left optic nerve carries information from both eyes describing the right visual field, and the right optic nerve carries information describing the left visual

field. This contralateral representation of the visual fields persists into the cerebral hemispheres, the optic nerve terminates on the lateral geniculate nucleus, whose axons project
via the optic radiation to the visual cortex. A smaller projection from the lateral geniculate
nucleus goes to the superior colliculus of the midbrain.

After terminating in the primary visual cortex of the occipital lobe, further visual
processing occurs through a series of projections that travel anteriorly over the cortex.
Visual processing continues from the occipital lobe to the parietal and inferior temporal
lobes. Forward, parallel, and backward projections interconnect the cells within these
territories, which in turn are interconnected with other areas of the cortex and the subcortical regions, such as the frontal eye fields and the thalamic nuclei.

Visual Filtering

Cells within the visual system respond selectively to different attributes of visual
stimulation of the retina. Different populations of neurons are "tuned" to specific types of
stimulation, similarly to the way that a radio can be tuned to different broadcast frequencies.
In this way, a particular neuron responds to a certain type of stimulation and filters out
irrelevant stimulation. Differentiation of the visual field into properties or features begins
in the retina and reaches exquisite levels of selectivity in the cortex.

Retinal Response

Even at the level of the retina, complex neuronal systems have developed that transform
the pattern of illumination on the visual receptors into a distributed and feature-sensitive
pattern of neuronal activity. In the retina, rod and cone cells respond to quite different
properties of illumination. Rod cells are sensitive to shorter wavelength illumination than
cones and are more sensitive in conditions of dim illumination. All rods show the same
sensitivity function across wavelengths, whereas three types of cones exist. The three types
of cones are maximally sensitive at wavelengths corresponding to blue, green, and red hues.
Cones, therefore, can subserve color vision, as each class of cones can encode a particular
hue. Finally, rods and cones are asymmetrically distributed over the surface of the retina.
Cones are concentrated in the center area of the eye, the fovea, and rods predominate in the
peripheral areas. Cones synapse on a single bipolar cell, whereas several rods synapse on a
given bipolar cell. This arrangement results in better spatial resolution for cones and more
reliable transmission for rods. These properties of the rods and cones result in different
general response characteristics across the surface of the retina. The fovea of the retina
provides good color and spatial resolution, whereas the periphery provides poorer color and
spatial resolution, but better contrast sensitivity, particularly in low illumination.

At the level of the ganglion cell in the retina, two populations of cells have been
identified that show very different response properties: small, parvocellular neurons and
large, magnocellular neurons. These cells initiate two streams of visual processing that
maintain their identity beyond the occipital cortex (for a review, see Zeki & Shipp, 1988).
Parvocellular cells show low-contrast sensitivity; slow, sustained responses; and wavelength
selectivity. Magnocellular neurons show high-contrast sensitivity; fast, transient responses;
larger receptive fields; and lack of wavelength selectivity. The parvocellular cells project in a
discrete stream to the lateral geniculate nucleus, to the primary visual cortex, and through a
series of connections to the inferotemporal cortex. Within the cortex, the parvocellular
stream is most sensitive to wavelength, orientation, texture, and disparity. It terminates
in the inferotemporal cortex, which is specialized for form perception. The magnocellular
stream is responsive to movement, direction, orientation, location, and disparity. It termi-

nates in the parietal lobe and is specialized for the detection of location, motion, and possibly depth discriminations. The parvocellular system appears designed to answer the question, "What is it?" whereas the magnocellular system seems to answer the question, "Where is it and which way is it going?"

Attentional Processes in the Visual System

Neurons in the visual system are responsive to specific properties of visual stimulation. In general, neurons early in a processing stream are associated with small receptive fields and are tuned to simple visual attributes, whereas neurons later in the processing stream are associated with larger receptive fields and may respond to specific conjunctions of visual attributes. Neurons early in the stream of visual processing not only send projections forward to "association areas" in the parietal and temporal cortex but also receive massive numbers of projections from neurons downstream in the visual stream, and from neuronal populations far removed from the sensory visual pathways. These "backward" projections imply that higher order processes modulate sensory processing. It is not surprising, then, that several types of attentional effects on neuronal activity have been repeatedly demonstrated in primates. These attentional effects appear to be modulated by neural populations widely separated over the cortex and the subcortex, and they include arousal, stimulus selection, surround inhibition, response generation, and adjustment to a visuomotor response.

Arousal

Execution of a demanding task may induce a global increase in the firing rate of visual neurons. This is the only type of attentional effect so far reported in the primary visual cortex (Robinson & Peterson, 1986; Wurtz, Richmond, & Newsome, 1984).

Response Initiation

Enhanced activity in the frontal eye fields and the superior colliculus appears to be involved in the initiation of saccadic eye movements toward visual targets within a cell's receptive field (Posner, Cohen, & Rafal, 1982; Wurtz *et al.*, 1984).

Responses to Visual Tracking

Cells in the medial superior temporal area may show enhanced firing when pursuit eye movements are engaged to follow a moving stimulus (Wurtz *et al.*, 1984).

Stimulus Selection and Spatial Attention

Both enhancement and inhibition of neural activity have been associated with tasks that require attention to objects in space. Attention to object properties enhances the response of neurons in the higher-level visual cortex (e.g., V4) and the inferior temporal cortex. When a discrimination task is made more difficult, and an animal is required to put forth more effort to maintain performance, activity (from V4 neurons in response to the target stimuli) are enhanced, and the receptive field become more selective for task-relevant stimulus attributes (Spitzer, Desimone, & Moran, 1988). Fixation on a spot of light constricts the receptive field of a neuron in the inferior temporal cortex (Robinson & Peterson, 1986; Wurtz *et al.*, 1984). Moran and Desimone (1985) found that responses of cells tuned to unattended stimulus features are attenuated. The neural response to task-relevant stimuli, therefore, is enhanced and sharpened by attention and effort, whereas responses to irrelevant stimuli and features are inhibited.

Unlike neurons in the frontal eye fields or superior colliculus, neurons in the posterior parietal cortex can respond to a target stimulus even when fixation is maintained elsewhere in space (Posner *et al.*, 1982). Parietal activity increases when stimuli are related to motivational value. For example, fixation on food targets is more effective than fixation on nonfood objects or pictures of food. Aversive as well as positively reinforcing objects produce parietal cell activation. Goal-directed arm movements produce activation of neurons, whereas the same movements made without a goal do not. Goal-directed arm movements to a point in space produce an enhancement of parietal responses even when the performer is trained not to fixate on the target of the motion (Robinson & Peterson, 1986). Cells in the parietal cortex also show a contrasting attentional effect: Visual fixation may increase rather than attentuate a response to extrafoveal stimulation (Mountcastle, Motter, Steinmetz, & Duffy, 1984). This effect may reflect the role of the parietal lobes in maintaining a contextual representation of the body's position and movements within visual space.

Shifting Visual Attention

Posner, Peterson, Fox, and Raichle (1988) reviewed experiments in primates and humans that demonstrate how a complete behavioral action—shifting attention to a new spatial location—is subserved by at least three widely separated neuronal ensembles: the posterior parietal lobe of the cerebral cortex, the pulvinar region in the thalamus, and midbrain regions contributing to eye movements. Posner *et al.* (1988) used a paradigm that required persons with and without brain lesions to respond to targets in cued and uncued locations. Patients with parietal lobe lesions have difficulty disengaging their attention from one location to move it to another. Midbrain lesions slow the movement of attention. Thalamic lesions slow eye movements to both cued and uncued targets, regardless of the time allowed to deploy attention to a cued location.

Summary

Visual selective attention is subsumed by multiple neural systems. Research has focused on sensory enhancement of the inferior parietal region, eye movement control of looking from the frontal eye, and thalamic integration. It is evident that the control of attention is determined by a matrix of neural systems.

Neural cells in certain brain regions seem to have attentional properties that allow them to focus through a process of sensory enhancement. The underlying mechanisms seem to involve complex neural computations. Various types of attentional effects are associated with different neuronal populations. The firing thresholds of cells in the *striate cortex* can be altered by arousal, without stimulus or spatially selective changes in the receptive fields of individual neurons. Receptive field properties of cells within the *prestriate area V4* and cells within the *occipital-inferior temporal pathway* associated with object recognition are selectively activated to enhance response to specific visual features or objects. Increased effort narrows receptive field specificity and enhances response to target features. These activation effects are complemented by the inhibition of cellular responses to irrelevant stimuli.

In the *parietal lobe*, which subserves the representation of spatial relations of the body and the space within which it moves, attentional enhancement can occur in cells with receptive fields peripheral to the fixation point. Reinforcing or aversive objects are associated with increased firing. Goal-oriented movements are also associated with neural activation. The parietal lobe also appears to show attentional effects in cells with extrafoveal receptive fields, so that these cells may subserve the spatial representation of the whole environment.

The *frontal eye fields* and the *superior colliculus* are involved in the initiation of movements or saccades required to shift attention across space. The performance of a complete behavioral sequence of shifting attention and responding to a target at a new point in space requires the integrated activity of neuronal populations located in widely dispersed areas of cortex and subcortex, including the midbrain, the pulvinar, and the posterior parietal region.

ATTENTIONAL MECHANISMS FOR OTHER SENSORY MODALITIES

The vast majority of research devoted to delineating the neural mechanisms of attention has focused on the visual system. There may be several reasons for this, including the fact that vision is probably the most dominant sense in humans. Also, the visual system operates with obvious spatial constraints and frequently requires attentional selection relative to spatial position. Furthermore, there has been considerable evidence for the existence of specific neural systems of attention in the visual system.

Yet, the attentional capacity is not limited to the visual system. In fact, many of the early cognitive studies of attention focused primarily on the auditory system (e.g., Treisman, 1964). Dichotic listening paradigms were frequently employed to demonstrate limitations on divided attention. Also, much of our knowledge of the characteristics of the orienting response comes from the measurement of autonomic responses to auditory stimuli.

That attention plays a role in other sensory systems should not be surprising. If one envisions being at a cocktail party, it is easy to recall situations in which attention is pulled to a particular voice in the crowd. Examples of attention are readily apparent for other sensory modalities as well. In a crowded room you may be completely inattentive to low-intensity tactile stimuli, such as brushing against another person. Yet in an open field such contact would be hard to ignore. Olfactory stimuli such as the smell of cookies baking is also likely to be noticed. However, the degree of attention to this stimulus is governed by motivational factors.

The neural mechanisms of attention undoubtedly vary greatly as a function of the sensory system that is being considered. Some sensory systems, such as audition, seem to have high-level cortical processing areas that perform integrative functions. Other sensory systems, like olfaction, are much more primitive in humans and seem to have direct access to subcortical-limbic structures, as well as cortical areas. While it is beyond the scope of this book to review each of these systems, we will discuss some of the likely neural mechanisms of attention across several different modalities.

Auditory Attention

Upon reaching the inner ear auditory signals receive initial processing in the cochlea, where initial frequency analysis occurs. Subsequently, information passes along the classical subcortical sensory pathways, where it is processed through a chain of subcortical nuclei including the inferior and superior colliculus and the red and olivary nuclei. After this initial processing, the auditory information reaches the lateral geniculate nucleus of the thalamus, where it is relayed to the primary auditory cortex (areas 41 and 42) of Heschl's gyrus of the temporal lobe. From this cortical area, auditory activation advances to higher cortical systems that integrate and/or perform specialized operations on this information. The superior temporal gyrus of the dominant hemisphere contains Wernicke's area, surrounding which are complex heteromodal association areas in the parietal and temporal lobes. The cortical auditory processing areas have access to limbic structures, including the hippocampus.

Unlike the visual system, which has very exact spatial characteristics relative to the two retinal fields, sound coming into the ears is not as well-lateralized. Yet, neurons in the primary auditory cortex of each hemisphere exhibit maximal response to sound coming from the contralateral side of the surrounding environment. Therefore, spatial localization of sound is possible, which is of obvious relevance to auditory spatial attention.

Benson, Hienz, and Goldstein (1981) provided one of the few demonstrations of neural enhancement of auditory attention, through recordings of neurons of the primary visual cortex. They used single-unit recording methods to measure neurons' responses and compared results when the animal was required to localize sound versus only detect whether a sound had occurred. Neurons in the primary auditory cortex showed increased response when sound localization was required. This finding not only illustrates the role of this system in sound localization but also the selective response of the system to different task demands (i.e., an attentional effect). In humans the relationship between sound localization and attention may be more complex.

Language is a dominant function in humans. Therefore, linguistic processing is one of the most obvious byproducts of auditory processing. Because of the importance of language, humans' attention is tuned to the verbal informational content of sound. As a result, auditory attention is principally governed by the semantic information conveyed by sound. When an auditory message is important, attention is enhanced. Auditory attentional enhancement is probably facilitated by high-order auditory association areas that interact with a network of neural systems similar to those described for visual attention. Neural enhancement would increase the processing resources (i.e., associative networks) allocated to particular auditory information. While there is little empirical evidence for the specific neural mechanisms that enable attentional enhancement of auditory input, this process could be governed by mechanisms similar to those described for visual processing.

In addition to the verbal semantic analysis of the dominant hemisphere, it appears likely that analogous nondominant cortical systems may facilitate attention based on nonlinguistic features of the auditory information, such as prosody (Benowitz, Bear, Rosenthal, Mesulam, Zaidel, & Sperry, 1983). Attention to the prosody of speech often provides important information for the listener, such as the emotional content of the message. This information seems to be selectively processed by nondominant temporal cortical systems in interaction with the limbic system, independent of the verbal linguistic analysis system of the dominant hemisphere.

Prior to the cortical auditory processing that was just described, subcortical auditory processes occur. It is likely that the OR is generated as a response to primitive auditory registration in subcortical auditory pathways. To the extent that subcortical processes influence the generation of the OR, they also play an important role in auditory attention.

Somatosensory Attention

Somatosensory information is probably not as relevant to attention as either auditory or visual attention for most cognitive operations. Yet, tactile stimulation is capable of producing reflexive behavioral responses. For instance, painful stimuli are among the strongest unconditioned stimuli (UCS) that humans experience. Stimuli that cause pain rapidly gain dominance over stimuli from other modalities. On the other hand, it is possible to learn to reduce pain intensity by directing the focus of attention away from painful sensations using meditation and hypnosis procedures. The neurophysiology of pain has been well investigated. Gating mechanisms exist which allow pain signals traveling to the cortex to be extinguished over time (Melzac & Wall, 1965; Melzac, 1973). This gating response illustrates a low-level neural response that provides a simple form of attentional control over pain signals. Of course, it is questionable whether the automatic and reflexive nature of pain gating truly qualifies this process as an attentional mechanism.

The majority of data regarding the neural mechanisms of somatosensory attention comes in part from studies of human neglect syndrome (see chapter 9). Failure to recognize one side of one's own body is occasionally reported in patients with right parietal lobe lesions. Somatosensory information contributes to the ability of humans to have spatial awareness (see chapter 19). However, as is the case for the auditory system, there are few neurophysiological studies applicable to the analysis of somatosensory attention.

The primary somatosensory system is located in the superior parietal lobe (area 3b) and receives ascending somatosensory stimulation from pathways that project from the thalamus. The primary somatosensory cortex contains neural areas that can be mapped in direct correspondence to specific body surfaces. Adjacent to area 3b are two other somatosensory areas (areas 1 and 2) which respond to specific informational characteristics of tactile and proprioceptive inputs. Secondary somatosensory areas also exist, including area 5 of the superior parietal lobule, which presumably perform modality-specific processing of tactile information. Tertiary association areas provide for integration of somatosensory information with other sensory modalities. Since somatosensory and visual integration plays an important role in visual-spatial behaviors, it is reasonable to assume some overlap of the attentional enhancement mechanisms for spatial attention.

Olfactory Attention

It is widely assumed that the olfactory system plays a diminished role in attention, as today's society provides a tremendous amount of information for visual and auditory processing. Yet, despite the dominance of these other sensory modalities, olfactory stimulation may be among the strongest elicitors of behavioral attention. Odors that are unpleasant cause immediate revulsion and behavioral withdrawal, while pleasant odors may elicit appetitive urges. As is the case for painful stimuli, strong olfactory stimuli often act as UCS. Strong odors are likely to dominate stimuli from other sensory systems, as olfactory stimuli frequently provide important organismic information. Therefore, it is obvious that even in humans the olfactory system has a direct influence on attention.

Olfactory receptors have direct innervation to the piriform cortex, a primitive neural region that projects to the paralimbic and limbic structures as well as other cortical association areas. As a result of this pattern of connectivity, olfactory stimuli gain ready access to systems that govern emotional response, memory formation, and the regulation of appetitive states. For this reason, olfactory stimuli may also have easy access to the attentional mechanisms. Interestingly, patients with partial complex epilepsy that involves limbic structures frequently experience strong olfactory auras, perhaps because of the close relationship of the olfactory and limbic systems.

SUMMARY

Although neuroscientists have focused primarily on mechanisms underlying simple behavioral processes, many findings have indirect bearing on more complex cognitive operations like attentional control. Recently, some neuroscientists have begun to study directly the neurobiology of attention. In this chapter, we have focused on two broad areas of neuroscience research that are of relevance to an understanding of the neural mechanisms of attention: neural plasticity during conditioning and visual selective attention. Admittedly, other areas are also relevant. For instance, the mechanisms of motor and premotor control also have a bearing on attentional operations. We focused consideration on conditioning and sensory mechanisms because these areas have yielded the greatest amount of information regarding the substrates of attention. The processes underlying conditioning and sensory processing have a direct influence on attention and also illustrate how the multiple neural systems contribute to attentional control.

We reviewed evidence for neural plasticity across different animal species, behavioral contexts, and levels of neural complexity. The identification of neural mechanisms for conditioning in simple organisms like *Aplysia* provide a conceptual link between attentional (habituation) and conditioning (LTP) events. Attentional control and memory formation may share neuronal substrates, particularly in simple cases of conditioning.

There is growing evidence that memory formation can be explained as a function of neurochemical changes producing long-term potentiation in individual neurons. Yet, there are many aspects of conditioning and information processing that are not adequately explained through this level of analysis. Learning requires more than a unitary process of associative formation. Attentional processes such as stimulus and response selection, although dependent on memory formation, are separate processes that seem to involve a large number of components. We built a case for attention and memory formation arising from common neuronal mechanisms. In doing so, we have simplified attention so as to make it somewhat analogous to the behavioral phenomena of orienting, sensitization, and habituation. In reality, attentional behavior in humans cannot be fully equated with these processes, even though they seem to be components of attention. Although attentional processes may depend on the same biochemical events that produce long-term potentiation in single cells, in isolation these single-unit responses do not adequately explain how humans attend. Attentional control seems to depend on the complex interactions of multiple neural systems in networks. The extent to which the types of plasticity discussed in this chapter pervade the systems governing attention still needs to be determined. In more complex animals like humans, even conditioning cannot be attributed to a unitary process, as there is evidence of multiple forms of learning with different neuroanatomical loci. Typically, sites that have the capacity for learning also exhibit response characteristics that implicate them in attentional operations. Sites of learning and attentional processing share a general characteristic: They exhibit neural plasticity, which enables an integration of new information with older memory representation. Attention can be thought of as the interface between current stimulus input and the encoding process.

The distinction between attentional and memory effects may depend on whether short- or long-term neurobiological modifications have occurred as a result of information processing. The presence of sensitization and habituation in the context of the conditioning of simple organisms bears out this point. Some sensory and motor neural systems seem to lack specific memory-encoding functions, but to exhibit short-term plasticity. This characteristic suggests that these systems have the capacity for short-duration storage, which is necessary for the integration of information and attentional operations. Neurons with short-term durability of plasticity are capable of modifying their response to new information, but most rely on encoding in other neural systems for permanent storage. Research effort has largely been directed at discovering the basis for the longer term potentiation that is essential for production of durable memory. Transient forms of plasticity have equally important implications for the neural control of attention.

The OR reflects the transient response of the organism before conditioning. For this reason, it is of great interest to students of attention. In simple organisms, the OR and habituation can be explained by a two-process model that includes components of sensitization and habituation. However, in humans, these responses are under the control of more complex interactions. We have discussed models that propose mechanisms for the maintenance of habituation in humans. The neural mechanisms for habituation and sensitization must be accounted for in any comprehensive model of attention.

Inhibitory processes seem to play a critical role in the process of habituation, as well as in other attentional control processes. Neural inhibition provides a means of accounting for the termination of one response over another, which enables the animal to control the direction of its behavior. Neural inhibition is apparent at all levels of the nervous system and therefore is an intrinsic aspect of behavioral control. In this chapter, we have focused specifically on the concept of inhibition for the purposes of illustrating how behavioral control is established. Of course, the brain also contains "activational" processes that facilitate further responding along a particular vector. Therefore, attention is controlled by the interaction of inhibitory and facilitatory influences at multiple levels of the nervous system.

Although attention is controlled by the dynamic interactions of multiple neural systems, it is also apparent that selective attention occurs at very early stages of processing soon after sensory registration. We have used the example of selective visual attention to illustrate this occurrence. Passive filtering and task-driven attentional effects are present at every stage of visual information flow within the visual system. Filtering on the basis of stimulus attributes such as orientation, contrast, color, movement, and disparity is largely automatic; specific populations of neurons encode specific visual attributes.

Selective attention to objects in the environment is subserved by a variety of mechanisms that are widely distributed within the brain and that have very specific functions. Our conscious experience of attending to one thing in a coherent environment represents the rapid integration of the outputs of these subsystems. It is as if the brain first breaks the two-dimensional visual field into many pieces, each containing a few attributes of a piece of the field, and then puts them all together again into a three-dimensional representation. Although the extent to which attention is controlled by the interaction of neural systems versus events occurring within individual neural cells is not yet established, it is clear that attentional operations occur at both neural levels. Yet, the way in which these fragmentary representations are reconstructed into an experiential whole in fractions of a second is utterly unknown.

Models and Mechanisms of Attention

A Summary

RONALD A. COHEN and BRIAN F. O'DONNELL

In the course of Part I, we have reviewed the evidence relating to many models of attention. These models have been associated with systems as global as consciousness and as molecular as the graded potential of a single neuron. In this chapter, we will develop a coherent framework to classify attentional components derived from these models, and to discuss the evidence for their theoretical viability.

Attentional mechanisms can be organized into four components that form a rough temporal sequence and, to some degree, an anatomical hierarchy. These four components are (1) sensory attention; (2) capacity; (3) response selection and control; and (4) sustained attention. Sustained attention presupposes the operation of the first three systems and reflects their operation over time. We maintain that the biological and behavioral evidence suggests that attention is a discrete category of mental operations, which is hierarchical, distributed, and modifiable. Because attentional mechanisms are usually spatially distributed within the brain and temporally extended, they can seldom be localized to a point in information flow such as a bottleneck, or to a single anatomical structure like the frontal lobes. The conscious experience of an attentional focus is an emergent property of a vast number of largely unconscious subprocesses.

We will summarize evidence for the attentional components of sensory selective attention, response selection and control, capacity, and sustained attending. The evidence comes from many sources and is described relative to research from the fields of (1) cognitive psychology; (2) behavioral psychology; (3) psychophysiology; and (4) neurophysiology.

SENSORY SELECTIVE ATTENTION

Sensory attention can be categorized into actively deployed processes (including selective or focused attention) and automatic processes (such as priming and the orienting responses). Shifts of attention can be motivated by top-down or bottom-up processes.

Selective attention occurs when some stimuli are given preferential treatment in terms of further information processing, whereas the influence of other stimuli on cognition or behavior is filtered or attenuated. On the basis of extensive research efforts beginning in the early 1960s, there is now strong evidence suggesting the importance of early sensory attentional selection. The existence and nature of sensory selection have been explicated by evidence from single-cell neurophysiology, surface-recorded event-related potentials (ERPs), studies of classical conditioning, cognitive psychology experiments, and introspection.

Cognitive Psychology

Introspectively based experiments during the 19th century suggested that selective attention operates by enhancing the awareness of a region of consciousness and inhibiting stimuli from other areas. These models were remarkably prescient regarding contemporary psychophysiological findings. Gestalt experiments showed how properties of the stimulus field itself induce an organization of figure and ground in sensory experience.

More recently, dichotic listening experiments have shown that humans are extremely effective in isolating a single message on the basis of simple physical features that discriminate between channels of information. In fact, special training is needed for a person to process any verbal information outside an attended-to channel. Focused or directed attention within the visual field results in the selective processing of a restricted spatial region and usually operates during the search for objects that are made up of conjunctions of simple features.

Several cognitive mechanisms may account for sensory selection. Filtering, the subject of much previous debate, now seems to be a viable basis for the early attenuation of sensory signals soon after perceptual registration. Filtering may occur as a result of the resolution of single sensory units or the interaction of multiple units. Sensory enhancement is a potential mechanism for attentional selection because it facilitates the focusing of attention. It may account for how attention is focused on narrower or wider frames of reference. Sensory selection seems to depend on complex neural computations performed after primary sensory registration.

The experimental techniques of priming provide additional evidence for sensory selection. Priming decreases response latency by creating a sensory expectancy. Although the neural basis for this effect remains obscure, it may represent faster processing induced by sensory enhancement resulting from the priming stimulus. However, several other factors may also contribute to priming effects. Priming produces a memory cue that may reduce attentional load. The expectancy that is created by the priming stimulus also reduces the demands on response selection and control. Unlike sensory filtering, priming can occur on the basis of complex or semantic features, rather than simple physical cues.

Behavioral Psychology

Although early behaviorists largely rejected the need for a construct of attention, the mechanisms proposed to account for classical conditioning led to behavioral explanations of attentional phenomena. Within classical conditioning, learning occurs independent of response control, as the response of the animal does not govern future presentations of the unconditioned stimulus (UCS). Therefore, conditioning depends largely on the associative relationship among stimulus factors. Neobehaviorists developed behavioral theories of attention that are grounded in the principles of generalization, discriminative learning, and stimulus compounding. These processes provide possible mechanisms for the components of stimulus selection that we have discussed. Two specific findings from classical conditioning research have direct implications for attentional selection: expectancy and the orienting response (OR). Experiments demonstrating that the presentation of conditioned stimuli (CS) creates a state of expectancy led some behavioral theorists to posit an attentional component within conditioning. The orienting response demonstrates a behavioral basis for automatic attentional shifts.

Psychophysiology

Both auditory and visual ERPs have provided physiological support for an early, task-related filter mechanism for specific auditory and visual channels. This selection may occur as early as 80 msec after stimulus onset in either modality of stimulation.

Changes in stimulus properties, or the introduction of novel stimuli, may result in an orienting response, which is often detected by autonomic measurement. The orienting response suggests that some sort of internal representation of the environment is maintained, and that the current environment is constantly being matched against this representation for incongruities. The orienting response, then, represents an automatic mechanism for shifting attention that is driven by sensory events. Attention may also be passively shifted by well-learned imperative stimuli, such as hearing one's name spoken.

Neurophysiology

In 1976, Neisser asserted that "shifts of attention are not reflected in quantitative reductions of the inflow along certain nerves as was once supposed, but by very general changes in cerebral activity" (p.87), and that there was no biological mechanism or system that carried out filtering. This position is no longer tenable. Since the early 1980s, overwhelming evidence has accumulated that establishes the filter properties of individual sensory neurons, as well as selective changes in neural activity associated with visual–spatial task demands. Within the visual system, filtering on the basis of sensory features is a pervasive mechanism for the segregation of object properties and location within the visual field. Moreover, the responses of single cells to visual features can be inhibited or disinhibited on the basis of attentional demands. These findings suggest that sensory neurons act as filters that carry out complex, hierarchical, and task-influenced visual characterizations of the stimulus field.

RESPONSE SELECTION

Response selection was not considered an important factor influencing attentional control in many of the early information-processing theories. Now, there are compelling reasons why response selection should be considered an important component of attention. Most important, the selection of environmental stimuli for further processing is often determined by the individual's behavioral goals. Without this goal-directed tendency, there would be no pressure to attend. Therefore, response production is essential to goal attainment, and both of these activities depend on response selection from the available alternatives.

The distinction that is now commonly drawn between controlled and automatic attention provides another reason for considering response selection an important attentional control process. As we have described in previous chapters, there is considerable experimental evidence supporting the distinction between controlled and automatic attentional processes. There is also evidence suggesting that attentional effort is often associated with premotor activation and the response demands of tasks.

Cognitive Psychology

Just as many behaviorists tended to minimize the need for an attentional construct, many cognitive psychologists tend to minimize the need for response factors in the control of attention. Within information-processing frameworks that use signal detection theory, attention is viewed as a sensory factor. However, the distinction between controlled and automatic attentional processes that has been demonstrated since the late 1970s, suggests that response factors may be important in certain types of tasks. When a situation has high response demands relative to a large set of stimuli that are not well engrained in long-term memory, attention cannot be automatically allocated. The controlled attentional processing required under these conditions is very effortful and taxes response systems. For instance, one can drive a car on a sunny day along a rural superhighway rather automatically. However, driving a car on icy roads in the winter requires very directed attention, as there are increased expectancies of exceptional responses (e.g., rapid maneuvering and braking to avoid an accident). In the latter situation, attention to sensory inputs is determined by the need to select and generate responses.

Of relevance to this discussion are findings pertaining to performance on multiple complex tasks. Because the capacity to perform such tasks depends on the extent to which the tasks are performed in an automatic or a controlled fashion, attention often involves fluctuations between automatic sampling and more effortful control functions. Human operators attending to multiple tasks rely on information derived from their sampling of the available stimuli to create response strategies. Stimulus sampling creates changes in response tendency. Conversely, response demands may influence the disposition of the operator, which may have an impact on the allocation of sensory selection.

Several other cognitive approaches are of theoretical significance in our consideration. The study of manual tracking led to models that postulated that the behavioral control of even the simplest forms of tracking requires both stimulus sampling and response feedback mechanisms. This topic is discussed in greater detail in Chapter 21. Recent studies of how visual attention and grasping are integrated have led to a more biologically based approach to the tracking problem (e.g., Wise & Desimone, 1988). Although it now is apparent that response demands influence selective attention, parametric studies of the relationship of response and stimulus factors still need to be conducted.

Behavioral Psychology

Operant learning theory postulates that responding may lead to reinforcement, which then perpetuates further responding. Even though most operant learning theorists do not acknowledge the need for an attentional construct, many of their research findings indicate how response mediation may influence attentional selection. The operant models of discriminative learning have provided a behavioral mechanism to account for the attentional control of responding. Discriminative cues provide information that may facilitate an animal's response selection, so that it makes an appropriate response to achieve reinforcement.

Classical conditioning fits more closely with sensory models of attention. However, the discovery that the response to the CS often contains anticipatory and preparatory components provided indications that response-related factors may influence attention, even when the response is inconsequential to the reinforcement that will be received. The CS that cues the animal to the impending UCS acts as an attentional signal, as well as a prompt to prepare for a reaction.

Psychophysiology

Several lines of evidence from the field of psychophysiology support the role of response systems during attention. The common finding of autonomic response changes during attention supports the notion that attending is closely associated with response production. Autonomic responsivity has been shown to differ according to the dimension of activity and passivity. The OR is most commonly associated with passive attention and reflects an automatic activation in response to a novel stimuli. Orienting produces a decreased heart rate as the animal prepares for further responding, and it may also include various muscular responses reflecting body positioning relative to the signal.

During directed attentional tasks, including tasks that involve sustained and effortful processing, there is generally a reversal of the heart rate response. Other physiological responses also reflect the intensity of attentional effort. Phasic autonomic responses (like skin conductance increases and pupilary dilation) and somatomotor responses (like EMG) provide indexes of attentional allocation. Although it can be argued that these responses are the by-product of rather than a basis for attention, the fact that directed attention results in motoric activation reflects the linkage between attention and the neural systems involved in response preparation, selection, and initiation.

Central electrophysiological measures are also influenced by response requirements. The N2–P3 complex of the event-related potential is activated by infrequent task-relevant events. As we discussed in Chapter 6, these components correspond to late, response-driven, pigeonholing mechanisms rather than to sensory filtering mechanisms. Intriguingly, the N2–P3 complex can be generated by task-irrelevant novel events, a finding suggesting that the same neural network may be activated by bottom-up or top-down processes. Unlike filtering mechanisms, response selection is usually goal-driven, categorical, temporally extended, and effortful.

Neurophysiology

There is both direct and indirect evidence supporting the role of premotoric neural systems in the control of attention. Three types of experimental findings that were described previously (Chapter 3) are of relevance, including studies of (1) eye movements and visual search; (2) the distinction between sensory attention and motor intention; and (3) executive control functions of the prefrontal cortex.

Eye movements are a fundamental component of attending. Animals produce certain types of saccades as a way of tracking objects across their spatial field. In recent years, intense research efforts have been devoted to the question of whether these movements are the basis for attentional selection or the result of a more primary mechanism. Various investigators have determined that attention is possible without eye movements. Yet, these studies do not go so far as to discount the importance of eye movements in normal visual attention. Although cortical sensory areas (e.g., the inferior parietal cortex) are involved in the enhancement of attentional responses, eye movements are necessary if the animal is to fixate its processing resources on a target. The parameters underlying saccadic eye movements during attending have been well demonstrated in numerous studies.

The analysis of eye movements during attention, as well as the discovery of a theoretical distinction between motor and premotoric neurophysiological responses has led to studies that have distinguished between the sensory selection and intentional components of attention. As we described in Chapter 7, investigators have demonstrated the presence of a behavioral enhancement of visual attentional responses in neurons of the frontal eye fields, in addition to the inferior parietal lobes. The superior colliculus was also found to be important in the initiation of saccades. Together, cells of these structures seem to provide a control system for visual attention by enabling a sequencing of saccades and a visual enhancement of targets that are salient. Furthermore, the existence of neuronal populations that are activated by sensory stimuli only when followed by a motoric response provides evidence for specialized neural systems mediating sensorimotor integration.

Additional support for the role of factors related to response selection for attentional control is evident in prefrontal cortical functions. The prefrontal cortex provides an important, though less direct, control over attention by exerting executive regulation over behavior. We previously described studies (in Chapters 3 and 7) that illustrate that neural cells of the frontal cortex are involved in response inhibition, switching, and other processes essential for behavioral control. One way that the frontal complex accomplishes this control is by inhibiting the pressures to respond produced by activation from the reticular, hypothalamic, and limbic systems. Damage to the prefrontal structures also causes disorders of the OR and habituation, responses that are closely associated with attention. We will elaborate on the role of the frontal limbic and subcortical systems in the control of attentional response selection in chapter 10.

ATTENTIONAL CAPACITY

The concept of mental capacity and its relationship to attention has been derived from several types of evidence. The most fundamental reason that a capacity construct is necessary is that humans are not capable of handling an infinite amount of information simultaneously. If this were possible, we would not need to be concerned with capacity or, for that matter, with attention. That we are forced to select among the stimuli in our environment illustrates that our capacity for information processing is limited.

Theoretically, it should be possible to specify the upper limits of performance of a particular individual. However, people usually do not function at optimal levels at all times. Attention depends on the available resources, which determine the optimal level of performance possible for a particular behavioral function. Attention also reflects the momentary functional state, which is determined by energetic factors that reduce performance from the optimum (Kahneman, 1973). Unfortunately, it is not easy to determine an optimal performance level that is universal across individuals, nor is it possible to specify one level that reflects optimal performance for an individual across all types of tasks and situations.

Attentional capacity has been associated with two different types of limitations which can be characterized as structural and energetic in nature (see Table 8.1). Structural capacity limitations are determined by the optimal processing characteristics of the system, including channel capacity, working-memory capacity, processing speed, and the temporal-spatial characteristics of the system. Variables that place limits on this capacity include (1) performance required on more than one task; (2) an increase in task complexity; (3) an increase in memory demand; (4) either an excessively high or excessively low rate of occurrence of target events; and (5) excessive task duration.

Capacity is also influenced by natural or imposed variations in the individual's energetics. Energetic properties include arousal, motivation, and generated effort. One of the most important indicators of the need for the capacity concept was the behavioral observa-

TABLE 8.1.   Components Influencing Capacity

Structural	Energetic
Memory/encoding	Arousal
Timing characteristics	Effort generation
Spatial characteristics	Motivation
Cognitive resources	
Processing speed	

tion that performance varies over time. The energetic properties that influence performance capacity seem to be a major factor accounting for this temporal variability. At times, attentional performance variability can be attributed to environmental changes or learning. At other times, performance variations seem to reflect fluctuations in intrinsic neurophysiological state and the influence of motivation, reinforcement, or other factors affecting task salience.

The influence of energetic factors on performance can be appreciated from both observational and experimental data. Neurophysiological effects of arousal have been noted at the single-cell level, as well as at the level of the autonomic response. Unfortunately, constructs like arousal and effort have resisted operational definition and reliable categorization. Some authors have even questioned whether such constructs have any utility whatsoever. Yet, their influence on human performance is so pervasive that many paradigms cannot easily be interpreted without recourse to these or similar constructs.

Performance varies over time on many tasks, even when task demands are held constant. For example, sensory thresholds may vary over successive trials, as a re-presentation of the same stimulus creates greater familiarity. Reductions in novelty and strengthening of memory of the stimulus influence sensitivity to the stimulus. As introspective psychologists pointed out in the previous century, attention constantly fluctuates over time, in both focus and intensity. This temporal character is a fundamental aspect of attention and helps to distinguish attention from other cognitive processes. For this reason, we have included the construct of sustained attention, a separate attentional function that we will summarize in the final section of this chapter. At this point, it is worth noting that a major determinant of sustained performance is the interaction of attentional capacity with sensory and response selection demands.

Cognitive Psychology

The emphasis of most of the early cognitive research was directed to specifying the structural mechanisms underlying capacity and resources. Structural models of attentional capacity such as those advanced by Broadbent (1952, 1958, 1971), Kahneman (1973), Shiffrin and Schneider (1977), and Norman and Bobrow (1975) address capacity in terms of the limitations within or between information-processing structures. Capacity is considered a function of the sensory selection capabilities of the individual. Because performance on one task often declines when a secondary task is added, a capacity limitation has been inferred, as humans can handle only a finite amount of information at one time. Without postulating a capacity construct, it is difficult to explain why performance on simple tasks varies over time if motivation and the cognitive structures are held constant. Although the above-named investigators alluded to the influence of effort on performance, energetic influences were not well integrated into their framework.

Subsequently, the importance of variables associated with memory and previous learning was demonstrated. For instance, the degree to which information placed a load on variable memory was shown to influence performance (e.g., Schneider & Shiffrin, 1977). This finding provided a true structural factor limiting capacity. Although memory is also a dynamic process, the limits of the short-term memory span and the consistency of material in the long-term memory suggest that the entry of material into memory influences the ability to attend to that information.

Although much emphasis has been placed on analyzing the relationship between memory and attention, some cognitive researchers have recently directed research to other structural factors that have a bearing on attentional capacity. The temporal and spatial characteristics of behavior seem to be particularly interesting to students of attention. Experimental data that have helped to establish the parameters and constraints of the spatial-temporal organization of cognition and behavior. These findings are beginning to be applied to the study of attention. In our view, the temporal-spatial organization of experience places important constraints on attention and limits its capacity. These issues are discussed in Part III of this book.

Perhaps the most troubling concept associated with cognitive or structural capacity in the common notion that people have some form of global capacity. This concept has been expressed historically through related constructs such as intelligence. Although there appears to be some relationship between global cognitive ability and attentional capacity, this relationship is inexact. If one were to compare individuals functioning in the moderate range of intellectual retardation with individuals in the superior range, the results would be rather unambiguous. The subjects with higher intellectual scores would most likely perform better on attentional measures. However, this relationship does not hold up in comparisons of the attentional characteristics of individuals with smaller differences in intellectual scores. Furthermore, difficulties arise when one attempts to draw a theoretical link between standard intellectual measures and global capacity.

Behavioral Psychology

The concept of capacity was not given much consideration by traditional learning theorists studying operant and classical conditioning. The work of Pavlov (1927) and subsequent researchers on classical conditioning illustrated the role of the OR. This provided groundwork for the concept of arousal, a fundamental component of energetic capacity. However, this concept was more fully developed in later psychophysiological approaches.

Hull (1943) and subsequent neobehaviorists operationalized constructs that accounted for an energetic factor (e.g., drives and motivation) to explain the pressures that catalyze behavior. They viewed drive as a hydraulic state function that varied in accordance with external factors like time of deprivation. Hull also postulated an oscillatory function that anticipated the need to account for attentional or energetic fluctuations. However these concepts were somewhat removed from our current concept of capacity.

Neobehaviorists have also placed an emphasis on the role of intervening variables, including excitation and inhibition. These two processes were also incorporated into neurophysiological models in the early part of this century, and served as a cornerstone in attempts to link neurophysiological activation and arousal with behavioral phenomena like attention. These efforts eventually led to the view that behavioral and neural energetics need not be considered a unitary function. Instead, the energetic state of the individual is a composite of the local patterns of activation (inhibitory and excitatory) across different neural systems.

Psychophysiology

The demonstration of the psychophysiological bases of arousal has had great impact on the study of attention, by providing a physiological index of attentional capacity. Physiological responses during attending reflect the momentary energetic state of the individual. However, as we discussed in Chapter 6, this relationship is not straightforward, as autonomic activation may not directly reflect cortical activation. Arousal and activational theories of attention have been plagued by both conceptual and methodological problems. Yet, we believe that there are compelling reasons why these concepts should not be abandoned. Recent neurophysiological data support the role of the reticular formation as an activating system causing the enhancement of specific sensory attentional pathways. Also, the concept of arousal has importance as a descriptive concept that characterizes the overall energetic state of the animal. There can be little doubt that, in the range of normal energetics, an animal that is asleep can be considered less aroused than an animal that is in an agitated state. These energetic states have obvious importance in determining attentional capacity.

Neurophysiology

There are now many experimental data related to the role of different neuroanatomical systems in regulating the energetic state of the animal, as well as in more specific behavioral functions. We will not elaborate on this evidence at this time. However, it must be emphasized that the capacity of the animal to respond to the reinforcing qualities of stimuli has direct bearing on its attentional performance. Furthermore, neurophysiological evidence pertaining to neural speed, spatial and temporal behavioral organization, and memory and encoding constraints has helped to validate these structural components of attentional capacity. These components will be reviewed later in this book.

SUSTAINED ATTENTION

Sustained attention requires the maintenance of sensory selection, capacity, and response selection over time. Therefore, it is vulnerable to deficits in any of these functions. Pinpointing the source of a breakdown in sustained attention remains a research question. Most studies of sustained attention have used vigilance paradigms, characterized by an infrequent occurrence of response-demanding events. Diminished arousal tends to cause a tonic decrease in stimulus sensitivity, which may cause a failure of sensory attention. Phasic changes in alertness are associated with faster reaction times and higher error rates, an association suggesting a response-based effect. Vigilance decrements over time appear to be the result of changes in response criteria.

Sustained attention is also influenced by reinforcement. Although information-processing studies of vigilance seldom include reinforcement schedules, animal studies demonstrate that different reinforcement schedules have a significant impact on response maintenance.

Cognitive Psychology

The discovery that, under certain experimental conditions, attentional performance declines dramatically as a function of time on task, even for short periods, led to a consideration of the characteristics of vigilance. Perhaps more than any other area of cognitive investigation, the study of vigilance led to a consideration of task demands and response-related factors. Mackworth's finding (1950, 1965, 1969) of a drop in false positive error rates after long periods of vigilance suggested an increased response bias toward conservative behavior over time. However, vigilance and fatigue vary greatly in accordance with task parameters. The rate of the target stimuli relative to the total stimuli that are presented influences vigilance and the tendency to fatigue. Therefore, cognitive investigations of vigilance have indicated that sustained attention is a complex behavior controlled by factors associated with the sensory, response, and capacity components that we have discussed.

Studies of the relationship between effort, the semantic qualities of the task, and task complexity illustrate that all of these factors influence the ability of subjects to sustain attention. The levels-of-processing effect that indicates that greater attention is directed toward more salient semantic tasks illustrates this point. Subjects tend to have difficulty sustaining attention on tasks that are overly complex and nonsalient, as well as on tasks that are too simple, uninteresting, and monotonous. Performance on tasks at both extremes can be modified by influencing the payoff to subjects.

Behavioral Psychology

In many ways, learning theory was devoted to showing how reinforcement contingencies and the relationship between different types of stimuli can perpetuate behavioral responding. Concepts related to sustained performance are at the heart of behavioral theories and therefore are self-evident. Yet, sustained attention and vigilance are underrepresented in neuropsychological models of attention, and need to be incorporated to a greater extent.

Psychophysiology

Studies of the physiological parameters underlying habituation and extinction provide the most direct psychophysiological support for mechanisms underlying sustained attention. Unfortunately, there have been few attempts to extend these efforts beyond relatively simple paradigms.

Neurophysiology

There is now an abundance of experimental data pertaining to the question of how reinforcement influences different neural systems, such as limbic and hypothalamic structures. Reinforcement produces a selective enhancement or inhibition of sensory and response signals, which influences the flow of information through the system. Although these relationships are being explored for specific structured tasks, how these neurophysiological mechanisms interact to create a behavioral flow is still not well understood.

SUMMARY

We have described four primary components of attention: (1) sensory selection; (2) response selection and control; (3) attentional capacity; and (4) sustained attention. Support for the existence of these components comes from several scientific domains, including the fields of cognitive and behavioral psychology, psychophysiology, and neurophysiology. These four attentional components must be considered when one is studying the neuropsychology of attention.

II

Neuropsychology of Attention

Neuroanatomical Disorders of Attention Affecting Sensory Selection

In this chapter, attentional disturbances resulting from damage to brain systems that govern sensory selection are discussed. Hemi-inattention and neglect syndromes are perhaps the most intriguing disorders of attention seen by clinical neuropsychologists. We begin with a discussion of these syndromes and continue with a more general consideration of temporal and parietal lobe influences on attention. The hemispheric asymmetries of attention are then considered. We conclude with a brief review of the role of the thalamus as an informational gateway in the control of attention.

HEMI-INATTENTION AND NEGLECT SYNDROMES

Neglect of and inattention to part of the environmental field, syndromes seen in some patients after focal brain lesions, are among the most exotic forms of attentional disturbance. Patients with these syndromes may even exhibit a striking lateral neglect of one half of a particular stimulus. A patient who is asked to draw a reproduction of the stimulus that has been presented may respond by copying only half the object.

Hemispatial neglect can be dissociated from primary sensory disturbances, such as hemianopia. After occipital lesions, there is frequently loss of part of the visual field. Yet, patients with hemianopia are usually able to direct their attention to scan areas of the visual field to which they are blind. In contrast, patients with hemineglect syndrome frequently have normal visual fields and yet exhibit an inattention to stimuli at certain spatial positions. They are able to perceive the entire field but do not consistently attend to all stimuli that are perceived. Therefore, a dissociation can be made of disorders of sensory registration and perception from disorders of sensory attention.

The phenomena of hemiattention have been of great interest to neuropsychologists for several reasons. Hemi-inattention is a dramatic demonstration not only of lateralized brain organization, but also of the fact that cognitive functions may be highly specialized in their spatial representation. Disorders of hemi-inattention illustrate that attention is not a unified cognitive phenomenon that is equally distributed across a particular sensory modality. Instead, attention seems to be spatially distributed, often across different modalities. Lesions that produce neglect cause a fragmentation or distortion of the spatial distribution of attention, as the probability and strength of the response to half the spatial field are diminished. Normally, there is an interaction and a rivalry between perceptual components and spatial positions, so that attention is balanced across spatial regions. This balance is lost with the occurrence of lesions that produce a hemi-inattention syndrome.

Clinical Presentation

One of the first cases of a focal hemineglect and inattention syndrome was first described by John Hughlings Jackson in 1876 (Jackson, 1932). Jackson's patient exhibited a number of unusual clinical features, including an inability to recognize objects, people, and other visually presented stimuli. Although she showed confusion in situations that required visual recognition, she was not impaired in her reasoning capabilities. The patient was able to see, yet failed to recognize the stimuli that were being presented. Most strikingly, this patient could not fixate on a central point, as she tended to gaze to one side. Eventually, the patient died, and a tumor was noted in the right posterior temporal lobe.

This case demonstrates many of the classical features of what is now known as the *hemi-inattention and neglect syndrome*. The most obvious component of this syndrome is the failure to attend to one side of the visual field. Associated features include a disorientation to place and person, agnostic problems, apraxia, and spatial disorientation. In Jackson's patient, there was also a motor impersistence, raising interesting questions about the role of motor control systems in this syndrome.

Since this initial report, many cases of lateral neglect have been described in the neurological literature. The fact that this disorder is so dramatically lateralized has certainly contributed to the interest in this phenomenon. Also, the fact that the nondominant cerebral hemisphere is often implicated has raised hopes that this syndrome may lead to an understanding of the role of the "other side" of the brain.

Although neglect syndromes were originally thought to be the product of lesions of the nondominant hemisphere, hemineglect is not exclusively a right-hemisphere brain disorder. Therefore, the interpretation of the phenomenology of this syndrome is not clear-cut. Although most researchers agree that there is a larger percentage of patients with neglect resulting from right-hemisphere lesions, the proportions have been estimated to be approximately 10–1 across different studies (Weinstein & Friedland, 1977).

Neurobehavioral Profile

Patients with hemi-inattention syndromes may fail to recognize stimuli presented in different modalities, although examples of visual and tactile neglect are most commonly described. In some clinical examples, patients cannot recognize body parts on one side of their bodies. When asked to draw or copy simple figures and objects, a patient with neglect may misrepresent features on the side contralateral to their cortical lesion. Hemi-inattention has also been described in other sensory modalities, including a unilateral loss of responsivity to olfactory, gustatory, and tactile stimulation. Within the somatosensory modality, an altered response to vibratory stimuli has been well documented.

The body position and direction of movement are often disturbed in disorders of neglect. Patients may direct their gaze or their entire body position away from the side contralateral to the region of the lesion. The ability to follow directions may also be lateralized. The patient who is able to respond appropriately by moving an arm on the intact side may flounder when asked to perform an identical task on the impaired side of their spatial frame of reference. A neglect of one side may also be evident in basic living skills, such as a patient's failure to dress on one side.

Although much emphasis has been placed on sensory inattention, unilateral neglect has also been demonstrated relative to emotional experience and memory performance. It is not uncommon for patients to show disturbed emotional experience relative to stimuli presented to the neglected side of the spatial field. A patient followed by our group showed such a disturbance, as he responded appropriately when approached from his intact side, but he became hostile and verbally combative when social interactions were initiated from the impaired side. Memory deficits may also reflect the side of neglect, as the patient may recall stimuli presented from one side, but not from the other. These examples illustrate that hemi-inattention syndromes cannot be conceptualized as simply sensory or motor deficits.

Patients with severe hemisensory disorders may have no signs of a neglect problem, as they may be able to read, write, and perform constructional tasks without lateral deficits. Even patients with dense homonymous hemianopia may be free of hemi-inattention. In contrast, patients with hemi-inattention may show relatively intact visual fields. Similarly motor deficits are not the basis of the problem. Although patients may fail to gaze to one side, they are usually capable of the necessary occulomotor movement through other means of stimulation. At times the relationship between the sensory disturbances present following damage to the visual cortex may be difficult to dissociate from hemi-neglect. For instance, Nadeau & Heilman (1991) recently described a patient with hemianopia who did not exhibit a hemi-spatial neglect. Yet, this patient's hemianopia was dependent on the direction of gaze.

While hemi-neglect syndromes are often difficult to dissociate from hemisensory disorders, hemi-neglect seems to best fit the criteria for an attentional disorder. The patient is often capable of sensory and motor processing and yet selectively attends in a unilateral fashion. The fact that neglect can be dissociated from primary sensory and motor processes is a strong reason for viewing it as affecting a separate cognitive system. Furthermore, the intensity and specificity of neglect often arise across contexts. The patient may show neglect in one situation and not in others. Such variability is also consistent with expectations about attentional phenomena.

One of the interesting characteristics of neglect is the tendency of patients to show indifference to, denial, or lack of awareness of their symptoms. Often, patients confabulate and produce elaborate descriptions that are complete fabrications about their neglected side. This syndrome may even take the form of a depersonalization of the affected body part. The alteration in affective response to the neglected side suggests an interrelationship between emotional experience and attention.

As described earlier, the neglect syndrome often coexists with other neuropsychological deficits. The occurrence of apraxia in these patients is most notable. Hecaen *et al.* (1956) demonstrated that, in 59 cases of unilateral spatial agnosia, a vast majority of the patients (95%) also exhibited constructional apraxia. A significant percentage of the patients (35%) also exhibited both unilateral neglect and "dressing" apraxia. Confusion in spatial orientation is often apparent, as the patient may not be able to follow a map or maintain a direction while traveling on a particular route. Of course, part of this impairment may relate directly to unilateral inattention.

Psychometric Characteristics

Many brain disorders result in subtle neuropsychological deficits that can be detected only by careful quantification. In contrast, the neglect syndromes are often so dramatic that it is relatively easy to demonstrate the disorder. Therefore, the evaluation of hemi-inattention can often be conducted solely on the basis of behavioral observation and bedside examination using qualitative measures. However, this is not always the case. The evaluation of hemi-inattention can be facilitated through careful psychometric assessment that includes the following types of measures.

Task Analysis

Assessment of the patient's response tendencies on routine tasks is often very informative. Observations may suggest a tendency to omit words or items from one side of material that the subject is asked to read. A similar pattern of response may be noted when patients are asked to describe the contents of a picture. Patients may fail in their spontaneous drawing or copying of simple objects; they may omit or distort critical features on one side of the drawing (see Figure 9.1).

Lateralizing Tasks

A failure to respond to stimuli from one side of the environment may be demonstrated. When a series of auditory stimuli are presented, there may be a failure to respond to sounds or even voices on one side. An inability to gaze in one lateral direction may provide another indication. Unilateral gaze deficits may occur either in pursuit response or to commands. Another visual task that may help to delineate the disorder involves the presentation of paired stimuli in the intact visual field. Often, patients with hemi-inattention shift their gaze away from the impaired side, even though the stimuli are actually presented in the intact field.

Body Part Identification

Deficits in response to commands to respond with a limb on one side may be demonstrated. For instance, the patient may be unable to follow a simple instruction with the left arm and yet will not have problems doing so with the right arm. An inability to identify body parts on one side may be seen. Similarly, problems with right–left orientation may be evident.

Line Bisection

A popular task for the detection of this disorder involves the bisecting of a large number of lines randomly placed on a sheet of paper. The patient may fail to bisect lines on one side of the paper. Also, there may be an inability to bisect the lines accurately, as the point of bisection may be consistently shifted to one side. The resulting asymmetry is highly suggestive of hemi-inattention.

Cancellation Tasks

A number of tasks have been developed that require the patient to scan through an array of stimuli and detect (cancel out) all of the items of a certain stimulus class (e.g., the letter *A*). This type of task was used in a large study of hemi-inattention by Diller and Weinberg (1977), who found that hemi-inattention was strongly associated with right-hemisphere brain lesions. Forty percent of their sample of patients with right-hemisphere lesions showed deficits on this task. It was also noted that the nature of the target stimulus

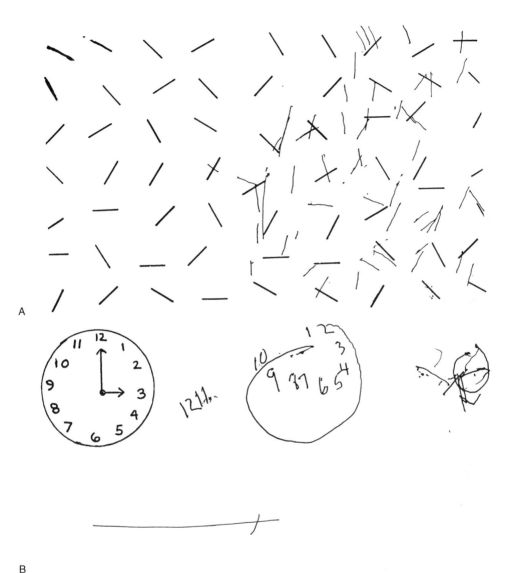

A

B

FIGURE 9.1. (A) Line bisection by a patient with visual neglect syndrome. The patient, W.M., was instructed to bisect all the line segments on the page but only marked the right hemifield. The patient was a 50-year-old man who had suffered a right-hemisphere cardiovascular accident 2 months before his neuropsychological evaluation. Formerly a carpenter and an amateur cartoonist, he was unable to copy or draw the simplest figures. His verbal skills were spared (VIQ = 92), but he was unable to perform any of the WAIS-R Performance tests. His mood was elevated despite his awareness of his deficits. (B) W.M. was asked to copy the clock and produced the middle figure. The numbers have become spatially dissociated from the circle around the clock. The drawing on the far right of the figure is the patient's attempt to draw a clock from memory, showing that his spatial disorganization was even worse when he attempted to use a remembered representation. At the bottom figure shows the patient's attempt to bisect a single horizontal line segment. Note how the line is bisected to the right of center because of a neglect of the left side of the line.

did not predict the quality of the performance, as patients performed at similar levels regardless of the type of stimulus that was presented (i.e., numbers, letters, or pictures). Diller and Weinberg also found that the errors, rather than being errors of commission, were always the result of a tendency to omit or neglect the stimulus.

Diller and Weinberg also found a tendency for patients to omit stimuli from the left side on various tasks. An "anchoring" effect was noted, as patients performed better when cues were given to direct their attention to the extreme left. Other techniques can also be used to override the tendency to neglect. Task performance also depended on the proximity of the stimuli to each other. When the stimuli were spaced farther apart, there was a decrease in error rates. This finding suggests that a rivalry in stimulus processing may account, in part, for the inattention phenomenon.

Double Simultaneous Stimulation

Double simultaneous stimulation (DSS) is perhaps the most theoretically based of the commonly used assessment techniques. DSS involves the presentation of two simultaneous stimuli over repetitive trials. The two stimuli may be presented either within or across modalities. Eventually, the patient may fail to respond to one stimulus, the conclusion being that a lateral extinction effect has occurred. Because this is an important experimental methodology with implications for understanding the mechanisms of this disorder, this technique is discussed in the next section. Some investigators have suggested a distinction between the phenomena of extinction and hemi-inattention (Weinstein & Friedland, 1977; Heilman, Watson, & Valenstein, 1985).

Hypotheses Regarding the Mechanisms Underlying Hemi-Neglect

Many hypotheses have been proposed to account for the neural mechanisms underlying the phenomenon of hemi-neglect since the syndrome was first identified. These hypotheses reflect several major theoretical perspectives that differ with regard to what they emphasize as the primary defect underlying hemi-neglect (Heilman, Watson, & Valenstein, 1985). Neglect and the other related disorders that we have discussed have been attributed to defects of (1) sensation, (2) perception, (3) spatial organization, (4) attention and arousal, and (5) interhemispheric inhibition.

Some of these hypotheses are no longer tenable in light of recent neuropsychological evidence, while other hypotheses have been supported. Each of these hypotheses has been favored by certain factions within the fields of behavioral neurology and neuropsychology at one time or another, and therefore are of both historical and scientific interest. We will briefly review the central tenets underlying each perspective, as this sheds light on current theories regarding the mechanisms underlying the neglect syndromes.

Sensory Defect Hypotheses

Many neurologists prior to 1950 did not distinguish disorders of neglect from other unilateral sensory disturbances. The neglect of one side of the body or environment that some patients with contralateral brain lesions exhibited was considered to result from deafferentation of sensory pathways and/or the sensory cortex. This position was supported by the high incidence of primary sensory disturbance in these patients. Patients with neglect syndrome frequently have a visual hemianopia or decreased somatosensory experience on one side of the body. Therefore, the unilateral quality of neglect seems to fit with the unilateral nature of many sensory disturbances, in which the ascending sensory pathways are disrupted unilaterally.

Proponents of sensory defect hypotheses generally argued that an altered mental state interacts with this sensory defect to produce neglect (Battersby, Bender, & Pollack, 1956). The basis for the sensory defect has been attributed to different causes, including loss of sensory input patterns to the neocortex (Sprague, Chambers, & Stellar, 1961). Others have proposed that asymmetry in sensory input to the two hemispheres accounts for the extinction phenomenon associated with neglect (Eidelberg & Schwartz, 1971).

Perceptual Defect Hypotheses

Alternatively, neglect has been considered by some investigators to be a disorder of perception. Proponents of perceptual defect hypotheses argue that the basis of neglect is not related to the integrity of sensory input, but rather to the quality of sensory integration that follows initial registration. Various mechanisms have been proposed that might underlie the perceptual defect that causes neglect. For instance, neglect has been viewed as a defect of spatial perception resulting from a failure of sensory synthesis (Denny-Brown, Meyer, & Horenstein, 1952; Denny-Brown & Chambers, 1958). This defect of sensory synthesis (amorphosynthesis) causes a failure of spatial summation, which in turn leads to neglect. Failure to process and synthesize multiple simultaneous stimuli (e.g., Double Simultaneous Stimulation) is predicted by this model. Since neglect is often associated with parietal lobe lesions, and the parietal lobes are known to be important to visual spatial processing, there is a logical basis for this hypothesis. While perceptual hypotheses do not consider neglect to be the result of primary sensory failure, perceptual hypotheses do emphasize that the perceptual defect underlying neglect involves a disturbance at the next level of cognitive operation following sensory registration (i.e., sensory synthesis).

Spatial Defect Hypotheses

In contrast to the perceptual hypotheses, spatial defect hypotheses propose that hemi-neglect results from a faulty spatial schemata. The abnormality of spatial schemata is viewed as the result of a defect of intrinsic spatial organization, resulting from alterations in the way the external environment corresponds with an internal spatial representation. Damage to the parietal lobe may produce a "spatial agnosia," as the patient tries to compare stimuli from the external spatial environment with this faulty spatial schemata. A failure to recognize part of the spatial field results. Unlike the perceptual defect hypotheses, which emphasize sensory integration as the basis of neglect, spatial defect hypotheses propose a fundamental distortion of spatial experience (Bisiach, Luzzatti, & Perani, 1979; Bisiach & Luzzatti, 1978).

Attention-Arousal Hypotheses

Advocates of attention-arousal hypotheses maintain that neglect is primarily a form of inattention arising out of a failure of arousal to activate neural systems responsible for spatial attention (Heilman and Watson, 1977; Heilman, Watson, and Valenstein, 1985). Attention-arousal hypotheses postulate that a defect in an actual attentional system of the cortex is at the root of neglect. Therefore, hemi-neglect is fundamentally related to hemi-inattention. The hypotheses discussed previously did not propose the involvement of an attentional system, or that neglect is fundamentally an attentional disorder.

Poppelreuter (1917) used the term "inattention" to describe neglect. Subsequently, the view that neglect was due to inattention was criticized because most patients with neglect cannot consciously override their neglect with concentration or conscious effort. However, this criticism was largely unjustified, since it is now apparent that attention is possible without conscious awareness, volition, or controlled effort. Therefore, whether attention is improved with concentration should not be used as a test for whether attention is involved in a cognitive operation. Furthermore, as we discuss later in this chapter, the severity of neglect apparent at any point in time can be modified by changing task variables.

While there continues to be some disagreement as to whether neglect is fundamentally a disorder of attention, most neuropsychological researchers now believe that attention is at least implicated in the neglect syndrome. Therefore, the analysis of attention has become a major cornerstone in studies of the neglect syndromes.

The attention-arousal hypothesis proposed by Heilman, Watson, and Valenstein (1985) maintains that hemi-inattention and hemi-neglect result from a complex interaction among neural systems that produce arousal or ascending activation and cortical systems that govern spatial selective attention. We will not consider all of the features of the model generated by the attention-arousal hypothesis at this point, as this model is described in greater detail in Chapter 14. However, an important feature of the attention-arousal model is that attention is dependent on a complex interaction of multiple neural systems, including limbic structures, the inferior parietal lobes which act as a multimodal sensory association area, and mesencephalic structures which govern arousal. Other neural models developed to explain the neglect syndromes have also proposed that attention is governed by multiple influences. For instance, Mesulam (1985) proposed a network model to explain neglect and related disorders.

Interhemispheric Hypotheses

The fundamental tenet of the interhemispheric hypotheses is that interactions between the cerebral hemispheres account for the neglect syndrome. The fact that the cerebral hemispheres are specialized for particular cognitive functions (e.g., the left hemispheric language dominance) led some theorists to argue that functional asymmetries between the hemispheres are either exaggerated after cortical lesions that produce neglect or that one hemisphere suppresses the other. For instance, Kinsbourne (1970, 1974) proposed that rivalry between the two hemispheres is the basis for hemi-neglect. After damage to the right hemisphere, the dominance of the left hemisphere is thought by some theorists to increase, which causes a shift of attention to the right side of the spatial environment.

Originally, cortical suppression was thought to occur as a result of this hemispheric imbalance, as one hemisphere dominates and inhibits the impaired side. Extinction would occur because of a suppression of response to the stimulus presented to one side of the spatial field. However, Birch, Belmont, and Karp (1967) proposed an alternative basis for the interhemispheric effect, not dependent on a suppression effect: that slowed information processing in the damaged hemisphere creates a vulnerability to the effects of interference for stimuli occurring on the neglected side of the environment. In contrast, Kinsbourne (1970) proposed that in cases of unilateral cortical damage, continual inhibition across the hemispheres through the corpus callosum may result in decreased trans-callosal activation from the damaged hemisphere to the intact hemisphere. Suppression of the damaged hemisphere by the overly active dominant hemisphere pulls the focus of sensory processing toward the side of space contralateral to the intact hemisphere.

Which Hypothesis Is Correct?

When inexperienced clinicians examine patients who have neglect syndromes, they are likely to interpret the observed disorder as sensory or perceptual. This interpretation arises from the fact that these patients fail to detect stimuli in one half of the environment. The occurrence of deficits across multiple sensory systems clouds this interpretation, as it is difficult to interpret the basis of a multimodal sensory disturbance. Yet, it could be argued that a multimodal sensory disturbance is possible if the neglect syndrome involves higher order sensory integration. However, the demonstration of numerous other clinical and experimental findings makes a pure perceptual or sensory hypothesis untenable. For instance, extinction with double simultaneous stimulation illustrates that neglect is not simply a sensory disorder, as patients who show abnormal extinction often respond well to unilateral stimulation.

There are many examples of findings that illustrate the attentional component associated with hemineglect, extinction, and other related disorders. Although space does not permit an exhaustive review of this evidence, several examples that illustrate the role of attentional parameters deserve address.

Experimental Evidence for an Attentional Mechanism

Perhaps the most compelling evidence that neglect syndromes are not simply sensory or perceptual disorders comes from studies that have considered the influence of nonsensory factors. While the manipulation of psychophysical stimulus dimensions such as loudness or stimulus duration affects the pattern of extinction, a finding supporting a perceptual hypothesis, there are also many nonpsychophysical variables that also influence the severity and the spatial characteristics of the neglect. In the following section we will review several findings that suggest an attention-arousal mechanism for the neglect syndromes.

Cueing to spatial position has been shown to affect the magnitude of deficits found in patients with unilateral neglect (Riddoch & Humphreys, 1983). Riddoch and Humphreys hypothesized an attentional mechanism to account for this effect. However, this study did not directly manipulate attention during the extinction paradigm. A similar effect was also described by Robertson (1989). When subjects were presented cue words on the left side before the bilateral presentation of the target symbols, they sometimes failed to report the symbol on the intact right side of the spatial field. This finding illustrates the role of expectancy in mediating neglect.

In a direct test of the effect of cueing on extinction, Birch, Belmont, and Karp (1967) demonstrated that, when the left-sided stimulus is presented less than a second before the stimulus on the right, extinction is dramatically reduced. They argued that slowed information-processing speed in the damaged hemisphere had created the extinction effect. When the duration between the two stimuli was increased, the effect of this slowing was reduced. However, it could also be argued that the first stimulus on the left side directed attention to that side of space and overrode the extinction effect.

Recently, Kaplan, Verfaellie, DeWitt, and Caplan (1990) tested the possibility that attentional factors mediate the extinction effect during DSS. Their findings demonstrated that task contingencies influence extinction during DSS in a rather remarkable way. Kaplan's patients, who suffered from neglect and extinction of the left visual field during DSS, were given a task in which a visual cue stimulus occurred before each extinction trial. Sometimes, the cue stimulus occurred in the neglected space, and at other times it occurred in the intact hemi-space. In one condition, stimuli were presented in strings of five successive presentations to the intact right side before each presentation to the left hemi-space. In a second condition, the cue stimulus was alternated between the right and left visual fields and in another condition, the cue stimuli were always presented on the left. Paradoxically, the patients showed much greater rates of extinction when the cue stimulus always occurred on the neglected side, whereas they showed the least extinction when a string of cues were presented to the right side.

As Kaplan *et al.* predicted, repeated presentation to the intact hemi-space, when there was expectation of a stimulus to the opposite, impaired hemi-space, decreased the severity of hemispatial extinction. In response to the expectancy of a left-sided presentation, the patients were able to override their tendency to extinguish on the neglected side of the spatial field. These findings illustrate that task demands and response expectancies may greatly influence symptom presentation. This result would not be expected if the neglect syndrome were simply a sensory defect.

By increasing the task demand on visual selective attention, it is also possible to affect the symptoms of hemispatial neglect. Rapcsak, Verfaellie, Fleet, and Heilman (1989) studied the performance of patients with right-hemispheric lesions on cancellation task performance. The difficulty in making a discrimination of target stimuli from distractors varied across the tasks. The patients had much greater difficulty with both the exploration of space on the left side and also visual discrimination performance when the task difficulty increased.

Perhaps the strongest evidence that neglect is not a sensory disorder comes from studies that demonstrate the role of motoric or response-dependent factors. Patients who exhibit spatial neglect fail to adequately scan the environment (Butter, Rapcsak, Watson, & Heilman, 1988). Although it is possible that this exploratory deficiency results from a unilateral defect in spatial representation, the result is a reduced motor response to one hemi-space.

Recent investigations have provided further evidence that neglect of left hemi-space involves a failure of response activation and/or arousal (Cohen, Smith, & Fisher, 1991; Coslett, Bowers, & Heilman, 1987; Coslett & Heilman, 1989; Coslett, Bowers, Fitzpatrick, Haws, & Heilman, 1990; Valenstein & Heilman, 1981; Valenstein, Van Den Abell, Watson, & Heilman, 1982; Verfaellie, Bowers, & Heilman, 1988; Verfaellie, Rapcsak, & Heilman, 1990). For instance, Coslett *et al.* (1989, 1990) demonstrated that patients with neglect caused by right hemispheric stroke not only exhibit a failure to detect stimuli in one hemi-space, but also typically have difficulty initiating movements in the contralateral hemi-space. Patients with right hemisphere damage even had greater difficulty moving their contralateral shoulder, reflecting a hemihypokinesia for a rather gross response.

A close relationship between response intention and sensory attention is often seen in patients with neglect. For instance, Cohen *et al.* (1991) demonstrated that a patient with a right anterior basal ganglia lesion exhibited both a failure in attention to stimulation and in initiating movement and planned responses in the contralateral hemi-space. Verfaellie *et al.* (1988) demonstrated a right hemispheric dominance for response preparation (i.e., intention) on a reaction time test in normal subjects. Ultimately, spatial selective attention probably depends on compatibility between stimulus and response processes (Verfaellie *et al.*, 1988).

Even in disorders that are usually attributed to sensory or perceptual defects, selective attentional impairments may exist. For instance, Verfaellie *et al.* (1990) demonstrated that a patient with Balint's syndrome benefited from attention cuing only when stimuli were presented in the upper visual field. The patient did not benefit from cuing to either the left or right visual fields. Balint's syndrome causes a bilateral failure of visual gaze and is due to bilateral parietal-occipital lesions. This finding illustrates that this perceptual disorder is influenced by attentional factors. However, conclusions about the role of attention in disorders affecting visual perception must be made with caution. For instance, patients with primary visual disturbance may exhibit gaze-dependent hemianopia without actually having a hemispatial neglect (Nadeau and Heilman, 1991).

Findings like those just described lend strong support to the position that hemi-neglect is caused by an attentional failure. Attention and intention reflect cognitive operations that extend well beyond the usual definition of sensory or perceptual phenomena. While some investigators separate attention from intention, we consider both sensory selective attention and response intention to be attentional components, as both influence the selection and control of stimuli and responses. At a minimum, the sensory and response components associated with neglect are so interrelated that it is meaningless to think of these syndromes as simply disorders of spatial organization. A close linkage between various aspects of information processing seems to be important in the production of neglect. Ultimately, neglect has perceptual, motoric, spatial, and interhemispheric characteristics.

In recent years, researchers have combined components of these different hypotheses. For instance, Heilman, Watson, and Valenstein (1985) provided an alternative to the original spatial, attention–arousal, and interhemispheric hypotheses by suggesting that neglect involves disturbances across these three functions. From the standpoint of the interhemispheric hypothesis, the intact hemisphere may be capable of orienting to either side of space. Yet, when simultaneous processing of multiple stimuli is required, the intact hemisphere becomes overloaded and decreased responsivity to the neglected side occurs.

In the next section, the neuroanatomical substrates of the neglect and hemi-inattention syndromes are discussed. Evidence that multiple brain systems produce neglect provides another strong argument against the notion that these syndromes are related to a primary sensory disturbance. Defects of systems normally associated with arousal, sensorimotor integration, and response selection and control have all been shown to produce disorders of neglect.

Neuroanatomical Evidence

Neglect and hemi-inattention provide one of the clearest examples of a disorder of attention caused by focal neuroanatomical damage. In fact, the most interesting aspect of the neglect and inattention syndromes is their unusual spatial distribution. Patients with global cortical damage may actually show a greater inattention to external stimuli. However, their inattention is of less neuropsychological interest because it does not tell us much about the distribution of attentional processes. The demonstration of hemi-inattention illustrates the specificity of attentional processes.

Nondominant Parietal Lobe

Early studies of unilateral neglect proposed that the nondominant parietal lobe was the principal site of the lesions producing this disorder. Hecaen, Penfield, Bertrand, and Malmo (1956) described unilateral neglect after surgical removal of the right inferior parietal lobule in a series of patients. Other studies have described neglect after infarctions in this region (Denny-Brown & Chambers, 1958; Heilman, Pandya, Karol, & Geschwind, 1971; Heilman & Valenstein, 1972) (see Figure 9.2). Recent studies have demonstrated that patients with parietal lesions have great difficulty disengaging from stimuli in right hemispace when they are required to orient covertly with a shift of attention to the left (Posner, Walker, Friedrich, & Rafal, 1984).

Although much of our knowledge of hemi-inattention syndromes comes from direct clinical observations of humans, there have also been experimental studies of neglect in other animals. In fact, the earliest evidence for neglect came from studies in which various anatomical locations were lesioned in animals. Recent studies of single-unit neural activity in the monkey's inferior parietal lobule indicate increased activation associated with scanning of and grasping toward motivationally salient stimuli (Bushness et al., 1981; Hyvanrinen, Poranen, & Jokinen, 1980; Mountcastle, Lynch, Georgopoulos, Sakata, & Acuna,

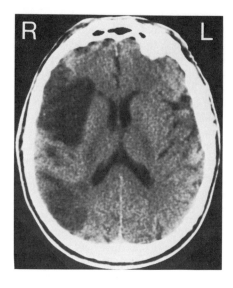

FIGURE 9.2. CT scan from a patient with a recent cerebrovascular infarction involving the right hemisphere. This individual exhibited the classic symptoms of hemispatial inattention, unilateral neglect, extinction, lack of body awareness, and orienting defects of the left side.

1975). This activation was found to occur even in the absence of motoric factors such as eye movements. Yet, these experiments also indicate that this region's activation is contingent on sensory, motoric, and motivational factors. Manipulations of any of these factors influence the firing rates of cells in this region.

Other Neuroanatomical Sites of Neglect

Although neglect is most commonly noted after nondominant parietal lobe damage, it has also been found in patients with damage to other cortical and subcortical lesions, including the cingulate gyrus, the lateral prefrontal cortex, the thalamus, and subcortical centers like the basal ganglia, the internal capsule, the nigral-striatal pathways, the reticular system, and the intralaminar nuclei.

Many of the earliest studies showed that lesions to structures of the frontal regions cause neglect (Bianchi, 1895; Welch & Stuteville, 1958). Lesions of the frontal eye fields produce contralateral neglect. Studies by Goldberg and Bushnell (1981) demonstrated that neurons of the frontal eye fields are activated before the onset of saccades, a finding suggesting an attentional response. Watson, Miller, and Heilman (1978) produced nonsensory contralateral neglect in monkeys by lesioning the frontal eye fields for motivationally relevant stimuli, suggesting that the lesions had produced a hemispatial attentional deficit rather than a hemisensory disturbance.

Neglect has been demonstrated through the experimental lesioning of a wide range of subcortical structures, including the brain stem, the reticular pathways, the cingulum, the superior colliculus and amygdala, and the basal and the nigral-striatal system. Although we do not provide here a detailed discussion of each of these findings, the diversity of the sites that can produce neglect is striking. The fact that lesions in these different structures are capable of producing neglect suggests that hemi-inattention depends on the interaction of limbic, sensory, and reticular inputs to the parietal lobes, which affects both covert orienting in space and overt motoric activity such as saccadic eye movement.

Split-Brain Influences

Studies of neurosurgical patients who have undergone commissurotomy have yielded a wealth of data regarding the importance of interhemispheric interactions in normal cognitive functioning. Following this surgery, most patients with a "split brain" can perform a task with one hand, while the actions of their other hand suggest a unilateral unawareness of what the other side is doing. Yet, some investigators have argued that this unusual behavior does not truly reflect an inattention (Joynt, 1977), as these patients often show an aware-ness of incorrect responses of one cerebral hemisphere by the opposite hemisphere.

Experimental studies of postcommissurotomy patients suggest that there may in fact be an inattention syndrome present. Levy and her colleagues (Levy, 1974; Levy & Trevarthen, 1976; Levy, Trevarthen, & Sperry, 1972) devised tasks in which simultaneous stimuli were presented tachistoscopically to each hemisphere. The subjects were asked to match the pictures on either graphic or semantic characteristics. Split-brain patients showed a fluctua-tion in performance, as the criteria that they used to make a match varied across trials. Levy *et al.* noted that patients never matched on the criteria of both semantic and graphic quality and therefore argued. This finding suggested that they were showing an alternating unilateral inattention.

Other studies have indicated that the instructional set may affect the bias to respond with either the left or the right hemisphere. Levy (1974) argued that this type of task illustrates that hemi-inattention phenomena may result not only from depressed activation of the impaired hemisphere, but also from an imbalance of activation between the hemi-spheres.

Kinsbourne's work (1970, 1971, 1982) also emphasized hemispheric effects in explaining hemineglect, as well as other attentional effects. For instance, when subjects were asked to swing their heads to the left, they responded with shorter reaction times on a spatial-pattern matching task. Kinsbourne argued that the lateralizing effects of task requirements orient the individual in a manner that will ultimately affect selective attention. These effects are considered a function of natural tendencies to orient to the right side, because of left-hemispheric dominance.

Comment: Although neglect and hemi-inattention are characterized by the presence of hemispheric asymmetries, ultimately one may question whether the laterality associated with these syndromes is the most interesting feature. The hemispatial character of neglect arises in large part because of the unilateral nature of the brain disorder. What happens if both cortical hemispheres are damaged?

Balint's syndrome is a disorder that arises from bilateral occipital damage. Patients with Balint's syndrome experience an inability to turn their eyes to a point in the visual field. They also can not grasp under visual guidance and show a general visual inattention. This condition has sometimes been described as a psychic paralysis of gaze. Although some patients with Balint's syndrome exhibit cortical blindness, it is possible for these patients to have primary disorders of spatial exploration and bilateral inattention.

As we described earlier, Verfaellie *et al.* (1990) demonstrated that a patient with Balint's syndrome failed to benefit from cues directed to the right and left hemi-space. Rizzo and Robin (1990) also demonstrated a defect of sustained attention associated with simultan-agnosia in two patients with bilateral superior occipital stroke. With simultanagnosia, a disorder in which individuals cannot report the occurrence of multiple stimuli presented simultaneously, patients describe their visual experience in a haphazard, unintegrated manner. The fact that this syndrome, often considered a form of primary perceptual dysfunction, has an attentional component leads to some interesting possibilities. First, it suggests that bilateral posterior cortical damage may influence attention with respect to the entire spatial frame. Second, these cases illustrate that attentional disturbance may be nested in more primary perceptual defects.

A fundamental question remains: Is the hemispheric asymmetry associated with the neglect syndromes a critical determinant of the underlying attentional disorder? It is possible that although neglect is lateralized because of the unilateral nature of the brain disorder, the accompanying unilateral asymmetry is merely a manifestation that makes the attention disorder stand out. With bilateral damage, more severe forms of inattention may exist, though this inattention is harder to measure because it is embedded in fundamental problems with perceptual detection across the entire spatial field.

Hemi-Inattention and the Orienting Response

The relationship between hemi-inattention and the orienting response (OR) is evident in the early models of this disorder. In particular, the concept of extinction was used to describe the effects of double simultaneous stimulation. The two stimuli have inhibitory effects on each other, so that the stimuli on the neglected side are more likely to be ignored. By using the concepts derived from experiments on the orienting response, Heilman and his colleagues (Heilman & Watson, 1977; Heilman, Watson, & Valenstein, 1985) developed an attention-arousal hypothesis of neglect.

Experimental tests of this hypothesis have indicated that a state similar to neglect can be produced in monkeys by lesioning the reticular formation of the mesenchephalon (Watson, Heilman, Miller, & King, 1974). Similar effects were noted in lesion studies using rodents. Marshall, Turner, and Teitelbaum (1971) produced neglect by lateral hypothalamic lesions that destroyed reticular-hypothalamic pathways. Destruction of other subcortical structures such as the nigrostriatal system has also been shown to produce neglect.

The attention-arousal hypothesis posits that neglect is fundamentally a disorder of the orienting response reflected by a failure to activate the nondominant hemisphere of the brain which controls attention. For instance, cues that are directed unilaterally have been shown to influence the effect of unilateral-neglect-inducing lesions on task performance. When animals were trained to perform tasks in hemispace that required the animal to respond following a cue, the effect of unilateral lesions is greatest on cuing to the ipsilateral side. Similar findings have been noted in human studies. This finding cannot be easily explained through a sensory hypothesis.

Studies of EEG activity associated with experimentally induced neglect have yielded interesting results. Although animals with bilateral midbrain lesions often show generalized slowing on EEG, animals that show neglect often have unilateral slowing (Watson et al., 1974). In studies of human neglect, similar findings have been noted. Watson and Heilman (1977) found that 22 of 23 patients with neglect had unilateral slowing on the side of their parietal lobe lesion. The late components of the event-related potential also appears to change following cortical lesioning, whereas the earlier sensory components are relatively unaffected.

Summary

Although extinction can be partially explained by means of a simple sensory model, a more comprehensive attentional model is necessary to explain the full range of findings related to extinction and neglect. Although we have emphasized the symptoms of neglect, extinction, and inattention in this review. We have discussed evidence that factors associated with expectancy, attentional task demands, response selection, and intentionality influence these disorders.

Neglect is a unilateral phenomenon and therefore, some interhemispheric mechanism seems to be implicated. Certainly, the incidence of neglect following right-hemisphere lesions supports this likelihood. However, arguments over whether these syndromes occur because of hypoarousal of the impaired hemisphere or because of a disinhibition of a suppressed hemisphere continue. This issue, although significant, may be less important than resolving the nature of the relationship between the neural systems governing spatial representation and other systems responsible for exploration, arousal, as well as the other components that comprise these syndromes.

The fact that neglect can be induced through subcortical lesions in animals indicates that the hemispheric effects maybe secondary to the changes in the mediation of normal activation by the reticular or other, associated systems. Ultimately, there appears to be a normal balance of cerebral activation, which is disrupted with lesions that cause neglect and that may occur at different anatomical levels. An examination of the spectrum of symptoms found in patients with neglect leads to the unavoidable conclusion that these syndromes reflect a hemiattention resulting from the interaction of a complex set of factors. There probably is not one isolated mechanism for neglect. Instead, neglect and hemi-inattention are attentional disorders of unilateral arousal and orienting, relative to a temporal-spatial frame of reference.

PARIETAL AND TEMPORAL LOBE INFLUENCES

The parietal and temporal lobes have traditionally been viewed as sensory association areas. Damage to certain temporal and parietal areas produces specific sensory or perceptual disturbances. These sensory areas contain a neuroarchitectural arrangement that is relatively fixed and that provides a concise environmental representation. In addition to the sensory systems are other areas that perform secondary analyses on sensory information. These secondary analyses may be limited to one type of information, or they may integrate multiple forms of information. Sensory integration and high-level associations require less specificity of function and the capacity to modify operations based on the information at hand.

Damage to the parietal and temporal regions is often associated with attentional disturbances or confusional states. The most striking examples are the neglect syndromes, which we discussed in the previous section. Although neglect is associated with damage to other regions, parietal damage is the most frequent cause of these syndromes. If the temporal-parietal areas are primarily involved in the creation of a sensory representation, how is it that they influence attentional processing? As Mesulam (1981, 1985) pointed out, the representational map provided by the temporal-parietal association areas is dynamic and shifting. Current templates of the external environment are modifiable based on new stimulus information. Attentional selection and focusing may emerge as a result of systemic integrative properties that create these modifications. This is best understood by considering the neuroanatomical arrangement of sensory association areas (see Figure 9.3).

Behavioral Geography

The parietal and temporal lobes contain many neuroanatomical regions. Located within each lobe are both modality-specific and multimodal association areas. Mesulam (1985) differentiated between unimodal (modality-specific) cortex that responds to one type of sensory input and heteromodal areas that integrate information from multiple modalities. Modality-specific areas perform second-order processing of input from specific primary

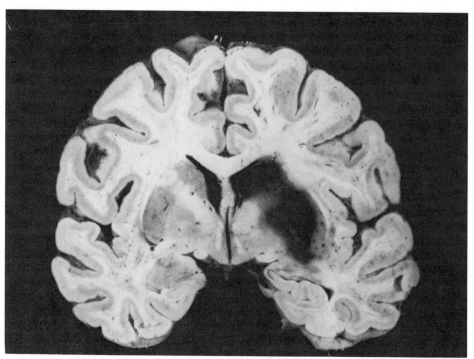

FIGURE 9.3. Coronal section of human brain from a 72-year-old woman who developed a profound neglect syndrome secondary to a hemorrhagic infarct affecting the right anterior basal ganglia. Her lesion involved the anterior limb of the internal capsule, caudate nucleus, putamen, and globus pallidus. The posterior limb of the internal capsule and thalamus were spared. The patient exhibited left hemineglect to visual and tactile stimuli, anasognosia, and failure to recognize the left side of her body. A failure to sustain motor and exploratory behavior on the left side of space was also noted. This case demonstrates that selective damage to an extrapyramidal structure may affect both sensory selective attention and intentional response control.

sensory areas such as V1, S1, and A1. The auditory cortex (A1) is found on Heschl's gyrus in the posterior temporal lobe. The somatosensory cortex (S1) is contained in the postcentral gyrus, the most anterior-superior parietal area.

Surrounding S1 and A1 are modality-specific association areas. Posterior to S1 is the superior parietal lobule, which performs processing of primary somatosensory input. The superior temporal gyrus is modality-specific for auditory input. The most posterior part of this gyrus is generally considered part of Wernicke's area and is critical in processing the auditory input of language.

The primary visual system (V1) is actually found in the occipital lobe, though many of the modality-specific association areas for this system are found in the temporal and parietal lobes. Following initial registration in V1 in primates, visual information is processed in the adjacent peristriatal cortex, where analyses of featural, spatial, and movement characteristics are performed. Visual information then progresses to anterior modality-specific regions of the temporal and parietal cortex. Experimental evidence indicates that in primates, visual information is processed along two pathways (Mishkin, Ungerleider, &

Macko, 1983; Ungerleider, 1985). A superior pathway projects to modality-specific areas of the superior parietal lobule and handles low-spatial-frequency input with information about spatial location. An inferior pathway projects to temporal visual association areas that perform high-spatial-frequency analyses regarding featural characteristics.

A number of multimodal association areas are also found in temporal-parietal regions. In the parietal lobes, the angular gyrus, the supramarginal gyrus of the inferior lobule, and the rostral and caudal superior lobules have multimodal functions. The temporal lobe contains many more modality-specific and paralimbic areas. However, some multimodal integration occurs in the medial temporal regions and in the superior temporal sulcus. The multimodal areas of the temporal lobe seem to integrate limbic information with visual and auditory input.

The multimodal areas of the parietal and temporal lobes are often considered higher order association areas because they are associated with cognitive operations somewhat removed from primary sensory analysis. The multimodal areas of the superior lobule receive somatosensory and visual projections and contain neural systems involved in somatospatial and visual-spatial integration. Aspects of the left inferior parietal lobule, as well as adjacent temporal regions, are involved in language and verbal associative processes. Damage to these heteromodal association areas produce complex language problems such as anomia, alexia, left–right disorientation, and Gerstmann syndrome. Nondominant parietal lobe damage is more likely to produce constructional apraxias, visual-spatial impairments, and confusional states (Benton, 1967, 1973; Benton & Fogel, 1962). Furthermore, damage to multimodal visual and somatosensory association areas

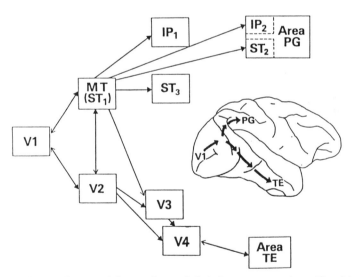

FIGURE 9.4. Visual cortical areas of the monkey and their known connections. Visual information diverges from the striate cortex (V1) along two pathways. The superior occipitoparietal pathway projects dorsally to the medial temporal (MT) and superior temporal ares (ST₁). From these areas information flows the the inferior parietal area (IP₁) and to the superior temporal area (ST₃). Visual information from MT also is directed to area PG, which contains the inferior parietal lobule (IP₂) and the superior temporal lobule (ST₂), where spatial processing is thought to occur. The inferior occipitotemporal pathway directs information through a series of visual neural systems (V2, V3, V4) and eventually reaches the temporal area (TE), where object recognition processes are thought to occur.

often results in alterations in body schemata and in the spatial organization of experience (Popelreuter, 1917; Ratcliff, 1982; Ratcliff & Newcombe, 1973). These systems seem to contain a template or "distributed associative network" of temporal-spatial information (long-term memory).

Attentional Operations of the Parietal Systems

Neural systems of the parietal lobes play an important role in many cognitive functions. Localized damage to specific areas of the parietal lobes produce differential patterns of cognitive dysfunction. As described previously, different areas of the parietal lobes have been implicated in language, visual-spatial and visual-integrative, somatosensory, and memory functioning. While all of these cognitive functions have at least indirect influence on attention, some, like visual-spatial analysis, play a significant role in establishing the parameters and constraints on attention. Since attentional processes control the selection of information from the external environment, the nature of spatial representation in the parietal lobe undoubtedly influences the way attention is allocated.

The parietal lobes also contain neural systems that are important for associative memory. Other brain systems, such as the hippocampus and paralimbic structures, have been shown to be essential for memory encoding and the formation of long-term storage (e.g., Zola-Morgan and Squire, 1986). Yet once encoded, memory is probably stored as a distributed associative network within heteromodal cortical areas in the parietal and temporal lobes (Mesulam, 1981, 1985; Rumelhart, Hinton, McClelland, 1986). Associative processes within temporal-parietal cortical areas are critical for attention, as they create a continually changing schemata upon which current information processing is referenced. The comparison of new stimuli to existing schemata has long been thought to be central to attentional operations. For instance, Sokolov (1960, 1976) proposed that such a comparison process was the basis of the orienting responses (OR). Even after the OR has occurred and the individual is actively attending to certain information, attentional allocation is governed by the salience or associative strength of the information. Therefore, associative networks within the parietal lobes have a direct influence on attention. The relationship between memory and attention will be further considered in Chapter 18.

Associative and visual-spatial representations within the parietal lobes seem to influence attention by providing a reference or schema for information being processed. However, there is also evidence that certain areas of the parietal lobe have an even more direct role in selective spatial attention. As we discussed previously, damage to the nondominant parietal lobe has long been associated with cases of unilateral neglect (e.g., Denny-Brown & Chambers, 1958). Subsequent researchers demonstrated that an attentional disturbance underlies hemi-neglect, since after right hemispheric brain damage many patients have difficulties directing attention to the left. This finding led to the development of attentional theories of neglect (Heilman, Watson, & Valenstein, 1985). Most attentional theories of neglect maintain that the nondominant parietal lobe contains a specialized area that governs attentional selection across the spatial environment.

Investigators have tried to distinguish which parietal regions are most critical for attention. Most emphasis has been directed toward characterizing the roles of the superior and inferior parietal lobules (e.g., Heilman & Watson, 1976; Heilman & Van Den Abell, 1979, 1980; Posner, Walker, Friedrich, & Rafal, 1980, 1987). While systems contained in the parietal lobe are not the sole determinant of hemi-neglect, parietal damage is the most frequent cause of these syndromes. Furthermore, as we discussed earlier, there have been numerous demonstrations of complex attentional operations under the control of neural systems of the parietal lobe.

Perhaps the strongest experimental evidence for attentional operations within the parietal lobes comes from studies of attention in primates. For instance, efforts directed to specifying which parietal and/or temporal areas are most responsible for attention in primates have indicated that specialized parietal areas for attention seem to exist (Desimone & Gross, 1979; Desimone, Albright, Gross, & Bruce, 1980; Goldberg & Robinson, 1977, 1980; Wurtz, Goldberg, & Robinson, 1980, 1982). The superior parietal cortex has been differentiated from the inferior parietal regions on the basis of the type of processing that is performed. Area PG of the inferior parietal lobule seems to respond when animals look at motivationally relevant objects. Single-unit recordings taken from this region in primates indicate that neurons activate before actual sensory analysis as the animal prepares for a target in the peripheral visual field (Bushnell, Goldberg, and Robinson, 1981). This region is responsive to complex object recognition and also enhances in its response when motoric response is required. The direction of visual gaze influences the response of inferior parietal neuron (Anderson & Mountcastle, 1980).

The inferior parietal lobule responds to the spatial position of the object that is processed and to abstract figure-ground relationship parameters. This responsivity is a fundamental aspect of sensory selection based on spatial location (Lynch, 1980; Ungerleider & Mishkin, 1982). The sensitivity of this region to task-relevant visual targets provides support for the idea that the inferior parietal lobule performs attentional operations (Goldberg & Robinson, 1977, 1980; Goldberg & Seagraves, 1987; Wurtz, Goldberg, & Robinson, 1980, 1982). Stimuli with greater motivational salience are likely to elicit greater neuronal responses, suggesting that the inferior parietal lobule is very sensitive to motivational signals and response demands. Furthermore, the attentional response of the inferior parietal lobule seems to occur independent of eye tracking movements, which illustrates that the spatial response of this area is not secondary to motor activation or pre-motor influences. Yet, neurons in this region show enhanced response when a subsequent motoric response is required.

Attentional Capacity of Temporal Neurons

The temporal cortex is an extremely complex neuroanatomical region that contains a multitude of heterogeneous functional systems. Contained within the temporal lobes are neural systems involved in visual associative operations, auditory processing, language, memory consolidation, and emotional-motivational processing (i.e., limbic and paralimbic structures). Because of the functional heterogeneity of the temporal lobes, it is difficult to characterize a simple relationship of this region to attention.

The associative and memory functions of the temporal lobe influence attention for the reasons we discussed previously for the parietal lobes. The temporal lobes seem to be part of a broad associative network, along with the areas of the parietal lobes, which form a distributed memory system. Associative information within the temporal cortex undoubtedly contributes to formation of schemata upon which new information is referenced.

The auditory processing functions of the temporal lobes also play a likely role for certain types of attention. For instance, short-term memory and attention span may be influenced by the auditory processing capacity of the individual. Contained in the temporal lobes are neural systems that are important for the timing and sequencing of information. Linguistic sequencing and syntax is often disrupted after lesions appear in temporal language structures. Therefore, it appears likely that while some parietal-temporal systems create a spatial representation (like a photographic snapshot), other neural systems contained in the temporal lobe piece together these single frames into temporal continuity. Syntactic and other language operations of the left temporal lobe probably influence the sequentiality and/or logic of serial attentional operations. However, relatively few investigations have been made into this relationship.

Limbic and paralimbic structures that are closely associated with medial temporal areas play an important role in attention. By modulating the salience or emotional-motivational value of information to be processed, the medial temporal lobes help to establish the focus of attention. Motivationally relevant information is enhanced through associative elaboration, while the response to irrelevant information diminishes. The limbic system's role in attention will be discussed in greater detail in the next chapter.

While the temporal cortex seems to influence some attentional processes, it does not appear to be critical for spatial selective attention. While some investigators have reported that monkeys have impaired eye movements during discrimination learning following inferior temporal ablation (Bagshaw, Mackworth, & Pribram, 1970), it is not clear that this effect was directly associated with an attentional dysfunction. Following temporal lobectomy, patients rarely exhibit neglect syndromes. Brain diseases such as herpes encephalitis may unilaterally damage major portions of the temporal lobe and dramatically impair memory without producing significant problems with selective spatial attention (see Figure 9.5).

Certain temporal areas play a significant role in visual processing. The inferior parietal lobule is less responsive to object recognition and discrimination demands and more responsive to information regarding spatial position. Conversely, the areas such as the superior temporal sulcus appear to be tuned to analyze featural characteristics of objects (Desimone & Ungerleider, 1986; Ungerleider & Desimone, 1986). Neurons of the superior temporal cortex also appear to be less responsive to motivational influences, though they may be very responsive to very specific types of stimuli with high motivational salience, such as faces (Bruce, Desimone & Gross, 1981). Lesions of the superior temporal sulcus disrupt object discrimination and featural analysis. However, there is also evidence that this region is rather heterogeneous in function, and that multiple visual areas exist in regions of the caudal superior temporal sulcus (Desimone & Ungerleider, 1986).

Attention as a Function of Two Visual Systems

Primates appear to process information along two separate visual processing pathways following initial sensory registration (Mishkin, Ungerleider, and Macko, 1983; Ungerleider & Desimone, 1986; Ungerleider & Mishkin, 1982). The superior visual system is more responsive to low-spatial-frequency information, while the inferior pathway seems to respond to high-spatial-frequency information. Neurons tuned to low spatial frequencies are not useful for providing information about an object's features, but are likely to be very sensitive to broad spatial characteristics, such as the position of an object. Conversely, neurons tuned to high spatial frequencies are likely to be very sensitive to featural characteristics, but not to spatial position. In terms of an old proverb, the high-spatial-frequency neurons cannot see the forest, only the trees. The high-spatial-frequency system reaches its most complex level of representation within the temporal lobe, while the highest level of low-spatial-frequency system is located in the inferior parietal lobule (area *PG*).

Other investigators have also shown that neurons of areas along each of these routes vary as a function of featural parameters. Not only is there a dissociation between the superior and inferior visual routes based on a spatial-frequency preference, but visual neurons also show preferences for different sizes and regions within the visual field (Mountcastle, 1978, 1979; Mountcastle, Anderson, & Motter, 1981; Mountcastle, Lynch, Georgopoulos, Sakata, & Acuna, 1975; Mountcastle, Motter, Steinmetz, & Duffy, 1984). Therefore, areas of the visual system seem to be tuned to different combinations of featural spatial frequency and visual field regional preference.

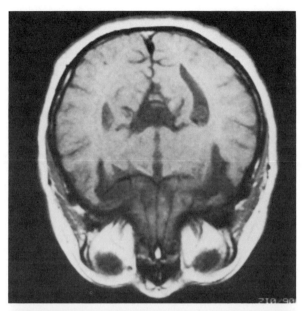

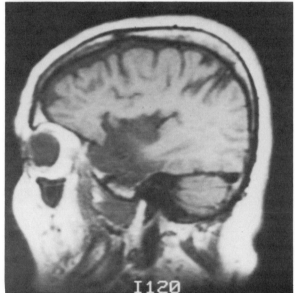

FIGURE 9.5. MRI scan of a woman with bilateral medial temporal lobe and basal frontal lesions. This 44-year-old woman developed a severe amnestic disorder at age 16. She continued to suffer from persistent anterograde amnesia and residual behavioral disturbances, including anosmia, compulsive eating, flat affect, behavioral inertia, and social withdrawal. Nevertheless, her verbal and visual integrative capacity remained well above average (VIQ = 117, PIQ = 125). Her performance on psychometric tests of attention were largely within normal limits. In contrast to the patient in Figure 9.2, this patient exhibited essentially intact attentional capabilities, even though her memory was severely disturbed. The limbic and basal forebrain damage appeared to be reflected primarily in motivational disturbance and impoverished affect. Her case illustrates that attention and memory dysfunction can be dissociated, and that a severe amnestic disorder can coexist with spared attentional functions. Attention does not seem to be undifferentially distributed across all temporal regions.

Based on the information-processing characteristics of each of these systems, one might predict that activation of neurons within each system prior to an actual stimulus presentation produces different attentional effects. The sensitivity of neurons for selection based on particular featural characteristics should vary based on the anticipatory information that is provided. Neurophysiological investigations have largely supported this prediction, as activation of neural systems in each of these areas before a target stimulus is presented produces different anticipatory effects. The modulation of visual selection biases following the presentation of anticipatory cues, but before the actual target stimulus presentation, has been labeled sensory enhancement.

Both inferior parietal and temporal neural systems activate in response to the expectancy of incoming information, though they do so relative to different stimulus characteristics (e.g., Desimone & Gross, 1979; Desimone, Albright, Gross, & Bruce, 1980; Goldberg & Seagraves, 1987). The occurrence of sensory enhancement seems to reflect an attentional process, associated with the focusing of processing resources for optimal performance. By enhancing or attenuating the response of neurons prior to actual sensory analysis, sensory focusing and selection during early stages of visual processing prior to later stage sequential operations becomes possible. Of course, attentional effect associated with sensory enhancement ultimately depends on expectancies that are created by previous behavioral experiences, response demands, and motivational influences. Furthermore, the act of attending to spatial locations enhances the perceptual sensitivity (Bashinski & Backrach, 1980).

Focal Attention and the Temporal Lobes

While the role of the inferior parietal lobe in visual selective attention in humans is well accepted, there is less agreement on how visual systems in the temporal lobe influence attention. There are relatively few neuropsychological investigations using human subjects that dissociate parietal and temporal functioning on the basis of the different types of visual tasks that we have just discussed. While clinical descriptions of visual spatial disturbance following posterior cortical damage are abundant, it is difficult to study patients using the methodologies of primate researchers. Furthermore, the high-spatial-frequency preference attributed to the temporal lobes is typically considered an aspect of visual perception, recognition, or synthesis, not attention. Yet, there are good reasons to ask how attention interacts with featural detection, recognition, and synthesis.

Although featural detection is largely a perceptual phenomenon, there must be a mechanism that directs attention to local features of objects. If we view spatial attention as a telescope scanning space, we can also form an analogy of perceptual attention as a microscope searching for the relevant fine featural characteristics of objects. In each case, we must account for a search component that directs the level and specificity of attentional focus. Therefore, it is reasonable to predict that the object recognition capacity of the temporal lobes is also influenced by attentional factors. Unfortunately, at this point the attentional processes underlying such object focusing are less well understood, though expectancy seems to be important to all attentional operations.

As we discussed previously, both parietal and temporal neural systems may be activated by the expectancy of incoming information, though their response to expectancy may be to different characteristics of information. Enhancing or attenuating the response of neurons prior to actual sensory analysis provides for sensory focusing and early sensory selection which occur before the sequential operations of subsequent response-driven processes. Furthermore, the attentional effect associated with enhancement may be influenced not only by expectancies arising from external stimuli, but also by expectancies created by previous behavioral experience and the results of different response alternatives. These factors should affect not only spatial attention, but also focused attention on object features.

Several recent studies have been conducted to examine differences between spatial attention to global spatial features and focal attention to featural characteristics. Robertson, Lamb, & Knight (1988) demonstrated that patients with large right hemispheric lesions affecting the temporal-parietal junction are likely to fail to detect the global form of stimuli. Conversely, patients with similar lesions of the left hemisphere more frequently failed to detect smaller (focal) features. When patients with left-sided lesions were subdivided according to site of lesion, those with inferior parietal lesions had difficulty attending to global and local features, while those with superior temporal lesions showed better reaction-time performance relative to global targets. Robertson *et al.* (1988) interpreted these findings as evidence that hemispheric asymmetries relative to the global-local feature distinction are due to a perceptual mechanism. In a subsequent study, Lamb, Robertson, & Knight (1989) provided further evidence for an attentional dissociation between inferior parietal and superior temporal regions on the basis of the global-local featural distinction.

The distinction between neuronal response to global and local object characteristics suggests that different types of attention may respond to different frames of reference. Neural systems of the inferior parietal lobule seem to have a very broad frame of reference, which enables these systems to be very sensitive to macroscopic variations in the environmental field. Other neural systems, including those of the superior temporal lobule, seem to have a much narrower frame of reference, which enables them to be sensitive to very subtle characteristics of stimuli. Attentional focusing on a narrow frame of reference (i.e., local features) is closely associated with the processes of featural analysis and perceptual synthesis. Therefore, neuropsychological researchers often do not consider this level of visual processing to be related to attention. Yet, the phenomenon of focal attention to local features exists, and probably should be distinguished from visual perception.

Summary

The association areas of the parietal and temporal lobes perform several different types of sensory-related functions. The most obvious functions are those connected with the secondary analysis of sensory information. The integrative functions of these areas are also obvious, as a host of neuropsychological findings illustrate that damage to temporal-parietal systems disrupt complex cognitive processes (e.g., reading) that require mixing multiple sources of information.

The visual-spatial representation of environmental and body schemata that are constructed from sensory experience is a particularly important form of multimodal information. This representation provides a spatial framework within which animals are able to direct their attention. When this spatial framework is distorted as a result of damage to these cortical areas, spatial attention relative to a spatial frame of reference is disturbed. This disturbance may occur as a result of the actual alteration of the spatial frame, as well as a failure of these cortical systems to modify their response to motivational and response-preparational information. Therefore, this attentional disturbance results from a breakdown of the interaction of multiple processes. Disturbances of attention associated with temporal and parietal damage reflect a failure of neural system to adapt to the spatial frame of reference created by sensory input. Furthermore, neural systems of the temporal and parietal regions seem to be specialized for different types of spatial analysis, which in turn is likely to influence different aspects of attentional behavior.

Many of the findings that we have discussed suggest a diminished role for the temporal lobe in sensory selective attention. One might argue that the types of perceptual processes that are engaged in at the level of the superior temporal lobule do in fact involve featural selection. However, as we discussed previously, attentional selection of this type is very difficult to dissociate from perception, as the relation of attention to the selection of local features is not yet well established.

On the other hand, the temporal lobe may have other roles relative to attention.

Contained in the temporal lobes are neural systems that are important in the timing and sequencing of information. Linguistic sequencing and syntax are often disrupted after lesions to temporal language structures. Therefore, it appears likely that the parietal-temporal systems create a spatial representation (like a photographic snapshot), whereas other systems contained in the temporal lobe piece together these single frames into temporal continuity. Temporal sequencing is influenced by limbic influences that coordinate the sequence of representations with external schedules of reinforcement.

ATTENTION AND THE CEREBRAL HEMISPHERES

The cerebral hemispheres are functionally asymmetrical. Hemispheric asymmetries are reflected in the performance of normal people. The left hemisphere is dominant for motor functions, as well as for many aspects of language. Functional asymmetries are apparent on many types of cognitive tasks. People normally show bias for information presented contralaterally to the hemisphere that specializes in that type of information processing. For instance, when verbal information is presented to the right visual field, it is usually processed more rapidly than when it is presented on the left. The advantages of right-hemispheric presentations have been described for faces and other types of visual spatial information (Kimura, 1967; Moscovitch, 1982). Research on hemispheric specialization has proliferated, so that there is now a large body of empirical studies regarding the lateralization of cognitive functions.

For some neuropsychologists, the characteristics of hemispheric asymmetries are the key to understanding many aspects of cognition. Other neuropsychologists acknowledge the existence of hemispheric asymmetries but reject the wide range of phenomena attributed to laterality. After all, the hemispheric effects produce only a dichotomous neuro-anatomical division (left vs. right). By making a hemispheric distinction, how much resolution of the brain's complexity is really achieved? Debates over the importance of hemispheric asymmetries continue, as do questions regarding the exact functional nature and structural locus of asymmetries and the relevance of cerebral lateralization to attentional processes. Therefore, we will briefly consider some neuropsychological evidence for hemispheric influences on attention.

Locus of Functional Asymmetries

Hemispheric asymmetries tend to emerge during the later stages of information processing. Studies have demonstrated that unilateral brain lesions of primary sensory systems do not produce significant hemispheric divergence in psychophysical performance (e.g., Corkin et al., 1970, 1973; Filby & Gazzaniga, 1969; Milner, 1962). Generally, lesions produce the same degree of sensory and perceptual dysfunction for primary informational features regardless of hemisphere. Yet, when higher order information is to be extracted (e.g., phonemes, facial features, and semantic information), hemispheric divergence is noted.

The information-processing approaches that have been applied to this analysis support this distinction according to processing stage. For instance, Moscovitch et al. (1976) found facial-processing asymmetries when a 100-msec interstimulus interval occurred between when the target was presented and when the response was required. This type of finding suggests that information is processed equally well by both hemispheres during the period when the sensory icon is present. However, during subsequent stages of processing, hemispheric advantages develop.

When different types of information are presented bilaterally, words are perceived better in the right field and faces in the left. This finding suggests that the hemispheres may act as dual information-processing channels under conditions of simultaneous stimulation. This possibility was tested in studies designed to detect interference effects (Moscovitch & Klein, 1977; Pirozzolo & Rayner, 1977). Material-specific interference was noted, as recognition of a target stimulus was most impaired when the interfering stimulus was compatible (e.g., face-face or word-word). The presence of hemispheric asymmetries in this material-specific interference effect suggested that competition between compatible stimuli for a limited capacity of hemisphere-specific processing accounted for the performance differences. In summary, hemispheric differences emerge at later stages of processing when information is synthesized, integrated, and prepared for output. The greater the attentional demands of a task, the more accentuated the asymmetry is likely to be.

Neuroanatomical Locus

It is apparent that the structural locus of hemispheric asymmetries in humans arises at sites following initial sensory registration. In the visual system, asymmetries arise subsequent to V1 in the prestriatal cortex or in the posterior temporal cortex. Neuropsychological findings provide some support for this, as asymmetries are noted for reading and complex verbal functions with left temporal and parietal damage, and for object recognition and spatial analysis with right temporal and parietal damage (e.g., DeRenzi, 1968; Warrington & James, 1967). However, these hemispheric differences for the processing of visual information are not always clear-cut. The evidence is clearer that auditory information processing is highly lateralized (Berlin & MacNeil, 1976; Kimura, 1967). Dichotic listening studies illustrate that, following unilateral temporal lobectomy and commissurotomy, unilateral performance is greatly affected.

Attentional disturbances are more common after damage to the right hemisphere rather than after damage to the left (DeRenzi, Faglioni, & Scotti, 1970). This fact has led some theorists to suggest that the right hemisphere is specialized for directed sensory attention (e.g., Heilman, Watson, & Valenstein, 1985; Mesulam, 1985). Support for this notion comes from several sources, including positron emission (PET) studies that show more activation in the right hemisphere during attentional processing, as well as from analyses of the performance of brain-damaged subjects. Right-hemisphere lesions are more likely to produce confusional states. They also show smaller galvanic skin response to stimulation (Heilman, Schwartz, & Watson, 1978) and bilateral rather than unilateral deficits in reaction time (Howes & Boller, 1975). After right unilateral brain injury, the loss of automaticity may be associated with perception of extreme effort (Brodal, 1973).

Attentional Priming and Interference

Structural information processing models of hemispheric asymmetries assume that hemispheric performance differences arise because each hemisphere is specialized and best handles certain types of information. An alternative explanation is that humans selectively process (attend to) certain types of information in each sensory field. Kinsbourne (1970, 1974, 1982) proposed that task expectations (i.e., verbal vs. nonverbal) "prime" attention to the contralateral sensory field. In one experiment, he presented verbal or nonverbal informational cues to each hemisphere before target stimulus presentations and found that hemispheric advantages could be obtained during the processing of material that would not normally have been lateralized. Subsequently, numerous studies tested this hypothesis with mixed results, leading many to conclude that perceptual asymmetries due to this type of attentional asymmetry are weak. Priming does induce expectancy according to task demands, as one hemisphere is activated for further processing.

The occurrence of interference decreases the efficiency of information processing within each hemisphere. When a task is presented to one hemisphere in order to "prime" performance, performance may be facilitated on a second task. For instance, verbal activation may facilitate a simple manual response made by the subject (e.g., Bowers & Heilman, 1976; Hicks, 1975). However, if the motoric response is complex, the concurrent verbal task interferes with performance. The impairment caused by interference is greatest when the tasks are mediated by the same hemisphere, perhaps because the tasks share common mechanisms, or because they compete for limited attentional resources. The bilateral visual presentation of two shapes produces interference, presumably because of the sharing of processing resources of the right hemisphere and because of the competition for access. The unilateral presentation of two shapes does not cause such competition, as access is more immediate.

The distinction between automatic and controlled processes also reflects interference effects on hemispheric asymmetries. When there is excessive interference, the capacity for automaticity diminishes. During dichotic listening, shadowing of verbal stimuli in the right ear causes a loss of automaticity of speech, and rhythmic tapping in the left ear is more disruptive than in the right ear (Bradshaw, Nettleton, & Geffen, 1971, 1972).

Split-Brain Analysis

Analysis of the processing characteristics of patients after commissurotomy (i.e., split-brain) for this treatment of seizure disorder has provided the richest sources of information on hemispheric asymmetries. In a series of well-known studies, Levy (1974; Levy, Trevarthen, & Sperry, 1972) presented to split-brain patients a chimeric visual stimulus consisting of two images joined at the vertical midline. The task required the subjects to match the chimeric stimulus to test pictures. When ambiguous instructions were given, the left hemisphere matched the stimuli based on functional properties, whereas the right hemisphere matched the stimuli based on appearance. When the instructions specified how the subject should match the stimuli, functional categorical tasks were responded to with the right hand, whereas structural categorical tasks were responded to on the nondominant side. Subsequent studies (e.g., Gazzaniga & Ladavas, 1987; Gazzaniga, 1970) have demonstrated that there are remarkable distinctions between the two hemispheres, and that the two hemispheres may actually exhibit rivalry on certain tasks.

Attention and the Split Brain

Levy et al. (1972) reported that the left hemisphere uses a sequential analytic strategy for learning facial recognition, whereas the right hemisphere processes complex spatial configurations as a "gestalt." This dichotomy has also been suggested by other studies (e.g., Zaidel & Sperry, 1973). The right hemisphere seems to perform a holistic featural analysis. This suggests advantages of the right hemisphere for cognitive operations that require a rapid gross analysis. Because attention can be viewed as a process of selective activation before more detailed sequential processing, the right hemisphere is a logical choice for this type of processing.

Recent studies of patients after callostomy have studied the characteristics of spatial selective attention (e.g., Dimond, 1976). Normally, there are costs in attending to wrong spatial positions. When attention must be directed across the vertical midline, the cost of inaccurate spatial attention is greater (Rizzolati et al., 1987). After complete section of the corpus callosum, the discrepancy between the location of the attentional cue and the target stimulus becomes even more critical (Reuter-Lorenz & Fendrich, 1990). When patients were required to cross a vertical midline, they showed disproportionate impairments in response time to the target. This finding fit with Gazzaniga and Ladavas's interpretation (1987) that the hemispheres of the brain compete, and that each hemisphere of the bisected brain is biased to orient contralaterally.

As we have discussed previously, the concept of hemispheric rivalry is one hypothesis regarding the mechanism of hemineglect syndromes. Although the results we have described show advantages of the right hemisphere for attention, they also illustrate that attention is bilaterally distributed. Both hemispheres interact to control attention in contra-lateral fields, although the right hemisphere may show some priority across fields.

Overview: Hemispheric Asymmetries of Attention

The lateralization of attentional functions has been suggested by studies that have indicated differences in the analytical and processing capacities of the two cortical hemi-spheres. We have discussed several lines of evidence that have a bearing on the question of asymmetries of attention, including (1) differences in processing strategy between the hemispheres; (2) hemineglect; (3) other findings of results of unilateral brain damage; (4) hemispheric differences in activation and arousal; (5) differential physiological activa-tion across hemispheres; and (6) attention after collosal separation.

It is clear that hemispheric asymmetries in cognitive functions exist, and that atten-tion is controlled differentially across hemispheres. The types of attentional deficits that are likely to be observed depend on the type of information to be processed, the nature of the interference, and other task-related factors. The role of the right hemisphere in directed attention is supported by the prevalence of hemineglect after right parietal brain damage and by studies of split-brain patients.

Neuropsychological studies of emotional experience (see Heilman & Satz, 1983) and the distribution of activation during attentional tasks provide another intriguing source of support for asymmetries of attention. Evidence that the nondominant hemisphere may modulate emotional arousal suggests another way that the nondominant hemisphere influ-ences attention, as emotional arousal relative to incoming stimuli would catalyze attentional processes. Differential cortical activation is apparent from a host of neurophysiological studies.

In general, right-hemispheric damage seems to cause greater attentional impairment. Yet, both cortical hemispheres perform attentional processing. Therefore, hemispheric asymmetries of attention reflect cerebral dominance, rather than a complete lateralization of attentional control.

THALAMIC INFLUENCES ON ATTENTION

The thalamus is composed of a large number of nuclei that serve as relays for information flow in the brain. A discussion of all of the thalamic nuclei is beyond our present scope, though their function can generally be specified according to the brain systems with which they interact. Most thalamic nuclei have reciprocal relationships with subcortical and cortical areas. Subcortical impulses are relayed to cortical areas, and cortical signals are directed through many thalamic nuclei to subcortical structures. Therefore, the thalamus acts as a gatekeeper for neural information.

Some thalamic nuclei relay primary sensory and motor information. For instance, visual information from the optic nerve arrives at the lateral geniculate nucleus, where it is directed to the visual cortex. Other thalamic nuclei respond specifically to a particular sensory modality but handle higher order information. Still other nuclei relay information between nonspecific multimodal cortical association areas and mesocortical and limbic system structures.

Although most thalamic nuclei serve cortical-subcortical communication, there are several special nuclei that do not project to cortical areas. The reticular nucleus and the intralaminar nuclei receive impulses from ascending reticular activation. These nuclei are then interconnected with other thalamic nuclei. This arrangement is uncharacteristic of other nuclei of the thalamus. Most thalamic nuclei exhibit little crosstalk, but rather communicate either with cortical or subcortical systems. The capacity of the reticular and intralaminar nuclei to communicate with other thalamic nuclei gives these nuclei special significance. Reticular activation provides for generalized arousal, which influences information flow in these other pathways. Therefore, these special nuclei associated with reticular activation have special significance in attentional processes. Attentional state is influenced by the reticular system and the associated thalamic nuclei.

Specific attentional disturbances are occasionally associated with lesions of other thalamic nuclei. For instance, damage to thalamic structures such as the pulvinar may produce neglect and hemi-inattention. The pulvinar interacts with the basal ganglia and visual association areas. The neglect syndrome resulting from this damage presumably occurs because of a unilateral disconnection between cortical and subcortical areas.

Thalamic Integrative Functions

Unilateral thalamic lesions have been shown to produce hemispatial neglect (Watson, Valenstein, & Heilman, 1981; Vilkki, 1984; Ferro, Kertecz, & Black, 1987). One explanation for neglect following thalamic damage is that a disconnection occurs between cortical areas that control spatial allocation of attention and subcortical systems that generate the arousal necessary to catalyze attention. However the thalamus may also play a more direct role in attentional control.

The rich network of reciprocal connections between the thalamus and other subcortical and cortical areas has important implications for the role of the thalamus in attention. By gating the flow of information across neural systems, the thalamus may also provide an integrative function. Crosson (1985) developed a model for thalamic integration for language functions. He suggested that the thalamus not only modulates arousal, but also performs preverbal semantic monitoring. If the thalamus exerts this type of monitoring, it is easy to see how attention would be influenced. The thalamus may function in a way analogous to the electronic mixing system used in the music recording industry. As the relative weight of associative information varies, the bias of the thalamus changes, thereby influencing what information flows through the system. Such a process would have attentional properties, as the act of informational gating provides for attentional selection.

In summary, the thalamus has three roles in modulating attention: (1) the thalamus receives reticular activation and serves to project this arousal to cortical processing systems. This is a generalized attentional effect resulting from the catalyzing influence of arousal. (2) The thalamus serves as a relay and gate for specific cortical-subcortical interconnections, which are critical for the coordination of sensory and motor functions. (3) The thalamus probably acts as an integration system, which influences the associative value of information, thereby governing the focus of attention. Ultimately, all of these factors interact in the control of attention.

SUMMARY

In this chapter, we have considered disorders that affect sensory selection. The neglect and hemi-inattention syndromes were discussed first. These syndromes are perhaps the most dramatic form of attentional disturbance in clinical neuropsychology. Patients who exhibit neglect on one side of the spatial environment usually exhibit a failure of hemispatial sensory selective attention. Therefore, the neglect syndromes provide a good illustration of the neural systems underlying sensory selective attention.

While early theories of neglect posited that failure to respond to stimuli on one side of space reflected either a sensory or perceptual defect, there is now overwhelming evidence that a failure of normal spatial attention underlies these disorders. Experimental findings illustrate that by manipulating attentional variables such as stimulus load and motivational state, the performance of patients can be altered, thereby demonstrating that attention is a critical determinant of neglect. Furthermore, manipulation of arousal levels in patients with neglect seems to influence their performance, suggesting that the attentional mechanism includes an arousal component.

Even though problems with sensory selection seem to be a central feature, neglect seems to involve a more complex interaction of attentional factors. Patients with neglect also may have hemispatial problems with response intention and directional hypokinesia. Therefore, neglect and hemi-inattention can only be explained by considering a network of neural systems. This fact is supported by clinical evidence that unilateral damage to many different brain structures can produce neglect.

In the second part of the chapter, we discussed the role of specific neural systems that appear to be important for sensory selective attention. We initially focused discussion on the role of parietal and temporal lobe structures in attention and considered experimental evidence for specialized attention areas within these structures. There is now strong evidence for a division of function within the visual system based on the characteristics of information that is processed. One system appears to be more tuned to spatial position, while the other seems to be tuned to featural characteristics. While the visual-spatial system is more obviously implicated in attentional operations, there is also reason to believe that the focused attention to fine featural detail that occurs is probably controlled by systems contained in the temporal lobe.

Beyond the specific attentional capacities of the parietal and temporal lobes, it is important to consider the associative networks that exist in these cortical regions. Distributed associative networks within the temporal and parietal lobes provide schemata against which new information is compared. Ultimately, there are many different frames of reference for information that is processed, so neural mechanisms must exist that are capable of providing attentional focus for different types of information.

We next considered the interhemispheric influences on attention. There is strong evidence supporting the role of the nondominant cortical hemisphere in producing neglect. Some theorists attribute neglect primarily to interhemispheric interactions. Others argue that while the neural mechanisms of attention are lateralized, interhemispheric interactions are not essential. Without restating all of the issues that were discussed earlier, it seems clear that hemispheric asymmetries exist that influence the spatial character of selective attention. The right hemisphere appears dominant for attention. Yet sensory selective attention is ultimately a function of neural mechanisms distributed across multiple neural systems.

We concluded our discussion in this chapter with consideration of the role of the thalamus in sensory selection. The thalamus was considered in this chapter for several reasons. First, the thalamus facilitates sensory integration, because it provides for relays which gate the neural transmission. Therefore, the flow of information within the brain is directly influenced by the integrity of the thalamus. Second, the thalamus contains many cortical-subcortical relays, which are important for certain aspects of selective attention. For instance, the coordination of eye movements with attentional direction depends on interactions between subcortical structures (e.g., the superior colliculus) and cortical structures, including the frontal eye fields and the inferior parietal cortex. Finally, the thalamus provides a gating mechanism for reticular activation (i.e., arousal), which initially catalyzes the overall attentional system.

The neuroanatomical distinction that has been made between disorders affecting sensory selection (chapter 9) and disorders affecting response selection and attentional control (chapter 10) is somewhat arbitrary. Attentional components like sensory selection and response do not correspond orthogonally to specific brain structures, as evidenced by the fact that lesions of parietal lobe structures may produce impairments of response intention, along with a failure of selective attention. Yet overall, the attentional functions controlled by the neural systems of the posterior cortex seem to be critical for sensory selective attention, and as we discuss in the next chapter, systems contained in the frontal cortex seem to be critical for response intention and control.

Attentional Control

Subcortical and Frontal Lobe Influences

In the last chapter, we discussed how neural systems of the parietal and temporal lobes influence selective attention to sensory information. Sensory selective attention occurs largely as a function of the spatial characteristics of information to be processed. The profound hemi-inattention and neglect that often results after damage to these neural systems reflects a failure of directed and selective attention relative to the temporal-spatial frame of reference within the environment.

While neural systems of the parietal lobe play an essential role in selective attention, they are by no means the only cortical areas that influence attention. In fact, neglect may result from unilateral lesions in many different neural systems. Therefore, attention is not under the control of a unitary neural system. Instead, attention depends on the interaction of neural systems, including the frontal lobes, limbic structures, and other subcortical systems, including the hypothalamus and mesencephalic reticular system.

In this chapter, we consider the contribution of the frontal lobes and several subcortical systems to the control of attention. We begin with a discussion of how the frontal lobes influence response planning, selection, and execution, all of which are critical determinants of attentional control. We then discuss the subcortical control of attention. The limbic system, hypothalamus, and reticular system have multiple influences on attention, as they control behavioral direction, salience, and reinforcement characteristics, as well as the behavioral energetics of the animal.

THE FRONTAL LOBES

The anterior region of the cortex is referred to as the frontal lobe. The frontal lobes perplexed researchers for many years. Unlike some cortical structures, which have relatively circumscribed functions, the frontal cortex has multiple functions and contains numerous heterogeneous subsystems. The functional and structural relationships within the prefrontal cortex and to other brain systems are still relatively unknown. However, it is now obvious that the neural systems that compose this region play a critical role in the control of attention and other "executive" functions.

Neuroanatomical Considerations

The prefrontal cortex is the most rostral aspect of the frontal lobes of the brain (see Figure 10.1). The frontal lobes make up those cortical areas that are anterior of the central sulcus and marked laterally by the Sylvian sulcus. Their surface contains three main sulci (the precentral, superior, and inferior frontal sulci) that create the boundaries of four gyri. While this gross topography exists in primates, the exact surface morphology of the frontal lobes varies across animal species and is a function of the overall size of the brain. The prefrontal cortex is demarcated by a lateral boundary (the presylvian fissure) that is present in most higher order mammals. Its posterior boundary is marked by either the medial or the inferior frontal fissure (Connolly, 1950).

Studies of the phylogenetic development of the prefrontal cortex (see Fuster, 1989, for a review) have suggested that two distinct primitive structures (the hippocampus and the

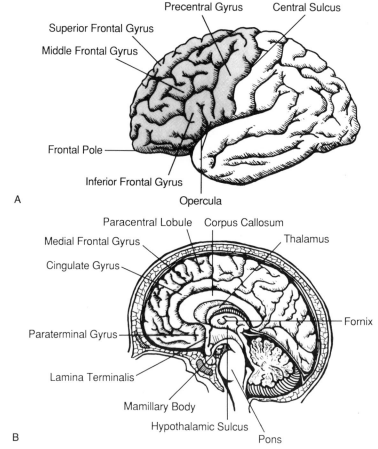

FIGURE 10.1. Two views of the cerebrum showing (A) the superior lateral surface and (B) the medial surface of the cortex. The area of the frontal lobe is shaded in gray. The relationship of the frontal lobe to subcortical, limbic, and posterior cortical structures is evident.

piriform cortex) were compressed as adjacent frontal cortex expanded and surrounded these structures in higher animal species. The presylvian areas exhibit this type of enlargement as a function of evolution in mammals. The frontal cortex of primates is characterized by the progressive development of the motor cortex as it expanded rostrally. Therefore, the prefrontal cortex seems to have developed from three primordial neuronal structures that expanded and converged to form an area of neocortex (Sanides, 1970).

The cell architecture of the prefrontal cortex is similar to that of the rest of the neocortex, as it contains seven stratified layers of tissue that differ by pattern of cell and plexus distribution. The characteristics of the prefrontal tissue vary across species. Fuster (1989) suggested that, by analyzing the prefrontal cortex as a function of the thalamic projections into this region, one can separate different architectural features. In rodents, the prefrontal cortex consists of two distinct areas (medial and orbital areas) that receive projections from the lateral and medial aspects of the mediadorsal nucleus of the thalamus. There is no granular layer (IV) in either area in rodents. As one analyses higher order mammals, there is an appearance of layer IV, but it does not necessarily contain granule cells. In primates, the prefrontal region is composed of homotypical isocortex that is laminated with a dense granular layer IV. This characteristic makes it different from other cortical regions. The significance of this granular layer seems to be its polymorphism. It is comprised of a multitude of Golgi Type II cells that have small dendrites that branch in various directions to make a rich network of interconnections with other cells of this region.

Afferent and Efferent Connections

As previously mentioned, a strong relationship exists between the prefrontal cortex and the mediodorsal thalamic nucleus. The prefrontal cortex receives most of its subcortical afferent fibers from this nucleus through anterior radiations from the thalamus and the thalamic peduncle. Nauta (1961, 1964, 1972) showed that this nucleus also relays impulses from other neural structures to the prefrontal cortex. These include input from the reticular system, the amygdala, the substantia nigra, and the inferior temporal cortex. The lateral portion of the mediodorsal thalamus primarily contains afferents from the prefrontal region.

In addition to the mediodorsal nucleus, several other thalamic structures have afferents to the prefrontal cortex, though many of these nuclei project to more caudal parts of the frontal lobes. Although thalamic afferents make up the most dense projections to the prefrontal region, several subcortical structures have direct input into this area. Investigators have demonstrated pathways to the prefrontal cortex from the brain stem, the pons, the hypothalamus, and several limbic structures, including the amygdala and the hippocampus. The projections from the limbic structures are distributed more diffusely than those originating from other subcortical structures.

The prefrontal cortex also receives important input from sensory and motor neocortical areas. Mesulam (1985) reported that these projections tend to originate from secondary sensory and motor association areas, instead of from primary isocortical regions. A multitude of interconnections also provide afferent interactions among networks of cells within the prefrontal cortex. Therefore, the prefrontal cortex receives inputs from most other areas of the brain, either through direct projection, or through pathways arising out of secondary associational structures.

Efferent projections from the frontal cortex innervate many of the structures that provide afferent input. The prefrontal cells tend to be organized in fields. These fields of neuronal cells generally correspond in a reciprocal arrangement with the structures with which they share efferent and afferent connections. The prefrontal cortex also has efferent input into the basal ganglia but does not receive afferent signals from this structure, so that the basal ganglia are the one primary exception to this rule of reciprocity. Input into the basal ganglia from prefrontal regions enables fine motor control.

The orbital areas of the prefrontal cortex have many projections to the hypothalamus, the septum, and subcortical structures such as the pons and the midbrain. Prefrontal efferents to the limbic system pass through the cingulate gyrus and transverse the corpus callosum, where impulses are distributed to other cortical regions. These efferents also reach the limbic system through the cingulate, parahippocampal, entorhinal, and retrosplenial cortex. The entorhinal and parahippocampal cortex are the primary relays of the impulses into the hippocampus, whereas the amygdala receives much of its input from orbital areas. Secondary sensory association areas are also efferently connected to the prefrontal cortex through thalamic and other subcortical innervation.

In summary, the prefrontal cortex has a multitude of interconnections that allow communication with most other areas of the brain. There are major efferent projections from the prefrontal cortex into the thalamus, the limbic and other cortical centers, the secondary sensory association areas, and the basal ganglia. There is also input from this region into subcortical centers at lower brain levels. Afferent input into the prefrontal cortex originates from many cortical and subcortical structures, though the mediodorsal nucleus is a primary relay center of projections to this region. The orbital prefrontal regions have particularly dense connections with the medial thalamus, parts of the caudate nucleus, and the amygdala. The dorsolateral prefrontal regions are more closely connected to the lateral thalamus, the hippocampus, and other cortical association areas. This dual level of organization seems to account for functional differences between subareas of the prefrontal cortex.

Clinical Manifestations

One of the first reports of the effects of frontal lobe injury to be described was the case of Phineas Gage, a railroad worker who sustained a puncture wound that resulted in unusual behavioral changes (Harlow, 1868). Although Gage's general cognitive abilities were relatively well preserved, he showed a striking impairment of complex behavioral control. This was characterized by disinhibition, as Gage would act on primitive drives without concern about the social consequences. An example was his tendency to defecate in the backyard of his home. He also showed changes in personality and emotional functioning. He vacillated in his mood and exhibited much impulsivity.

Since the case of Phineas Gage, there have been many other reported clinical cases of frontal lobe dysfunction in patients with damage resulting from various disease states. There are numerous etiological bases for frontal lobe lesions in neurological patients, which include open and closed head injury, tumor, lobectomies, vascular disorders such as stroke, and some CNS diseases that have focal frontal effects (e.g., Pick's disease). Most of these disorders do not produce lesions that are isolated in specific frontal regions, and therefore, the data derived from case studies often contain much artifact. Perhaps the best source of evidence about the effects of frontal lobe damage is patients with shrapnel wounds obtained in war, as their lesions are fairly well circumscribed. However, such patients are not always available, and the traumatic consequences of such wounds pose other problems. Therefore, clinical knowledge of the effects of frontal lesions must ultimately be pieced together from the convergence of a large sample of imperfect case studies.

Over the years, there have been a variety of ideas regarding the role of the frontal lobes. Fifty years ago, neuroscientists even suggested that the frontal lobes had little or no functional significance (Hebb, 1945; Hebb & Penfield, 1940). The significance of the frontal lobes has become more apparent as single-case and larger scale studies have demonstrated impairments after damage to these regions (Hecaen & Albert, 1975a,b; Fuster, 1989). Patients often show a change in their ability to respond emotionally to everyday events. Problems with the control of impulses often occur. Patients may have difficulty inhibiting sexual, aggressive, or other urges (Rylander, 1939). Judgment under stress is often affected, even though in a nonstressful situation individuals may demonstrate an awareness of the correct course of action. Furthermore, the planning and organization of behavior often become quite impaired. Patient behavior may become very erratic, as they fail to respond when there are strong environmental cues to do so, or they may fail to change responses when other cues indicate that such a change is appropriate. This failure to change may have consequences in goal-directed activities, as well as in the ability to initiate or sustain consistent responses.

The observation that some patients become restless, hyperactive, or even manic after frontal lobe dysfunction, whereas others become docile, inactive, or even akinetic, illustrates one of the difficulties in predicting the effects of damage to this region. In an early description of bilateral frontal damage reported by Brickner (1934), the patient became increasingly hypomanic and aggressive, and at the same time showed a diminished sexual drive. This apparent paradox points to the fact that behavioral control is a phenomenon that cannot be specified in a single dimension (e.g., activity-passivity). Instead, a patient may alternate between behavioral extremes in a dimension, failing to inhibit or modulate strong impulses.

Recent studies have also found a paradoxical array of deficits following frontal lobe damage. For instance, Eslinger and Damasio (1984) described a patient who had functioned very well before developing an orbital frontal meningioma. Following surgery, he continued to show above-average performance on intellectual and memory measures, yet could not hold a job because of a lack of reliability in his work. A breakdown in interpersonal functioning was also noted, which eventually led to his wife's divorcing him. The effects of this orbital frontal tissue loss appeared to be reflected almost exclusively in emotional and social functioning, with an associated breakdown in the reliability (temporal consistency) of his performance. Obviously, the consistency of his behavior was disrupted.

In our laboratory, we have had the opportunity to evaluate a number of patients who have undergone a cingulotomy for the relief of chronic pain (Cohen, McCrae, Phillips, & Wilkinson, 1990). This surgical procedure severs frontal-limbic pathways through the medial cingulate gyrus. These patients exhibit fairly characteristic changes, which include emotional blunting, increased passivity, and decreased levels of agitation associated with their pain. They do not show major neuropsychological deficits, but they do exhibit slowing on information-processing tasks, motor tasks, and tasks requiring an alternation in response between different sets. Instead of problems with impulse control and behavioral disinhibition, these patients exhibit problems of initiation, and they seem to become hypokinetic.

At first glance, the wide range of behavioral expression that is evident in patients with damage of the frontal lobes may seem paradoxical: Why should some patients show increased lability and disinhibition, while others are very perseverative and have great difficulty initiating responses? However, if we consider the fact that the frontal lobes are not one homogeneous morphological unit, these findings may be more interpretable. Commonalities do exist among the various forms of frontal lobe dysfunction. There is usually an obvious disruption of the ability to regulate and switch responses. In hypokinetic patients, there is an inability to initiate new responses, resulting in excessive rigidity or a perseverative quality. Other patients may exhibit the opposite tendency; hyperactivity, impulsivity, or even agitation. A response regulation problem is also evident, though the consequence is a failure to inhibit responding. Patients may show a bias to respond prematurely to new stimuli, even when the strength of the stimulus is not great.

In some patients, both tendencies coexist. These patients may have trouble generating responses to stimuli that are not emotionally salient, strong signals, or associated with a momentary drive state. However, when the salience or strength of a stimulus is stronger (e.g., has sexual content), the opposite response tendency may be expressed, as these patients lack the inhibitory capacity necessary to stop their response. As a result, patients with frontal lobe damage often respond with inappropriate behaviors in social situations but are more passive and lacking in initiative when alone or unstimulated.

Patients with lesions of the frontal lobes usually show changes in their pattern of activity (see Figure 10.2). Reductions in activity levels are common and have been described by clinicians for many years (e.g., Hecaen & Ajuiaguerra, 1956; Kleist, 1908; Rylander, 1939). These patients may also be easily distracted by irrelevant stimuli. Therefore, although they may be generally inactive, they often show an increase in attentional variability.

Ablation Studies

The first behaviorally controlled studies of the affects of induced frontal lobe lesions indicated deficits in learned procedural motor behavior and problem solving across a number of animal species (Franz, 1907).

Ablation of the prefrontal cortex often causes an increase in spontaneous movements. However, following surgery, animals usually show random patterns of activity that lack direction toward normal goals (e.g., Jacobsen, 1931; Miller & Orbach, 1972). However, the nature of these changes may vary across animal species. Also, hypoactivity may be noted immediately after surgery, which may later change to hyperactivity or, in other animals, may remain as a reduced state of activity. The time since the damage is a determinant of the animal's activity level.

Removal of the prefrontal cortex may cause a paradox of behavioral hypoactivity and hyperactivity within a particular animal (Kennard & Ectors, 1938; Kennard, Spencer, &

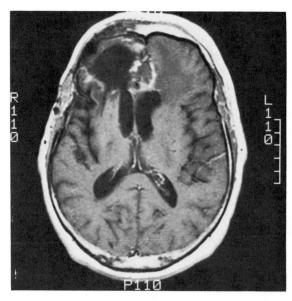

FIGURE 10.2. MRI scan of a 42-year-old male exhibiting a large right frontal neoplasm. Although his general cognitive functions were largely spared, he exhibited moderate problems with sustained and focused attention and executive control. His behavior was mildly disinhibited with affective dysregulation.

Fountain, 1941). Classically conditioned responses may be disinhibited or omitted. The ability to delay responses in certain conditioning paradigms is also disrupted. The orienting response is typically altered, so that the animal may show increased responsivity to novel stimuli but diminished response to less salient stimuli (Grueninger & Pribram, 1969). Problems with habituation are usually noted, with a failure to inhibit orientation to new stimuli.

Exploratory behavior is usually diminished in animals with frontal lesions. They may show a bradykinesia (a general failure to search the environment), or they may engage in a disorganized and poorly directed search. The affective response, to environmental stimuli are characteristically impaired after ablation. Animals show inconsistent aggressive and defensive behavioral responses to stimuli encountered during their search.

Failure to inhibit or delay responding in accordance with changes in environmental information is a central component of syndromes resulting from damage to the prefrontal cortex (Mishkin, 1957, 1964; Pribram, Mishkin, Rosvold, & Kaplan, 1952; Stepien, 1972). Animals that have undergone frontal ablation continue to perseverate in a response tendency, even when cues suggest that shifting to a new strategy could be beneficial. They also fail to delay responding to an immediate alternative, when such a delay would enable them to respond to a more favorable alternative (Kennard, 1939; Watanabe, 1986a,b). Studies have indicated that these syndromes are associated with selective damage to orbital areas. Behavioral discontrol arises from a disinhibition of inappropriate motor behaviors, drives, and emotional behaviors, and from attention to irrelevant stimuli.

In contrast to the effects of ablation, electrical stimulation of frontal brain regions causes an increase in orienting behavior, including the elicitation of physiological orienting responses. Such stimulation may also elicit a directed sequence of action. Stimulation of the frontal lobes creates a more vigilant attentional state, as well as an increase in goal-directed behavior. These effects provide further illustrations of the role of the prefrontal cortex in regulating behavioral state.

Impact on Arousal and Activation

Different behavioral presentations occur depending on the specific site of frontal lobe damage. Luria (1966) described a distinction between the effects of lesions of the medial and orbital surfaces of the frontal lobe, and lesions of the dorsolateral regions. Disturbances of the medial and orbital areas are likely to cause problems with the orienting response, as well as with many associated responses, such as the defensive reaction and the expectancy component of classical conditioning. Affective and personality changes accompany lesions to this area.

Lesions of the dorsolateral regions are likely to affect expressive language, and sensorimotor and motor output. Cognitive functions such as logical processing, problem solving, and abstraction are likely to be impaired. Luria (1966) distinguished between the specificity of lateral frontal lobe impairment and the nonspecific disregulation of activation associated with medial-orbital damage. To illustrate this distinction, Luria (1966) contrasted groups of patients with both types of frontal damage and compared them with normal control subjects and a group of non-frontal patients with brain damage. The autonomic and central electrophysiological responses (EEG) to informative and uninformative stimuli were studied. Patients with medial-orbital lesions failed to show physiological activation to verbal stimuli (words). This effect was not evident in patients with lateral frontal lesions or other nonfrontal lesions.

In a second experiment (Luria, 1966), the effects of sustained intellectual effort on these same electrophysiological measures was investigated. The normal subjects showed a change in EEG activation as measured by signal asynchrony during such simple tasks as sustained serial addition. Patients with medial and orbital frontal lesions did not show the same changes in EEG asymmetry, whereas patients with lesions in other locations showed a normal physiological response pattern.

As we have previously discussed (Chapter 6), arousal probably should not be considered a unitary physiological process. Therefore, it is important to demonstrate the aspects of arousal that are affected by frontal lobe damage. Khomskaya and Luria (1977) demonstrated a distinction between a generalized activation associated with overall task demands and a more specific activation based on the type of task to be performed. In event-related potential (ERP) paradigms, normal control subjects showed specific areas of regional activation for a given task (e.g., left-hemisphere activation during a verbal memory task), as well as a small change in generalized EEG activity. Patients with medial and orbital lesions had severe disorders of activation of the event-related potential (ERP) on tasks that required directed attention and selection among stimuli. In contrast, patients with brain stem lesions had generalized activation problems; yet they did not show the same ERP abnormalities on attentional tasks.

Orienting behavior and habituation are disrupted following prefrontal lesions. After damage to this region, animals show a very slow rate of habituation. They also show a decline in the amplitude of autonomic orienting responses (Butter, 1964; Kimble et al., 1965). Extinction of classically conditioned responses is often impaired following experimental frontal ablation (Butter, 1969). In all of these studies, damage to the prefrontal cortex was associated with disruptions in normal physiological arousal and response activation.

A distinction among the different physiological correlates of attentional control was made by Pribram and his colleagues (Pribram, 1955, 1961, 1967, 1969, 1971; Pribram & McGuinness, 1975). He demonstrated that removal of the frontal lobes in monkeys causes a disruption of the normal expectancy response. The expectancy response is linked to physiological activation that is specifically related to the anticipation of response production. Pribram and McGuinness (1975) argued for a distinction among arousal, activation, and effort as control mechanisms for attention. Findings regarding the role of the frontal lobes in the maintenance and allocation of neural activation were supported by Pribram's experimental work (1961) on the expectancy response in primates. After removal of the frontal lobes, monkeys show a deterioration in the quality of this response. Fuster, Bauer, and Jervey (1982) have demonstrated task-specific variations in cellular response of the dorsolateral prefrontal cortex. This suggests that activation patterns associated with frontal lobe control of behavior may be heterogeneous and very dependent on the nature of the response that is required.

Distinctions between the physiological reactivity associated with generalized expectancy and the sensory and response components of tasks has also been demonstrated in studies of normal humans (Cohen & Waters, 1985). Using autonomic measures such as heart rate and skin conductance, Cohen and Waters dissociated the arousal associated with stimulus processing from activation related to response production on a levels-of-processing task. Such studies confirm the fact that attentional control is determined by multiple interacting processes that differentially affect physiological arousal and activation.

In summary, the medial and orbital frontal regions serve to control the selective activation of the brain by task demands, as well as changes in the salience of the information that is being processed. Furthermore, these areas seem to exert more generalized control over the level and quality of behavioral activity. The anatomical interconnection of these regions and subcortical systems, including the limbic structures (e.g., the hippocampus and the amygdala), the hypothalamus, and the reticular activating system, seems to be important in defining the functional basis of this control. Damage to these frontal regions usually causes both a disruption of response activation in specific types of tasks and changes in the overall behavioral activity of the individual.

Movement, Action, and Attention

The close anatomical relationship between the prefrontal regions and the motor systems of the frontal cortex is well established (Porrino & Goldman-Rakic, 1982; Sanides, 1970). In fact, a number of early researchers considered the frontal lobes a higher order control center for movement. Although it is now evident that the prefrontal regions are not responsible for motor generation and control, these cortical areas do influence the normal production of "voluntary" movement and actions.

Patients with focal lesions of the orbital and dorsolateral prefrontal cortex maintain a normal range of movement. They can move their limbs on command, and they are usually not severely apraxic. If a ball is thrown to them, they respond by trying to catch it. If asked to throw the ball back, they probably can respond by doing so. Yet, patients with frontal lobe damage may fail to initiate a variety of actions spontaneously. Their ability to execute a chain of movements is typically impaired. They can execute individual motor responses but lack the ability to direct a series of such responses toward a goal. Disregulation of motor and action programming is common in patients with frontal lobe lesions. This clinical phenomenon provides a conceptual bridge between simple motor behaviors that can be explained without consideration of the prefrontal regions and more complex forms of responding that involve intentional actions that require a secondary or tertiary motor system.

The disruption of voluntary movement accompanying frontal lobe disorders is of theoretical importance, as it illustrates the relationship between motor sequencing and the generation of a program of action in the environment. If animals respond only to signals from incoming stimuli, it is difficult to see why motor sequencing is critical to planning goal-directed actions, or to other higher cognitive phenomena. However, if responding is seen as a more active process that is initiated by organismic needs or pressures, then the programming of a sequence of actions is critical for the animal to explore and seek out stimuli that will yield the desired reinforcement.

When an animal generates a program of action, it must also be capable of monitoring and modifying the plan in response to changes in the environment during execution of the plan. This may be accomplished through a selective inhibition or facilitation of steps in the program sequence. Such monitoring would require feedback after each step in the action program to provide information about the consequences of the response. Monitoring would also depend on a mechanism for response modification, through a process of selective amplification or attenuation of previous responses. The frontal lobes may fill this role.

The coupling of the feedback and response control mechanisms of the frontal lobes probably is the basis for "higher cognitive" functions such as abstraction, planning, and hypothesis generation. These processes can be seen as the by-product of second-order or higher-order feedback arising out of either overt or covert action sequences. For example, Skinner (1938) viewed problem solving as a form of rule-governed behavior, in which a person generates a series of questions or response alternatives (second-order rules) that lead to the construction of a solution. Although Skinner would not have suggested a basis for this operation in covert processes, it is now evident that many humans can test response alternatives without making overt responses. A system of higher order feedback is necessary for hypothesis testing to occur covertly, as higher order feedback provides information about the potential consequences of rule-governed hypotheses about future behavior. This could occur only through a mechanism by which covert response constructions are generated and then tested before the production of an overt response.

Eye Movements and Attention

One of the clearest examples of the connection between systems governing response control and stimulus selection is the control of eye movements. Traditionally, visual perception has been considered a function of the occipital and other posterior sensory brain regions. Damage to the visual projections or striate cortex results in cortical blindness or the loss of some part of the visual field. After a cerebral vascular accident, there is often a loss of vision in the field contralateral to the site of the damage. However, the remaining visual areas usually continue to operate (Teuber, 1960), and patients compensate for their visual field loss by directing their gaze accordingly. The eye movements of patients with this lesion are generally intact.

In contrast, damage to the frontal lobes does not cause a loss of the visual field; rather, it results in a breakdown of visual scanning and attentional search (Luria, Karpov, & Yarbus, 1966). This deficit has been well defined in experimental studies in which eye movements are recorded through light reflectance or photoelectric recording techniques (Butter, Rapcsak, Watson, & Herman, 1988; Goldberg & Bruce, 1986; Yarbus, 1965). A tracing of scanning movements is generated for the time of a visual analysis task, and the results are compared for normal and brain-injured subjects.

The results of such experiments demonstrate a failure of scanning with massive frontal lobe lesions. Patients with frontal lobe damage tend to fixate on one pictorial feature rather than to search the entire stimulus. The result is a failure to attend to the whole picture. Frontal lobe patients often report fewer details from pictures that are presented. There are also associated disturbances in motion perception; "inertia of gaze" is often reported in these cases. The patient is not able to shift attention according to changes in the environment. As a result of these problems, there may be a tendency to miss features of a visual scene, leading to the conclusion that the patient has responded impulsively, when in fact the problem was a failure to scan completely.

The ocular scanning impairment described above illustrates the role of active motor responding in the control of visual analysis. Patients with a lesioned frontal lobe are still capable of seeing an entire visual field. Yet, they do not respond consistently to the content of the entire field. Visual search is carried out by a "motor act" of directed gaze. With frontal damage, patients can see but do not always look. For instance, Butter *et al.* (1988) demonstrated impairments of sensory attention, motor neglect, and "release" of fixation after a unilateral frontal lesion. Their patient failed to move his eyes when a stimulus on the left required rightward movements, but he had no difficulty moving his eyes to a stimulus on the right. This patient's directional motor neglect was characterized by an abnormality in his eye movements. The prefrontal cortex facilitates spatial sensory attention as neurons in this area are sensitive to spatial discriminative information (Kojima & Goldman-Rakic, 1984).

Neuroanatomical studies have indicated the presence of "frontal eye fields" in cortical area 8. These fields constitute a specialized frontal region that regulates ocular movements. Area 8 integrates multimodal sensory inputs and associations. The posterior regions of area 8 also have characteristics of the motor association cortex. Therefore, this cortical area is critical in sensorimotor integration. Lesions of area 8 cause disruption of the orienting response and of saccadic activity (Goldberg & Bushnell, 1981; Schiller, True, & Conway, 1979). Unilateral lesions of the frontal eye fields in monkeys cause a failure to orient toward the contralateral hemisphere (neglect). Problems with motor guidance and avoidance behavior is commonly observed in laboratory animals (Crowe, Yeo, & Russell, 1981).

Single-unit recordings made from the frontal eye fields indicate activity bursts before visual scanning or the production of saccadic movements. Goldberg and Bushnell (1981) were able to predict the direction of saccades by mapping the visual field associated with the particular neuron. This finding suggests that the initiation of eye movements is triggered by attentional activation and enhancement. These findings are discussed in greater detail elsewhere in this book.

The fact that the frontal eye fields are closely connected to other areas of the premotor cortex and to both thalamic and subthalamic nuclei illustrate why the frontal eye fields are important to visual selective attention. This region also processes limbic system inputs. Therefore, it is capable of responding based on reinforcement or the motivational properties of the given setting.

Temporal Disruptions

Frontal lobe damage often produces memory impairments. Jacobsen (1936) used a delayed-response test to demonstrate this phenomenon in rhesus monkeys. The delayed-response test requires an animal to learn where a reinforcer (i.e., food) is placed. After a delay (ranging from several seconds to long durations), the animal is retested on a task requiring it to select the correct placement. Correct selection results in the animal's receiving the reward. In a modification of this procedure (delayed alternation), the animal must change its responses based on a predetermined rule (e.g., alternating between choices to one side or the other). Following bilateral prefrontal ablation, animals are impaired on both tasks when delays are long (e.g., Meyer & Harlow, 1952).

Performance on the delayed-matching-to-sample task is also impaired following frontal damage (e.g., Glick, Goldfarb, & Jarvik, 1969). This task is similar to the other delayed-response tasks, except that the animal is required to choose a spatial placement from several alternatives during the testing. Greater experimental control is possible with the use of this procedure. The poor performance that is found across all of these tasks was originally accounted for by a failure of immediate memory. These deficits have been demonstrated to be a function of the increased level of distraction occurring during longer delays (e.g., Bartus & LeVere, 1977; Malmo, 1942). Furthermore, performance can be facilitated by increasing the salience of the cues used during the learning procedure, a finding indicating that attentional factors account for much of the memory dysfunction. If the level of hyperactivity and nonrelevant motor behaviors is reduced, an improvement in task performance can also be obtained (Mishkin, Rosvold, & Pribram, 1953; Pribram, 1950).

The temporal characteristics of performance following prefrontal damage are relevant to an understanding of attention, as attentional control problems occur as a function of time. Tasks of long duration typically result in greater deficits for patients with impaired attention. If these deficits are directly related to memory problems, many of the other attentional effects found after frontal lobe damage could be accounted for as a by-product of an underlying memory disturbance. However, if the memory impairment results from a failure of temporal organization due to a sequencing problem, a different set of explanations for these effects emerges. The relationship between attention and memory is addressed in greater detail in Chapter 18 of Part III.

Executive Control

The frontal lobes have often been characterized as the center of executive functioning. The term *executive* refers to the role of these systems in response execution and control. The frontal lobes influence performance on complex tasks involving abstraction, planning, and problem solving. Although this diverse set of cognitive functions seems to reflect a very diverse and complex set of processes, ultimately these processes may be controlled by primary response-control mechanisms. Hypothetically, executive regulation can be accomplished by a mechanism that is similar to the "and" and "or" gate controls of a computer. Patterns of limbic activation, along with sensory associational signals, are processed through the frontal regions and are sequenced with regard to the anticipated response possibilities. Within such a system, the complex hypothesis testing that is necessary for problem solving depends on mechanisms similar to those involved in simple motor-response selection. This mechanism involves a series of binary decisions with reference to the signals being processed. These binary decisions take various forms: act-halt, go–no-go, search-focus, or intake-execute. Decisions either to widen or to narrow the categorical parameters of a search may also be controlled by this type of decision process. These choices of response made by the frontal system dictate whether the individual will continue with a particular vector of responding or will shift to other response alternatives. Therefore, this brain system has an important function in regulating the flow of behavior.

As we have discussed, a fundamental role of the prefrontal cortex is the sequencing of sensory, associational, and response alternatives. Sequencing creates a temporal flow or stream of behavior and cognition. Without the executive control of this region, mental experience seems to be composed of a rather random collection of sensory associational frames. Each individual frame may be relatively well integrated, but there is no continuity between frames. The prefrontal cortex seems to be a critical force that enables the system to move from a single frame to multiframe temporal organization. As children mature, so does their ability to project into the future. They begin to base their behavior on future consequences. With damage to the prefrontal region, temporal experience is greatly impaired, and people have great difficulty orienting their behavior toward future goals. They lose the capacity to project their sequencing toward hypothetical response paths that may occur in the future. The extent to which sequencing without the frontal lobes is possible needs to be determined in future studies.

A cortical mechanism that promotes switching across response alternatives and sequencing based on decisions made on these alternatives would have to be very sensitive to changes in the environment. Sensitivity enables the information from these stimuli to trigger changes in response pattern. The prefrontal cortex seems to have an important role in adjusting this sensitivity. It may do so by setting momentary response biases in accordance with variations in the affective-motivational values that are assigned to the information being processed through other brain systems. As a consequence, the animal selects from the response alternatives based on the reinforcement associated with new stimulus alternatives, or as a result of associations activated during processing. Through the actions of the prefrontal cortex, the process of response influences future sensory selections. In neural systems with highly developed frontal lobes, there is less demand for sensory system sensitivity at all times. The frontal systems can direct the sensory selection systems of the temporal and parietal cortex to enhance or reduce their featural or informational resolution and accuracy in accordance with momentary response demands. As a result, executive response control plays a pronounced role in governing attentional control. It appears unlikely that stimulus sensitivity, filtering, and selection accounts for all aspects of selective attention. The frontal lobes account for the sequential direction, the selection process, and the capacity to sustain or attenuate energetic-motivational states.

Summary

The disturbances in attention that occur after damage to neural systems contained in the frontal lobes illustrate that attention cannot be interpreted as simply an extension of sensory processing. Although the nature of the neuropsychological impairment varies as a function of the specific frontal region that is lesioned, attentional impairment seems to be common in most forms of frontal lobe disorder.

Lesions of the prefrontal cortex disrupt a number of functions that relate to attentional control, including performance on learning tasks involving discrimination and delayed response, motility, visual search, and social-emotional functioning. Deficits in many of these functions is related to failures of inhibition and the suppression of interfering stimuli. Disinhibition impairs the ability of the animal to sequence and sustain a multiframe flow of responses, as well as the capacity to suppress responding to irrelevant stimuli. The abnormal orienting responses of monkeys with prefrontal ablation is an indication of this problem, as these animals show indiscriminate responses to external stimuli. Disorders of spatial selective attention are most striking with damage to the frontal eye fields, although impairments may be noted with lesions in other frontal regions. The failure to persist with a particular stimulus may account for the affective and social abnormalities following this damage. In addition to causing inattentiveness to affective and social cues, orbital lesions seem to impair the ability to enhance affective states, and this impairment leads to an impoverishment of emotional experience.

In this section, we have described a number of ways in which the prefrontal cortex exerts control over attention. Visual spatial attentional selection is influenced by scanning processes, which are controlled by the frontal eye fields. Scanning contributes directly to attentional search by enabling the processing of all features from visual input. Although selective attention is possible without eye movements, it is clear that damage to the frontal eye fields severely hampers normal attention.

Ultimately, damage to prefrontal systems interferes with the ability to self-regulate and to exert control over response selection. Feedback arrangements between the prefrontal regions and the limbic, reticular, and other cortical centers provide a mechanism for reprocessing sensory, motor, and associational information. As a function of this feedback, individuals are able to alter their response patterns. The prefrontal cortex also appears to be capable of generating higher order feedback (i.e., feedback about previous feedback). This arrangement may be the basis for "metacognitive" phenomena, including humans' capacity for self-awareness.

The prefrontal cortex acts to delay or inhibit response tendencies that originate in more primitive brain structures, such as the hypothalamus. With damage to the frontal lobes, this capacity is compromised, and patients may act "impulsively" (Kojima & Goldman-Rakic, 1982; Kojima, Kojima, & Goldman-Rakic, 1982; Kojima, Matsumara, & Kubata, 1981). This role in delaying responses is critical in attentional control, as impulsive responding does not allow an adequate consideration of the response alternatives. The generation of long-term goal-directed behavior, which depends on the capacity to delay responses, appears to be determined by this region. The prefrontal areas serve an important role in response sequencing. With damage to this region, the ability to organize responses temporally is impaired, and this impairment affects goal-directed behavior. Goal attainment depends on the maintenance of a vector of response planning and selection over a period of time.

The prefrontal cortex appears to be capable of generating hypotheses about possible response outcomes based on previous learning, which facilitates pursuit of the goal. Therefore, the attentional component of "intentionality" is influenced by this region.

The conditions of hyperactivity and hypoactivity that accompany frontal lobe damage create attentional inefficiencies. These are caused by changes in the tendency either to respond or not to respond. These response biases may occur regardless of whether a salient stimulus is present, but they reduce the capacity to respond appropriately when a truly important stimulus is present.

The orbital prefrontal cortex modulates impulses originating in limbic structures such as the amygdala and the septum, as well as in the hypothalamus. These impulses reflect "primary motivational" value to incoming information and ultimately governs the organismic importance attributed to this information. Damage to the prefrontal cortex disrupts emotional experience and, ultimately, the salience that is attached to stimuli and events. The animal's ability to extract organismic relevance from the information it processes is reduced. The motivational changes that occur as a function of this disruption affect attention, as an animal attends only if it interprets information as meaningful.

CINGULATE CORTEX

The cingulate cortex is a mesocortical (paralimbic) region that is highly interconnected with many different subcortical, limbic, and cortical regions. In primates and humans, the cingulate cortex is frequently divided into anterior (Broadman areas 24 and 32) and posterior (area 23) (Baleydier & Mauguiere, 1980). The posterior cingulate cortex projects to upper and deep laminae of the cortex, including parietal, temporal, and frontal regions. The posterior cingulate cortex also projects to subcortical systems, including thalamic nuclei, the pons, and the basal ganglia. It receives projections from cortical areas and thalamic nuclei as well. The posterior cingulate is also highly interconnected with the anterior cingulate regions.

In contrast to the posterior cingulate, the anterior cingulate cortex receives most of its projects from the superior temporal sulcus and the frontal lobe. It also receives projections from the posterior cingulate and from certain thalamic nuclei. The anterior cingulate has more limited projections to cortical areas, but receives inputs primarily from the lateral frontal cortex and posterior parietal cortex. Like the posterior cingulate, it is well connected with basal ganglia structures. An unusual feature of the anterior cingulate is that it has rich projections to limbic structures, including the nucleus accumbens and the amygdala.

To summarize, the cingulate cortex is organized into two apparently distinct systems: (1) A posterior system that receives input from and projects to many cortical systems and the thalamus, and (2) an anterior system that receives input from fewer cortical areas, but processes thalamic and frontal-parietal signals, with rich projections to limbic structures.

Cingulate Influences on Cognition

As a result of the posterior cingulate's interconnection with many cortical and subcortical systems, damage to this region tends to produce impairments of memory and episodic recall of temporal sequence (Mesulam, 1985). In contrast, the anterior cingulate cortex was once thought to play a little role in cognitive processing, as early investigations of intellectual functioning following cingulotomy indicated few impairments (Barris & Schuman, 1953; Corkin, Twitchell, & Sullivan, 1979; Vasko & Kulberg, 1979). Even so, alterations in affective and personality characteristics were noted, which served as a rationale for this surgery in psychiatric patients (Ballentine et al., 1977). While subsequent investigations generally supported the idea of a limited cognitive role for the cingulate cortex, findings of subtle cognitive changes following cingulotomy were described by Corkin et al. (1979). Most noteworthy are reports of akinetic mutism immediately after bilateral cingulate damage (Laplane, Degos, Baulac, & Gray, 1981), a problem that tends to be transient. There is some evidence that the more lateral the lesion in the cingulate, the greater the expressive impairments (Cohen et al., 1990).

Investigators using positron emission tomography (PET) techniques demonstrated increased activation in the cingulate region during the condition of increase focused attention to processing of a single word (Petersen, Fox, Posner, Mintun, & Raichle, 1989). In a separate study, these investigators also reported that the anterior cingulate cortex became activated when demands for sustained attention were present.

We studied 18 patients with bilateral cingulate damage who underwent cingulotomy for treatment of chronic intractable pain (Cohen et al., 1990). Immediately after surgery, these patients exhibited impairments of several components of selective attention, including sustained and focused attention as well as intentional behavior. In fact, the most notable deficit observed in these patients immediately after surgery was an impairment of controlled verbal fluency. Over time, most attentional deficits improved; however, most patients continued to have significant deficits of self-generating responding. This deficit was evident in several ways: (1) decreased spontaneous verbalizations during the natural context of the evaluation; (2) a decreased quantity of productivity on tasks requiring creative generation of multiple solutions; and (3) reduced levels of effort generation on tasks. While deficits in self-generated responding persisted, patients tended to perform well when the attentional task had specific response demands that were not dependent on the patient's generative capability. Subsequently, Janner and Pardo (1991) described similar findings in a well-controlled single-case study of a patient treated with cingulotomy for depression. These neuropsychological findings suggest that the anterior cingulate cortex plays an important role in the intensive aspect of attention, particularly self-generation of attentional effort (see Figure 10.3).

Interestingly, after surgery, cingulotomy patients frequently continue to experience pain, but they express less interest in the pain. Approximately 40% of our sample indicated that the pain did not bother them as much. This change tended to be associated with changes in affective–personality presentation that were reported by the patient's family. In many cases, cingulotomy patients were described as less brooding and more passive. While they would react emotionally when appropriate, their emotional responses tended not to persist as long as they had before surgery. These altered emotional tendencies are interesting in the context of the attentional findings just described. The cingulate cortex seems to play a role in the modulation of affective-motivational state relative to the direction of attention.

Cingulate Effects on Habituation

In another study of this same patient population, we demonstrated that maintenance of habituation of the orienting response is also impaired following cingulotomy (Cohen, Meadows, Kaplan, & Wilkinson, 1992). Further, these alterations in habituation were related to processes that govern attentional modulation.

Findings of altered physiological activation secondary to cingulate damage are of particular relevance to understanding the control mechanisms underlying attention. The cingulate cortex provides a potential bridge between neural systems of limbic cortex, which are involved in affect and the determination of salience, and frontal systems involved in executive-response regulation. Alterations in arousal and attentional activation have been reported in various patient populations following brain damage (Heilman & Van Den Abell, 1979; Heilman et al., 1978; Holloway & Parsons, 1978). Luria (1966) characterized abnormalities of arousal and the OR response, as one of the essential features of frontal lobe dysfunction. Studies of neurophysiological response in primates with frontal ablations have confirmed the importance of the anterior cingulate and frontal cortices to the maintenance of habituation (Bagshaw et al., 1965; Pribram & McGuinness, 1975). Subcortical and limbic brain systems have also been shown to play an important role in the elicitation of the OR and maintenance of habituation, as ablation and electrical stimulation of these structures produce differential effects on habituation (Ursin, Wester, & Ursin, 1979). The amygdala has

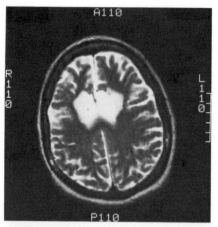

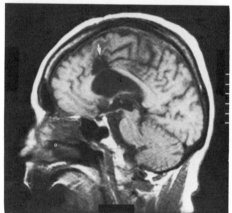

A

B

FIGURE 10.3. MRI scans showing bilateral lesions of the anterior cingulate gyrus produced by surgery to alleviate a chronic pain disorder in a 54-year-old female patient. (A) An axial (T1 weighted) slice illustrates the bilateral symmetrical spherical lesions in the cingulate cortex. (B) A sagittal (T2 weighted) slice, 2.5 mm to the right of midline, illustrates the position of the lesion in the anterior cingulate gyrus relative to the corpus callosum and intact cortical structures. Post-cingulotomy, patients exhibited mostly intact cognitive performance. Mild sustained and selective attentional impairments noted immediately after surgery improved over time. However, greater impairments of intentional behaviors were found that affected response initiation, self-generated behavior, and spontaneous verbal discourse.

been identified as an important structure underlying these responses. In humans, reduced galvanic skin response has been demonstrated following focal limbic lesions, and patients with Korsakoff's syndrome and Huntington's disease exhibit marked reduction in the amplitude of the OR and abnormal habituation (Oscar-Berman & Gade, 1979). In contrast, patients with posterior brain damage, such as aphasics, frequently exhibit intact OR and habituation, but may exhibit abnormal activation during more salient tasks (Meadows & Kaplan, 1992).

While impairments of habituation following frontal, limbic, and subcortical brain damage and preservation of the OR and habituation following posterior brain lesions have been demonstrated in studies employing traditional psychophysiological methods to elicit the OR, investigators have had discrepant results. For instance, Tranel and Damasio (1989) reported that autonomic reactivity remained intact in a patient with bilateral amygdala damage, as normal levels of autonomic reactivity associated with presentation of the patient's name was interpreted as indication of an intact OR. The OR, however, is usually considered to be a response to nonsalient unconditioned stimuli, which readily habituates. Therefore, normal autonomic reactivity in this patient may have reflected a response to salient conditioned stimuli (CS), rather than an OR per se. Other investigators have demonstrated hypoarousal following posterior brain lesions (e.g., Heilman *et al.*, 1978), though, again, these studies used salient stimuli to elicit a physiological response, a condition that differs from traditional OR–habituation paradigms. A distinction must be made between alterations in physiological activation associated with cognitive operations and/or the processing of salient conditioned stimuli and alterations in physiological response associated with the OR. The OR concept often has been extended beyond its original definition. Yet, these studies illustrate the difficulties encountered when considering the relationship between neuropsychological parameters, the neurophysiological mechanisms underlying OR and habituation, and the constructs of arousal, activation, and attention. When all previous neuropsychological evidence regarding the OR and habituation is considered, a rather complicated and somewhat confusion picture emerges, as the effect of brain damage on these responses depends on the site of the lesion in interaction with the specific task requirements used to elicit the OR (which varies according to how one defines an OR).

In light of these previous findings, we analyzed the OR and habituation characteristics of our patients with bilateral anterior cingulate lesions, using a traditional habituation paradigm. We used nonsalient stimuli to elicit the OR that were not already conditioned (CS) or unconditioned stimuli (UCS). Our goal was to determine whether bilateral cingulate lesions produce alterations in habituation of the skin conductance response (SCR), which could be related to either disruption of an underlying inhibitory mechanism or an impairment of a second competing process of sensitization. We used an extended "below-zero" habituation paradigm in which habituation training is given beyond the point of complete habituation to test whether habituation is controlled by inhibitory processes. Theories that habituation results from increased inhibition of the OR over successive stimulus presentations generally predict that habituation should be strengthened by extending below-zero training. The effect of extended below-zero training was tested by evaluating subsequent spontaneous recovery of the OR. Spontaneous recovery of the OR should be attenuated if extended training strengthens habituation. If the cingulate region influences habituation by modulating such an inhibitory process, then patients with cingulate lesions should exhibit more spontaneous recovery, as they fail to adequately inhibit the OR. Therefore, the present study extends previous findings regarding the effect of below-zero training in normal subjects to patients with lesions of the cingulate, a brain region considered to be important for normal habituation. We also tested the effect of a dishabituating stimulus on recovery of the OR and subsequent habituation to determine whether cingulate lesions differentially affected habituation and sensitization.

Our study demonstrates that bilateral anterior cingulate damage affects habituation of the orienting response. Following cingulotomy, patients required more trials to reach the criterion of complete habituation. This finding is consistent with previous investigations that have reported impairments of habituation following frontal lobe lesions and indicates that the anterior cingulate is also important for normal habituation.

While our results clearly demonstrate an impairment of habituation, they also suggest a rather complex and paradoxical relationship between cingulate damage and the processes underlying habituation. While the overall rate of habituation (trials to complete habituation and the slope of the regression line across total trials) was diminished postcingulotomy, the initial rate of habituation in the first three trials was actually greater in the cingulotomy patients. In effect, patients with cingulate damage began to quickly habituate with re-presentation of the stimuli, but then failed to maintain this rate of habituation. Several explanations for the cingulotomy patient's failure to maintain their initial habituation rate were considered, but then dismissed.

Arousal Hypothesis

The least plausible explanations are that a defect of tonic arousal or an abnormality of OR elicitation affected the habituation rate. The cingulate patients did not exhibit increased SCRs during the baseline period, the two rest periods, or the habituation–rehabituation trials. Infact, the only observed effect that could be interpreted as an indication of altered arousal was the finding of an increased number of spontaneous activations during habituation training for the cingulate patients. Since there was not an overall difference in SCRs between groups during this same period, it is unlikely that these spontaneous activations reflect increased tonic arousal. Instead, the increase in spontaneous SCR activity during habituation training appears to be related to either autonomic lability or irritability. Since the cingulate patients exhibited greater spontaneous activity only on the habituation training trials, it is unlikely that this effect relates to a general autonomic lability, which would produce greater spontaneous activity on all conditions. Therefore, the increased rate of spontaneous activations during habituation training for the cingulate group seems to be task dependent. Orienting response elicitation also appeared intact for the cingulate group, as neither SCR to voice instructions not SCR-OR to the first stimulus presentation of the habituation series differed between groups. Furthermore, amplitudes for spontaneous recovery of the OR following habituation were similar between groups.

Habituation Hypothesis

Another hypothesis that we ruled out was that cingulate lesions disrupted the underlying neural process of habituation. While the cingulotomy group clearly had a habituation abnormality, it seems unlikely that this abnormality reflects a disturbance of the neural habituation process per se. Cingulate lesions produced a time-dependent habituation abnormality, as habituation rates on early trials (trials 1–3) of initial habituation training differed from habituation rate across total trials. If the habituation abnormality associated with cingulate damage was caused by dysfunction of the primary neural systems that decrease the OR (e.g., type H neurons), then there would be no reason to assume different habituation rates between the initial trials and the later ones.

Sensitization Hypothesis

We next considered an alternative hypothesis: that habituation was affected by sensitization abnormalities. Unfortunately, our data do not suggest a simple relationship between sensitization and the habituation abnormalities secondary to cingulotomy. Sensitization was tested in two ways in this study: (1) by evaluating the effect of extended training on subsequent spontaneous recovery, and (2) by evaluating the dishabituation effect caused by presentation of a dishabituating stimulus. Neither test revealed an increased sensitization response for the subjects with cingulate lesions. In fact, the opposite was true.

Some previous theories of habituation have predicted that extended training should produce below-zero habituation, strengthening the habituated state as a result of additional exposures to inhibitory influences (Thompson & Spencer, 1966). Yet, investigations of habituation in normal subjects have revealed the opposite effect, as extended habituation training produces a slight increase in subsequent spontaneous recovery (Waters & McDonald, 1974, 1975, 1976). Our present results are consistent with these findings, as extended training did not strengthen habituation in either group, but instead increased the amplitude of spontaneous recovery, particularly for the normal control subjects. The simplest explanation for this effect is that extended training produced an increase in sensitization, which competes with the habituation. However, since the cingulotomy patients exhibited less spontaneous recovery relative to the control subjects as a result of extended training, our findings do not indicate that cingulate damage caused increased sensitization. If cingulate damage produced a tendency for increased sensitization, then extended habituation should have produced greater spontaneous recovery in the cingulotomy patients.

Evidence against the explanation of increased sensitization after cingulate damage also emerges from the dishabituation paradigm. The control subjects exhibited larger SCRs to the dishabituating stimulus and larger ratios when the SCR to the dishabituated stimulus was compared with the SCR for the initial OR on trial 1 of the habituation series. Therefore, our findings indicate that greater habituation occurred in the control subjects rather than the cingulotomy patients. Since the effect of dishabituation is most easily explained as a by-product of sensitization, the smaller response of the cingulotomy patients to dishabituation provide further evidence that sensitization was not increased following cingulate damage. In summary, findings regarding the effect of extended habituation training and dishabituation weaken the hypothesis that habituation abnormalities after cingulate damage are a simple function of excessive competing sensitization.

Neural Inhibition Hypothesis

While extended training did not strengthen habituation beyond the point of complete habituation, one might still argue that habituation is generated by inhibitory processes that simply do not have an effect beyond the point of "zero" response. If so, then the cingulate cortex may serve in the production of this inhibition and cingulate damage could disrupt the inhibitory process required for normal habituation. Unfortunately, the results of this study do not support this possibility. If habituation results from inhibitory processes that suppress the OR, then spontaneous recovery of the OR following habituation can be attributed to a release from inhibition after a time delay (i.e., disinhibition). If damage to the anterior cingulate causes disinhibition, then increased spontaneous recovery would be expected. As we discussed previously, we found the opposite effect, as spontaneous recovery after habituation training did not differ between groups and extended habituation training produced greater spontaneous recovery in the normal control subjects. The ratio of spontaneous recovery following extended habituation to spontaneous recovery following initial habituation was greater for the normal control subjects compared with the cingulotomy patients. Furthermore, while the control subjects consistently required fewer trials to rehabituate after spontaneous recovery and dishabituation compared with the cingulate group, both groups exhibited a decreased number of trials to rehabituate compared with their initial habituation rate. Also, ratios of the rate of rehabituation to initial habituation did not differ between groups. Even the ratio of habituation rate for the newly presented dishabituating stimulus and the rehabituation rate to the initial stimulus on the final habituation series did not differ significantly between groups. Taken as a whole, these findings fail provide any evidence that the cingulate region affects habituation through a simple neural inhibitory process or that cingulate damage causes a breakdown of such inhibition.

An Alternative Hypothesis

To summarize, the results of this study enable us to rule out several explanations for the abnormal habituation observed after cingulotomy, as our findings cannot be attributed to abnormal tonic arousal, faulty OR elicitation, failure of a unitary neural habituation process, or a simple increase in sensitization. While we are able to rule out a number of explanations, we are still left with the problem of how to account for the habituation abnormalities postcingulotomy.

Three findings from this study provide information that may help to resolve how the cingulate region influences habituation:

1. Increased interatrial variability following cingulotomy.
2. The distinction between initial and overall habituation rates.
3. Increased spontaneous activations during habituation training for the cingulotomy patients.

Findings from our work with cingulotomy create interpretative problems for habituation theories that propose that only the two competing processes of habituation and sensitization (Groves & Thompson, 1970) are necessary to account for behavioral habituation in humans. Cingulate damage does not cause a major disruption of initial habituation rate, nor does it enhance sensitization. Yet, the cingulotomy patients exhibited a temporal inconsistency of habituation, characterized by a tendency to fluctuate between large and small ORs over the course of successive trials. Their response on a particular trial has less bearing on how they would respond on adjacent trials. Furthermore, the cingulotomy patients exhibited an increased occurrence of random spontaneous activations that were noncontingent on the stimulus train during habituation training. This finding suggests that over time their attention became more diffused and was not consistently allocated to the tone stimulus.

The essential features that characterize the habituation abnormalities after cingulotomy are a breakdown in the temporal inconsistency of the habituation process and a decoupling of physiological activation and attention from stimulus occurrences. Therefore, it is possible that the primary role of the cingulate cortex in the habituation process is to maintain temporal consistency to behavioral responding and to integrate attentional responding relative to the ongoing flow of affective impulses and stimulus occurrences. In this capacity, the cingulate cortex may serve to integrate a host of interacting inhibitory and excitatory influences within the cingulate cortex, which ultimately modulates the temporal consistency of behavioral habituation and attention.

Perhaps findings of this study can best be reconciled by considering what is known about the functional role of the cingulate cortex. The cingulate is a mesocortical "paralimbic" region that is intricately interconnected with the limbic system and the prefrontal cortex. Neuropsychological theories of attention have increasingly included the cingulate cortex as a part of a multicomponent neural attentional system. The cingulate cortex appears to have a modulatory influence on limbic outflow. We have previously demonstrated that cingulate damage interferes with intentional activation, including the capacity for spontaneous response generation and response persistence. This finding is supported by findings from our group, the single case study by Janner and Pardo (1991), and evidence of intentional hemineglect in a patient with unilateral cingulate damage (Watson *et al.*, 1973). Cingulotomy has also been shown to produce a decrease in the obsessive components of affective experience and complaints of pain (Ballentine *et al.*, 1977). Following cingulotomy, patients frequently continue to experience affective impulses and/or pain, yet report diminished attention to or concern with these experiences (Cohen *et al.*, 1990). Cingulate lesions seem to disrupt the tendency to respond consistently to affective impulses, suggesting that the cingulate cortex plays a modulatory role in processing affective signals from the limbic system. The cingulate cortex may exert influence over feedback and/or feedforward mechanisms that enable recursive processing of limbic impulses, a hypothesis with some neurophysiological support. While additional research is needed to demonstrate how the cingulate cortex accomplishes these modulatory functions, the present findings provide evidence that it does so through a complex interaction of multiple processes.

Summary

The anterior cingulate cortex is a paralimbic brain region that is richly interconnected with limbic structures, including the amygdala and cortical areas, particularly the frontal cortex. It appears to exert significant influence over attention. While several different attentional deficits occur immediately after cingulotomy, the most pervasive and lasting deficits appear to relate to the intensive aspects of attention. The greatest impairments tend to occur relative to the capacity for self-generated behavior. While the attentional deficits associated with cingulate damage seem to be correlated with habituation abnormalities, the habituation impairments observed after cingulotomy do not seem to reflect a primary dysfunction of either neural habituation or sensitization. Instead, the anterior cingulate seems to play a role in modulating and creating a temporal continuity for affective-motivational impulses relative to ongoing stimuli that arouse attention.

SUBCORTICAL INFLUENCES ON ATTENTION

The cortex has long been considered the center of higher cognitive functions. For this reason, most of the early neuropsychological studies of brain dysfunction were concerned with the affects of cortical lesions that resulted in syndromes like aphasia, agnosia, and apraxia. The subcortical regions were often seen as less relevant to understanding cognitive processes like language, as these areas seemed to be concerned with more primitive organismic functions.

The subcortex is a remnant of the "old brain," common to both humans and lower animal species. Early neurophysiological investigations demonstrated that structures like the hypothalamus were important to the regulation of drives and appetitive states. The relationship of these "organismic" functions to cognition is not self-evident, and there was a tendency to place these functions at different phylogenetic levels. Yet, there has been an increasing awareness among neurophysiological researchers that the behavioral responses controlled by subcortical systems play an important part in more complex cognitive operations. The processes of attention are very dependent on subcortical influences. The subcortex, in particular the limbic system, integrates higher cognitive functions with more primary organismic pressures (McLean, 1959).

Less is known about the clinical neuropsychological effects of subcortical lesions on attention, whereas there is a wealth of existing knowledge about the effects of cortical damage, in part because of the assumption that the cortex is the primary center of cognition. Perhaps a more important reason is the methodological difficulties encountered in attempts to study these regions in humans. Lesions to subcortical structures due to stroke are less common than lesions to cortical regions. Also, higher mortality is associated with damage to the subcortical systems that are necessary to maintain peripheral physiological regulation. In those patients who are available for study, the subcortical lesion is often produced by a tumor or other disease process that does not have complete specificity with regard to the regions of involvement. It is extremely difficult to find cases in which a specific structure has been lesioned without effects on the surrounding areas. This problem is magnified by the fact that most of the subcortical structures of interest are very small and difficult to study without a direct observation of brain tissue. Neuroradiological data are often not sensitive enough to provide good resolution in many of these regions.

Much of our knowledge about subcortical influences on cognitive processes like attention has come from studies of animals in experimental paradigms. In the laboratory setting, discrete lesions can be made in specific neural structures, a procedure that avoids the pitfalls that were previously described. It is now well established that subcortical structures play a key role in such phenomena as memory encoding and emotional behavior. Attentional dysfunction is also common after damage to subcortical brain structures, although the characteristics of these disturbances is somewhat more difficult to characterize, as attention is relatively difficult to measure in nonhumans.

The term *subcortical* oversimplifies the neuroanatomy of the brain, as it implies a dichotomy of brain organization. Although the cortex is morphologically distinct from most of the brain systems referred to as subcortical, this division is not always clear-cut. The subcortex actually consists of numerous discrete neural systems which are heterogeneous in structure and function (see Figure 10.4). To a large extent, the cortical and subcortical distinction serves as a heuristic to account for the brain's role in both cognitive and lower behavioral functions. However, this may not be an accurate representation of how cognition is organized. It is useful to subdivide the subcortical regions of the brain into smaller structural-functional system.

Several subcortical systems have been identified that have particular relevance to our consideration of attention. These include the limbic, the reticular, and the hypothalamic-pituitary systems. There is some disagreement over which anatomical structures make up each of these systems. For instance, some neuroscientists argue that the hypothalamus is actually a limbic structure, whereas others choose to consider it separately. These considerations are determined in part by whether one emphasizes the anatomical or the functional relationships of a structure to other components of a particular system. For the purposes of our discussion of attention, consideration is given to the limbic and reticular systems, and to the hypothalamic-pituitary axis, as three separate systems. Although these systems are not independent of each other, they seem to have relatively selective behavioral roles. Damage to these systems affects attentional control in different ways.

Limbic Influences on Attention

Perhaps the most intriguing area of the subcortex is the limbic system, with its broad impact on various critical processes, such as memory and emotion. The limbic system is generally regarded as including the following structures: the hippocampus, the amygdala, the septal area, the substantia innominata, the piriform cortex (olfaction), and a variety of nuclei, including the nucleus basalis and the mammillary bodies. A number of mesocortical areas exist that have been described as "paralimbic" (Mesulam, 1985). These include the temporal pole, the insula, parts of the orbitofrontal cortex, and the parahippocampal cortex. The cingulate and retrosplenial cortex are also typically described as limbic or paralimbic structures.

Some investigators do not consider the limbic system a true subcortical system, as it contains several cortical structures and is intimately interconnected with other areas of the cortex. Regardless of one's position on this argument, it is widely accepted that the limbic system is the point of interaction between cortical processes such as language or visual integration and impulses arising from the hypothalamus and other lower systems.

The Hippocampus

The hippocampal formation receives input from paralimbic areas and forms a circuit with the amygdala, the mammillary bodies, the thalamic nuclei, the cingulate gyrus, and

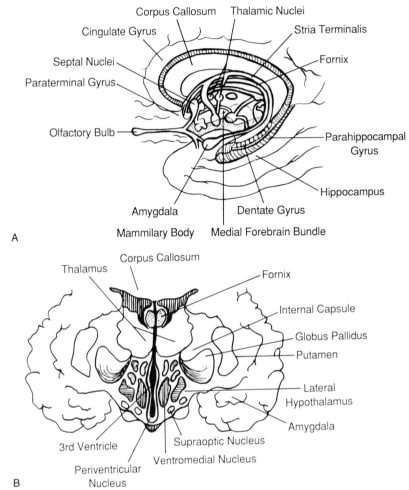

FIGURE 10.4. Two views of the rhinencepahlon illustrating the relationship of the limbic system to cortical and subcortical structures: (A) depicts the relation of the hippocampus, the amygdala, the septal nucleus, and other limbic structures to the basal ganglia, the temporal lobe, the cingulate gyrus, and the corpus callosum; (B) a section through the hypothalamus, showing the relationship of this structure to the basal ganglia, the thalamic nuclei, the amygdala, and other periventricular (third ventricle) structures.

the entorhinal areas (Papez, 1937). The hippocampus is also reciprocally connected with the septum. It is well established in animal studies that damage to the hippocampus results in impaired memory. Lesions of the hippocampus in rodents result in severe impairment of learning. Similar effects are noted in primates, though hippocampal lesions by themselves seem to produce only moderate amnestic syndromes (Mahut, Moss, & Zola-Morgan, 1981).

Mishkin and his colleagues (1978, 1982) demonstrated that the combined effect of hippocampal and amygdaloid lesions far exceeds the amnestic effects of isolated hippocampal lesions. Mishkin (1978, 1982) had monkeys perform a delayed-nonmatching-to-sample task after lesions were produced in order to show this effect on visual recognition memory. Mishkin *et al.* demonstrated a dissociation-of-memory disturbance based on selective lesioning of the hippocampus or the amygdala. Zola-Morgan and his colleagues (Zola-Morgan & Squire, 1985a, 1985b, 1986; Zola-Morgan, Squire, & Mishkin, 1982) demonstrated that damage to the amygdala may not be as critical a determinant of memory formation. Their investigations implicated the hippocampus and the entorhinal cortex.

Studies of human amnesia also indicate that the hippocampus is very important in memory processes. The most classic illustration of a focal lesion of the hippocampus producing amnesia is Milner's famous case of H.M. (1959, 1967, 1968), who suffered bilateral temporal lobe damage as a result of surgery for seizure disorder. Although H.M.'s amnesia was originally related to hippocampal destruction, most investigators now believe that he also had destruction of surrounding cortex. Squire (1984) reported evidence from a larger patient sample that further implicates the hippocampus in memory processes.

There is relatively little direct evidence from humans regarding the role of the hippocampus in attentional control, as there are few human cases of isolated hippocampal damage. Much of what is known comes from experimental investigations of lesioned animals. Isolated hippocampal lesions reportedly do not cause major problems in focused or selective attention (Isaacson, 1982a,b). In fact, animals with hippocampal lesions are often less distractible on goal-directed tasks (Wicklegren & Isaacson, 1963). However, subsequent research has suggested that this might only apply to very salient stimuli, as animals show greater reactivity to unexpected events (orienting response), and poor attentional performance on discrimination tasks with low-intensity, low-salience stimuli (Bauer, 1974). Furthermore, the relationship of target to background stimuli greatly influences performance after hippocampal damage (Kaplan, 1968). Performance is much more impaired when the stimuli and the task are part of a complex behavioral sequence than when the animals are inactive. Behaviors that require the formation and extinction of hypotheses are often impaired (Kimble & Kimble, 1970).

Attentional performance is influenced by the salience and distinctiveness of cues. After hippocampal damage, animals have difficulty with performance when there is less contrast among stimulus cues. Also, the reinforcement value of stimuli influences distractibility. Hippocampal damage produces greater problems with attention to negative stimulus cues. In compound stimulus paradigms, these animals do not exhibit normal interference or "blocking" effects (Kamin, 1968, 1969).

Animals with hippocampal damage have great problems with spontaneous alternation (Douglas, 1967, 1975), inhibition (Kimble, 1968), and perseverative behaviors (Dalland, 1970, 1976; Kimble, Kirby, & Stein, 1966). Exploratory behaviors are also affected (Kimble & Green, 1968), though this effect may be due not to a decrease in searching activity, but to the efficiency of the search (O'Keefe & Nadel, 1978). Animals tend to become hyperactive, though this reaction is environment-dependent: they are hyperactive in large open spaces, but not on more focused tasks like the running wheel (Douglas & Isaacson, 1964). Impairments of exploration are usually evident (Suess & Berlyne, 1978) and are a function of stimulus complexity and novelty.

Because hippocampal damage results in severe amnestic disturbances, animals have great difficulty adopting a consistent and effective strategy on tasks, as they have few new memories to work from. As a result, they may show greater variability in their response selection, because they do not benefit from learning. One would expect greater impairments on attentional tasks that tax memory. When the memory demands of a task increase, there is a decreased capacity for automaticity, which results in demands for attentional effort. Therefore, the capacity for controlled attentional processing should decrease when there is a severe amnestic disorder resulting from damage to the hippocampus or other critical structures involved in memory formation. Unfortunately, this relationship between attentional effort and performance following hippocampal damage has yet to be well established in humans.

The Amygdala

The amygdala has a reciprocal feedback arrangement with the hypothalamus and is also closely connected to the rest of the limbic system (Nauta, 1961; Nauta & Haymaker, 1969). Stimulation of the amygdala produces changes in autonomic activity (Bonvallet & Bobo, 1972) and emotional response (Delgado, Roberts, & Miller, 1954). Destruction of the amygdala results in striking changes in normal emotional response and drive state (e.g., Fonberg, 1973; Pribram & Bagshaw, 1953). After surgical sectioning of the forebrain commissures and unilateral lesioning of the amygdaloid body, monkeys that would normally be agitated respond passively to humans in the visual field consistent with their damaged side. In contrast, they react in their normal aggressive way to humans in the opposite visual field, which is associated with the intact amygdala. These findings illustrate the specificity of the amygdala's response to emotional input. Rodents show an increase in blood flow in the amygdala in response to conditioned fear response (LeDoux, Thompson, Iadecola, Tucker, & Reis, 1983). The amygdala's response to emotional stimuli is influenced by hypothalamic activation.

Animals with amygdala disconnected from cortical input often show Klüver-Bucy syndrome, which is characterized by indiscriminate sexual behavior, decreased aggressive and aversion responding, and a failure to distinguish edible from nonedible foods. In humans, the best evidence of the role of the amygdala in emotional experience comes from studies of patients with temporal-limbic epilepsy who have depth electrodes implanted for study of the electrical activity associated with their seizures (e.g., So, Gloor, Quesney, Jones-Gotman, Olivier, & Andermann, 1989).

Like the role of the hippocampus, the role of the amygdala in the control of attention is not yet well defined. Yet, the amygdala has a number of indirect influences on attention. The amygdala plays a role in the maintenance of autonomic tone (Anand & Dua, 1956). Electrical stimulation produces different autonomic responses, depending on what site is stimulated (e.g., Reis & McHugh, 1968). Presumably, the amygdala influence attention by controlling the range of physiological responsivity that will occur relative to changes in external environmental input or internal associative signals. The relationship between autonomic reactivity and attentional demands is well established (e.g., Cohen & Waters, 1985; Kahneman & Beatty, 1966). Therefore, the amygdala is critical in mediating the effects of emotionally charged signals on physiological activation. Ultimately, it may determine which inputs are relevant, thereby allocating further responding.

The amygdala has also been shown to play an important role in the maintenance of the orienting response (OR). The rate of habituation is impaired, as animals do not reduce their OR following repeated presentations of a nonreinforcing stimuli after lesions to the amygdala. Experiments have demonstrated that animals become inattentive after ablation of the amygdala (Pribram, 1969). They are able to orient to new stimuli but fail to consistently do so. This is particularly true if the stimuli are not rewarded. This deficit is most notable for visual stimuli. A subsequent study revealed that sensory inputs into the amygdala provide selective associational information (Turner, Mishkin, & Knapp, 1980).

The amygdala also acts in a reciprocal arrangement with the hypothalamus and may serve to gate impulses from this center. As a mediator of hypothalamic impulses to act, the amygdala serves a critical role in attention by establishing the salience of the signals that are being processed. Damage to the amygdala causes dramatic changes in appetitive behaviors, including the creation of bulimic animals (Pribram & Bagshaw, 1953). Lesions and stimulation of the amygdala also produce different effects on hypothalamic regulation of endocrine functions (Zolovick, 1972). Recent studies have indicated that several regions of the amygdala have different influences on behavior. However, the amygdala seems to have an overall role in the regulation of the drive associated with both affective and appetitive behavior. The amygdala influences animals' ability to increase responding under conditions of reward and to inhibit responding with nonreward. Animals lose this capacity after amygdaloid damage and tend to perseverate (Henke, Allen, & Davidson, 1972; White, 1971).

This relationship is evident in the analysis of human seizure patients, as well as in animals with induced seizures involving the limbic system. The phenomenon of "kindling" is thought by some researchers to serve as a basis for the generation of partial complex seizures. Kindling refers to a neurophysiological phenomenon whereby neuronal discharges develop in response to weak electrical stimulation occurring in neural regions that are vulnerable to seizure activity. Some neurological investigators have proposed that kindling may be a precursor for the development of seizures, including partial complex seizures involving the limbic system (Wada, 1986). Kindling, which has been demonstrated under experimental conditions using laboratory animals (e.g., McIntyre, 1979), may explain some of the unusual disturbances of attention, affect, and behavioral response that are apparent during the interictal and preictal periods (auras) in some patients with partial complex epilepsy. Most patients with partial complex limbic seizures experience alterations in attentional state during or even just prior to their seizures.

Selective attention may be impaired with amygdaloid damage because of a failure to assign value to stimuli in an adequate manner. As a result of this failure, sensory information is not correctly gated. The filtering of signals based on their organismic salience serves as a cornerstone of attentional processing. Although there is now considerable evidence that the amygdala plays an important role in attention, much empirical study is still needed to specify the relationships between emotional regulation, salience, sensory filtering, and attention.

Limbic Nuclei

Several important limbic nuclei have been isolated that play critical roles in limbic functions, including the nucleus basalis, the septal nuclei, the nucleus accumbens, and the substantia innominata. These structures are well connected with other limbic structures, such as the amygdala and the hippocampus, as well as to various cortical regions. The septal nuclei and the substantia innominata are part of the basal forebrain and therefore serve as another bridge between cortical and subcortical areas. The fact that these structures are rich in cholinergic cell bodies suggests their importance in behavioral functions such as memory.

Again, there is not an abundance of human clinical data regarding the effects of focal lesions to these structures. There is evidence to suggest the breakdown of functioning in these areas with Alzheimer's disease (Whitehouse, Price, Clark, Coyle, & DeLong, 1981). However, this evidence is not clear-cut, as Alzheimer's disease is known to affect a number of subcortical structures.

In rats, damage to the nucleus basalis impairs performance on passive avoidance tasks (e.g., Flicker, Dean, Watkins, Fisher, & Bartus, 1983; Grossman, 1976). These structures also seem to play a critical role in emotional reactivity and responses to appetitive stimuli. They respond to signals for reward and therefore act as another mediator of stimulus salience. Damage to the septal nuclei often results in severe rage reactions or hyperemotionality (Moore, 1964). In contrast, electrical stimulation of the septum produces the experience of pleasure in schizophrenics (Heath & Mickle, 1960). Self-stimulation of the septum can be induced with little training (Olds & Milner, 1954). In many respects, the septal nuclei have an opposing relationship to the amygdala with regard to emotional responsivity and other behavioral response tendencies (Corman, Meyer, & Meyer, 1967). Septal lesions produce complex alterations in behavior that depend on task demand and reinforcement dynamics in the situation (Cherry, 1975; Corman *et al.*, 1967).

The nucleus accumbens also appears to be a critical structure for the mediation of positive reinforcement. Stimulation of this nucleus has been associated with the experience of pleasure. Furthermore, the action of many neurochemical substances that reduce pain and produce pleasure, such as morphine and cocaine, seem to be mediated within this structure. Obviously, a neural structure with profound effects on the quality of reinforcement should greatly influence attention.

The behavioral response of animals after lesions of limbic nuclei varies according to the reinforcement properties of the situation, as avoidance behavior tends to be greatly affected (McCleary, 1966). As in the case of the other limbic lesions, effects on various appetitive, locomotive, exploratory, and other behaviors important in attention are often noted.

Although the specific relationship of these responses to human attentional control is not entirely clear, it would appear that these nuclei act as another bridge between the salience of stimuli and the tendency to continue a certain response tendency. There are some indications that, along with the amygdala and the hippocampus, the septal nuclei create a system for responding to different types of stimulus values (e.g., reward vs. aversion). Also, the relevance of these nuclei to memory functioning has implications for attentional phenomena.

Mesocortical Influences

The mesocortical tissue surrounding the limbic system receives inputs from a variety of other cortical regions (Van Hoesen & Pandya, 1975; Van Hoesen, Pandya, & Butters, 1972). Mesulam (1985) referred to these structures as "paralimbic," as they act as a bridge between the limbic system and higher cortical centers. Because the mesocortical region is made up of many different structures with input from a variety of sensory and motor association centers, it is difficult to delineate a single function for these structures for attention. For instance, the temporal poles and the insula act of sensory signals from posterior brain regions, and the cingulate gyrus appears to handle signals from the prefrontal areas. One thing that all of the mesocortical structures share is their role in integrating multiple signals from different domains for further processing by the limbic system.

Mesulam suggested that the paralimbic areas act as a buffer between the complex association information from the cortex and the more primary stimulus–response tendencies of lower brain systems. Thus, the structures of the mesocortex serve to inhibit normal response urges by allowing for a modification of responses based on the internalized information or goals that exist in cortical association areas. As in the case of the limbic structures, the mesocortex presumably acts as a "gate" to modulate response tendencies. If this hypothesis is accurate, the role of these regions in attentional control is self-evident.

Several lines of evidence reflect on the role of these structures in attention. With respect to the cingulate gyrus, there are considerable data from studies of the effects of cingulotomy. In the past, neurosurgeons used this procedure to treat severe psychiatric disorders. It was found that lesioning of medial regions of the cingulate gyrus has its greatest effect on disorders of chronic pain and obsessive-compulsive personality. In both cases, the disruption of impulses through this structure seems to diminish the tendency to ruminate (Ballentine, Levey, Dagi, & Diriunas, 1977; Cohen *et al.*, 1990). It appears that disrupting signals in this region short-circuits a feedback system between limbic and prefrontal systems. Normally, this feedback arrangement seems to result in the recursive processing of messages. Patients who have tendencies to obsess may experience this recursive feedback in a very detrimental way, as they are unable to break from a particular association or behavioral pattern. Cingulate lesions reduce the degree of recursiveness. Significant impairments of other aspects of selective attention have been described in patients following cingulotomy (Cohen *et al.*, 1990; Janer & Pardo, 1991), though some of these impairments recover over time.

Besides the role of the mesocortex in maintaining feedback arrangement, there appear to be other, related functions for these structures. The direction of affective responses relative to the ongoing context of the stimulus or response set seems to be regulated by these areas.

Memory disturbance occurs with damage to various mesocortical structures (Bachevalier & Mishkin, 1989; Murray & Mishkin, 1983; Phillips, Malamut, Bachevalier, & Mishkin; Zola-Morgan, Squire, & Mishkin, 1982). However, in humans, it is difficult to attribute the amnesia solely to damage to these regions, as the hippocampus is often also damaged in cases of tumor and cerebral vascular disorder.

Hypothalamic Influences

The hypothalamus is a heterogeneous anatomical structure containing many subsystems and nuclei. The hypothalamus is highly interconnected with other neural centers including the thalamus, the midbrain, the limbic structures, and the paralimbic cortex. Important efferent pathways projecting from this structure are contained in the medial forebrain bundle, the mammillary peduncle, and the hypothalamotegmental tract. Afferents project along the stria terminalis and the ventral amygdalofugal fibers (Reichland, Baldessarini, & Martin, 1978).

There are two mechanisms by which the hypothalamus effects neuronal activity. It can exert hormonal pressure by changing the biochemical milieu relative to particular physiological systems (endocrine role). It can also facilitate the activation of specific brain structures through direct neural interconnection (nonendocrine role). These functions of the hypothalamus are not independent of each other, as endocrine and nonendocrine influences interact in the control of most behavior (Reichlan *et al.*, 1978). As the center of neuroendocrine control, the hypothalamus contains cells that specialize in the neurosecretion of hormones that affect a wide range of functions, from physiological regulation to control over specific behavior. Several releasing hormones (e.g., corticotropin-releasing hormone, gonadotropin-releasing hormone (GNRH), and somatostatin) direct the release of other hormones from this gland. There are also numerous neuropeptides (e.g., endorphins, angiotensin II, neurotensin, and substance P) that act as chemical signals and have specialized roles in mediating certain networks of neurons.

In addition to its role in endocrine function, the hypothalamus also serves a number of nonendocrine roles. Different functions are anatomically distributed within the hypothalamus. The preoptic anterior hypothalamus contains thermal and olfactory receptors, structures involved in sleep onset, and parasympathetic pathways. The tuberal hypothalamus contains numerous endocrine pathways, as well as the lateral and ventromedial nuclei, which are involved in caloric regulation and the sense of thirst and hunger. The posterior hypothalamus has receptors that establish thermal set point, as well as nuclei involved in sleep regulation. Pathways from this posterior area also interact with the reticular activating system, and with limbic centers, including the septum, the amygdala, and the hippocampus.

The hypothalamus is closely interconnected with the limbic system. Although all cortical regions receive projections from the hypothalamus, only the structures of the limbic system have major input from the hypothalamus. The limbic system also appears to have descending pathways that affect hypothalamic function. These two systems form a functional circuit through which reciprocal communication is possible. Some researchers consider the hypothalamus a part of this system.

Descending pathways from the hypothalamus allow it to exert regulatory influence on a variety of peripheral physiological responses. It was considered the "head ganglion of the autonomic nervous system" by some investigators (Hess, 1969). Some evidence suggests that instead of being a ganglion, the hypothalamus serves as a point of integration of autonomic signals (Korner, 1971). Both sympathetic and parasympathetic impulses emanate from the hypothalamus and descend through the brain stem to effect target systems throughout the body. Signals from the hypothalamus also have reciprocal arrangements with the reticular system.

Behavioral Implications

The experimental literature on the physiology and behavioral influences of the hypothalamus is very rich. In fact, more may be known about this structure than about any other structure in the brain. However, the way in which hypothalamic function affects cognitive processes is still not well understood. The hypothalamus is known to control various appetitive behaviors and states of drive, including hunger, thirst, and sexual drive. For instance, the relationship of the lateral and ventromedial nuclei to eating and drinking behavior was well established in some studies, in which these structures were selectively lesioned or stimulated (Hetherington & Ranson, 1942; Hoebel & Teitelbaum, 1966). As we have discussed earlier in this text, the hypothalamus also plays a central role in the creation of drives and the establishment of reward and punishment (Olds, 1955, 1958a,b; Olds & Olds, 1958, 1965).

The hypothalamus also plays an important role in sexual and territorial behaviors (Ferris, Singer, Meenau, & Albers, 1988). Damage to caudal regions can produce hypersexuality, and ventromedial lesions often disrupt sexual desire. This disruption has been associated with gonadotropin deficiencies due to lost secretion of luteinizing-hormone-releasing hormone (LHRH). Behavior associated with maintaining thermoregulation is also disrupted with certain lesions of the posterior hypothalamus (Reichlan *et al.*, 1978).

The hypothalamus is critical to the maintenance of arousal and consciousness. Stimulation of the anterior hypothalamus has been shown to produce narcoleptic states of unresponsiveness, whereas arousal is generated by posterior stimulation. Lesioning of each of these areas produces the opposite effect (Nauta, 1946; Ranson, 1939; White, 1940). Normal arousal depends on signals from an intact reticular system. Von Economo (1931) first noted insomnia secondary to anterior hypothalamic damage in humans. Since that time, a number of single-case studies have been reported that indicate different sleep disorders according to the site of damage. Recent investigations have implicated the suprachiasmic nucleus (SCN) as a center for the control of circadian rhythmicity. The SCN is a small structure that sits in the anterior basal section of the hypothalamus above the chiasm. Lesions of this structure have been shown to disrupt normal sleep–wake activity and to cause an associated chaotic pattern of arousal (e.g., Albers, Lydic, Gonder, & Moore-Ede, 1984). Cohen and Albers (1990) reported a single-case study of a human patient (A.H.) with SCN damage due to craniopharyngioma (see Figures 10.5 and 10.6). This patient not only showed major arhythmicity of sleep and arousal but also exhibited major difficulties in behavioral and attentional control.

Autonomic functions are also disrupted with hypothalamic damage, and it is now widely accepted that this structure serves as a bridge between higher cognitive states and peripheral physiological responsivity. Because of its importance in regulating all of these

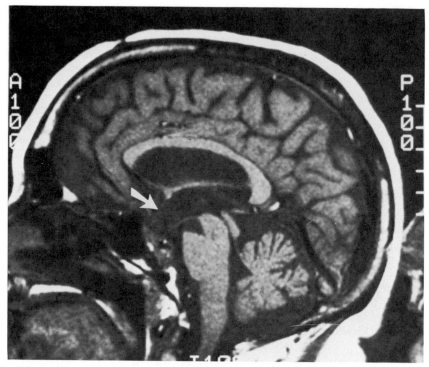

FIGURE 10.5. MRI scan of A.H., a patient with anterior hypothalamic damage in the area of the SCN resulting from surgical removal of a craniopharyngioma. She exhibited striking dysfunction of the temporal dynamics of attention, with marked fluctuations of arousal and attentional capacity. Her attentional variation corresponded with a disruption of normal daily biological rhythms (Cohen & Albers, 1991).

core physiological and behavioral functions, the hypothalamus has typically been considered the seat of primitive animal drives and impulses. These drives serve as a catalyst for more complex behaviors.

The effect of hypothalamic damage on primary physiological and behavioral states is quite evident from the large number of experimental studies of hypothalamic lesions in laboratory animals. As a general rule, hypothalamic damage results in impaired endocrine function and has potential effects on other neural circuitry that depends on the site of the lesion. In humans, bilateral damage to the hypothalamus is necessary to produce major symptoms. For this reason, lateral hypothalamic damage is less likely to cause functional impairment than medial damage. A common basis for hypothalamic lesions in humans is tumor, such as craniopharyngioma and pituitary masses. Subarachnoid hemorrhage, hydrocephalus, and encephalitic conditions also cause hypothalamic disorders in some patients.

As previously described, alterations in normal states of arousal are common after damage to the hypothalamus. Although this has often been studied relative to the existence of sleep–wake disruptions, it is apparent that the hypothalamus and the reticular system are both involved in the maintenance of the full spectrum of arousal. During intermediate states between sleep and consciousness, the individual may be aroused, but incapable of adequate

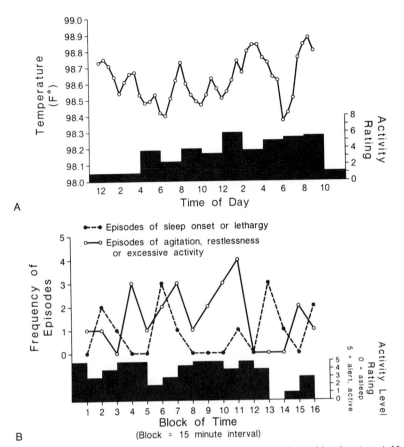

FIGURE 10.6. (A, B) The temperature, activity, and arousal variable of patient A.H.

cognitive functioning. Damage to the hypothalamus can affect arousal by creating either hypo- or hyperarousal. Such damage may also create an erratic and fluctuating state of arousal which in turn would cause broad fluctuations in cognitive performance and behavioral control. Such a situation was seen in the case of A.H., whose SCN damage seemed to facilitate a state of behavioral lability.

Because the hypothalamus is closely associated with both the limbic and the reticular systems, one might expect damage to the hypothalamus to affect memory processes. Learning and memory disturbance is found after lesions to both the lateral and the ventromedial regions (e.g., Gold & Proulx, 1972). This disturbance affects encoding more than storage, as previously learned behaviors are retained. In humans, the effects of damage to the ventromedial hypothalamus is more difficult to determine, as very few patients exhibit lesions specific to this nucleus. Generally, patients with hypothalamic damage resulting from tumors or other neurologic diseases have significant disturbances of arousal, attention, and new learning. Given the degree of interconnection between the ventromedial hypothalamus and other limbic structures, it is likely that lesions of this nucleus have a secondary effect on other aspects of limbic function. Disorders of memory are common with hypothalamic damage (de Wied & Boltus, 1979; Cohen & Albers, 1991).

Emotional behavior has been considered a function of the hypothalamus for many years (Cannon, 1929). Experimentally induced "sham rage" can be produced after hypothalamic damage. There have been numerous studies demonstrating the linkage between the hypothalamus and emotional behavior. Although on the surface this relationship seems simple, emotional behavior is actually the by-product of complex regulatory and behavioral control mechanisms of the hypothalamus. As the hypothalamus exerts control over a wide range of appetitive behaviors, such as eating, sexual response, and sleep, it elicits excitatory and inhibitory impulses that create the reactions of pleasure and aversion within the animal.

The hypothalamus affects behavior by generating and/or modulating a wide range of biobehavioral responses. It does so in correspondence with environmental signals that adjust the physiological state to the external conditions that are present. In turn, the hypothalamus elicits a wide range of impulses that catalyze responding, create "drive" states, and provide a direction to behavior.

Attentional Effects

There are few neuropsychological studies of the attentional effects of hypothalamic lesions in humans. Most patients who sustain damage to the hypothalamus become gravely ill and experience a large number of endocrine problems that cloud interpretation of their attentional impairments. Damage to the lateral hypothalamus impairs the active avoidance response to aversive stimuli (e.g., Olds, 1962; Olds & Frey, 1971; Olds & Olds, 1962). The animal seems to not register or maintain reinforced behavior. Unilateral lesions of the lateral hypothalamus create attentional neglect, as animals fail to display behaviors on one side of the spatial environment, but not on the other side (Grossman, Dacey, Halaris, Collier, & Routtenberg, 1978; Marshall, Turner, & Teitelbaum, 1971). After such lesions, animals fail to show an OR to stimuli from any modality presented from the opposite side. The occurrence of sensory and intentional hemineglect after hypothalamic lesions provides perhaps the strongest evidence that the hypothalamus is important for attention. Unilateral damage to the hypothalamus seems to disrupt the ability to selectively direct and catalyze behavior.

Single-case human studies have also yielded information regarding the specific effects of hypothalamic lesions on attention. Cases of hemi-inattention and neglect syndrome have been reported (see Heilman, Watson, & Valenstein, 1985, for a review). In cases of bilateral hypothalamic damage, the attentional effect depends on which hypothalamic nuclei are damaged. For instance, the patient A.H., who had damage to the SCN region, exhibited circadian abnormalities and disruption of the temporal organization of attentional behavior (Cohen & Albers, 1991).

Because the hypothalamus contains many subsystems that control a large number of different behaviors, it is possible that specific lesions of the hypothalamus would produce behavior- or task-specific disturbances. For instance, lesions of areas involved in feeding control may create inattention to food, but not to other stimuli. However, under normal clinical conditions, hypothalamic damage is not this selective, as tumors and other neurological diseases produce imprecise lesions. Therefore, when humans survive hypothalamic damage, they often experience dramatic impairments of consciousness, awareness, and arousal, with disturbances of general attentional tone.

The hypothalamus appears to exert control over attention, because of the complex array of primary behaviors that are under its control. Not only does the hypothalamus respond to and modulate generalized arousal, it also enables very selective response activation. The hypothalamus is made up of many different nuclei that exert control over the basic forms of animal behavior, including eating, drinking, sexual response, aggression, escape responses and pleasure. Some nuclei of the hypothalamus actually act in reciprocal relationship with one another, to provide a high degree of behavioral specificity. Although many of the behaviors under the control of the hypothalamus appear to be very primitive (e.g., feeding), the interactive influence of the many appetitive and simple behaviors that enables exhibit constitute the building blocks for more complex cognitive processes.

As the hypothalamus creates behavioral pressures to eat, sleep, fight or do some other act, it increases the salience of the information related to that behavior. A hungry animal's behavior is directed to eating; therefore, attention is biased toward cues that will produce food. Because the hypothalamus is involved in primary organismic functions, there is sometimes a tendency to dismiss this type of behavioral control as being separate from the cognitive aspects of attention. Yet, this level of control is fundamental to the generation of directed and sustained attention. By modulating the behavioral response tendencies of other neural systems, the hypothalamus influences the animal as it maintains, stops, or switches its behavior. These processes are central to attentional control.

The Reticular System

The reticular system of the brain is composed of a core of nuclei and pathways originating in the brain stem, with broad distribution through the midbrain. The intra-laminar nuclei of the thalamus are also considered part of this system because of their electrophysiological relationship to these lower centers. The reticular system initially received much investigative attention, as it was determined that the brain stem reticular system served as a pacemaker underlying EEG rhythmicity (Moruzzi & Magoun, 1949). Because this system is important in the maintenance of levels of cortical arousal, it has become known as the ascending reticular activating system (ARAS). The reticular formation and the intralaminar nuclei have patterns of activation that increase during wakefulness, and that decrease during deep sleep. Bilateral lesions to the midbrain reticular centers result in coma or severe states of lethargy and reduced sensorium.

The modulation of states of activation is the primary task of the reticular system. At the extremes of activation, the organism is faced with conditions of hypoarousal to the extent of coma, or with conditions of hyperarousal in which the organism may have a generalized tendency to be overly responsive to stimuli or to be hyperactive. These extreme states can be produced through pharmacological intervention. Barbiturates and other CNS depressants tend to suppress reticular activation, whereas stimulants tend to cause increased excitabil-ity of these structures (Rapoport, Buchsbaum, Zahn, Weingartner, Ludlow, & Mikkelsen, 1978). The influence of these substances on reticular activity illustrates that neurotransmit-ters such as norepinephrine, serotonin, and acetyl choline play critical roles in the mainte-nance of optimal arousal. Noradrenergic input arises from the locus coeruleus, whereas the raphe nucleus serves as a locus for serotonergic pathways.

Reticular activation seems to be broadly distributed via the thalamus across cortical areas. Therefore, it appears to be nonspecific in its functional impact. For years, many investigators postulated that the ascending reticular activating system was the center of attention. However, the nonspecificity of this activation makes it difficult to account for attention solely on the basis of the function of this system. Groves and Thompson (1970) and Sokolov (1963) both suggested models that consider this system central to attention (see Chapter 7). In the case of Groves and Thompson's model, reticular activation contributes to the OR and catalyzes continued responding, while a second system produces habituation. While the exact mechanisms underlying the OR, habituation, and sensitization are not yet well understood in humans, the fact that these responses are influenced by reticular activations and that they influence attention seems certain.

The degree of activation generated by the reticular system has a direct impact on the quality of attentional performance. When monkeys were trained to perform response alternation, as in the go–no-go task, they showed an activational burst approximately 0.5 sec before the presentation of the stimuli and returned to baseline after the task was completed (Ray, Mirsky, & Pragay, 1982). This finding suggests that the reticular system is capable of producing a phasic anticipatory activation. In another study, Goodman (1968) demonstrated a relationship between activation in these regions and reaction time to a discriminative cue during operant learning. An inverted-U function similar to that suggested by Yerkes and Dodson (1908) was found, with the shortest response times generally occurring with midlevel arousal. Thus, the degree of activation generated by the reticular impulses has a direct impact on attentional performance.

In humans, empirical data relating mid-brain reticular structures to performance comes in part from sleep–wake studies. During states of lethargy occurring after sleep deprivation, a decrease in attentional performance is associated with fatigue. Lesions to the brain stem and the midbrain typically have severe consequences, so that it is difficult to delineate subtle attentional effects. Patients with damage to the brain stem and the reticular formation who survive are often disoriented and confused and show severe problems maintaining vigilance or cooperation for even very short periods (Lindsley, 1950, 1962). Often, they are abulic, as they tend to drift between states of sleep, drowsiness, and extreme lethargy. All other cognitive functions may appear to be impaired, although it should be clinically apparent that their difficulties are, to a large extent, produced by an inability to maintain vigilance. These patients can often be differentiated from patients with other brain syndromes on the basis of their ability to perform well for brief time periods; then they lapse into periods of confusion and delirium.

Damage to the reticular system may be caused by a number of different factors, including tumor, vascular infarct, or insult to the brain stem. The attentional disturbance that is noted in patients with posttraumatic head injury can often be attributed to damage to these activational centers (see Chapter 11). In many head-injured patients, the primary symptom following recovery from coma is a reduced arousal level that is coupled with bradykinesia and an amotivational syndrome. This is often believed to be secondary to frontal lobe damage. However, a common basis for these symptoms may be damage to white matter pathways in brain stem and midbrain. Shearing forces associated with traumatic injury may tear these fibers and cause a failure of normal reticular activation (Adams & Victor, 1981).

Summary

Attention is influenced by three subcortical systems: the limbic system, the hypothalamus, and the reticular system. As Mesulam (1985) suggested, they form a systemic matrix for the regulation of the "state functions" necessary for the control of attention. These systems interact and create a network that is essential for normal attention. Each system exerts a relatively specific influence on attention, though these influences are integrated to create an attentional tone.

An essential feature of damage to the reticular system is disruption of normal arousal and abnormalities of consciousness. Patients with reticular damage often fail to react effectively to stimulation. They may also exhibit fluctuations in behavioral states with variations in accordance with arousal level. The effects of reticular activation on attentional control are quite evident both in experimental animal studies and from clinical data on human patients. The relationship of reticular activation to attention appears to be nonspecific. However, the generalized activation produced by this region leads to changes in sensory sensitivity and in the thresholds for response production. The reticular systems interact with limbic and higher cortical areas (via the thalamus) to produce more specific patterns of activation according to the prevailing task demands. The reticular system modulates general levels of arousal across different brain regions, but it has particular impact on the limbic system structures and the hypothalamus, and it catalyzes behavior.

The hypothalamus modulates this energetic state in accordance with existing biological pressures that create a drive state. The hypothalamus provides the fuel for emotional experience and is important in behavioral approach, withdrawal, and avoidance. However, it is the higher subcortical centers of the limbic system that provide the linkage between these impulses and the sensory signals, associations, and response intentions from cortical centers.

The limbic system and the mesocortical areas of the brain play an important role in attentional control, though it is more difficult to establish a direct one-to-one relationship between damage to particular structures and a specific type of attentional disturbance. Three functions that can be attributed to these systems are critical components of attentional control: (1) memory formation and retrieval; (2) modulation of affective value for stimulus and response salience; and (3) the integration of multimodal signals and associations for further processing.

Disturbances of Attention

Neurological Disease

RONALD A. COHEN and BRIAN F. O'DONNELL

In the last chapter, the impairments in attention associated with lesions of specific brain structures were discussed. We now discuss how attention is affected in several common neurological disorders. Neuropsychological investigators have devoted much effort to the analysis of patterns of cognitive performance associated with a wide variety of brain disorders. The goal of this work is often to demonstrate how the deficit pattern associated with a particular disease compares with that of other brain diseases. By making dissociations based on variables such as the anatomical location of the lesions, the size of the lesion, the type of neuronal damage, and the progressive nature of the disease, the researcher hopes to gain insights into brain–behavior relationships.

Although attentional disturbances are common by-products of neurological diseases that affect the brain, they typically receive less emphasis than other cognitive dysfunctions, perhaps because attention is more difficult to measure in a clinical situation and is also more difficult to localize to a specific site of damage.

LOCALIZED AND NONLOCALIZED DEFICITS

Brain diseases sometimes produce a deficit pattern that reflects a clear relationship between structure and function. For example, cerebral vascular disorders often produce damage to a circumscribed cortical region, with effects on a specific cognitive function. The great interest in the aphasias among early neuropsychologists was undoubtedly due in part to the dramatic and unmistakable nature of these disorders, and to the possibility of localizing aphasias to discrete cortical sites. A clear interpretation of the relationship between anatomical structure and cognitive function was possible.

A distinction between specific (localizing) and nonspecific (nonlocalizing) deficits is often made in neuropsychology. As discussed previously, focal brain lesions produce specific disturbances of attention such as hemineglect. However, attentional disorders are not usually that well localized. After generalized brain damage, patients exhibit conceptual impairments, slowness of ideational process, reduced scope of attention, and reduced memory efficiency, which vary as a function of how much damage has occurred (Goodglass

255

& Kaplan, 1979). This relationship corresponds with Lashley's principle of mass effect (1929). That inattention and confusional states are often nonspecific affects of brain damage has been the basis of a "so what" attitude regarding attentional phenomena among some neurological researchers.

Yet, there is good reason to analyze the disturbances of attention as they occur with different neurological illnesses. Such an analysis can yield useful information about the variations of normal and abnormal attention. There are both commonalities and differences in the attentional dysfunction that is exhibited across different neurological diseases. We review here the attentional deficits observed in several common neurological disorders in order to characterize these variations.

MULTIPLE SCLEROSIS

Multiple sclerosis (MS) is one of the most common neurological diseases affecting young adults. It is characterized by a multifocal demyelination of the white matter of the brain and the spinal cord. Lesions of varying size develop from destroyed myelin and leave plaque, which can be observed on pathological examination.

The lesions of MS often affect long fiber tracts. Therefore, spinal nerves are often involved causing motor weakness and parasthesias. The optic nerve is also a common site of lesions that result in visual impairments. Other common symptoms include dysarthria, diplopia, nystagmus, tremor, ataxia, loss of bladder control, and alterations in affective and cognitive state. The occurrence of specific symptoms appears to depend on the neural structure that is lesioned. Because the site of lesion varies across patients, it is difficult to predict a specific pattern of dysfunction. Also, the course of the illness is quite variable. Some patients show a chronic and progressive course of symptoms, and others show a relapsing and remitting course or even a benign pattern.

The cognitive presentation of patients suffering from MS was not given much consideration in early clinical studies. Investigations of this disease often emphasized the prominent sensory and motor symptoms. Because MS is not a disease that directly affects the gray matter of the brain, it was believed that higher cognitive functions were spared. This view has given way to increased evidence of significant neuropsychological deficits in MS patients. These deficits often occur quite independently of the presence of other neurological symptoms (see Rao, 1986, for a detailed review).

Approximately 10% of patients with MS exhibit a progressive deterioration of global cognitive abilities that may resemble a cortical dementia. These patients have great difficulty on a wide range of neuropsychological tasks. Often, as the disease progresses, there is severe memory dysfunction, which may be related to the development of lesions in the subcortical tissue surrounding the third ventricle. Neuropsychological studies have suggested that the cognitive impairments of MS differ from those seen in cortical dementia, as the symptoms of aphasia, apraxia, and agnosia are usually not present in MS dementia (Grant, McDonald, Trimble, Smith, & Reed, 1984; Heaton, Nelson, Thompson, Burks, & Franklin, 1985; Rao, 1986; Cohen & Fisher, 1989). The term subcortical dementia, which has been used to describe the cognitive disorders of Parkinson's and Huntington's diseases, seems also to characterize the cognitive deterioration observed in MS. Learning, memory, and executive control often become markedly impaired. Problems with perceptual-motor speed are usually evident that seem to be related primarily to significant psychomotor slowing. Attentional impairment is also usually apparent in these patients, though it is difficult to disentangle deficits of attention from the psychomotor slowing that is prominent.

Patients with MS who do not exhibit a progressive global deterioration of cognitive functioning may still experience neuropsychological dysfunction (see Figure 11.1). Heaton *et al.* (1985) reported that 46% of the MS patients in their study could be classified as exhibiting neuropsychological dysfunction. Cognitive impairments were common in patients with even mild physical disability. MS patients were found to have the greatest impairments on measures of memory encoding and perceptual-motor integration, whereas broader intellectual abilities were less compromised. Interestingly, Heaton *et al.* did not find attentional dysfunction to be significant, as the presence of attentional deficits could be accounted for by psychomotor slowing. This conclusion was based on a covariance analysis in which performances on tests such as Trail Making, the Stroop Interference Test, and a distraction test were compared. Problems on these tasks were associated with slow performance on other tests without strong attentional demands.

In contrast to this finding of minimal attentional involvement, Cohen and Fisher (1989) found that problems with sustained attention were evident in patients with MS. A significant percentage of patients with MS had difficulty completing Trail B and the Stroop color–word-naming test, whereas none of the normal control subjects had such difficulty. Furthermore, patients with MS had significantly greater difficulty on a continuous performance test. This could not be due only to their slow response times, as during one of the tasks the interstimulus interval was sufficiently large (0.4 sec) to allow the subjects enough time to make a response. MS patients also showed greater inconsistency across trials than normal control subjects, which appeared to be related to fatigue.

Although the problems with sustained attention that have been noted with MS may be partly related to psychomotor slowing, it would be a mistake to assume that impaired psychomotor functioning indicates that attention is intact, or that psychomotor slowing precludes the existence of a fundamental attentional disturbance. In fact, psychomotor inefficiency may reflect the basis of attentional disturbances of MS. The psychomotor slowing that is pervasive in MS patients seems to correspond to problems with performance on a variety of tasks that require attentional capacity. These patients show problems with the speed of information processing that affect their ability to maintain consistent

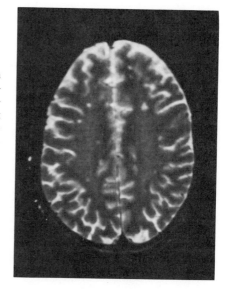

FIGURE 11.1. MRI scan of a 42-year-old woman with multiple sclerosis. Severe white matter disease is evident. This patient exhibited intact language, perceptual, visual–spatial, and conceptual and reasoning abilities. She exhibited mild memory deficits that primarily affected acquisition. Yet memory storage was largely unaffected. In contrast, she exhibited severe deficits of sustained, focused, and selective attention. Significant psychomotor slowing was evident, along with disabling fatigue. This case illustrates that attention depends on an intact information-processing system and the ability to communicate efficiently across neuronal systems. With multiple sclerosis, there is often disruption of information-processing efficiency, which in turn greatly affects attentional capacity, but not necessarily conceptual functioning.

performance. Therefore, perceptual-motor slowing and attentional difficulties may reflect a common source of dysfunction.

The problems with memory encoding that are noted also seem to be correlated with psychomotor slowing and problems with sustained attention. Patients with MS often report that they cannot maintain consistent effort on tasks. Under conditions of increased information load, they typically show a greater decrement in performance on memory tasks than would be seen in normal individuals. They also show slowing in their response times on a variety of information processing tasks.

Psychomotor slowing may be partly related to more primary motor impairments. However, it is unlikely that gross motor slowing can by itself account for the effects on information-processing speed. Cohen and Fisher (1988) found that the motor impairments of MS patients could be dissociated from the attentional difficulties of these patients. Difficulties with sustained effort and fatigue were more highly correlated with performance deficits on attentional tasks than with the level of motor dysfunction. Motor dysfunction was assessed by performance on a Grooved Pegboard test. Even though performance on this motor task correlated with the level of attentional difficulty and of reported fatigue, the strength of this correlation was not as great as that between performance on tests of attention and executive control and subjective measures of fatigue. For instance, poor performance on the Stroop Interference Test, Trail Making B, and a continuous-performance task tended to be more highly correlated with levels of subjective fatigue that was reported in a diary maintained each day (see Table 11.1).

Fatigue and Inattention

Although progressive cognitive decline is not noted in all patients with MS, the presence of problems with fatigue is a frequent symptom occurring in as much as 92% of this clinical population (Freal, Kraft, & Coryell, 1984). Fatigue is of theoretical interest in our discussion of attention, as the term *fatigue* is often used to refer to an inability to persist after

TABLE 11.1.   Subjective Fatigue Reports in Multiple Sclerosis

	MS fatigue patients[a] (Mean ± SD)	Normal controls[a] (Mean ± SD)
Diary items		
Overall energy level	3.00 (0.9)	4.2 (0.8)
Motor stamina	2.75 (0.8)	4.5 (1.1)
Ability to persist	3.02 (1.1)	4.0 (0.9)
Motivation	2.98 (1.2)	3.6 (1.3)
Concentration	2.98 (0.6)	4.5 (0.7)
General well-being	2.90 (0.8)	3.9 (1.0)
Overall fatigue	2.96 (1.3)	4.5 (0.7)
Sleep (night before)	2.10 (1.9)	3.3 (1.3)
Fatigue factors[b]		
Concentration/ sustained attention		
Motor stamina		
Motivational state		

[a]Scores reflect rating of 1–5 (1 = poor, 5 = excellent).
[b]Standardized factor scores.

long periods of sustained activity. As we discussed in Chapter 3, fatigue is a difficult symptom to characterize. In many neurology texts, fatigue is given mention as an important and troubling clinical phenomenon. For instance, Adams and Victor (1981) described two types of fatigue; one involving a feeling of lassitude and reduced energy, and the other being due to reduced motor strength. Relatively little attention is given to fully characterizing the physiological and psychological manifestations of this symptom, perhaps largely because of the difficulties encountered when one attempts to investigate fatigue.

Fatigue is often used as a concept to describe the subjective experience of the individual, who feels that she or he cannot continue with a task. By this criterion, fatigue reflects a self-perception of the individual's state of tiredness, decreased energy, or reduced motivation. The term *fatigue* can also refer to the patient's feeling of decreased motor capability.

The concept of fatigue has also been used to characterize the behavioral and physiological changes occurring over long periods of responding. In most neurology texts, the term *fatigue* refers to a neuromuscular event. With prolonged and/or rapid responses, the capability of the neuromuscular junction to initiate an action potential diminishes. This phenomenon was described as *neuromuscular fatigue*.

In behavioral studies the term *fatigue* has been used to refer to a decreased level of performance that occurs under conditions of sustained performance, or under conditions of altered CNS capacity due to sleep deprivation and other extreme conditions. Unfortunately, there was little correspondence between these different uses of the word *fatigue*. Neuromuscular depletion cannot be shown to be the basis of these other forms of fatigue in most cases. Instead, behavioral and subjective fatigue seem to reflect the state of the CNS.

Behavioral fatigue can be distinguished from neuromuscular fatigue. An individual exhibiting neuromuscular fatigue can no longer generate a muscular response when fatigue occurs. The neurological disease myasthenia gravis represents an extreme example of such a condition. Under conditions of neuromuscular fatigue, the electrophysiological characteristics of the action potential change, and the muscle ceases to react normally. Neuromuscular fatigue is not common in healthy individuals, except under conditions of extreme physical exertion. In contrast, behavioral fatigue is a common occurrence that happens to most people when they engage in a demanding activity for long durations. It is characterized by a decline in the quality of performance, but it is not due to neuromuscular depletion.

Under conditions of behavioral fatigue, the individual is still usually able to respond for short intervals at any given time. However, there is an inability to persist in responding. The primary manifestation of this type of fatigue is an increased inconsistency, as the individual fails to respond optimally for much of the time. There may be an increased variability of performance over time.

Such inconsistency was demonstrated by Cohen and Fisher (1989) in their study of MS patients. The declines in performance that were found on neuropsychological measures over the performance of certain tasks could be considered behavioral fatigue. The origin of this fatigue seems to be the CNS, rather than events occurring in the periphery. Furthermore, this fatigue is pervasive across a variety of different types of tasks and is manifested with increasing task demand (i.e., task length, information load, and memory demands).

Behavioral fatigue may be considered a manifestation of the inability to sustain attention. When the individual persists on a demanding task, eventually there is a decrement in performance that can be called *fatigue*. In this definition, fatigue is the end product of attentional failure under conditions in which the person cannot escape from a task in which he or she must persist.

The term *fatigue* may also refer to an underlying neurophysiological state that results in inattention. The pilot who becomes exhausted after long durations of flight may experience problems due to the need to sustain focused attention (behavioral fatigue). However, underlying the fatigue state may be the fact that the pilot has also remained sleepless for long durations. Therefore, the internal biological demands on the individual may set the conditions for fatigue. In the case of MS, there are changes in the tendency to fatigue that depend on biological factors that may vary as a function of the time of day or even the season of the year. The phenomenon of fatigue is governed by both behavioral demands and the neural resources that can be devoted to the task at a given time.

In summary, the neuropsychological impairments that accompany MS illustrate the intricate relationship between cognitive performance and the underlying processes of attention and the symptoms of fatigue. The effects of this disease on central white matter is such that it can cause a major breakdown in the communication of information across associational areas that are otherwise unaffected. This breakdown in information-processing capacity causes severe dementing conditions if certain regions of the brain are involved. However, even when dementia is not present, this decreased ability to transmit nerve impulses often causes a compromised information-processing system, as evidenced by response slowing, attentional variability, and difficulties with executive regulation. Fatigue may be the most obvious consequence of these effects.

HEAD INJURY

Head trauma is a frequent consequence of the human inclination toward high-velocity transport and physical aggression. In the United States and Britain, between 200 and 300 per 100,000 of the population are admitted to the hospital each year for head injuries (Jennet & Teasdale, 1981). Any experience that results in a sudden acceleration and deceleration of the head can produce damage to the brain, even when the head does not strike an object. For example, an occupant of a car that comes to a sudden stop may suffer head injury, even though she or he is strapped into the car, because the brain is thrown back and forth against a rigid object: the skull. Primary brain damage results from the immediate consequences of the impact on the brain caused by sudden acceleration. Secondary brain damage, on the other hand, appears because of the changes in the brain environment that occur because of the initial trauma.

Teasdale and Mendelow (1984) described two different types of primary brain damage: contusions and diffuse axonal injuries. Contusions are hemorrhagic lesions caused by the impact of the brain on the rough surfaces of the skull. Most frequently, contusions occur on the basal surfaces of the frontal lobes and the poles of the temporal lobes, regardless of the site of the external impact on the head. Diffuse axonal damage occurs owing to the shearing of axons as they are stretched by the movement of surrounding brain tissue. The axons tear or break and then degenerate. Axons of the brain stem and the cerebral hemisphere are both affected by this type of injury, which is probably more attributable to rotational than to linear movement of the brain. The most consistent effect of primary brain damage is unconsciousness. The duration of unconsciousness is due primarily to the severity of the axonal damage; cortical contusions can occur without any loss of consciousness. Loss of consciousness probably reflects brain stem damage, possibly due to damage to the reticular activating system.

Teasdale and Mendelow (1984) listed a host of factors that can result in secondary brain damage. These are of two types: intracranial and extracranial. Intracranial factors include hematomas, brain swelling, infection, hemorrhage, and hydrocephalus. Extracranial factors include respiratory failure and hypotension. The mechanisms by which these factors affect brain damage are hypoxia and ischemia, and the distortion or compression of brain tissue.

Clinical Presentation and Sequelae

The level of consciousness shown by the victim after head trauma is one of the best measures of the severity of brain damage. The level of unconsciousness is most frequently quantified by means of the Glasgow Coma Scale, which measures eye, verbal, and motor responsiveness (Teasdale & Jennett, 1974). The depth and duration of posttraumatic coma are reliable indicators of the severity of brain damage and the probability of long-term recovery.

Recovery from coma is heralded by opening of the eyes and by eye movements. These may be followed by the patient's uttering words and following simple commands. What follows may be a period of traumatic delirium, when the patient shows confused, aggressive, and generally disinhibited behavior, for which there is a subsequent amnesia. The patient's behavior gradually becomes more appropriate, although disorientation and inertia persist. After discharge, personality changes are frequent, and the patient may be apathetic, emotionally labile or blunted, and socially disinhibited and may show psychomotor retardation for an indefinite period (Jennet & Teasdale, 1981). Because the frontal lobes are the most likely to suffer contusions from head trauma, the prevalence of personality change is not surprising. The neurological sequelae of severe head injury include hemiparesis, brain stem syndromes, cranial nerve injuries, and seizure disorders.

After a less severe head injury, a patient may experience a postconcussional syndrome. Symptoms include headache, dizziness, and, more variably, nervousness, memory problems, fatigue, insomnia, irritability, sexual dysfunction, and alcohol intolerance. In the majority of patients with mild concussions, the intellectual and emotional symptoms show good recovery, and these patients are able to return to former social and occupational responsibilities within a few months. A minority of patients continue to exhibit a postconcussional syndrome long after the initial injury. These patients often show no objective neurological signs or impairment on neuropsychological assessment. Although for many years these symptoms were considered primarily psychological in origin, it has been found that even mild concussions produce brain damage. Mild concussions can result in long-term disability in the absence of medically apparent signs of significant brain damage. In a study of 538 patients with minor head trauma, defined by 20 minutes or less of unconsciousness and a hospital stay of less than 2 days, many of the patients experienced severe problems in returning to normal levels of function (Rimel, Giordani, Barth, Boll, & Jane, 1981). Of these patients, 79% reported headaches, and 59% experienced memory problems; 34% had failed to return to employment. Significantly, after litigation, the compensation to the patients bore little relationship to the symptoms and the subsequent unemployment. This finding suggests that the failure of these patients to recover from head trauma was influenced by factors other than economic contingencies. After reviewing longitudinal studies of patients with persistent postconcussional problems, Dimken, Temkin, and Armsden (1989) cautioned that patients who show poor psychosocial recovery from mild head injury may be influenced by personality, social, or economic problems that predate the injury. The specific psychosocial factors that influence recovery remain to be identified, however, if they exist.

Neuropsychological Effects

General Effects

The effects of head trauma vary greatly with the severity of the injury, and with the specific cause and loci of the damage. Mild injuries may result in a postconcussive syndrome. More severe injuries are often associated with marked impairments. Such patients typically experience mental and motor slowing; memory deficits, especially the ability to learn new information; difficulty in sustaining effort or attention; and difficulty with mental arithmetic. Patients are usually more impaired on visuoconstructive tasks than on verbal tasks and have more difficulty with complex than with simple tasks (Brooks, 1984; Conkey, 1938; Levin, Benton, & Grossman, 1982). Performance slowing and impaired learning tend to be the most persistent deficits (Brooks, 1984).

Attentional Disturbances

Disturbed attention in head trauma patients has been noted since the turn of the century. Persistent distractability, forgetfulness, poor concentration, apathy, and fatiguability are prominent clinical sequelae of head trauma and are reported as problems by many patients (Gronwall, 1987; Van Zomeren & Van Den Berg, 1985). Nevertheless, neuropsychological characterization of attentional disturbances in these patients has been neglected, and the results of studies have frequently been inconsistent. In part, the reason has been the minor role that attention played in the evolution of psychology and psychometrics the first half of this century; tests of language and memory disturbance, by contrast, received far more neuropsychological investigation. Second, the severity of the head trauma, the type of brain damage incurred, and the stage of recovery of the patient being tested should be considered in tests for attentional deficits, but studies usually contain a small sample that represents only one type of patient at a specific stage of recovery. Therefore, the results of studies are difficult to compare, as the patient samples show great differences in clinical characteristics.

Head trauma patients as a group perform poorly on most tests of mental control, concentration, and performance speed. Timed tests are particularly sensitive to head trauma. Vigilance performance is often impaired. The classic tests of attention from the Wechsler Intelligence and Memory scales (Digit Symbol, Digit Span, and Mental Control) are often depressed (Gronwall,1987). The basis for such deficits remains speculative. Deficits in arousal, selective attention, divided attention, processing speed, and frontal executive failure have all been advanced as explanations for functional syndromes. Correlation with noninvasive or postmortem measures of pathology, however, has seldom been attempted. One such study (Langfitt, Obrist, Alavi, Grossman, Zimmerman, Jaggi, Uzzell, Reivich, & Patton, 1987) described serial findings from a broad range of imaging methods and neuropsychological assessments in two patients with head injuries. Langfitt *et al.* found that different techniques were often sensitive to quite different aspects of neuropathology. MRI was superior to CT in delineating hemorrhagic and edemic territory during the acute stage. Areas of decreased density, probably representing encephalomalacia, were detected by both CT and MRI. PET scans showed additional regions of dysfunction associated with decreased glucose metabolism as well as dysfunction in regions of structural damage detected in CT and MRI. Unfortunately, the neuropsychological data from these two patients was not presented in any detail. One patient returned to work as a laborer and showed residual apraxia and recall problems, though his family considered him normal. The second patient retained a high average IQ and performed within normal limits on tests, but he was impaired by inattention, rapid mental fatigue, slowing, and impoverished ideation in his everyday life. The neuropsychological battery was surprisingly insensitive to focal lesions in the temporal regions in both patients.

Focal Frontal and Temporal Lobe Deficits

The frontal and temporal lobes frequently suffer contusive damage in head trauma. Stuss (1987) argued that such damage suffered by head trauma patients may produce subtle deficits similar to those observed in classic frontal and temporal lobe syndromes. Stuss, Eli, Hugenholtz, Richard, LaRochelle, Poirier, and Bell (1985) studied 20 patients who had shown good recovery from closed-head injury. Although lacking definite neurological signs of severe residual CNS dysfunction, the patients all complained of difficulty in concentration, fatigue, irritability, and decline in everyday task performance, complaints typically seen in postconcussive syndromes. Their performance on a set of neuropsychological tests was compared with that of a group of control subjects matched for age, gender, handedness, education, language, and IQ. Although the patients and the controls were matched on IQ, they showed marked deficits on the Brown–Peterson test of memory under interference and paired-associates memory after a delay period ($p < .01$). Tests showing mild deficits included Stroop color time, tapping speed, Wechsler Logical Memory delayed recall, Wisconsin Card Sorting perseverative errors, and Wechsler visual reproductions ($p < .05$). Other timed tests showed a tendency toward slowing ($p < .10$). The patients showed no marked differences on the remaining Wechsler Adult Intelligence Scale-Revised (WAIS-R) subtests; on the Orientation, Information, or Mental Control subtests from the Wechsler Memory Scale; on aphasia evaluation; or on the generation of word lists. Even when head trauma patients showed good clinical recovery and retain IQ scores in the normal range, tasks that demand rapid processing, resistance to interference, and learning sometimes caused a breakdown in performance. Stuss *et al.* interpreted these findings rather broadly as being indicative of a divided attention deficit reflecting reduced overall information-processing capacity. In a later review of these results, Stuss (1987) also considered the possibility that these performance failures reflect focal brain syndromes, although the patients did not receive adequate imaging assessment to allow a test of such hypotheses.

Experimental Findings

Van Zomeren, Brouwer, and Deelman (1984) attempted to categorize attentional deficits by using three experimentally defined approaches: selectivity, speed of information processing, and arousal.

Selectivity

In defining selective attention deficits, Van Zomeren and colleagues emphasized response selection rather than sensory filtering. Selective deficits should occur if head trauma patients are less able to suppress automatic or habitual responding to information irrelevant to the current task. This then interferes with the maintenance of attention and with responses to the channel or message of interest. This deficit was referred to as a focused-attention deficit by Shiffrin and Schneider (1977). Such deficits occur in everyday life when stimuli provoke well-rehearsed but inappropriate responses, for example, when a person attempts to manipulate the light switch on a newly purchased lamp and gropes briefly in a habitual attempt to find the switch in the same location as on the previous lamp. Neuropsychologically, focused-attention deficits due to response competition have been most commonly investigated by means of the Stroop test, in which a person is required to suppress a well-learned response in favor of a new response dictated by the task. Selective attention can also be defined from the perspective of a sensory filtering of information. A selective attention deficit in this case occurs if a person is unable to attend efficiently to a given stimulus because of distraction by irrelevant stimuli or is unable to maintain attention to a given channel of information (vigilance deficit). The classical experimental protocol for investigating selective attention processes is the dichotic listening paradigm, in which a person attempts to follow one of two messages, each message being presented to a different ear. After an extensive review of the literature, Van Zomeren *et al.* (1984) concluded that head trauma patients do not show focused attention deficits that cannot be attributed to a slowing of processing speed.

This conclusion stands in frank contrast to the subjective reports of patients and the impressions of clinicians and patients that distractibility by task-irrelevant information is a major problem. For example, Lezak (1978) reported that, in a series of 51 patients seen for research evaluation, 76% of whom had traumatic brain damage, 87% showed distractibility. Van Zomeren and Van Den Burg (1985) reported that, two years after a severe head injury, 33% of patients reported difficulties in concentrating, and 21% reported an inability to do two things simultaneously. These results suggest that current tests of selectivity, or vulnerability to distraction, may fail to capture difficulties posed by task demands in the patient's natural environment. Van Zomeren *et al.*'s conclusions discount some of their own findings of an interaction between the number of distracting stimuli in a task and the degree of deficit shown by head trauma patients, as well as the poor performance of head trauma patients on vigilance tasks. This may be due to Van Zomeren *et al.*'s emphasis on defining selective attention deficits on the basis of response conflicts generated by prior exposure to distracting stimuli. A second possible explanation of these discrepant clinical and experimental findings is that experimental tasks of selective attention are too easy and therefore lack sufficient discriminating power to detect interactive effects. Most experimental tests of attention use simple, explicit task demands, and brief, highly structured stimulus–response periods and require focusing on only one task at a time. In everyday life and work, however, task demands are rarely explicit, multiple tasks must be performed over extended periods of time, and task priorities must be constantly reevaluated.

Processing Speed

Van Zomeren *et al.* (1984) argued that slowing of processing speed in head trauma patients accounts for most of the cognitive deficits that have been experimentally associated with head trauma. Speed-of-processing deficits should be especially apparent on tests that demand controlled processing, as described by Shiffrin and Schneider (1977). Controlled processing occurs when task-specific strategies must be used to supplement automatic processing. Because controlled processes make demands on operations and storage systems that are limited in capacity and that are frequently serial in operation, divided-attention deficits can occur if the processing speed is inadequate to keep up with the stream of relevant information arriving from the environment, or with the tendency of the contents in short-term memory to decay. For example, most people have difficulties carrying out complex arithmetic problems mentally because the intermediate steps are forgotten before they can be integrated (try to mentally multiply 4,532 by 8,964; the process is trivial if a paper and pencil are available to reduce the load on the working memory). The speed of information processing in head trauma patients is slower on many tasks, particularly those in which there are many stimulus alternatives, or in which there is stimulus–response incompatibility. Performance is delayed on both simple and choice reaction-time tasks (Gronwall, 1977). Van Zomeren *et al.* (1984) interpreted these results as indicating a slowing of controlled processing or, in Shiffrin and Schneider's terminology, a divided-attention deficit. Slowing of processing speed would have an obvious impact on the performance of deadline-related tasks in the real world. Simply by executing tasks slowly, patients tend to constantly fall behind in attempting to carry out their premorbid work load.

An ambitious study by Stuss, Stethem, Hugenholtz, Picton, Pivik, and Richard (1989) investigated the effects of head trauma on a set of reaction time measures varying in task demands for several groups of closed-head-injury victims. These patients had varied in the severity of the initial injury and their stage of recovery. Tests of simple visual reaction time and choice visual reaction time were included. Choice reaction time (RT) included an easy discrimination condition in which the target and the distractors shared no attributes, a complex condition that required selecting responses on the basis of multiple attributes, and a redundant condition that required the subjects to ignore uninformative attributes in the distractor stimuli. Three groups of subjects with injuries of varying severity were tested. The severity of the patients' injuries ranged from those who had received a mild concussion and no hospitalization to patients with severe neurological damage who had received inpatient treatment. The patients were slower than the controls on all choice RT tests. Slowing in simple RT was less consistent. The patients were less able than the controls to maintain performance by filtering out redundant information. A group of head injury patients who had required hospitalization showed greater RT variability, and more variation in performance levels between testing sessions, than the controls. These results suggest that head injury victims may exhibit several types of attentional deficits. In general, head trauma patients show slowing of information processing on choice reaction-time tasks suggestive of mental slowing. In addition, more severely injured patients may show problems with focused attention, or with the ability to filter out irrelevant information. Finally, the patients showed inconsistency in performance across trials, suggesting a deficit in sustained attention. Fatigue effects, characterized by reaction time measures at the beginning and after an hour of testing, were not significant in any of the groups.

Mild-head-trauma patients frequently show normal performance on traditional psychometric testing. It is possible that tests using tasks specifically designed to detect the attentional deficits associated with a slowing of processing speed are more sensitive to subtle deficits due to head trauma. Gentilini, Nichelli, and Schoenhuber (1989) reviewed the results of two studies of mild-head-injury patients, one using traditional psychometric tests, the other using tests of selective, sustained, divided, and spatially distributed attention. Traditional neuropsychological tests were ineffective in discriminating between controls and mild-head-trauma patients 1 month after the head injury. Tests of reaction time during attentionally demanding tasks, on the other hand, showed response slowing in the head injury group that was present at 3- and 6-month follow-ups. These findings suggest that attentional tests of processing speed may be much more sensitive measures of head injury effects than traditional neuropsychological measures.

Arousal

Head trauma patients frequently seem to have a disorder of arousal on clinical evaluation, characterized by lack of energy, mental slowness, or an inability to sustain effort. In reviewing the small number of studies of arousal-relevant performance, Van Zomeren *et al.* (1984) found little evidence that head trauma patients show more rapid decline in alertness or arousal during task performance than control subjects. Their performance was impaired on both continuous RT tasks and vigilance tasks, a finding suggesting that if an arousal or alertness deficit existed, it was a chronic rather than a phasic deficit. EEG and autonomic data did not document lowered arousal in head trauma patients during task performance. In fact, there is some evidence from EKG and EEG studies that head trauma patients are hyperaroused, both in a resting state and during performance. Van Zomeren *et al.* suggested that head trauma patients, because of their deficits in memory and processing speed, must constantly put forth great effort to cope with everyday demands. This constant effort results in the fatigue, stress disorders, and reactive emotional disturbances commonly experienced after initial recovery from mild head trauma. Van Zomeren *et al.* put forth a coping hypothesis, which predicts that head trauma patients will show stronger physiological signs of mental effort on cognitively demanding tasks. Although there is modest evidence for this coping hypothesis, it seems concordant with subjective resorts by patients and with clinical impressions of their struggle to cope with the demands of daily living.

P3 Response in Head Trauma

The P3 response of the evoked potential in head trauma patients has been reported to be both slowed and of diminished amplitude (Curry, 1981; Pananicolaou, 1987; Squires & Olle, 1986). Slowing of P3 latency is consistent with other evidence of slowed mental speed in head trauma patients. Pananicolaou (1987) reported that patients with a history of posttraumatic amnesia had slowed P3 responses, whereas patients in an amnestic period had P3 latencies that were within normal limits. The P3 response in this study, however, was not evoked within the context of task demands. Therefore, it may have reflected passive rather than active attentional processing. Diminished amplitude of the P3 response may be indicative of underresponsivity to task-relevant stimuli, perhaps reflecting problems in maintenance of arousal.

Remediation of Attention Deficits

The cognitive rehabilitation of head trauma patients has had limited success in remediating attention deficits. The generalization to other tasks of performance improvements on computer-based attentional tasks has been poor. Several authors have suggested focusing on remediating, or providing coping strategies for, specific difficulties encountered by patients in daily life, rather than attempting to alter attentional function as a mental process (Ponsford & Kinsella, 1988; Wood, 1987).

Summary of Deficits after Closed-Head Injury

The prevalence of attentional deficits in head trauma patients has been documented from the vantage point of subjective reports, neuropsychological investigations, experimental tests, and psychophysiological responses.

Several major findings have emerged from the literature. First, even mild head injury can result in a persistent slowing of mental processing speed, particularly on tasks making attentional demands. Whether this slowing is the result of declines in overall cognitive capacity or in specific attentional mechanisms is not known. Second, vigilance performance may be impaired. Finally, although neuropsychological and experimental tests seem relatively insensitive to these problems, many head injury patients experience problems with fatigue and distractibility in everyday life.

The underlying basis of these performance deficits and their relationship to pathophysiology and stages of recovery remain poorly understood. There is a need for studies that use a multivariate approach to assessment, including the use of both psychometric and experimentally derived measures of attention deficits to evaluate well-characterized clinical samples over the course of recovery. At a minimum, research evaluation should test for distraction effects by relevant and irrelevant stimuli, fatigue effects, vigilance deficits, and deficient planning or organization in response to complex task demands. Responses should be scored for speed as well as accuracy, as mild-head-trauma patients may be accurate but slowed in performance. Neuropsychological tests that capture the sustained and multiple demands on performance characteristic of the naturalistic environment remain to be applied to this patient population.

SEIZURE DISORDER

Seizure disorders are typically accompanied by significant changes in the level or duration of consciousness. The electrical disturbance that constitutes the seizure may produce alterations of cognitive, behavioral, and emotional functioning. Impairments vary according to the sites of the brain lesions responsible for the seizure's locus and for the type of seizure disorder (e.g., partial vs. generalized). Seizures produce transient changes associated with the ictal event, which usually affect the ability of the patient to carry on normal activities during that time. Functional impairments may also be observed in both pre- and postictal consequences. During the times between seizures (interictal periods) patients vary considerably in their neuropsychological presentation. Therefore, when describing the effects of seizures on attentional functions, it is important to specify the time period of interest (e.g., ictal vs. interictal).

The Ictal Period

The actual seizure usually produces dramatic changes in the characteristics of consciousness and attention. Some seizures involve primarily momentary attentional lapses in which the patient seems to be staring off into space (i.e., absence phenomenon). Ictal events can be either very specific in their behavioral or cognitive manifestation, as in the case of partial simple seizures, or very global in their effect. For instance, partial simple seizures may produce specific sensory, motor, or physiological responses, whereas grand mal seizures involve a convulsion of the entire body. The attentional disturbance accompanying the ictal event relates to the location of the seizure's generator and to the degree to which various brain regions are involved.

Interictal Manifestations

There is much debate regarding the neuropsychological features of patients between ictal events. The cognitive impairments that are noted tend to correlate with the neuroanatomical site of the lesion or the abnormal brain tissue. However, this relationship is quite variable, as there is not necessarily a direct relationship between the severity of the seizures and cognitive deficits. Memory impairments are often noted in patients with epilepsy (Deutsch, 1953; Loiseau, Stube, Broustet, Batteleochi, Gomeni, & Morselli, 1980; Rausch, Lief, & Crandall, 1978). The type of memory deficit detected correlates with the side of the lesion in patients undergoing unilateral craniotomy (Milner, 1965), but may correspond only moderately with the exact sites of seizure foci (Fedio & Mirsky, 1969). In general, cognitive impairments vary as a function of the localization of seizure loci in partial complex epilepsy (Trimble & Thompson, 1987).

The attentional disturbances of the interictal period are also difficult to characterize because of the heterogeneity of the brain disorders that can cause seizures. Mirskey *et al.* (1960) found that patients with generalized epilepsy had greater problems on the continuous performance task, than those with focal seizures. Other researchers have found mixed results that depend on the subject inclusion criteria used in a particular study. Glowinski (1973) found all seizure patients to be impaired on divided-attention tasks. Impairments of attention in patients with epilepsy may be related to a slowing in mental processing speed. This possibility is supported by findings from several research groups (e.g., Arena, Menchetti, Tassinari, & Tognetti, 1979; Bruhn & Parsons, 1977).

Attentional disturbances in some patients with focal epilepsy may be related to associated affective and personality characteristics, particularly if the medial temporal and limbic systems are involved (Bear & Fedio, 1977). Although there continues to be debate over the existence of a specific "temporal lobe personality" associated with seizures generated from this region, most investigators agree that personality and affective disturbances are common. Furthermore, patients with seizures of the temporal-limbic system often seem to have problems with obsessive behaviors and impulse control. Attentional dysfunction is an obvious cognitive manifestation of this type of behavior tendency, although it is likely that the patient will show strikingly good attention to some tasks, while ignoring others that it may be appropriate to attend to. Therefore, seizure disorders with temporal-limbic loci illustrate the relationship between affective and motivational control and the regulation of attention.

METABOLIC DISEASES

Alterations in the level and quality of consciousness are a hallmark feature of the changes that occur secondary to metabolic encephalopathy. Metabolic disorders differ from other diseases that we have discussed in that their effect on the brain is usually secondary to the failure of some other peripheral organ system. In some cases changes in metabolic state can cause permanent damage to CNS structures. More frequently, the biochemical disregulation that accompanies these states results in transient alterations in the functional capability of neural systems.

In Table 11.2 some of the metabolic disorders that affect the processes of attention are listed. Some of these disorders cause primary disruptions of consciousness, resulting in confusion, lethargy, or even coma. Other disorders produce effects on higher cognitive processes.

Metabolic disorders affect consciousness by altering amounts of oxygen and glucose, or the balance of electrolytes, proteins, or other biochemicals. Generally, the change in consciousness that occurs is proportional to the degree of disruption from the normal metabolic state. For instance, in mild cases of hypoxia, there may be a transient period of

TABLE 11.2.   Metabolic Disorders That Often Affect Attention

Acquired disorders	Metabolic disorders
Hypoxia	Wernicke–Korsakoff's disease
Hypercapnia	Nicotinic deficiency
Hyperglycemia	B_{12} deficiency
Hypoglycemia	Inherited diseases
Hepatic failure	Hepatolenticular degeneration
Uremia	Family progressive myoclonus
Diabetes mellitus	Polysaccharide encephalopathy
Hepatocerebral degeneration	Polyneuropathies
Hypoparathyroidism	
Hyperthyroidism	
Hypothyroidism	
Cushing's disease	

inattentiveness. During this period, patients may show a slight breakdown in their ability to reason. They may also show a short period of motor discontrol. These effects are usually temporary. However, as the duration of anoxia increases, permanent changes may result owing to ischemic effects on the brain. With prolonged periods of anoxia, cerebral functions are reduced to complete unawareness, and coma results from the reduction in the level of arousal that is generated by the pons and the reticular systems. Eventually, death results when brain stem functions cease.

Hypoglycemic encephalopathies produced by changes in insulin levels or liver diseases that affect glycogen storage cause a variety of symptoms, including anxiety and hyperactivity. Eventually, drowsiness and confusion may result. Chronic hypoglycemia causes lethargy and reductions in psychomotor activity. These may lead to generalized intellectual deterioration.

Chronic hepatic insufficiency also produces similar symptoms with a wide variation in symptoms of altered arousal and sensorium. Delirium and confusional states are common features of liver dysfunction, as well as renal disease. Fatigue, apathy, and inattentiveness are key features of uremic encephalopathies. Following hypothalamic damage, there may be severe disregulation of sodium levels associated with a condition of diabetes insipidus. Metabolic disturbances which produce hypernatremia, hyperosmolarity, and hypercapnia may also produce dramatic deterioration in the overall quality of behavioral functioning, since these conditions are likely to cause stupor, lethargy, and diminished arousal, which in turn reduces attentional capacity. As sodium and other electrolyte levels are likely to fluctuate following such damage, there may be wide alterations in behavioral state. Such variability may also be evident with various forms of toxicity from drug effects.

Thyroid function has obvious effects on many aspects of cognitive and behavioral functioning. In fact, abnormalities of thyroid function can produce encephalopathies that can mimic depression and even dementia. Hyperthyroidism often produces agitation, anxiety, and fluctuations in affective state. In contrast, hypothyroidism usually causes apathy, psychomotor slowing, and inattentiveness. The relationship between thyroid activity and behavioral state has interesting implications for the role of metabolic activity on attention and arousal. When the metabolic rate is increased, symptoms associated with excessive arousal result, whereas the hypothyroidism produces symptoms associated with decreased behavioral activation. The inattention that occurs secondary to thyroid dysfunction mirrors the activational deficits that were just described.

Given the scope of this text, it is not possible to cover all of the metabolic syndromes that affect attentional processes. However, it is safe to say that changes in the metabolic state of the individual are likely to cause changes in the quality of consciousness and arousal of the individual. Inattention is often the manifestation of these changes. The type of attentional disturbance that is observed depends in part on the behavioral and activational effects that are induced. An individual who becomes more hyperactive and fidgety as a result of a metabolic influence is likely to show increased distractibility and excessive shifting of attention. Psychomotor retardation and lethargy are likely to be associated with a decreased tendency to attend to any relevant stimuli, resulting in problems with vigilance and errors of omission. With increased severity, there is often a more generalized effect on other aspects of cognition.

The variable nature of attention performance associated with many metabolic diseases illustrates the critical role that biochemical modulation plays in attentional regulation. When metabolic disorders are not treated, severe chronic conditions may result. Eventually, permanent structural brain damage may occur. In such cases, the original attention variability may develop into a more stable deficit with characteristics that depend on the brain regions that are involved. Therefore, the metabolic disorders represent a bridge between the anatomical and biochemical bases of neurobehavioral regulation.

HYDROCEPHALUS

The condition of hydrocephalus occurs when there is an abnormality of ventricular fluid flow in the CNS. Frequently, the pressure exerted by the cerebrospinal fluid (CSF) in the ventricles of the brain increases to cause hydrocephalus. In other instances, the CSF pressure is normal, but the flow is interrupted. Hydrocephalus can be caused by infection, metabolic changes, or structural abnormalities that disrupt CSF flow. The cranium, the dura, and the vertebral canal from an inelastic container that restricts cerebral volume; the result is increased pressure when the amount of fluid in the ventricles is increased. Normally, an equilibrium of fluid pressure is maintained through CSF absorption and circulation and metabolic action. However, certain diseases that disrupt venous outflow or that increase CSF volume change this equilibrium. Tumor, brain swelling, and clots of blood are common causes of increased intracranial pressure (Adams & Victor, 1981).

When the CSF is obstructed, tension hydrocephalus occurs. Although the sites of obstruction vary, obstruction is commonly seen at the foramen of Monro, the Silvian aqueduct, and the basal foramina of Magendie and Luschka. The subarachnoid spaces in lower brain regions of the midbrain, the pons, and the medulla may also be the point of obstruction. The ventricular enlargement that follows this obstruction exerts pressure on surrounding brain tissue, that can cause neural destruction. Often, the effects of such pressure are transient, as dysfunction is greatest at the time of maximal pressure. However, the age of onset of the problem also determines the functional outcome. Infants with congenital hydrocephalus may be very retarded in cognitive functioning as a result of massive enlargement of the ventricles that destroys much cortex.

Occult tension hydrocephalus, which occurs owing to tumor or some other acute obstruction, tends to produce a more specific clinical syndrome. Patients often exhibit marked inattention, distractibility, and problems with planning and response organization. In this sense, they appear to have the symptoms of a bilateral frontal-lobe disorder. However, they may also show an increase in motor dysfunction, with increased clumsiness, gait difficulties, and ataxia. These difficulties may suggest a parkinsonian presentation. With further progression of the illness, incontinence may be noted.

Normal pressure hydrocephalus (NPH) is similar in its presentation, as a triad of symptoms is usually found: progressive gait disorder, sphincter incontinence, and changes in cognition (similar to those described above). The main distinction between NPH and other forms of hydrocephalus is the nonprogressive nature of NPH, which is due to the establishing of an equilibrium between CSF production and absorption. NPH can be caused by trauma, hemorrhage from a ruptured aneurysm, and diseases such as meningitis.

The fact that symptoms are often relieved through treatments such as shunting illustrates that cognitive symptoms often reflect transient effects of pressure on critical neural structures. Patients with hydrocephalus usually show a variable pattern of cognitive performance. This variability is sometimes considered a hallmark feature of "subcortical" disorders. With NPH, considerable pressure is exerted on the central white matter and frontal horns, while the central gray matter, the thalami, the basal ganglia, and the brain stem are less affected (Adams & Victor, 1981). The central white matter disruptions may account for the presence of extrapyramidal symptoms and difficulties with response control. The problems with executive control found in patients with hydrocephalus may also be the result of disruption of these pathways, as the frontal lobes may become dysfunctional owing to expansion of the frontal horns (Benson, 1975).

Neuropsychological Impairments

Hydrocephalus is characterized by the presence of neuropsychological impairments on measures of visual-motor ability, attention, learning, and fine motor control. Typically, patients with this disorder do not show aphasia, agnosia, or apraxia. Therefore, their primary visual and verbal processing abilities remain uneffected. Memory is only mildly impaired in the early stages of hydrocephalus, although the rate of learning may be greatly reduced. The fact that executive regulation, attentional control, and motor functioning are selectively affected points to the interrelationship among these functions.

The attentional dysfunction that is found with NPH is noteworthy because of the characteristic variability that is usually found. Patients with this disorder are able to perform tasks at certain times and fail at other times. Presumably, this variation occurs as a result of changes in ventricular pressure over time. These attentional variations probably reflect alterations in information-processing capacity secondary to the effect of this pressure on critical pathways and structures.

ALZHEIMER'S DISEASE

Alzheimer's disease (AD) is a common, progressive dementing disorder. Its prevalence increases with age, with a striking increase in incidence after the age of 60. The disease is typically characterized by lapses of recent memory, occasionally accompanied by subtle changes in personality and mood. The memory disorder is progressive, and by the time a patient is brought to medical attention, a marked anterograde amnesia is apparent. Patients frequently lack awareness of their memory problems and are bewildered regarding a caretaker's insistence that they receive clinical attention. As the disease progresses, all areas of higher cognitive function deteriorate, and eventually, the patient is rendered mute and unresponsive. Depression, agitation, and personality and behavioral disorders (paranoia, hallucinations, and aggression) are common. The disease usually shows a rapid progression, with an average interval of 7 years between diagnosis and death (Khachaturian, 1985).

Although there are rare instances of families with a dominantly transmitted form of the disorder, the etiology of the disease is usually unknown. The neuropathology is remarkable for neuronal cell loss, senile plaques, and neurofibrillary tangles within the body of deteriorating neurons. This pathology is most severe in the hippocampal regions but can usually be observed in the frontal and parietal cortex as well (Kemper, 1986).

Patients usually show deficits in sustaining attention early in the disease course, but this deficit appears to be secondary to their amnesia. A patient will begin a task or sentence, suffer a distraction or pause to find a word, and then forget the task requirements or the thread of discourse. The span of apprehension as measured by Digit Span Forward is often within normal limits in the early stages of the disease. Psychomotor slowing on tasks like Digit Symbol and Trails is usually seen, probably reflecting a global deterioration of information-processing capacity. Very soon in the course of the illness, performance on any task demanding effortful processing is impaired (Storandt, Botwinick, Danzinger, Berg, & Hughes, 1984). Sensory attention, capacity, and response generation are soon affected. Possibly the only area of attentional performance that is spared is arousal. Although little systematic work has been done in this area, AD patients are usually alert, energetic, and motivated during testing.

PARKINSON'S DISEASE

Parkinson's disease (PD) is a neurological disease characterized by bradykinesia, rigidity, and tremor. The etiology of PD is usually unknown, but its core neuropathological features are consistent. PD is associated with the degeneration and loss of dopaminergic neurons of the substantia nigra. This loss results in the degeneration of the nigrostriatal system, a reduction of dopamine levels in the striatum, and secondary facilitation of cholinergic activity. The damage to the dopaminergic system results in a loss of the normal function of striatal and brain stem nuclei and results in abnormal muscle tone, disturbance of movement and posture, and possibly the inertia and depression commonly seen in PD (Hassler, Mundinger, & Reichert, 1979; Marsh, Markham, & Ansel, 1971; Pfeffer & Van der Noort, 1978). PD is usually associated with some degree of intellectual impairment, especially memory deficits and psychomotor slowing, and often leads to dementia. The incidence of dementia in PD is estimated to be 20%–40% (Mortimer, Christensen, & Webster, 1984).

Neuropsychologically, the deficits observed in PD are quite variable and change with disease severity. Mildly affected patients typically have mild problems with recent memory, mild visuospatial disturbance, and marked psychomotor slowing. The verbal fund of information is typically spared (Marsh, Markham, & Ansel, 1971; Pirozzolo, Hansch, & Mortimer, 1982; Sahakian, Morris, Evenden, Heald, Levy, Philpot, & Robbins, 1988). P3 latency of the auditory evoked potential is prolonged in PD, an effect showing that the slowing of mental processes is not confined to those tasks making demands for motoric response. Moreover, the degree of P3 prolongation is inversely related to the severity of the intellectual impairment, especially on tests of recent memory and concentration (Hansch et al., 1982; O'Donnell et al., 1987).

The most prominent attentional disturbances in PD, then, are psychomotor slowing, response maintenance, and concentration deficits on tests such as digits backward. The psychomotor slowing in PD is more marked than that in AD when patients are matched for disease severity (Huber, Shuttleworth, & Freidenberg, 1989). The degree of slowing in PD is correlated with the severity of the dementia, a finding suggesting that it indexes the global decline of mental capacity as well as specific disturbances of nigrostriatal motor systems.

BRAIN NEOPLASM

There are few controlled empirical studies of the attentional characteristics of patients with brain neoplasm. Brain tumors differ from structural lesions produced by stroke and other cerebral vascular diseases, as they produce dynamic lesions that change over time. The distinction between the effects of static and dynamic serial lesions on behavioral function has been well described by investigators studying neural plasticity (for a review, see Finger & Stein, 1982). Recht, McCarthy, O'Donnell, Cohen, & Drachman (1989) studied the development of aphasic symptoms in patients with dominant-hemisphere brain tumors. These changes were correlated with factors including the age at disease onset and the speed of tumor growth. Both factors were shown to be highly correlated with the presence of aphasic symptoms. This finding illustrates that the outcome of dynamic lesions is harder to predict.

It is well known that near the end stage of tumor progression, patients often show severe disturbances in mental state, including periods of reduced sensorium, delirium, disorientation, and diminished arousal. Eventually, many of these patients lapse into coma, a state reflecting the pressure effects on brain-stem-activating systems. The fluctuations in global state of attention associated with these changes are usually obvious.

At earlier stages in the disease process, it is very common for patients to become easily fatigued, and to have significant problems with sustained attention. Unfortunately, it is very difficult to dissociate the influence of specific brain-related changes on these symptoms from other causes associated with having a severe medical disease. Patients may also show fatigue from radiation treatment and chemotherapy, coexisting systemic disease, and depression or grief reaction. These confounds are not isolated to brain tumor. Patients with other disorders, including acquired immune deficiency syndrome (AIDS) and multiple sclerosis, often exhibit fatigue as a result of secondary factors not directly related to brain dysfunction resulting from their disease. This represents an intriguing problem for investigators interested in the basis of disordered attention and fatigue in these disorders (Cohen & Fisher, 1988, 1989).

SUMMARY

The neurological diseases that we have discussed in this chapter differ greatly in their neuropathology, their clinical course, and the resulting cognitive impairments. All of these diseases produce significant attentional disturbances, although the specific characteristics vary. Most neurological diseases that affect the brain produce a variable attentional state. Performance fluctuates in accordance with the demands placed on the individual and as a result of interactions with changing neurological status.

Some neurological diseases produce their greatest effects on attention, whereas in others, the attentional problem is a component of impairments affecting other cognitive domains. The attentional dysfunction that is present in most of these disorders may serve as a basis for more generalized problems with cognition. An exception is the case of Alzheimer's disease. The cortical dementias produce dramatic changes in a large number of cognitive operations, including associative processing, memory formation, and response control (frontal lobe functioning). Therefore, in the case of Alzheimer's disease, attentional dysfunction is probably subsumed under a broader range of deficits. With Alzheimer's disease, attentional variations may be inconsequential relative to the devastating effects of the generalized deterioration of cognitive resources. In fact, the attentional deficits seen in Alzheimer's disease may be the byproduct of a more primary breakdown of cognitive ability in areas such as memory, language and visual integration. Yet, patients with Alzheimer's disease also usually exhibit significant problems with executive control. Although this executive control dysfunction can be explained in part by the impairments in other cognitive domains, patients with Alzheimer's also usually exhibit problems with response production and control associated with frontal lobe pathology.

Attention dysfunction is clinically evident in most of the other neurologic diseases that we have discussed. While the basis of the attentional impairment may vary as a function of the specific disease that is considered, several common features seem to exist. Many of the neurological diseases discussed in this chapter produce attention deficits with associated alterations in psychomotor and energetic capacity. Diseases that affect subcortical functioning (e.g., MS and Parkinson's disease) frequently produce abnormalities in the production and maintenance of arousal and/or activation relative to prevailing task demands. Subcortical damage often impairs information processing ability by disrupting mechanisms that control the flow, gating, switching, and integration of information. As a result, effortful controlled attentional operations are often impaired, while automatic attention is often preserved.

Although there are many commonalities in these deficits of attention, distinctions can be made across the different disorders. Multiple sclerosis produces attentional deficits that are characterized by an associated problem with fatigue, and by reaction time slowing that is evident on a wide range of tests. The attention deficits of MS are probably related in part to the breakdown in neural transmission that occurs as a result of demyelination and associated problems in the integrity of signals that are processed. Specific disruptions of important subcortical systems, particularly in the periventricular region, may also be implicated.

The attentional deficits of hydrocephalus also involve systems that control responding, though there is a greater likelihood of significant problems in the gating and control of responses. Executive dysfunction is often apparent that is associated with frontal lobe dysfunction, as well as with the disruption of critical subcortical systems. In this regard, there may be a commonality with the executive disturbances in Alzheimer's disease, although the patient with hydrocephalus may show much greater variability in performance, as the pressure exerted on these regions fluctuates.

The metabolic disorders may produce a variety of different symptoms depending on the specific biochemical effects that are produced. However, common to many metabolic disorders is an alteration in the quality of consciousness and arousal. Metabolic disorders appear to have primary effects on the brain centers that control arousal and the energetics of the individual. Therefore, the attentional disturbances that occur in these disorders are likely to have a strong arousal or energetic component. Of course, with prolonged states of metabolic abnormality, there is a likelihood of disruption in other specific cognitive processes.

The nature of attentional disturbances varies as a function of the type of neurological disease that is considered. Although there are some common features in the attention deficits seen across neurological disorders, there are also distinguishing characteristics. Perhaps future neuropsychological investigations should be directed at characterizing the attentional characteristics of these disorders, as these may indicate much about the neurophysiological impact that different brain diseases have on the processes of attention.

Attentional Dysfunction Associated with Psychiatric Illness

RONALD A. COHEN and BRIAN F. O'DONNELL

In this chapter, we consider attentional disturbances that are commonly observed in patients presenting with four psychiatric conditions: (1) affective disorders; (2) schizophrenia; (3) attention-deficit–hyperactivity disorder (ADHD); and (4) anxiety/stress disorders. For each of these disorders, we review the characteristics of the attentional disturbance and the brain mechanisms that have been proposed to account for this attentional problem.

AFFECTIVE DISORDERS

Complaints of a diminished ability to concentrate and to sustain attention are common clinical features of patients with affective disorders. In fact, the presence of these symptoms are among the key determinants for making the diagnoses of both major depression and bipolar affective disorder (American Psychiatric Association, 1987). In the past, patients who reported attentional difficulties or other cognitive changes were often viewed as having "functional" symptoms arising out of subjective experience, without an actual neurophysiological basis. The tendency of some clinicians to minimize the cognitive impairments associated with psychiatric conditions was due in part to the apparent lack of neuroanatomical damage found in patients with affective disorders and other major psychiatric illnesses. Also, the obvious relationship of motivation to the affective disorders led to an assumption that these patients could perform well if they only had stronger willpower. Although there are major differences between the impairments in the affective disorders and those noted in patients with neuroanatomical damage, it now appears that the severe affective disorders have neurophysiological substrates. Furthermore, the cognitive symptoms found in patients with affective disorders are correlated with actual declines in performance on certain neuropsychological measures. The endogenous physiological changes that accompany severe states of depression and mania suggest that the subjective and behavioral characteristics of these disorders may have a common neurophysiological origin.

The clinical presentations of patients experiencing major depression and mania often reflect opposite states of energetics and motivation (see Table 12.1). Depressed patients are apt to lack motivation, normal interests, and goals. They often exhibit social withdrawal,

TABLE 12.1. Symptoms Associated with Affective Disorders

Major Depression	Mania
Depressed mood	Grandiosity
Blunted affect	Disinhibited affect
Psychomotor retardation	Psychomotor agitation
Distractibility	Concentration problems
Hyporeactivity	Hyperreactivity
Slowed thinking	Racing thoughts
Diminished interests	Excessive involvement in pleasurable activities
Decreased motivation	Increased goal directedness
Indecisive	Flight of ideas
Social withdrawal	Pressured speech
Fatigue	Energized
Sleep disturbance	Sleep disturbance

decreased talkativeness, and extreme fatigue. Manic patients are usually very energized, a state that is reflected in flights of ideas, pressured speech, and increases in goal-directed behavior. Whereas depressed patients have difficulty deriving pleasure from their involvements, manic patients gain much pleasure and seek pleasure through risk taking. They often act in a disinhibited manner and engage in activities with little social discretion. Their subjective cognitive experience is also quite different, as manic patients are likely to have grandiose ideas, with a feeling of heightened states of perception, mental acuity, and creativity. Depressed patients who are melancholic often report dulled thinking, dulled perception, and a feeling of slowed thoughts and functioning. Some depressed patients exhibit symptoms that are more similar to mania: irritability, racing thoughts, and other complaints suggesting an agitated state. Whereas the major depressions produce a more mixed symptom profile, mania and depression are relatively "bipolar" with regard to their presentation.

Clinical Studies

Much clinical research effort has been directed at the diagnostic problem of differentiating between "organic" and psychiatric disorders based on neuropsychological measures. In fact, neuropsychological studies occasionally have contrasted patients with documented brain lesions to psychiatric patients. This methodological approach has been used because of an assumption that psychiatric populations have functional rather than brain disorders. Studies that have made such a comparison have often found that psychiatric patients (excluding chronic schizophrenics) can be differentiated from brain-injured patients with approximately 75% accuracy (for reviews, see Heaton & Crowley, 1981; Heaton, Baade, & Johnson, 1978). A number of methodological problems exist in these studies, including a lack of control over many critical diagnostic variables. For instance, it is often difficult to separate patients with psychotic depression from those experiencing schizophrenia. Variables such as chronicity, age, education, and the exclusion of brain disease have often not been controlled for. The difficulty in obtaining clear-cut diagnostic groups continues to be a source of problems, even in recent studies.

Taylor, Abrams, and Gaztanaga (1975) conducted a study that controlled for many diagnostic variables, and that compared schizophrenic patients and manic-depressive patients by using the Halstead–Wepman Aphasia Screening and the Trail-Making Test. The schizophrenics were found to be more impaired on the language measure, but there was not a significant difference on the Trail-Making Test, as both groups were impaired relative to the norms for normal subjects. In a larger study, Taylor, Greenspan, and Abrams (1979) again demonstrated that patients with affective disorders do not show as great an impairment as schizophrenics on screening measures of language dysfunction, although both groups were found to make more errors than normal control subjects.

In a more comprehensive study, Taylor, Redfield, and Abrams (1981) compared 52 affective-disorder patients with schizophrenics and a small group of patients with "chronic brain dysfunction" on a large number of measures. Again, the schizophrenics were found to be impaired across a wide range of measures, whereas the affective-disorder group was primarily impaired on nonverbal measures. Flor-Henry and his associates reached similar conclusions in their studies of affective-disorder and schizophrenic patients (Flor-Henry, 1983; Flor-Henry, & Yeudall, 1979). Both groups were comparably impaired on "nondominant-hemisphere" indices, such as the Memory for Designs Test, Constructional Apraxia measures, Tactual Formboard (global), and Purdue Pegboard. The schizophrenics showed much greater impairment on language-based measures, as well as on tactual and motor tasks involving the dominant hand. These results were interpreted as indicating that nondominant cerebral dysfunction is associated with affective disorders. The investigators made the inference that impairment on these nonlanguage measures reflects reduced functioning in certain anatomical regions. Although reduced performance on nonverbal tasks may be associated with nondominant cerebral functioning, there may be other reasons for these findings. For instance, most of the tasks that were used to indicate nondominant brain functions also require more effort for adequate performance.

Cohen, Fennell, Bauer, and Moscovitch (1984) demonstrated that patients with affective disorders show the greatest impairments on tasks that are normally associated with executive and psychomotor functioning. Furthermore, their error types often corresponded with their diagnostic category. Depressed patients tended to make a greater number of errors of omission and had slowed response times that accounted for their weak performance on both constructional and executive control tasks. Patients who were manic showed the opposite tendency, with a larger number of errors of commission, short latencies before they made responses, and an impulsive response pattern that was reflected in a tendency to respond without considering alternative response possibilities. This response tendency was more apparent on tasks that required greater effort, as well as on tasks requiring the processing of new information. Affective-disorder patients performed adequately on most measures of "crystallized" ability and on tasks that assess core cognitive functions such as visual perception and language. Therefore, it is possible to account for the reduced performance of patients with affective disorders without postulating a hemispheric hypothesis. The reason for the "nondominant" effect in these patients may be more related to the behavioral demands underlying tasks that require visual-motor integration, effortful and sustained attention, and psychomotor speed. Certainly, the attentional demands of particular tasks seem to play a large role in determining how the patient with an affective disorder will respond.

Attentional Disturbance

Disturbances of attention in patients with affective disorders are commonly noted by clinicians and reported by patients or their families. However, there are relatively few empirical studies of the characteristics of attentional disturbance in these populations. As described by Cohen and his colleagues (1984), patients with severe depression and mania show a pattern of performance that mirrors their behavioral state. Apathetically depressed patients tend to respond by saying, "I don't know," to many questions. Likewise, they give up on tasks prematurely. Patients who are manic at the time of assessment show the opposite pattern. They respond too quickly without fully appraising all of the alternatives. They are easily distracted by irrelevant stimuli and may show a tendency to shift out of a "winning" response approach. These response styles can be demonstrated on tasks that measure information-processing capacity.

Byrne (1977) found that the performance of depressed patients on a lengthy vigilance task involving auditory signal detection was directly proportional to the degree of depression. The most depressed subjects had the greatest number of errors on this task. Malone and Hemsley (1977) also found that performance on a signal detection task was most impaired during severe states of depression and that patients showed improved performance when their depression had resolved. Similarly, Frith, Stevens, and Johnstone (1983) found that scores on a continuous-performance task improved after both sham and real electroconvulsive therapy (ECT) treatment. Therefore, the attentional disturbance associated with affective disorders seems to be state-dependent.

Learning and memory impairments are often evident in both depressed and manic patients (Breslow, Kocsis, & Belkin, 1980; Cohen et al., 1984; Cronholm & Ottosson, 1961; Stromgren, 1977). Often, the basis for these memory problems is not entirely clear. For instance, Stromgren (1977) used the Wechsler Memory Scale to study memory impairments in depressed populations and found that their performance on the "mental control" tasks was generally impaired, along with their performance on the logical memory and visual reproduction subtests. This finding was also supported by Breslow et al. (1980), who found impaired performance on mental control tasks such as Digit Span and Serial Addition. Interestingly, memory performance on the paired-associates learning subtest of the Wechsler Memory Scale was not impaired relative to that of control subjects, which raises questions about the extent of memory impairment in these patients.

Weingartener, Gold, and Ballenger (1981) conducted a series of tests of memory in depressed patients. They found that depressed patients did not show stronger memory performance on semantic tasks than in their recall of acoustically processed words without semantic context. In a second study, when depressed patients performed semantic sorting tasks on a set of 32 stimulus words, they generated fewer semantic categories than phonemic categories and ultimately recalled fewer of the words from the semantic category following this task. In contrast, when clustering was required of subjects on a semantic task, they performed at a level similar to that of the normal control subjects. These findings indicated that the memory performance of depressed patients is very dependent on the quality of the initial processing. Depressed patients seemed unable to generate the level of semantic organization that is necessary to improve the quality of encoding.

When the results of memory studies of depressed patients are interpreted in light of findings by Cohen and Waters (1985) regarding the performance of normal subjects in the levels-of-processing paradigm, it would appear that depressed patients are unable to generate sufficient effort to facilitate adequate encoding. In this regard, it is noteworthy that a strong relationship has been demonstrated between motor effort on dynamometer squeezing and memory performance on a consonant trigram task. This relationship varies inversely with the degree of mood impairment (Cohen, Weingartner, Smallberg, & Murphy, 1982).

Other investigators have also demonstrated reduced performance on motor tasks in patients who are severely depressed. Slowing on finger-tapping measures has been correlated with impaired performance on the Stroop Interference Test, as well as on other measures of mental control (Raskin, Friedman, & DiMascio, 1982). Again the ability to sustain effort, attention, and cognitive "flexibility" was found to be impaired in these patients. This finding is consistent with the reports of other investigators (Caine, 1981; Cohen et al., 1984). Depressed patients' inability to exert sufficient effort may account for problems in performance across a range of tasks; these problems range from difficulties with learning and memory to actual decrements in motor strength. As we suggested in Chapters 3 and 6, the ability to allocate effort on tasks seems to be a critical component of attentional control.

In summary, patients with affective disorders often experience significant neuropsychological dysfunction. They show sparing of most intellectual, language, and perceptual measures, a finding suggesting that their cortical systems are largely not affected. Tasks that make strong attentional demands give individuals suffering from affective disorders the greatest difficulty. Their attentional impairment can be traced to a failure to initiate adequate levels of effort. Problems with effort can ultimately be linked to alterations in normal levels of arousal and response-related activation.

The memory problems that are noted in these patients are typically caused by ineffective encoding, particularly under conditions of increased demand. Depressed patients lack the capacity to handle large quantities of information during memory encoding. This problem is associated with the attentional deficits that these patients experience. Their failure to use effective strategies during encoding points to the reduced capacity for executive control that accompanies these disorders.

Depressed patients also have problems with the retrieval of remote information. Their greatest difficulty is often encountered with information that was processed during the period of depression. This retrieval problem may be due either to their initial encoding difficulties or to problems with efficiency of retrieval during states of depression.

Memory formation and storage mechanisms do not appear to be greatly impaired by affective disorders. Yet, memory performance is typically diminished in patients who are depressed. This impairment seems to result from a failure to efficiently direct the encoding and retrieval processes. As we have suggested in previous discussions, the control of both encoding and retrieval is strongly influenced by attentional factors. Therefore, it is likely that most of the neuropsychological impairment noted in the affective disorders can ultimately be attributed to problems with the control of attention. These attentional problems probably relate to factors associated with the regulation of drive and motivation and the registration of reinforcement.

Neurophysiological Mechanisms

The attentional problems associated with the affective disorders have been attributed to a dysfunction in the systems that control arousal and response activation, as well as to factors related to motivation and drive states. Patients with major depressions often do not find reward in situations that previously provided reinforcement for them. The neural systems that serve to regulate emotion and the registration of the value of reinforcement include the hypothalamus, limbic structures such as the amygdala, the septal nuclei, and associated mesocortical and cortical areas. The neuroanatomical and physiological characteristics of these systems were discussed previously.

There is an intuitive basis for considering these same neural systems when considering the neurophysiological factors underlying the affective disorders. A fundamental component of the affective disorders is the disruption of normal emotional experience and associated changes in behavioral functioning that involve drive, motivation, and behavioral energetics. Although the emotional changes that accompany the affective disorders may occur as a reaction to life events, it is difficult to account for the "endogenous" behavioral responses without postulating an underlying neurophysiological mechanism. Presumably, the neural systems that have been shown to be involved in the control of these primary appetitive behaviors in animals are also implicated in the affective disorders.

Experimental and clinical evidence supporting the role of specific neural systems in the affective disorders has been difficult to establish. Most patients with affective disorders do not have focal brain lesions that can be analyzed and correlated with symptoms. Studies of patients with neurological diseases that cause secondary affective disorders have been more abundant (see Heilman, Watson, & Bowers, 1983, for a review). Patients with right-hemisphere brain dysfunction have greater problems with emotional perception and expression. They often show indifference in their response to situations, whereas patients with left-hemisphere lesions are more likely to show catastrophic reactions. Studies have suggested that right-hemisphere damage is also more typically associated with states of hypoarousal, whereas patients with left-hemisphere damage may show increased levels of arousal (Heilman & Van Den Abell, 1979; Heilman, Schwartz, & Watson, 1970). However, the neurophysiological basis of the affective changes accompanying hemispheric damage is not clear. Furthermore, the relationship between the affective changes associated with lateralized brain damage and more typical presentations of the affective disorders is not obvious.

Analysis of subcortical disorders, such as the basal ganglia diseases, has yielded another source of neurophysiological data relating to the affective disorders. Patients with Parkinson's disease commonly exhibit major depression that in many cases precedes the onset of other neurological symptoms (Mindham, 1970). Mayeux, Stern, Rosen, and Leventhal (1981) showed that neuropsychological deficits in inattention, calculation, and learning are often associated with these affective changes. Patients suffering from Huntington's disease, progressive supranuclear palsy, and Sydenham's chorea also show significant affective and behavioral disturbance, although the presentation varies from that seen in Parkinson's disease. Although there is not much direct evidence, alterations in monoamine metabolism may be a likely basis for these affective changes.

Focal lesions affecting the prefrontal cortex and the limbic structures often cause affective disturbances. A more detailed account of the effects of such lesions on attention was given in chapter 10. The relationship between orbital frontal damage and changes in emotional experiences has been studied extensively in experimental investigations of primate behavior (e.g., Butter, Mishkin, & Mirsky, 1968; Butter, Snyder, & McDonald, 1970). Humans also exhibit marked changes in affective behavior following frontal lobe damage (Damasio & Van Hoesen, 1983).

Subcortical damage, especially involving limbic structures, produces striking impairments of affective behaviors (Mayeaux, 1983; Damasio & Van Hoesen, 1983). In fact, abnormalities of affective behavior and personality in patients with partial complex epilepsy has been attributed to either hyper- or hypoactivity of critical limbic structures (Bear & Fedio, 1977). Disorders affecting the basal ganglia produce psychiatric disturbances (Mayeaux, 1977), while the hypothalamus is also critical to normal emotional experience. Hypothalamic damage that impairs attention and circadian functioning also causes a disorder of affect (Cohen & Albers, 1991).

When one considers neuropsychological evidence regarding the neural systems involved in emotion, it is apparent that disorders of emotional behavior arise when damage occurs to a fairly broad set of brain structures. Damage to the hypothalamus, the limbic system, the basal ganglia, the frontal cortex, and the posterior cortical areas. Furthermore, the areas that seem to be involved in emotional behavior correspond closely with neural systems that we have implicated as important for the control of attention.

Neurotransmitter and Endocrine Hypotheses

Neurochemical changes are thought to accompany severe depression and mania. Consideration of the neurochemical bases of affective disorders was spurred on by the fact that the affective disorders tend to be transient disorders. Therefore, when searching for a basis for these disorders, it was necessary to consider neural mechanisms that are relatively "plastic" in their ability to change their response tendency in short time periods. Biochemical modulation in the brain may more easily fit this requirement, as it is more difficult to account for temporary changes in "hard-wired" neuroanatomical systems. Also, neurotransmitter alterations are potentially reversible, whereas deficits that are due to brain lesions typically result in more stable patterns of impairment.

A number of hypotheses have been proposed to describe potential neurochemical mechanisms that underlie the major affective disorders. These hypotheses have emphasized the role of particular neurotransmitters, peptides, or endocrine systems. The original impetus for considering neurochemical bases for depression came from analyses of pharmacological actions on behavior and mood. Certain drugs diminish the action of catecholamines in the brain and induce states of depression, whereas others, such as monoamine oxidase (MAO) inhibitors, increase the concentration of monoamines and tend to decrease depression.

The effect of reserpine in producing depression has been well documented (Bunney & Davis, 1965) in studies of patients being treated for hypertension. Two amine systems have been implicated in depression: the indolamines and the catecholamines. Other neurochemicals, including peptides, corticosteroids, and hormones, have been considered possible influences on depressive state (Kety, 1970). Although it is beyond the scope of this book to review all of the neurochemical models of depression, it is useful to consider several of the mechanisms that have been proposed. Several of the neurophysiological models of the affective disorders are relevant to our discussion of the dysfunctions of attention that accompany the affective disorders.

Monoamine Hypotheses

The disregulation of monoamine metabolism has been proposed as a mechanism underlying the affective disorders. The observation that certain drugs affect the levels of particular CNS amines contributed to the development of neurochemical models of depression. Schildkraut (1965) proposed that abnormalities in norepinephrine (NE) activity may account for some forms of depression. This proposal led to the catecholamine hypothesis of affective disorders. The cornerstone of this hypothesis is that 3-methoxy-4-hydroxyphenylglycol (MHPG), a metabolite of NE was found in lower quantities in the urine of manic patients than in that of unipolar depressed patients. MHPG levels were unrelated to symptoms of agitation or retardation. In subsequent studies, several urinary catecholamine metabolites were assessed concurrently by means of a discriminant-function analysis (Schildkraut, 1977). Again the bipolar and unipolar patients could be discriminated on the basis of MHPG excretion. The measurement of platelet MAO activity also served to discriminate patient groups.

Studies of urine metabolites established an indirect link between the catecholamines and the affective disorders. Cerebrospinal fluid metabolites (3-hydroxyphenylglycol, 3-methoxy-4-hydroxymandelic acid) have also been shown to occur in decreased concentrations in depressed patients (Gordon & Oliver, 1971; Jimerson, Gordon, Post, & Goodwin, 1975). The changes in these metabolites have been shown to be correlated more highly with motor retardation than with the emotional aspects of depression. Postmortem studies have generally failed to show reduced catecholamine levels in the subcortical regions of depressed patients who committed suicide. Therefore, although there is a demonstrated relationship between peripheral levels of catecholamine metabolites and depression, direct evidence pertaining to levels in the brain has not been found.

Pharmacological evidence supports the role of catecholamines in depression. Tricyclic antidepressants affect the reuptake of norepinephrine in the nerve synapses of the brain and produce the clinical benefits of increased psychomotor activation and elevations in mood state. Monoamine oxidase inhibitors also have activating qualities and influence affective states by inhibiting the actions of MAO in breaking down excessive norepinephrine (Post & Ballenger, 1984). Lithium, which is therapeutic in bipolar disorders, increases norepinephrine turnover (Post & Ballenger, 1984) and also increases the release of catecholamine metabolites (Schildkraut, 1965, 1977).

Indolamines have also been implicated in another major theory of depression. The suggestion that serotonin (5-hydroxytryptamine) may be a regulator of mood was first proposed after observations of the effects of LSD on affective behavior. LSD is a pseudo-transmitter that mimics serotonin. Serotonin is synthesized by tryptophan, which is found both centrally and, in larger proportions, in the peripheral blood circulation. Studies of the relationship between free peripheral and central tryptophan levels in depressed patients have not suggested that a simple deficiency of this substance is responsible for affective change. The metabolite of serotonin (5-HIAA) has been demonstrated to exist at reduced concentrations in the cerebrospinal fluid of depressed patients (Ashcroft & Sharman, 1960), although this finding has not been uniform across other studies (see Post & Ballenger, 1984, for a review). Investigations of postmortem brain concentrations have also failed to reveal consistent serotonin deficiencies in depressed populations. As in the case of the catecholamines, the best evidence for the role of serotonin as a causitive agent in depression comes from pharmacological investigations of the effects of tricyclic antidepressants, MAO inhibitors, and the other drugs that are known to affect affective states.

Recent findings suggest that the brain metabolism of patients with major affective disorders may differ from that of normal individuals. These studies have used positron emission tomography (PET) with radioactive labeling to detect the activity of specific chemical systems (e.g., Farkas, Wolf, Jaeger, Canero, Christman, & Fowler, 1981). PET findings have indicated hypometabolism in anterior brain systems, with some lateral asymmetries (right < left). Regional cerebral blood flow measures also suggest that the distribution of the cortical metabolic demands of depressed patients differs from that of normals.

Neuroendocrine Influences

There has been considerable research directed at the possibility that affective disorders result primarily from a neuroendocrine dysfunction (see Ballenger, Post, Gold, Robertson, Bunney, & Goodwin, 1980, for a review). Neuroendocrine hypotheses have been developed based on the observation that the hypothalamus, which is important for emotional behavior, also is the seat of endocrine control.

The hypothalamus has long been assumed to be the seat of primitive impulses related to appetitive drive states. Its control of basic drives was established as the foundation for explaining other aspects of emotional experience. The hypothalamus exerts influence through endocrine control and through nonendocrine neural effects on the limbic and higher cortical centers. In this regard, hormones appear to serve as modulatory substances that mediate behavior in a more tonic fashion (de Wied, 1974).

In general, endocrine effects are much slower in their rate of action than direct neural transmission. Functionally, this characteristic enables different forms of modulation that would not be possible through direct nerve action. The fastest forms of transmission, along long myelinated axons, are typically capable of the least amount of modulation, as these nerves fire in an all-or-nothing manner.

The rate of secretion of anterior pituitary hormones depends on driving mechanisms within the hypothalamus and on negative feedback from target organ hormones. For instance, the release of adrenocorticotropic hormone (ACTH) depends on circadian pulses originating from certain nuclei and on the levels of glucocorticoids from the adrenal gland. The release of these glucocorticoids is associated with increases in peripheral catecholamine levels and ultimately with the psychological experience of stress. Stimulation of the hypothalamus and other limbic structures can trigger changes in adrenal activity. Furthermore, the activity of the hypothalamic–pituitary–adrenal axis has been shown to vary as a function of induced behavioral stress (Carroll & Davies, 1970; Mason, 1971).

Thyroid function, cortisol, and ACTH have all been implicated in depression. The fact that patients with endocrine disorders often experience affective changes is evidence of this relationship. However, it does not confirm that endocrine dysfunction is the basis for depression, as many patients with major depression do not have obvious endocrine abnormalities. One line of direct evidence of a neuroendocrine basis of depression came from a study of cortisol levels in depressed patients (Carroll, Curtis, & Mendels, 1976; Carroll, 1978) which indicate disregulation of cortisol and ACTH in depression. Dexamethasone, which normally suppresses cortisol release, was also found to result in a different suppression level in depressed patients (Carroll & Davies, 1970). This finding spurred a large number of clinical investigations of the use of dexamethasone suppression as a test for endogenous depression.

The circadian and circannual characteristics of endocrine activity further implicate it as a mechanism underlying depression. Patients with major affective disorders often show considerable variability in their behavioral state as a function of time of day. Sleep is often disrupted, as are normal patterns of arousal. The suprachiasmatic nucleus (SCN) has been shown to play a fundamental role in these forms of circadian disregulation. Rosenthal and Blehar (1989) described a relationship between the development of an affective disorder and time of year. Endocrine activity varies as a function of time of year, a fact that has led investigators to study the role of light in the regulation of pituitary-hypothalamic function.

Neurochemistry, Affect, and Attention

Disregulation of the brain's neurochemistry seems to underlie the affective disorders. As previously described, neuroendocrine and neurotransmitter influences have been suggested as possible mechanisms for depression and mania. The cognitive and behavioral symptoms that occur with the affective disorders may be attributed to variations in the individual's ability to be activated by task demands. The problem with response activation seems to be strongly related to disruptions in the way that reward is interpreted by the brain. Signals from the environment that might normally drive the individual to engage in rewarding behavior cease to generate this effect. Therefore, the neurochemical disregulation that accompanies these disorders may be the basis of a wide range of behavioral and cognitive changes.

The fact that alterations in levels of catecholamines and indolamines in the CNS can drive the organism toward states of either increased or decreased behavioral activation illustrates the modulatory effect of these substances (Mason, 1981). Subcortical structures such as the hypothalamus, the amygdala, and the reticular system provide the neural circuits that are necessary for affect. Neurochemical mechanisms control the window of activation that is possible within these systems. Because the neurochemical milieu of the brain varies as a function of time, behavioral activation has a temporal character. Neuro-chemical modulation enables the organism to change behavioral response tendencies in accordance with the endogenous variations that occur both because of systemic biological factors and because of a changing environment.

Attentional control is obviously under the influence of these same neurochemical influences. Variations in behavioral activation may even be considered the overt manifesta-tion of attentional experience. Certainly, in the case of the affective disorders, there is a strong correspondence between the symptoms of increased or decreased activity level, the subjective experience of "having" or "not having energy," and the ability to concentrate. We also know that we can directly alter attentional performance through drugs that change the brain's activational state.

Caffeine and other stimulants tend to increase vigilance, whereas alcohol and other CNS depressants decrease attentional capability. Drugs such as cocaine may have differen-tial effects by producing states of hypomania and increased vigilance, and at the same time, they may decrease higher cortical activation. Thus, certain substances do not appear to produce uniform activation throughout the brain. It also seems likely that the various components of attention may respond differently to neurochemical modulation, and that these differences may reflect neuroanatomical areas of neurochemical distribution in the brain. However, this level of specificity has not yet been empirically demonstrated.

If neurochemical disregulation is a major factor in the development of the affective disorders, several issues arise that relate to traditional neuropsychological interpretations. The attentional and activational difficulties that accompany these disorders cannot be explained solely on the basis of the neuroanatomical organization of the brain. Although certain cognitive disorders, such as aphasia, have been studied extensively by localizing the sites of lesions in the brain, it would appear that such cortical localization is less relevant to the study of affective disturbances. Even though studies have shown that lesions to one cerebral hemisphere or the other result in different forms of affective disruption, such studies do not seem to account for most cases of depression.

Neuropsychological studies have demonstrated deficits in both depressed and manic patients that have been interpreted to reflect right-hemisphere dysfunction. However, as we have previously argued, many of the "right-hemisphere" effects can be explained by the greater response and effort needed to perform visual organizational or constructional tasks. Similarly, the visual-motor deficits that are noted in manic patients are often correlated with disinhibition and impulsivity, factors associated with heightened behavioral activation.

The most consistent neuropsychological feature of both depressed and manic patients is the disruption of attention and response production. Therefore, future neuropsychological investigations of these disorders may benefit from a greater emphasis on the study of these attentional disruptions. An understanding of how the parameters of attention change as a function of the severity and type of depression would enable a more precise quantification of symptoms. Attentional measurements may also provide a more sensitive indicator of the subtle neurochemical variations occurring in patients with affective disorders.

SCHIZOPHRENIA

Diagnosis

Since the classic descriptions by Bleuler (1950) and Kraepelin (1931) there have been many attempts to develop reliable and meaningful diagnostic criteria for schizophrenia, and to define subtypes of the disease (Neale & Oltmanns, 1980). Unfortunately, schizophrenia remains a poorly defined disorder. After nearly a century of clinical practice and research, no set of diagnostic criteria has been universally, or even nationally, adopted. We shall review the DSM-III-R (American Psychiatric Association, 1987) diagnostic criteria for schizophrenia, primarily because they provide a standard for the categorization that is generally used within U.S. psychiatric services.

The DSM-III-R stresses the observable features of the disease and eschews criteria positing etiological mechanisms. The diagnosis of schizophrenia is made when the patient's symptoms have persisted as least 6 months, when the patient is functioning below the highest level previously achieved, and when the symptoms are not due to organic brain disease, mood disorder, or schizoaffective disorder. Characteristic symptoms include disorders of the content (e.g., delusions) or the form of thought (e.g., loose hallucinations); disturbances of perception, such as auditory or somatic hallucinations; flat affect; disturbed sense of self or volition; impaired interpersonal function; and deviant psychomotor behavior. Age of onset may range from childhood to late adult life, although adolescent and early-adult onset are most common. Subtypes include catatonic, disorganized, paranoid, undifferentiated, and residual types.

The symptoms of schizophrenia are frequently classified into two types: negative and positive. The negative symptoms are those that can be characterized as the absence of normal behavior or affect and include features such as social withdrawal and flat affect. The positive symptoms are behaviors or experiences that are not found in healthy individuals, such as hallucinations, delusions, and psychomotor disturbances.

Etiology

The etiology of schizophrenia remains unknown, as does its pathogenesis. After many years of vigorous debate, there seems to be increasing recognition that the expression of schizophrenia is influenced by both genetic and environmental factors (Kety, 1980; Mirsky & Duncan, 1986). Children of a schizophrenic parent are 10–15 times more likely to develop schizophrenia than children without a schizophrenic parent (Gottesman & Shields, 1982). The influence of genetic factors in this increased vulnerability has been documented by studies that have shown that children of schizophrenic parents who are raised by nonschizophrenic parents remain more likely to develop schizophrenia. Conversely, children of nonschizophrenic parents adopted and raised by a schizophrenic parent do not show a greater likelihood of developing schizophrenia (Heston, 1966; Rosenthal, Wender, Kety, Welner, & Schulsinger, 1971; Wender, Rosenthal, Kety, Schulsinger, & Welner, 1974). Monozygotic twins show a higher concordance rate for schizophrenia than dizygotic twins (Neale & Oltmanns, 1980, pp. 184–192).

The familial and social environment of children at high genetic risk of developing schizophrenia may contribute to its expression. Singer and Wynne (1966) noted that families with a schizophrenic parent were characterized by deviant communication between parent and children, which might influence the development of thought disorder. Risk factors in subsequent studies reviewed by Mirsky and Duncan (1986) showed that deviant, negative, or neurotic patterns of family interaction and communication are associated with a greater likelihood of high-risk children's developing schizophrenialike symptoms. In an intriguing study by Mirsky, Silberman, Latz, and Nagler (1985) of high-risk children raised within a kibbutz or by their own parents in towns or cities, high-risk kibbutz children were more likely to develop schizophrenia than those raised in towns (26% vs. 13%). Moreover, they were much more likely to develop affective disorders (39% vs. 4%). Thus, the kibbutz proved to be a more stressful environment for these children than their families, which typically included a schizophrenic parent. Mirsky and Duncan (1986) speculated that the kibbutz functioned as a hypercritical extended family, intolerant of deviant behavior, which exacerbated schizophrenic responses in at-risk children.

Neuropathology and Pathophysiology

Many neuropathological abnormalities have been reported in schizophrenic brains, although few findings have been consistently replicated. In a review of this literature, Kleinman, Casanova, and Jaskiw (1988) found that the most reliable neuropathological change found in schizophrenia is an increase in the number of dopamine Type II receptors. This increase is apparent in the basal ganglia, the nucleus accumbens, and the substantia nigra. Unfortunately, these studies postdate the introduction of neuroleptic treatment, which can increase the number of dopamine receptors. Because most schizophrenic patients now receive neuroleptic treatment, it is impossible to determine whether the increase in receptors observed in their brains is due to the primary disease process or to neuroleptic treatment.

Enlarged ventricles in many schizophrenics have been observed both on CT scan and in autopsy studies of brain structure (Shelton & Weinberger, 1986). Cerebral atrophy and cranial asymmetry have also been reported in these patients. Schizophrenics with enlarged ventricles or atrophy have been reported to be more severely affected than schizophrenics without signs of atrophy. Schizophrenics with these CT abnormalities have been reported to show greater chronicity, poorer treatment response, more severe negative symptoms, more severe autonomic dysfunction, and greater intellectual dysfunction (Mirsky & Duncan, 1986; Zahn, Van Kammen, Schooler, & Mann, 1982).

The Schizophrenic Deficit

Many hypotheses have been proposed to account for the deficits observed in schizophrenic performance on real-world tasks and laboratory tests of mental function (see Neale & Oltmanns, 1980, for an excellent historical review). Since the time of Bleuler and Kraepelin, schizophrenia has been a favorite ground for theoretical and clinical thinking, and there are models and tests that describe the primary deficit or deficits in schizophrenic ideation derived from the associationist, psychoanalytic, biological, behaviorist, information-processing, psycholinguistic, and psychophysiological schools of psychology. Schizophrenia, in fact, has served as a kind of mirror of the current *Zeitgeist* in clinical thought since the turn of the century. None of these models has gained sustained support from experimental investigation, and the quest for a robust model of the schizophrenic deficit continues with unabated vigor.

Why has it been so difficult to characterize the basic deficits in schizophrenia? There are, of course, the problems posed by the elusive nature of the disease itself. Schizophrenics show great variations in symptom presentation, severity, course, and response to treatment. Because the diagnostic criteria for schizophrenic patients have varied over time and between countries—in fact, between laboratories—it is usually impossible to confidentially compare different studies. The presentation of the disease itself varies over time in an individual. Most schizophrenics in clinical settings receive neuroleptic and other powerful psychopharmacological agents, which themselves induce acute and chronic changes in mental function.

As if these often intractable problems were not enough to confound investigators, there are profound problems in the measurement of a specific deficit in schizophrenia, which have been eloquently summarized by Chapman and Chapman (1973, 1978). These problems stem from the observation that schizophrenic patients show a generalized performance deficit. That is, on virtually any task that requires a voluntary response, schizophrenics perform more poorly than normal individuals. Researchers generally attempt to show that schizophrenics show a differential deficit, that is, a deficit on one task that is greater than that on other tasks. This deficit is typically related to the mental process that the investigator thinks is awry in schizophrenics. Chapman and Chapman have pointed out, however, that when two (or more) tests are used to measure the performance of a group with a generalized deficit, the group will show a greater deficit on the task with greater reliability and variability. Therefore, differential performance between tests may be due to differences in the psychometric characteristics of the tests, rather than to a differential deficit in ability. Both the reliability and the variability of a test are influenced by its difficulty level. It is not enough to avoid obvious ceiling and floor effects in test construction. A test that has an error rate of 50% has a greater true-score variance than a test with an error rate of 75%. The more difficult test, in this case, will discriminate better between schizophrenics and normal subjects than the less difficult test.

In order to deal with this confound, investigators must match tasks on reliability and true-score variance to make them psychometrically equivalent. These principles hold for both traditional psychometric tests and cognitive tests. Chapman and Chapman recommended matching items by using a group of at least 100 normal subjects and cross-validating these results on a second normal sample.

The demands that this strategy of task-matching makes on the investigator have resulted in a paradoxical situation. Although Chapman and Chapman's arguments are frequently cited, their recommendations on test development are seldom followed. Chapman and Chapman (1978) have used their approach to address several hypotheses regarding the schizophrenic deficit. Their results were frequently at variance with standard findings in the literature with the use of unmatched tests.

Disturbed Attention as a Hallmark of Schizophrenia

Attentional deficits in schizophrenics have been intensively investigated, partly because attentional processes have been considered by many theorists a prime candidate as a core deficit in schizophrenia. In addition, attentional disturbances are grossly evident in encounters with schizophrenic individuals. Both Kraepelin and Bleuler noted attentional disturbances in their patients, including perseveration in thought and action, tangentiality, inability to initiate actions or sustain attention, rapid fatigue, and orienting to trivial stimuli. Bleuler (1950) felt that the consciousness of these patients was nonselective, and at times, his patients seemed to be conscious of two things at once, such as the conversation and an unrelated, inward train of thought. Bleuler attributed some of those attentional problems to flat affect. Since attention is motivated by affect, individuals with flat affect show little ability to direct and sustain attention as a function of emotionally meaningful goals or emotional impulses. Bleuler characterized this deficit as a disorder of active (volitional) attention. He also noted that these patients' passive attention was disturbed as well, in that autistically withdrawn patients seemed little aware of the outside world and attended to stimuli in the environment almost randomly. Bleuler concluded from these observations that both the inhibiting and the facilitating components of attention were disturbed by the disease. In terms of high-level executive function, Bleuler considered the disruption of the associative organization of mental activity a fundamental symptom in schizophrenia. Bleuler was referring to schizophrenics' inability to purposefully organize thought and discourse. The subjective experience of schizophrenia, documented in more contemporary studies, also highlights attentional disturbances. Interviews with schizophrenics document difficulties in focusing attention, in concentration, in the integration of new information, and in following speech (Freedman & Chapman, 1973; McGhie & Chapman, 1961).

Models of Attention Deficit

Contemporary models of the attention deficit in schizophrenia can be categorized into those that investigate disturbances in the information-processing structures that direct and sustain attention and those that focus on disturbances of arousal. Gjerde (1983) characterized the information-processing models as having a perspective rooted in "cold cognition." Information-processing models typically attempt to localize the stage at which a deficit occurs and seldom account for the influence on performance of affect, arousal, or effort. Gjerde contrasted these "cold" models of schizophrenic cognition with models that postulate a deficit in arousal or effort in schizophrenics, which would be associated with disturbances in any stage of information processing that makes demands on effortful processing in short-term storage. Neither the information-processing nor the arousal models provide a means of considering the possibility that schizophrenic attentional deficits are due to distraction by internal events, such as auditory hallucinations, obsessional ideation, or emotional turmoil. Given that such covert events may capture a share of the conscious resources needed for the consideration of external stimuli, performance on attentionally demanding tasks will be impaired. This possibility is supported by studies that show that the degree of distractibility on information-processing tests shown by schizophrenics is correlated with the presence or severity of thought disorder (e.g., Oltmans, Ohayon, & Neale, 1978; Wielgus & Harvey, 1988). In a study of reaction time (RT) variability, schizophrenics reported that internal distractions, such as hearing voices and transient loss of set, often interfered with RT performance on a trial-to-trial basis (Schwartz, Carr, Munich, Glauber, Lesser, & Murray, 1989).

The overwhelming majority of information-processing experiments use tasks that require the active deployment of attention in response to task demands. Much of the initial work was directed by the hypothesis that schizophrenics had a defective sensory filter, and therefore, that task-irrelevant stimuli would frequently intrude into later stages of processing (Payne, Matussek, & George, 1959). Although schizophrenics were more distractible than controls, particularly on demanding tasks, the locus of this problem remains unclear because schizophrenics show problems in many areas of information processing that may influence selective attention. The accumulation of evidence from information-processing paradigms testing iconic memory, working memory, processing speed, attentional shifting, selective attention, perceptual judgments, and encoding strategies shows that schizophrenics demonstrate pervasive performance deficits. Slowing of reaction time is a ubiquitous feature in schizophrenic patients (Nuechterlein, 1977). Moreover, reaction time is more variable in schizophrenics than in patients with affective disorders, including those with an affective psychosis (Schwartz, *et al.*, 1989). It is unlikely that disturbances in any single information-processing structure account for the range of problems that have been experimentally identified. Consequently, there is an increasing consensus among investigators that the schizophrenic information-processing deficit is better characterized as a disorder of attentional capacity that is reflected in the performance on any task making great demands on conscious, controlled, limited-capacity, or effortful processes. Conversely, tasks that rely on automatic, well-practiced, unconscious, or parallel processing are performed normally by schizophrenics (Callaway & Naghdi, 1982; Neale & Oltmanns, 1980; Nuechterlein & Dawson, 1984). This dichotomy derives from the capacity models of information processing reviewed in the first section of this book (e.g., Hasher & Zacks, 1979; Kahneman, 1973; Posner & Snyder, 1975; Shiffrin & Schneider, 1977). Investigators using information-processing models have come, then, to the conclusion summarized by Chapman and Chapman (1973, 1978): Schizophrenics perform less well than normal subjects on almost any task that requires a voluntary response. The reason for this general deficit remains unknown, but its pervasive influence suggests that continued efforts to define an isolated cognitive deficit in schizophrenia may be of limited value. Arousal models associate the deficit that schizophrenics show on volitional, effortful performance to problems in modulating arousal levels to meet external task demands (Gjerde, 1983). The strongest evidence for arousal deficits comes from studies of skin conductance in schizophrenia, which are reviewed in the next section.

There are at least two major problems with the hypothesis that schizophrenics have problems with demanding, effortful processing and not with automatic processing. The first involves the relationship of such tasks to a generalized deficit. Because effortful tasks are, by definition, more difficult than automatized tasks, it is not surprising that effortful tasks discriminate between normal and schizophrenic persons more effectively than automatic tasks. It is therefore not clear on a methodological level how automatic and effortful tasks can ever be made comparable. The other problem with this conceptualization is that one of the best replicated biological abnormalities in schizophrenia, an abnormal or absent orienting response, occurs in the absence of task demands. This finding suggests that schizophrenics have a problem with passive as well as active attention, as suggested by Bleuler.

Significance of Attention Deficits

The clinical significance of attentional deficits in schizophrenia has been reviewed by Nuechterlein and Dawson (1984). They considered information-processing and attentional deficits in terms of their relationship to the trait of schizophrenia, as well as the state of the patient with respect to active psychotic symptomatology. Children at risk for the development of schizophrenia, children who later develop clinically diagnosed schizophrenic syndromes, and patients in remission after a schizophrenic episode often show deficits on cognitive tests. Such tests can be considered sensitive to the trait of schizophrenia, even though overt psychotic symptoms like delusions and hallucinations may not be in evidence. Other tests that are impaired only during an actively psychotic episode.

Trait markers include deficits in attention-sensitive tasks such as vigilance with high-processing loads, the forced-choice apprehension of large arrays, and the serial recall of items that involve active rehearsal. Performance on such tasks is impaired in high-risk samples, actively symptomatic schizophrenic patients, and relatively remitted schizophrenic patients. These deficits may reflect changes in schizophrenic mental function that precede, and are relatively unaffected by, active signs of the disorder. State markers include virtually all tests that require effortful, conscious processing. In addition, actively symptomatic patients also show problems with some more automatized tasks, such as the recognition of single letters or numbers.

Psychophysiology of Attention in Schizophrenia

Autonomic Responses in Schizophrenia

Forty to fifty percent of schizophrenics fail to produce a skin-conductance orienting response to novel stimuli (Dawson & Nuechterlein, 1984; Gruzelier & Venables, 1972). This finding, which has been found in schizophrenics sampled in the United States, Britain, and Germany, may indicate a severe impairment of passively elicited attention. Zahn (1988) cited work from his laboratory as demonstrating a variety of differences between schizophrenic and control subjects. In general, acute, unmedicated schizophrenics showed high baseline levels of autonomic activity on electrodermal measures; slow rates of adaptation to new stimuli and situations; and reduced reactivity during task performance and to task-related stimuli. Chronic elevation of autonomic indices argues against an explanation of schizophrenia based on chronic hypoarousal. Gjerde (1983) has suggested that schizophrenics are characterized by chronic hyperarousal rather than hypoarousal. Hyperarousal in normal subjects tends to bias a person to respond to dominant rather than nondominant information sources; to limit the breadth of attention, perhaps by restricting the range of cue utilization (Easterbrook, 1959); and to limit memory search to readily accessible information. Consequently, many of the information-processing failures demonstrated by schizophrenics may be due to the general effects of hyperarousal on performance, rather than to deficits in specific information-processing structures. Reduced reactivity to task demands and task-related stimuli, on the other hand, does indicate that schizophrenics show phasic disturbances of arousal related to variations in cognitive demands.

Not all schizophrenics show a severe disturbance in autonomic reactivity. Typically, patients who fail to show an electrodermal orienting response are called *nonresponders*, whereas those who show a normal orienting response are called *responders*. There have been some attempts to correlate the degree of autonomic disturbance with symptoms or pharmacological effects. Electrodermal nonresponders have been reported to show more severe negative symptoms, such as withdrawal, depression, and blunted affect, than responders. Responders typically show more agitated or hostile behaviors (Venables, 1984). These relationships have not been consistently replicated, however (Green, Nuechterlein, & Satz, 1989). Green *et al.* (1989) studied a large group of medicated schizophrenics and found no differences between responders and nonresponders in terms of negative and positive symptomatology. Negative symptoms as well as levels of anticholinergic medication were associated with lower tonic levels of skin conductance. Schizophrenic patients with cortical atrophy show more severe autonomic disturbances than schizophrenic patients without cortical atrophy (Zahn, *et al.*, 1982). In an interesting experiment with normal subjects, Zahn, Rapoport, and Thompson (1981) found that dextroamphetamine produced autonomic changes similar to those seen in schizophrenia, including increased arousal, slow habituation, and reduced tonic response in task performance. Prolonged use of dextroamphetamine can produce a paranoid psychosis. Zahn (1988) speculated that these common patterns of autonomic disturbance in schizophrenics and dextroamphetamine-influenced normal subjects may be a marker for a dopamine psychosis. In summary, patients who fail to show an orienting skin-conductance response are more likely to show negative symptoms and cortical atrophy. Dextroamphetamine, which can produce psychotic symptoms in normal subjects with chronic administration, also produces schizophreniclike changes in autonomic activity and response.

P3 Response of the Evoked Potential

The amplitude of the P3 response of the auditory-event-related potential is reduced in schizophrenia (Levitt *et al.*, 1973; Roth, Pfefferbaum, Horvath, Berger, & Koppell, 1980; Verleger & Cohen, 1978). Most investigators have reported that P3 latency is unaffected by schizophrenia, but some have found delayed P3 latency in schizophrenics (Pfefferbaum, Wenegrat, Ford, Roth, & Kopell, 1984).

Baribeau-Braun, Picton, & Gosselin (1983) examined the evoked-potential responses of medicated schizophrenics in a dichotic listening experiment. By using a dichotic listening paradigm, they were able to compare the N1 or Nd response enhancement associated with channel selection to the P3 response associated with target detection within a channel. The results were interpreted in terms of Broadbent's contrast between stimulus set (selection of a channel of information characterized by a simple physical attribute) and response set (selection of stimuli requiring a specific response within a channel). Schizophrenics attempted to detect target tones in either one or both ears, and at slow and rapid rates of presentation. Schizophrenics showed diminished N1 amplitude and P3 amplitude; prolonged reaction time; and poorer target detection. Unlike the control subjects, the schizophrenics showed enhancement of N1 amplitude at fast, but not at slow, stimulation rates, a finding suggesting that they were able to focus attention but had difficulty maintaining it on a channel at slow rates of stimulation. Moreover, dividing attention by listening for targets in both ears did not increase N1 amplitude in schizophrenics. P3 amplitude was diminished in schizophrenics in all conditions, even when only correct responses were considered. These results suggest that schizophrenics are able to deploy a selective attention strategy but are unable to maintain it at slow stimulation rates, or to deal with multiple input channels. Their diminished P3 amplitude suggests that schizophrenics are also impaired in their maintenance of a response set, showing less reactivity to informative stimuli, and being less able to detect informative events reliably. These data document a generalized deficit of attentional processes, coupled with a slowing of processing, in schizophrenia.

The clinical correlates of P3 abnormalities in schizophrenia are little understood. Duncan, Morihisa, Fawcett, and Kirch (1987) reported that improvement in clinical state as a result of neuroleptic medication was associated with increased P3 amplitude to visual stimulation, but that the auditory P3 response was uncorrelated with medication. Duncan (1988) proposed that the auditory P3 response may be a trait marker for schizophrenia, whereas the visual P3 response may be responsive to fluctuations in clinical state.

Electrical Sources of P3 Amplitude Reduction in Schizophrenia

The neuroanatomic or neurophysiological changes associated with P3 amplitude reduction in schizophrenia have recently been investigated. McCarley, Faux, and colleagues have reported that the scalp-recorded P3 component shows greater reduction over the left temporal scalp compared with the right temporal scalp region in right-handed male chronic schizophrenic patients (Faux, Shenton, McCarley, Nestor, Marcy, & Ludwig, 1990; McCarley, Faux, Shenton, Nestor, & Adams, 1991). They argued that this might reflect greater involvement of the left compared with the right temporal lobe. Using quantitative MRI image-processing techniques to quantify temporal lobe gray matter changes in schizophrenia, Shenton *et al.* (1992) reported gray matter reductions in the left superior temporal gyrus, left anterior hippocampal gyrus, left parahippocampal gyrus, and right parahippocampal gyrus. The volume of the left posterior superior temporal gyrus was correlated with both the amplitude of the P3 component over the temporal region and the severity of thought disorder in the patients (McCarley, Shenton, O'Donnell, Faux, Kikinis, Nestor, & Jolesz, 1992). These findings suggest that P3 amplitude may be specifically affected by abnormalities of left posterior superior temporal gyrus in schizophrenia and that this same anatomic region may be involved in the genesis of thought and language abnormalities in the disorder.

Summary

Tests of attentional processes, particularly those posing a high, information-processing load, show that these processes are impaired in schizophrenia. Reaction time is slowed and extremely variable. Vigilance performance is poor. Both stimulus set and response set phases are disturbed. The pervasiveness of the attention deficit in schizophrenia and the presymptomatic appearance of deficits on some tests of attention suggest that the attention deficit in schizophrenia may be a primary cognitive symptom of the disorder. Nevertheless, there is little strong or well-replicated evidence that this ubiquitous attention deficit is distinct from the generalized deficit that schizophrenics show on virtually all tests that demand effortful, conscious processing.

Psychophysiological evidence suggests that the attention deficit in schizophrenia has specific biological correlates. The skin-conductance orienting response is frequently absent in schizophrenics, and patients show signs of hyperarousal on this measure as well. A disturbed or absent orienting response has been associated with more negative symptomatology and more severe brain atrophy. P3 amplitude is consistently depressed in schizophrenia, and one study has also documented disturbances in electrophysiological measures of selective attention. These findings support the notion that schizophrenics are hyperaroused and show poor coordination of phasic arousal in response to stimulus events or task demands. Moreover, the lack of an orienting response argues against the hypothesis that schizophrenics show impaired attention only on tasks requiring effortful processing. The sensitivity of psychophysiological measures to schizophrenic psychopathology suggests that further investigation of their symptomatic and biological significance is warranted.

DEVELOPMENTAL DISORDERS OF ATTENTION

The Development of Normal Attention

Attentional processes develop over the course of infancy and childhood. Orienting to stimulus introduction and change occurs very early in development. The transition from passive, stimulus-driven responses to active, goal-oriented responses occurs later in development. In elementary school, children show significant variation in their ability to sustain attention over time. The ability to use attentional strategies to delay gratification and obtain long-term rewards shows development into the teenage years.

Orientation and Habituation

Infants show attentional responses to stimuli soon after birth. Within the first 4 months of life, both autonomic and motoric orienting responses are present. Using heart rate deceleration as a measure of stimulus response, Bowes, Brackbill, Conway, and Steinschneider (1970) found that infants oriented to auditory stimuli at 2 days after birth. Children whose mothers had been heavily medicated during birth took more trials to habituate to the stimuli, and this difference persisted at 1 month after birth. In a review of attentional processes and individual differences in infancy, Lewis and Baldini (1979) argued that rate of habituation provides a good measure of information processing in infants. In terms of Sokolov's model of the orienting response and habituation (1963), a novel stimulus elicits an ensemble of autonomic, motoric, and EEG responses that gradually habituate (diminish) with repeated presentations of the stimulus. If the stimulus is altered (e.g., in intensity), or if a new stimulus is introduced, the orienting response reappears. Sokolov interpreted the orienting response to be the result of a discrepancy between the current representation in memory of the environment and the novel stimulus. With repeated presentations of the stimulus, a model or representation of the stimulus is generated in the nervous system, and the stimulus is no longer discrepant from the internal representation of the environment. Therefore, the orienting response habituates. If a new stimulus is introduced, the orienting response is reinvoked until a new CNS representation evolves. Because the rate of habituation reflects how quickly an organism can assimilate new information cognitively, it may provide a means of measuring the efficiency of attentional processing and cognitive structures in infants.

In reviewing the literature regarding infant attention and habituation, Lewis and Baldini (1979) summarized several consistent findings:

1. Novel stimuli elicit attention more effectively than familiar stimuli. This difference takes several months to fully appear, however.
2. The rate of habituation to stimuli accelerates with development.
3. Slower rates of habituation and a reduced preference for novel stimuli have been associated with birth trauma and CNS dysfunction in infants.

Motoric orientation to the spatial location of auditory, tactile, and visual stimuli occurs within the first few months of life (Dodwell, 1983). Within a few days after birth, newborns can orient to and track a moving visual target. This tracking activity is accompanied by variations in heart rate concomitant with the appearance and disappearance of the target in the visual field (Bullinger, 1983). Motoric orientation responses seem to fade during the third month of development, then reappear with greater precision in the fourth month. This has been hypothesized to reflect the emergence of cortical influences on motor responses in the third month, which interfere with the more innately controlled subcortical orienting responses.

Passive versus Active Attention

In infancy, children's attention has been described as stimulus-bound, passive, or exploratory. As a child grows, attentional processes develop that support efficient, goal-oriented behavior. Attention becomes purposeful, active, and selective. With increasing age, children improve in extracting task-relevant features from stimuli (Hale, 1979). Gibson and Rader (1979) described attention as "perceiving in relation to a task or goal, internally or externally motivated (p. 2). Children become better able to select information from the environment on the basis of task demands. Moreover, children become more flexible in their direction of attention over time. They can switch attention fluidly between one stimulus and another as a function of changing task demands. They become better able to attend to nondominant features of a stimulus if the task requires such a shift (Hale, 1979).

Vigilance

The natural development of vigilance, or the ability to maintain attention when there are long periods between task-relevant signals, has not been well described. By grade school, however, there are significant differences between children on vigilance tasks; these differences have a profound impact on children's performance in the academic environment. Normal grade-school children perform well on the continuous-performance test, for example, whereas children diagnosed as hyperactive have great difficulty with such tests (Barkley, 1988).

A study by Cornblatt, Risch, Faris, Friedman, and Erlenmeyer-Kimling (1988) contrasting adolescent and adult performance on continuous-performance tests produced some surprising findings regarding developmental effects on vigilance performance. Adult and adolescent subjects were obtained from the same families, so that the correlation ("heritability") of attentional performance could be examined. The adolescents showed better performance on spatial than on verbal stimuli, whereas the adults showed similar performance levels on both tests. The adolescents, in fact, performed better than the adults on spatial processing. This interaction between age and performance was due to differences in accuracy unrelated to response strategies (β'). Both the adults and the adolescents improved their performance levels on retest. The adults were unaffected by distraction during the test. The performance levels of the adolescents, on the other hand, actually improved when distracting stimuli were introduced. This improvement in performance was reflected in a higher d' and a shift toward a more conservative response strategy.

Self-Control and Goal-Oriented Behavior

Infant behavior is often characterized as impulse-driven and is primarily responsive to immediate reinforcement. In the course of development, children learn methods of self-control that enable them to inhibit responses to immediate reinforcers (to delay gratification) and to maintain behavior that obtains reinforcers only after a long period of time. Mischel, Shoda, Rodriguez (1989) reviewed and summarized a variety of experiments that suggest the attentional and cognitive processes underlie the goal-directed delay of gratification. Their conclusions are summarized below.

Individual differences in the delay of gratification are apparent by age 4. Moreover, these differences are associated with long-lasting differences in behavioral style. In the protocols described by Mischel *et al.* (1989), children were typically offered a less valued reward whenever they wanted it or got a better reward if they forwent the less valued reward and waited an unspecified interval of time. Both types of rewards were in view during the waiting period. The children, who varied in their ability to delay gratification at age 4, were evaluated a decade later. The children who at age 4 could delay gratification longer were more academically and socially competent, better able to cope with frustration and stress, better able to maintain concentration and make plans, and more fluent verbally than the children who had been less able to delay gratification.

Attentional strategies affect a child's ability to delay gratification. When a child is shown the rewards while waiting, he or she is typically less able to delay gratification. When the children in Mischel *et al.* thought about the rewards, they were less able to delay gratification than when they thought about or engaged in distracting activities.

Paradoxically, looking at *pictures* of rewards or maintaining mental representations of pictures of rewards helps children to delay gratification. Somehow, symbolic representations of rewards, whether presented visually or maintained internally, help delay gratification, whereas viewing the actual rewards reduces self-control. In addition, the attributes of the imagined reward influenced self-control. Mischel *et al.* (1989) hypothesized that stimuli can be represented both in an arousing (consummatory) and in an abstract (nonconsummatory), informative manner, based on a distinction first advanced by Berlyne (1960). Concentrating on arousing, "hot" aspects of a stimulus (e.g., the taste of candy) disinhibits response, whereas concentrating on abstract, "cool" qualities (the length and shape of candy) enables a child to delay gratification. In fact, an abstract representation of the reward is more effective than an abstract representation of an irrelevant object. In a further analysis of longitudinal data, it was found that children's ability to delay gratification was predictive of adolescent characteristics only when the experiment was conducted with the rewards visibly present. When the rewards were not visible, the delay times had no relation to subsequent characteristics. These results suggest that individual differences may be most apparent when a child is required to develop active strategies to cope with a present temptation.

As children become older, they are able to articulate effective self-control strategies. They try to distract themselves from temptation and to use self-instructions to focus on the contingencies of the situations. The recognition that abstract representations are effective aids in delaying gratification does not occur until late in development, around ages 8–11.

Summary

The development of attentional processes takes place over a long time course from infancy to adolescence, reflects a number of different mechanisms, and is associated with significant individual differences. Infants are initially characterized by attentional responses that are provoked by stimulus change. Typically, new stimuli, or variations in stimulus features, evoke an orienting response. With development, the rate of habituation of the orienting response increases. Motoric orientation to the spatial location of auditory, visual, and tactile stimuli becomes apparent within the first few days to months after birth. As a child develops motor control, her or his perception becomes more selective, and her or his attentional capacity increases. A child attends to stimuli, or components of stimuli, that are task-relevant. A child's capacity to attend to multiple features of a stimulus improves. Attentional flexibility increases with age. The ability of children to sustain attention, particularly in the absence of immediate reinforcement, is quite variable. Severe difficulties in sustaining attention on vigilance tasks is characteristic of hyperactivity, or attention deficit disorders, and can interfere with a child's academic performance. By adolescence, spatial vigilance performance peaks. Verbal vigilance performance, in contrast, peaks in adulthood. Children's ability to resist short-term temptations to obtain long-term rewards depends in part on attentional strategies, which may have long-term implications for a child's social competence and achievement.

Attention Deficit and Hyperactivity Disorders

Attention disorders are frequently diagnosed in children. The DSM-III-R (American Psychiatric Association, 1987) provides for the diagnosis of an attention-deficit–hyperactivity disorder (ADHD), as well as of an undifferentiated attention-deficit disorder without hyperactivity or other significant psychiatric or neurological disturbances. In addition, attention deficits and hyperactivity are common attributes of other childhood disorders, such as developmental disabilities, learning disabilities, and conduct disorder.

The DSM-III-R regards as the essential features of ADHD developmentally inappropriate degrees of inattention, impulsiveness, and hyperactivity. The DSM-III-R diagnostic criteria for ADHD are listed in Table 12.2.

The prevalence of ADHD is estimated in the DSM-III-R to be up to 3% of all children. Boys are affected three to nine times more frequently than girls.

Because attention deficits may occur in the absence of hyperactivity or other major disturbances, the DSM-III-R includes a diagnosis of "undifferentiated deficit disorder." The inclusion criteria for this category are not specified in detail, and its diagnostic status is tentative.

Clinical Characteristics of ADHD

Disorders of attention, impulse control, and hyperactivity are common in children. The syndrome commonly referred to as hyperactivity includes some combination of hyperactivity with attentional and impulse control problems. Barkley (1988a,b) noted that ADHD children also have difficulty using rules to guide task behavior; their behavior is more influenced by immediate contingencies. The influence of immediate contingencies and the difficulty in formulating and carrying out goal-oriented search strategies have also been observed in laboratory studies (Douglas, 1983). The diagnosis of such disorders is obviously age-related: What is normal for a 2-year-old is clearly abnormal for a 5-year-old. The

TABLE 12.2.   Attention Deficit–Hyperactivity
Disorder Criteria

---

1. Fidgetiness or restlessness.
2. Difficulty remaining seated.
3. Easily distracted by extraneous stimuli.
4. Difficulty waiting turn in group situations.
5. Blurts out responses before questions are completed.
6. Difficulty with sustained attention.
7. Does not follow through or fails to finish tasks.
8. Shifts among uncompleted activities.
9. Difficulty with quiet play.
10. Excessive verbosity.
11. Often interrupts or intrudes on others.
12. Does not seem to listen.
13. Often loses objects necessary for task.
14. Engages in many risk taking activities.

---

[a]Must meet eight criteria for 6 months for DSM-III-R diagnosis
(American Psychiatric Association, 1987).

diagnosis is also heavily influenced by cultural expectations of what constitutes the range of age-appropriate behavior. Disorders of attention are most evident in cultures requiring attendance in schools for long periods of the day, where a child must stay seated and must sustain attention on highly abstract tasks with minimal ongoing reinforcement. Even in cultures as similar as the United States and Great Britain, the frequency with which this syndrome is diagnosed shows surprising variability. Rutter (1983a) cited evidence that the diagnosis of hyperactivity is made nearly 50 times as often in North America as in Britain. Differences persist even when standardized rating scales are used to compare prevalence between countries or within different regions of a country. In terms of epidemiology, parents or teachers may report that anywhere from 15% to 20% of children are hyperactive or inattentive. Problems such as restlessness, hyperactivity, inattention, impulsiveness, and distractibility are common in many childhood psychiatric syndromes, and it is not clear that hyperactivity defines a distinct syndrome (Rutter, 1983b).

Etiology

The etiology of ADHD and other attentional disorders remains problematic. Numerous twin and family studies suggest that a genetic component is involved in some cases (Shaywitz & Shaywitz, 1987). Because attentional problems are frequently observed in the aftermath of brain damage, their presence in children was thought by some to indicate some sort of low-grade brain damage, and the syndrome "minimal brain dysfunction" was coined to describe such unfortunate individuals. The lack of convincing evidence of brain damage in the majority of such children, the failure to establish a set of defining features for the syndrome, and the lack of an identifiable etiology have led to a retreat from this diagnostic label (Rutter, 1983b). The influence of stimulants that affect the catecholaminergic systems on ADHD behaviors, as well as indirect evidence of lower levels of dopaminergic and noradrenergic activity in ADHD children, has led to the hypothesis that the catecholaminergic function is disturbed (Shaywitz & Shaywitz 1987).

Treatment

The efficacy of stimulant medication in the relief of symptoms of ADHD has been established by many investigations (Cantwell & Carlson, 1978). Stimulants like methylphenidate decrease restlessness, decrease impulsive behaviors, and improve attention span. Performance improvements on attentional measures are also observed when normal children and adults are given stimulants. Academic achievement and peer relationships are less influenced by stimulant treatment. Few long-term studies have been carried out to compare treated and untreated ADHD children. In a review of long-term outcome in ADHD, Weiss (1983) concluded that ADHD children continue to have problems with impulsivity, restlessness, and poor social skills, and that long-term treatment with stimulant medication does not result in improvement in these areas or in academic performance.

Behavioral interventions, carried out by parents or teachers, have been used to increase the on-task behavior of these children, and to diminish off-task or disruptive behavior. Typically, behavioral studies are characterized by small numbers of subjects, often with individualized treatment programs, over a short time period (Sprague, 1983). Behavior modification does appear to be effective in reducing off-task behavior. More interestingly, behavioral interventions are often associated with improvement in academic performance, which are unaffected by stimulant medication alone. Few long-term studies of the relative efficacy of stimulant medication and behavioral interventions have been conducted. Studies carried out by Gittleman, Abikoff, Pollack, Klein, Katz, & Mattes (1980) suggest that methylphenidate and behavior modification are the most effective therapy for ADHD, followed by stimulant medication alone; behavior modification alone was found to be least effective. Sprague (1983) argued convincingly for a more rational approach to treatment combinations, using interventions in a complementary way. For example, stimulant medications would be used to deal with the attention deficit *per se*, behavior modification to shape specific study and social behavior, and remedial education to address academic deficiencies.

Neuropsychological Assessment

ADHD and related attentional disorders in children have not been well characterized in terms of traditional neuropsychological tests. The most widely used method of assessment of attention deficit in children has been parent or teacher rating scales, used to identify naturally occurring behaviors suggestive of hyperactivity, impulsiveness, distractibility, or attentional lapses (Barkley, 1988). In behavioral studies, direct observation of children in different environments, especially in the classroom, has been used. It should be stressed that there is often great situational variation in the behavioral manifestations of an attention deficit. A child may appear hyperactive and impulsive in school and not at home, and vice versa. Children who manifest ADHD behavior are said to show situational hyperactivity, and those who manifest hyperactive behavior across several environments are said to show pervasive hyperactivity. Children with pervasive hyperactivity have been reported to show more severe classroom attention deficits, cognitive deficits, and behavioral disturbance, and to have a worse prognosis (Barkley, 1988b).

On the Wechsler Intelligence Scale for Children-Revised (WISC-R) attention deficit is associated with depression on three subtests: Digit Span and Arithmetic from the Verbal section, and Digit Symbol from the Performance section; in general, verbal and visuospatial performance remain at normal or near-normal levels (Kaufman, 1979). This pattern is not unique to children with ADHD. Rather, it is found in any disorder that affects concentration, working memory, or processing speed.

Errors of omission and commission by children with attention deficits can be observed in a clinical go–no-go paradigm. Trommer, Hoeppner, Lorber, and Armstrong (1988) tested children with attention deficits. These children were further divided into those with hyperactivity and those without hyperactivity, and their performance was compared with that of normal children. The children were tested with a go–no-go paradigm developed by Mesulam (1985, p. 81). The task requires a child to raise and lower an index finger when the child hears a single tap ("go"), and to do nothing when two taps are heard ("no-go"). Children with attention deficits made more errors than controls. Initially, the nonhyperactive attention-deficit children made a high number of commission errors (responding to a no-go signal), but they improved with practice. The hyperactive children's performance did not differ from that of control subjects in the number of commission errors made initially, but they failed to improve with practice as did the control group and the nonhyperactive group. Errors of omission were very rare in the nonhyperactive and control groups. The hyperactive group showed the most frequent occurrence of omission errors. These findings were interpreted as showing that children with attention deficits without hyperactivity make impulsive errors but can improve with practice, and that attention deficit children with hyperactivity are impulsive as well as more likely to go off-task entirely. This is one of the few neuropsychological studies that contrast children with ADHD and children with nonhyperactive attention deficits.

In summary, children with attention deficits have been characterized primarily by observational behavior scales, usually scored by parents and teachers. The Digit Span, Digit Symbol, and Arithmetic subtests of the WISC-R are sensitive to attentional deficits. Go–no-go paradigms may have promise in the detection and characterization of attention deficit in the clinic.

Experimental Evidence

Laboratory Studies

Although ADHD children have been poorly characterized in terms of norm-based neuropsychological tests, they have been heavily scrutinized by means of laboratory tests of attentional, cognitive, and memory functioning (for excellent reviews, see Douglas & Peters, 1979; Douglas, 1983).

One initial hypothesis attributed the attention deficit in ADHD children to their higher susceptibility to distracting stimuli in the environment. In terms of filter theories of selective attention, affected children are unable to filter task-irrelevant stimuli during performance, and the processing of irrelevant stimuli interferes with efficient task execution. In a review by Douglas and Peters (1979) of numerous laboratory studies, it has rarely been found that hyperactive children or children diagnosed as having minimal brain dysfunction show performance decrements greater than those shown by controls when distracting stimuli are added to a task.

Although there is little evidence that ADHD children are unable to filter out irrelevant information, there is compelling evidence that they have difficulty sustaining attention, particularly on tasks in which informative or response-demanding stimuli are infrequently present. Vigilance tests, in which a person is required to make a response to an infrequently appearing target, are quite difficult for ADHD children. The vigilance test most frequently used with these children is the continuous-performance test, developed by Rosvold, Mirsky, Sarandon, Bransome, and Beck (1956). This test presents a subject with a sequence of letters one at a time, either spoken over earphones or displayed on a screen. The subject is required to press a key whenever a target stimulus appears, or after the last letter of a specified sequence of stimuli (e.g., press the key when a letter *A* appears if it has been preceded by the letter *X*). A variety of measures can be derived from the continuous-performance test, including reaction times and error types. Errors can be of two types: errors of omission (failure to respond to a target) and errors of commission (responding when a target is not present). Errors of omission are due to failures of sustained attention, or attentional lapses; errors of commission may be due to impulsivity, or a failure of response inhibition. Hyperactive children have been reported to make more errors of both types than normal children and to show more rapid deterioration of task performance over time (Sykes, Douglas, & Morganstern, 1973). Responses on continuous-performance measures by both hyperactive and normal children are usually improved by the administration of stimulant medication (Barkley, 1988b).

The most common research measure of impulsivity is the Matching Familiar Figures Test (Kagan, 1986). This test requires that a child choose a figure, from a set of pictures, that matches a target figure. The test includes 12 trials. Two scores are derived: the latency to the first response to each set of pictures and the total number of errors. Both measures discriminate ADHD children from normal children (Barkley, 1988b).

In summary, experimental tests of attention suggest that ADHD children are able to resist distracting stimuli about as well as controls, but that they show frequent errors on tasks that require sustained attention. In addition, they have difficulty in carrying out an adequate decision or search process before generating a response.

Psychophysiological Evidence

Although the literature related to autonomic measures of arousal is difficult to summarize easily because of the diversity of methods used to measure arousal, there is a consensus among recent reviewers that ADHD children are not chronically underaroused or overaroused. Rather, they appear to be less responsive to stimuli than normal subjects, a finding suggesting that they are unable to modulate arousal levels effectively in response to transient task demands (Douglas, 1983; Rosenthal & Allen, 1978). Evoked-potential paradigms eliciting the P3 response typically show reduced amplitude of the response. If P3 amplitude indexes reactivity to task-relevant stimuli, these results also support the hypothesis that ADHD children are underreactive to informative signals, at least in the types of simple, repetitive tasks used in P3 paradigms. The Nd or N1 response, associated with sensory filtering, has also been reported to be decreased in amplitude in hyperactive children (Satterfield, Schell, Nicholas, & Backs, 1988).

An intriguing study by Lou, Henriksen, Bruhn, Borner, and Nielson (1989) investigated the neurophysiological systems affected by hyperactivity by examining cerebral blood flow distribution with xenon-133 inhalation emission tomography. The children in the study all showed ADHD symptoms but were heterogeneous in terms of other medical and neurological characteristics, and some had definite CNS dysfunction. The control group was poorly described. Children with ADHD tended to show hypoperfusion of the striatal region of the brain, as well as hyperperfusion of the primary sensory and sensorimotor regions. This finding suggests that the striatal region in these children is underactive, whereas the neuronal activity in the sensory and sensorimotor regions is increased. The investigators speculated that this pattern may represent less of inhibition of the sensory system by the caudate nucleus. They also noted that animals with striatal lesions show deficits in delayed response, in delayed alternation, and on go–no-go tasks, as do ADHD children. The administration of methylphenidate to the children in the study increased blood flow to the striatum but had less impact on hyperperfusion of the sensory and sensorimotor regions.

Models of Attention Deficit Disorder in Children

It is clear that children diagnosed as having ADHD, hyperactivity, or minimal brain dysfunction perform more poorly than other children on many behavioral, academic, and interpersonal measures. Several investigators have attempted to develop models based on a few deficits that may account for the wide range of disturbances that develop in these children. Deficits may be considered primary because they appear in most children diagnosed with ADHD; because they may underlie a broad spectrum of concurrent deficits; or because they appear earlier and appear to cause other deficits. For example, ADHD children may show an increasing disparity in academic performance in comparison with normal children as they progress through grade school, because their attention deficit interferes with their learning basic skills and in turn prevents the acquisition of more complex skills in later grades.

Barkley (1988b) used a behavioral model to describe the problem performance of ADHD children. He noted that the primary symptoms of inattention, hyperactivity, and impulsiveness distinguish ADHD children from other children, but that each of these primary symptoms describes a wide range of behaviors that may vary from child to child. Moreover, all of the primary symptoms may not be present in every child, a fact recognized by the revised diagnostic categories and criteria in the DSM-III-R. Barkley put special stress on the observation that ADHD children may have a primary deficit in rule-governed behavior. He used a behavioral definition of rule-governed behavior as the ability of language or other symbol systems to serve as discriminative stimuli for behavior. Barkley pointed out that most laboratory tests for attention deficit require compliance to rules provided by the examiner. The results could be interpreted as indicative of difficulty in sustaining compliance with test instructions in the absence of strong reinforcement. He also proposed that the problems that ADHD children often have with problem solving may be construed as a difficulty in generating and implementing rules covertly (second-order rules). He argued that ADHD children are contingency-shaped in their behavior, rather than rule-governed. Consequently, they have difficulty doing any academic, social, or laboratory task that requires adherence to rules rather than immediately occurring natural consequences.

Douglas (1983) stressed the role of defective attention, inhibitory, arousal, and reinforcement processes in the cognitive and behavioral performance of ADHD children. Their difficulties in sustaining attention have been well documented. They are less able than other children to inhibit their responses, perhaps because of behavioral control by immediate reinforcers and because of the lack of intrinsic value of the stimuli. Douglas also noted that their search strategies seem to be compromised by the developmentally earlier tendency to explore a situation with little regard for task demands. Instead of searching through stimuli and identifying task-relevant information to guide their behavior, they are influenced by the sensory salience or idiosyncratic interest of the stimuli. Arousal deficits are most apparent on psychophysiological measures of stimulus reactivity, and in the difficulty that ADHD children have in using warning cues to modulate their arousal before the onset of a signal.

Most characterizations of ADHD deficits have an interesting developmental aspect. The behavioral and attentional problems experienced by these children are not deviant in the sense that psychotic behaviors are deviant. Rather, their behaviors are age-inappropriate. All young children initially use exploratory rather than task-oriented search strategies to interact with the environment; are more influenced by immediate contingencies rather than rules or long-term goals; and have short attention spans and show more impulsiveness than older children. What is different about ADHD children is that they behave younger than their peers and often fail to catch up. Their deficits are not intractable, however. Even without treatment, many ADHD children grow up to function normally in the adult world (Weiss,

1983). It remains an open question whether ADHD children grow up to be effective adults by developing effective coping strategies for their attention deficit, or whether the deficit itself sometimes disappears with maturation. With a better understanding of this process and more effective remedial treatment, it is possible that the great majority would develop age-appropriate behavior.

Evidence for Attention Deficit–Hyperactivity Disorder Subtypes

Since many children with attention deficit disorder (ADD) exhibit a symptom constellation that includes hyperkineses, impulsivity, and restlessness, ADD has often been linked to hyperactivity (ADD+H). The clinical characteristics of ADD+H are well established, and many researchers believe that ADD+H is a neurobehavioral disturbance. ADD+H children share many of the clinical characteristics observed in patients with frontal lobe brain injuries. This fact has led some investigators to propose that frontal lobe dysfunction may underlie ADD+H (Chelyne et al., 1986; Benson, 1991; Heilman, Kytja, Voeller & Nadeau, 1991). There is now converging empirical evidence associating ADD+H with frontal lobe dysfunction from neuropsychological studies (Trommer et al., 1988; Barkley, Grodzinski, & DuPaul, 1992), as well as neurophysiological studies of cerebral blood flow (Lou et al., 1984, 1989), positron emission tomography (Zametkin et al., 1990), and magnetic resonance imaging morphology (e.g., Hynd et al., 1990).

While comorbidity of ADD+H is very common (Shaywitz & Shaywitz, 1991), not all children with ADD exhibit hyperactivity (Loney et al., 1978; Lahey et al., 1984; Carlson et al., 1986; Barkley et al., 1991). Children with attention deficit disorder without hyperactivity (ADD−H) often exhibit a different clinical presentation from ADD+H children, a fact that led some investigators to propose that ADD−H actually is a different disorder than ADD+H (Barkley et al., 1991; Hynd et al., 1991a,b). While the existence of ADD subtypes is not universally accepted, there is at least some evidence that ADD−H and ADD+H are different neurobehavioral disorders. The clinical features associated with ADD+H and ADD−H differ in several ways. Children with ADD−H are less likely than ADD+H children to exhibit aggressive, or oppositional-defiant behaviors. However, ADD−H children appear to exhibit greater problems with social withdrawal, cognitive sluggishness, lethargy, and comorbidity with other learning disabilities (Edelbrock et al., 1984; Lahey et al., 1984). Therefore, while both ADD−H and ADD+H are characterized by impairments of vigilance, concentration, and other attention-related functions, these subtypes seem to differ in their comorbidity with other clinical features.

Neuropsychological Evidence

There is compelling neuropsychological evidence for an attentional disturbance in ADD+H. ADD+H has been shown to be associated with low scores on three subtests from the WISC-R: Digit Span, Arithmetic, and Coding (Kaufman, 1979). However, this pattern of test results is not unique to children with ADD+H, as it occurs with many disorders that affect concentration, working memory, and processing speed. Interestingly, other tasks commonly used to measure attentional functions have not reliably discriminated ADD. For instance, the hypothesis that ADD+H results in higher susceptibility to distracting stimuli was not supported by laboratory studies of divided attention (see Douglas & Peters, 1979).

Tests of sustained attention and vigilance provide greater sensitivity to ADD. The continuous performance test (CPT) (Rosvold et al., 1956) is particularly useful, since hyperactive children have been shown to make more errors of all types and to exhibit more rapid response decrease than normal children (Skyes et al., 1973). Also, CPT performance improves with methylphenidate treatment (Barkley, 1977; Rapoport *et al.*, 1978). The go–no-go paradigm also reliably discriminates ADD from normal children. Like the CPT, this task requires the patient to either respond or inhibit responding based on stimulus criteria. The go–no-go paradigm is particularly sensitive to response control deficits associated with frontal lobe dysfunction. The fact that only measures of sustained attention and response control (i.e., go–no-go) reliably discriminate ADD from normal children supports the hypothesis that ADD results from frontal lobe dysfunction. The performance of ADD children varies as a function of specific task and situational parameters across experiments, a fact that led Barkley (1988) to postulate that ADD reflects difficulties in using rules and behavioral consequences to guide task behavior. Douglas (1983) reached a similar conclusion regarding ADD performance inconsistencies after demonstrating that immediate situational behavioral contingencies produce impairments of formulation and performance of goal-oriented strategies in ADD+H. Swanson *et al.* (1991) demonstrated that ADD+H children were impaired with respect to overt shifting of spatial selective attention, but normal for covert shifts of attention on a visual–spatial cuing task such as the Posner (1980) paradigm. These findings support hypotheses that link ADD+H with anterior brain dysfunction.

While ADD+H appears to be associated with frontal brain dysfucntion, it seems less likely that this is the primary basis for ADD−H, since children with ADD−H have a different clinical presentation. While ADD−H has a high comorbidity with learning and emotional disorders (Edelbrock *et al.*, 1984; Hinshaw, 1987; Hynd *et al.*, 1991b), several studies failed to differentiate ADD+H from ADD−H on the basis of learning disorders (Barkley *et al.*, 1991; Carlson *et al.*, 1986). Unfortunately, ADD+H and ADD−H have been contrasted in only a small number of formal neuropsychological studies, many of which contain methodological problems that cloud interpretation. Most studies employing neuro-psychological measures have not differentiated ADD+H and ADD−H (Carlson *et al.*, 1986). Yet, Trommer *et al.* (1988) demonstrated differences between ADD+H and ADD−H on the go–no-go paradigm, as children with ADD−H initially made a high number of commission errors and improved with practice. ADD+H children did not initially differ from control subjects with respect to number of commission errors, but did not improve with practice, and also made more errors of omission by failing to respond to the "go" stimulus.

Recently, Barkely, Grodzinski, and DuPaul (1992) found that while the performance of ADD+H and ADD−H was similar on most neuropsychological measures, children with ADD−H had greater impairments on the Rey-Osterreith Figure. This finding suggests that ADD−H children may have greater difficulty with visual–motor integration. Few studies to date employ attentional paradigms designed to specifically dissociate deficits of sensory selective attention from impairments of response intention and/or executive control. Yet, such a dissociation might be expected based on these neuropsychological findings and also differences in clinical presentations for these subtypes.

Electrophysiological Approaches

Both the autonomic and evoked potential (EP) responses of ADD and normal children have been shown to differ. In this section, EPs, heart rate (HR), and skin conductance response (SCR) of ADD+H and ADD−H children on tasks with different attentional demands will be contrasted.

Autonomic Indices. Children with ADD syndrome are neither chronically hypoaroused or hyperaroused on autonomic measures, but instead have been found to be less responsive to stimuli than normal subjects, suggesting activational difficulties relative to transient task demands (see Hastings & Barkley, 1978; Douglas, 1983; Rosenthal & Allen, 1978). Since autonomic reactivity provides a good index of attentional allocation (e.g., Cohen & Waters, 1985), diminished autonomic reactivity is likely related to the underlying attention disturbance in ADD. The orienting response (OR) and its habituation provide particularly good indices of decrements in attentional response to repeated presentations of a nonsalient stimulus. Habituation rate is frequently impaired in patients with frontal lobe damage (Luria, 1966) and subcortical disorders such as Huntington's disease (Oscar-Berman & Gade, 1979). Cohen and Albers (1991) demonstrated that cingulate lesions produce habituation deficits that are more related to abnormal sensitization, rather than a failure of neural habituation. While a number of neural models for habituation have been developed, habituation in humans is still not well understood. There are few data regarding the mechanisms affecting abnormal OR elicitation, habituation, or sensitization in ADD or ADD subtypes.

ERP Abnormalities in ADD. Previous investigations of ADD suggest that usually ERP amplitude rather than latency is impaired, though in one study P3 latency was also greater for ADD children compared with the control subjects (Holcomb, Ackerman, & Dykman, 1985). Diminished P3 amplitudes to repetitive target stimuli have been reported in ADD (Loiselle *et al.*, 1980), and ADD subjects have been found to exhibit smaller P3 amplitude differences between targets and nontargets compared with the reading disability subjects (Holcomb *et al.*, 1985). Dykman *et al.* (1983) found ERP response gradients to be inconsistently related to reaction time, when ADD children were divided as EP augmenters or reducers based on their response to different stimulus intensities, and concluded that the N2-P3 gradient is an index of sensory registration rather than response strength. Satterfield *et al.* (1988) found the N1 component associated with sensory processing to be of reduced amplitude in ADD children. The Nd response associated with attentional processing was also reduced in amplitude, whereas the P3 response was found to be of normal amplitude. These results were interpreted as indicating an arousal dysfunction related to hyporeactivity to salient informative stimuli in ADD, since the Nd is a mismatch negativity to the target stimulus, and thought to be an OR component. Problems related to both automatic and controlled attentional processing were implicated. Satterfield *et al.* (1990) also reported abnormalities in the P3b and slow-wave potentials (SP1-3) in ADD boys, since these components were reduced in amplitude to the target stimuli in the attend channel rather than enhanced to the distractor stimuli in the ignore channel, though the effect depended on the child's age. Unfortunately, previous ERP findings are not conclusive, as inconsistencies have been reported across studies. For instance, Holcomb *et al.* (1985) reported that both an ADD and a reading disorder contract group had reduced P3b amplitudes. Harter, Diering, and Wood (1988) demonstrated that reading disorder children have reduced amplitude of ERP components at 240 msec over the left central hemisphere and at 500 msec over the right central hemisphere; they also found very little abnormality of the P2 or P3 components of ADD+H subjects without reading disorder.

ERPs and ADD Subtypes. Relatively few studies have directly compared subtypes of ADD and generally yielded mixed results. For instance, Holcomb *et al.* (1985) reported no differences in P3 amplitude between ADD+H and ADD−H children on a task that required attending to a target stimulus with 16% probability, while ignoring distractor stimuli, though all clinical groups had reduced P3 amplitudes. Klorman *et al.* (1990) used an oddball EP paradigm to study ADD children with and without aggressive features. While N1 amplitude was found to be increased to visual rather than auditory stimuli, no differences in N1 response as a function of ADD subgroup were found. However, their subgroups were not equivalent to the ADD+H–ADD−H distinction. In contrast, Dykman *et al.* (1983)

reported different patterns of augmentation of the N2-P3 response for ADD+H and ADD−H, since hyperactive children showed steeper augmentation gradients as a function of stimulus strength. Yet, when previous ERP studies of ADHD are considered together, one is met with considerable ambiguity and interpretive difficulties. While most studies have demonstrated differences between ADD and normal children on ERP measures, the specific components that distinguish groups differ across investigations. Since the paradigms employed to distinguish ADD often differ across studies, it is difficult to compare results. Also, the method of classification of subjects into groups is often quite different across investigations, which may account for the failure of some studies to distinguish ADD or subtypes. Better dissociation of ADD subtypes based on ERP response characteristics requires careful classification of subjects into subtypes, as well as the use of paradigms that may be sensitive to the different component processes underlying attention.

Neuroanatomic Abnormalities in ADD

If ADD+H and ADD−H are distinct neurobehavioral disorders, then it should be possible to identify neuroanatomic abnormalities involving different brain systems. While neuropsychological and behavioral findings suggest that ADD is associated with CNS dysfunction, there is little direct evidence of structural impairments of specific brain systems in ADD. Children with ADD rarely exhibit obvious structural impairments on neuroimaging, as cortical lesions or any other gross neuropathology on CT or MRI are rare in ADD. The absence of neuropathological findings in ADD is not surprising, as ADD is a developmental disorder, not associated with an acute neurologic event or disease process.

Even though gross structural impairments are unexpected in ADD, subtle neuro-anatomic variations in brain morphology may exist. Digitizing techniques for magnetic resonance imaging region of interest have proved to be very useful in quantifying the subtle brain lesions and morphologic abnormalities. For instance, investigators have used these techniques to demonstrate a relationship between the quantity of periventricular white matter plaques and cognitive dysfucntion in multiple sclerosis (Rao et al., 1986). Recently, investigators have reported abnormalities of certain brain regions in ADD children (Hynd et al., 1990). Children with ADD exhibited symmetry between the right and left frontal lobes compared with normal children, who tended to have larger volume in the right frontal lobe. Regional cerebral blood flow studies have also provided evidence of right striatal hypoperfusion in ADD (Lou et al., 1989). In another study, Hynd et al. (1991a) reported abnormalities of corpus callosum morphology in ADD, with smaller callosal volumes in the region of the genu and splenium compared with normals found. While these studies provide initial evidence of subtle neuroanatomic differences in ADD, there are still relatively few neuro-anatomic data on which to draw conclusions and no studies that correlate neuroanatomic findings with neuropsychological and/or neurophysiolgoical indices in a source analysis.

ANXIETY AND STRESS DISORDERS

The effects of anxiety and "stress" on attention are clinically obvious, but have not been systematically studied by neuropsychological investigators. Excessive levels of environmental demands eventually create informational interference and may tax attentional limitations. On the other hand, moderate task demands may actually facilitate performance by boosting "arousal" to optimal levels. This is the basis of the Yerkes–Dodson law (1908). Therefore, the effects of stress depend on a wide variety of task and organismic factors.

Anxiety also may have a beneficial effect on attentional performance, if the levels are moderate. However, when the anxiety level becomes extreme, performance invariably suffers. Interestingly, the effect of high anxiety levels is often to create hypervigilance to either external or internal events. Therefore, anxiety may adversely affect performance by narrowing the focus of attention beyond an adaptive level. The individual then becomes fixated on certain stimuli, while ignoring the rest.

The recursive quality of the obsessions experienced by certain patients with anxiety disorders supports the idea that these patients may actually exhibit heightened attentional states. They exhibit self-directed attention to an extreme. Surgical lesioning of the cingulate gyrus often disrupts the recursive nature of obsessive thinking, but it may also alter subtle aspects of attention control (Cohen, McCrae, Phillips, & Wilkinson, 1990).

The paradoxical excess of attentional processing in patients with anxiety disorders is interesting, as it reflects the relationship of attentional capacity, psychophysiological response, and subjective states (Weinberger, Schwartz, & Davidson, 1979). However, this topic has received little formal neuropsychological address.

Neuropsychological Assessment of Attention

The clinical assessment of attention usually depends on three sources of information: (1) psychometric tests designed to measure other cognitive functions, which provide indirect information about attention; (2) specific neuropsychological tests of attention; and (3) direct behavioral observation and measurement. As attention is a multifaceted process, the assessment of attention requires that the clinician obtain information about the characteristics of the patient's performance under different conditions. Therefore, to adequately assess attention, it is usually necessary to use more than one test. In this chapter, we discuss some of the approaches to the clinical assessment of attention, taking into consideration these three sources of information. The initial discussion focuses on the traditional methods of assessing attention. The reader is encouraged to review Lezak (1983) for a more detailed account of the actual test procedures and norms for tests of attention and executive functioning. At the end of the chapter, we discuss several experimental assessment methods.

PSYCHOMETRIC ASSESSMENT OF ATTENTION

Neuropsychological assessment has historically relied on tools and techniques developed within the clinical and psychometric traditions. Although some neuropsychological tests have been derived from classical experimental psychology paradigms (e.g., word list learning), the adoption of paradigms based on information processing and cognitive psychology by neuropsychological researchers is a recent phenomenon. The use of psychometric assessment and interpretive strategies has led neuropsychologists to measure and discuss attention quite differently from academic psychologists.

Clinical Assessment

Clinicians first consider mental performance from a diagnostic standpoint. In the case of attentional performance, a clinician asks whether a patient's performance is within normal limits for the patient's age, educational background, occupation, and so on, or if it is impaired. If it is impaired, the clinician considers whether the impairment may be due to a specific medical or emotional disorder, such as depression, dementia, or drug abuse.

Clinicians often make inferences regarding the role of attentional factors when they interpret the results of various tests of cognitive and behavioral functioning. In fact, some of the tests that we have previously described were not originally developed for the measurement of attention. For example, the Word Generation Test is an indicator of language fluency that has been shown to be sensitive to the broader domain of response generation capacity. It is safe to say that most tests of cognitive functioning require intact attentional processes for optimal performance to occur. Yet, it is often difficult to extract the contribution of attention on tasks that were not developed to directly measure attentional dysfunction.

Inferences about the role of attention in cognitive performance are often based on clinical interpretation of the behavior of the patient during the evaluation. A patient who is well directed, who makes eye contact, and who is oriented to a task is usually considered attending. As discussed earlier, the psychometric analysis of test results may provide another means of extracting information about the role of attention in cognitive performance. Such analysis has been used extensively in the study of performance on intellectual tests such as the Wechsler Adult Intelligence Scale (WAIS).

Another clinical determinant of the role of attention is the finding of excessive inter-task or interitem variability. When a series of test items is designed to measure the same capacity, and a patient shows adequate performance on a given trial and then fails on another, performance inconsistency is evident. It is difficult to account for this inconsistency on the basis of diminished cognitive ability, as performance of the task on certain occasions indicates that the particular faculty is present. An attentional explanation is often used.

Caution should be used when drawing conclusions about the role of attentional dysfunction in performance variability. First, the clinician must be certain that the test itself is reliable. Unreliable tests may have excessive interitem variability, so that what appears to be variability in the patient is actually due to the nature of the test. Even if a particular test has been found to be highly reliable, there may be other confounds when one is interpreting the role of attention.

Performance variability may be caused by a suboptimal processing of information by a particular functional system. For instance, cortical damage to posterior brain regions may cause visual problems that become apparent only when task demands increase. On a simple visual discrimination task, the patient may appear to be intact. With increased task complexity, the patient must exert greater effort to compensate for a subtle processing deficit, which results in greater attentional demand. Therefore, attentional variability may occur secondary to the increased requirement of effort resulting from a subtle primary processing defect. The clinician must rule out this possibility before concluding that attentional dysfunction is the basis of the variability.

The clinician, therefore, is very interested in tests that are sensitive to individual differences in performance due to attentional factors. An academic psychologist, on the other hand, is interested in how test performance is affected by experimental manipulations, such as the sensory properties of stimuli, the interstimulus intervals, the instructions, and the task complexity. As the experimental psychologist is minimally interested in the interaction between these manipulations and individual differences, he or she is content to use university students as subjects, who show considerable homogeneity in age, education, and life experiences. The experimental psychologist seeks to explicate the mental processes that mediate performance in normal persons; the clinical psychologist determines how mental illness and brain damage influence mental performance. These two traditions had little to say to each other until neuropsychologists became interested in the processes involved in test performance from a theoretical perspective, and experimental psychologists became interested in the biological bases of mental performance.

The clinician is very interested in the qualitative aspects of a person's behavior. Is an individual distractible? Obsessed by an image, action, or belief? Dulled or apathetic? Weakly responsive to stimuli or events? The clinician attempts to get a description of the patient's behavior in the natural world, preferably corroborated by reports of family members, friends, or co-workers. Many occupations require sustained attention to tasks, in spite of their repetitive nature. It is frequently a co-worker or supervisor who first notices a problem with sustained attention. Psychiatric or neurological disorders that affect a person's ability to maintain a thread of thought may be first noticed by family members because of increased difficulty in carrying out a discussion with the patient. Again, the approach of an experimental psychologist to a subject is quite different from that of a clinician. The experimental psychologist seldom assesses the qualitative and naturalistic aspects of an individual's behavior.

PSYCHOMETRICS AND NEUROPSYCHOLOGY

In contrast to the paradigms of experimental psychology, the methods and tests developed for the psychometric measurement of intellectual performance have had a great impact on neuropsychology. Psychometrics uses a normative approach to characterize individual differences in intellectual performance. As a normative approach places the performance of individuals on a test in relation to a broad sample of peers, it is suited to characterizing a patient's performance as being within or outside normal limits, and to rating the severity of a deficit in terms of the normal range of variation on a test. Psychometricians have long been interested in the empirically derived types of intellectual performance. Psychometricians such as Terman (1916) and Spearman (1927) conceptualized intelligence as a unitary attribute that affected all complex behaviors (commonly referred to as factor g in factor-analytic studies). Empirically, the existence of a single factor for general intelligence was supported by the finding that performances on a wide variety of mental tests show positive correlations. This effect was referred to as the positive manifold among mental tests. However, the correlation between tests, although typically positive, varied in magnitude. This variation suggested that, in addition to a general intelligence factor, other ability-specific factors were influencing test performance and varied with some independence. Even without positing innate differences in the distribution of mental abilities, it is obvious that educational and occupational experiences would result in very different patterns of performance on mental testing. A test battery that included tests of reading comprehension, mechanical ability, spatial puzzle solving, interpersonal skills, and business judgment would provide different profiles if administered to a professor of linguistics, a psychoanalyst, a manager, and a machinist.

Because people varied in terms of test performance, statistical approaches were developed to group tests by their natural covariation. One simple way of approaching this problem is to examine a matrix of correlation coefficients generated by a group of people who have taken a diverse set of tests. Typically, natural groupings emerge. Two such groupings that commonly emerge from such an approach are verbal and spatial performance. In a group of people, performance levels within a domain such as verbal tests tend to covary, as does performance from the domain of spatial performance. For example, a person who does well on a test of vocabulary typically performs well on another test of verbal performance, such as reading comprehension. A test of verbal performance, however, provides only a rough estimate of performance on a test of spatial problem solving.

Another approach to characterizing test performance groupings is called *factor analysis*. This statistical technique uses the correlation matrix (or some other measure of covariation among a group of measures) and identifies groupings of tests related to underlying "factors" (Thurstone, 1938). Factor analysis does not derive a unique solution from a given set of test intercorrelations, however, so the number of factors and their relationship can vary between studies, depending on the factor-analytic procedure used by the investigators. Nevertheless, factor-analytic studies of test performance have replicated a set of factors that appear to describe natural categories of mental skills. Some categories that have been extracted from many sets of tests are verbal abilities, spatial abilities, perceptual speed, and freedom from distractibility. One sweeping dichotomy contrasts crystallized intelligence (*Gc*), which is evident in the performance of tasks that entail the application of well-learned knowledge, rules and skills; and fluid intelligence (*Gf*), which comes into play when tasks require the generation of new solutions, concepts, relationships, and strategies (Cattell, 1963; Horn & Cattell, 1967). Unfortunately, for many years, psychometric studies failed to include tests that placed specific demands on attention. The existence of an attentional component in intelligence became clear, however, when the performance of brain-damaged individuals was considered.

Psychometric Patterns of Brain Dysfunction

Different types of mental performance as measured by psychometric tests covary among normal individuals. In normal individuals, however, these groupings are intercorrelated, and this intercorrelation appears to reflect something like the unitary intelligence factor posited by early researchers in the field. A very bright individual, for example, tends to do well on many types of tasks, whereas a dull person struggles with any type of complex task. When the brain has been damaged, however, one or another aspect of performance often shows a striking difference from other aspects, in part because different areas and systems within the brain appear to be associated with different types of mental performance. The left hemisphere, for example, apparently plays an essential role in language processes. Damage to the left hemisphere, then, produces a disproportionate level of language deficit compared to damage to other parts of the brain, and this difference is reflected in test performance. In an individual with a left-hemisphere stroke, performance on tests of verbal performance is usually depressed, whereas performance on tests of spatial performance typically remains near normal.

Psychometric studies of neuropsychological performance in brain-damaged individuals have consistently isolated a mental performance factor associated with attentional performance. This factor has emerged in studies using the WAIS-R—Wechsler (1981) and the Wechsler Memory Scale (Wechsler, 1945), two of the most widely used test ensembles in the neuropsychological literature. Ryan and Schneider (1986) factor-analyzed the WAIS-R performance of 100 heterogeneous brain-damaged patients and found that the tests were associated with three different factors: verbal abilities, performance (spatial) ability, and freedom from distractibility. Although the WAIS was originally divided into verbal and performance sections, the Digit Span and Arithmetic tests of the Verbal section and the Digit Symbol test of the Performance section usually form a third factor that has been related to concentration or freedom from distractibility. Similar results have been found with the Wechsler Memory Scale. Prigatono (1978) reviewed the factor-analytic literature relevant to the psychometric organization of subtests from the Wechsler Memory Scale. Two subtests from the Wechsler Memory Scale, Mental Control and Digit Span, were consistently identified as a concentration factor. O'Donnell, Drachman, Lew, and Swearer (1988) carried out a factor-analytic study of subtests from the WAIS-R, the Wechsler Memory Scale, and tests of verbal performance on 82 demented outpatients of heterogeneous etiology. A concentration factor was again identified and was associated with Arithmetic, Digit Span Forward, and Digit Span Backward from the WAIS-R; Mental Control and Digit Span from the Wechsler Memory Scale; and Sentence Repetition from the Boston Diagnostic Aphasia Examination (Goodglass & Kaplan, 1979). Even in dementing disorders, which are usually associated with a global deterioration of cerebral structure and function, concentration or freedom from distractibility appears to maintain its functional identity. The tests associated with this factor demand transient mental retention of several pieces of information (words or numbers) and the performance of mental operations on such strings of numbers or words. Distraction would interfere with performance on any of these tests, as information in immediate or working memory is usually lost if it is not used or rehearsed.

Attentional Factors

Although it is evident from neuropsychological studies that attention can be selectively impaired by brain damage, the definition and operationalization of the attentional mechanisms as neuropsychological phenomena remain in a primitive stage of development. Horn and Cattell (1967) reported that fluid intelligence declines with age, whereas crystallized intelligence increases through adulthood. This may be attributable in part to the demands that *Gf* tasks place on effort and sustained concentration. This relationship was formally investigated in an ambitious study by Stankov (1988). Stankov studied the relationship of different types of attentional processes to other measures of intelligence and described the relationship of attentional performance to normal aging. Stankov studied 100 people between the ages of 20 and 70. Each subject received 19 psychometric tests and 17 measures of attentional processes. The attentional processes tested included (1) concentration, or sustained attention; (2) search or perceptual speed; (3) divided attention; (4) selective attention; and (5) attention switching. He then carried out a factor-analytic strategy to categorize attentional performance empirically.

The factor analysis identified three types of attention: (1) search, or perceptual speed; (2) concentration; and (3) attentional flexibility. *Search*, or *perceptual speed*, was best characterized by tests that required a person to search a set of items for a target, or to compare strings of numbers or letters for their similarity or difference. The best correlate of this factor among the psychometric tests was Digit Symbol. *Concentration* was associated with tests requiring sustained attention. Digit Symbol again appeared as a psychometric correlate of this factor. *Attentional flexibility* was reflected in the ability to change sets over the course of a task. Tasks making heavy demands on *working memory* were related to separate factors, including Digit Span and Arithmetic from the WAIS-R. These attentional factors were strongly associated with a broad fluid intelligence factor and were dissociated from measures of crystallized intelligence. Greater age was associated with poorer performance on all the attentional factors, as well as on other measures of fluid intelligence. The decline in fluid intelligence was largely attributable to the influence of attentional deficits associated with increased age. Performance on measures of crystallized intelligence, on the other hand, improved with age. These results probably reflect the likelihood that a person's store of knowledge increases with age, even if her or his attentional abilities and speed in dealing with new situations decline. A factor-analytic study by Mirsky (1978, 1989) using eight measures of attention yielded a set of similar test groupings, which Mirsky labeled as tests of *focus and execution*, composed of tests heavily dependent on perceptual speed; *vigilance*, or sustained attention; *numerical-mnemonic* (Arithmetic and Digit Span), which made heavy demands on encoding and working memory; and *flexibility*, which loaded on a test requiring attentional switching.

NEUROPSYCHOLOGICAL TESTS OF ATTENTION

Span of Attention

Span-of-attention tasks measure the capacity of the individual to process different loads of information. These tests vary the quantity or complexity of information that must be handled in a short period of time. As the information to be processed is not already stored in memory, span-of-attention tests put a demand on short-term memory storage. Performance depends on the ability to hold a string of items for a short period of time, until a response is called for. Encoding of the information into more permanent memory storage is not necessary to the completion of these tasks. Typically, individuals are unable to recall information from such tasks soon after it is initially presented. Span-of-attention performance bridges the areas of attention and memory. Some investigators have considered these tasks measures of working memory.

Digit Span

Repeating a string of digits in exact order is probably the most common test of attention span. In an early cognitive investigation, Miller (1956) found that normal individuals were almost always able to recite on immediate recall between five and nine units of information. Subsequently, the limits of short-term span has been tested for different types of information, including digits, words, and spatial positions. The span of 7 ± 2 appears to be relatively invariant across subjects for different types of information. As severely amnestic patients can usually perform this test, it is a good measure of short-term attention span, and not of memory. However, digit span also indicates the capacity to process verbal information through the language system and therefore is correlated with aphasia screening tests that measure the ability to repeat phrases of varying length. Inconsistency in performance on digit span tasks gives an indication of temporal variability in attention that may occur under conditions of increasing stimulus load.

The Digit Span Backward test is a more sensitive measure of brain damage and attentional dysfunction than Digit Span Forward. While the Digit Span Forward task requires repeating a string of numbers in exact order, it is possible to perform this task with minimal attentional effort when the number of digits to recite does not exceed the span of short-term memory. When the number of digits to recite is not excessive, the digit span task requires only automatic language processing. Reasonable performance on this test is possible even in patients with rather severe brain damage, when the language systems of the brain are intact. In contrast, Digit Span Backward requires a cognitive operation of reversing sequential order that cannot be performed automatically. Working memory must be used on this task, as the subject must be able to hold the original order of digits covertly, so that reversal before recitation is possible. There is often a large discrepancy between the number of digits recited forward and backward, which may serve as a clinical indicator of dysfunction. The inability to recite letters in reverse order is another indicator of brain dysfunction. The capacity to spell words of varying length in reverse order correlates with backward digit span but allows for a comparison of performances with a different domain of stimuli.

Several attention span measures have been developed that do not depend on direct verbal processing. These include the *Corsi Block Test* (Milner, 1971) and the *Knox Cube Test* (Arthur, 1947). Both tests measure span of attention for spatially presented material. As spatial sequence span usually correlates highly with digit span performance, there is some suggestion that the attentional constraints measured by both types of tests are not solely accounted for by a language-mediated mechanism. On the other hand, correlations have been found between performance on the spatial-sequence-span test and the location of brain damage. Patients with visual field defects of the right side had a much greater level of impairment on the *Corsi Blocks Test* than patients with left-hemisphere visual defects (DeRenzi, Faglioni, & Previdi, 1977). Therefore, tests of attention span for both verbal and visual spatial material are sensitive to domain-specific lesion effects. They may also reflect a common attentional capacity that can be determined when domain-specific effects are accounted for.

Attentional Persistence and Vigilance

Tests of attentional span do not require the performance of a task over a long duration. In order to assess persistence and the ability to maintain vigilance, it is necessary to use a task that requires processing over long time periods. The effect of attentional variability that is independent of information load can best be assessed by using tests that place a limited stimulus load on the subject, but that require sustained attention. By definition, such tests should be relatively easy to perform (they make limited cognitive demand) but difficult to sustain because of their repetitive and lengthy nature.

The *Continuous Performance Test* (CPT) was developed to measure sustained attention and vigilance (Rosvold *et al.*, 1956). In its original form, the patient is instructed to respond whenever a particular target letter is presented. The target letter is presented along with distractors, so that, on a given trial, there is a predetermined probability that a target or distractor will be presented. As these probabilities can be predetermined, the signal detection characteristics of the task (i.e., misses, false alarm rate, and operator characteristics) can be determined. In its original form, the test took 10 minutes. Since its original development, the *CPT* has been modified so that it controls for various parameters, such as interstimulus and intrastimulus interval, number of trials, and type of stimuli (e.g., auditory stimuli).

Task complexity was varied on the original *CPT* by setting up a second condition in which the subject was to respond only when a target letter was preceded by another anticipatory stimulus (e.g., the letter *A* preceding the letter *X*). Rosvold and his colleagues found that patients with brain dysfunction showed a significant decline in performance when the more complex version of the test was used. Other variables, such as the number of stimuli to be processed on a given trial, the interstimulus interval, and the memory load of the task, can affect performance. The fact that performance is sensitive to these variables suggests that task duration is not the only relevant attentional factor that is assessed by this test.

The original versions of the *CPT* purposely limit the weight of variables such as stimulus complexity and memory load, so that the main demand of the task is its sustained duration. Under these conditions, the *CPT* actually measures the ability to sustain responding on a simple task that is likely to be of little inherent interest to the patient. This task characteristic has both positive and negative qualities. The *CPT* provides information about performance on specific task parameters with demand created by task duration and low information load.

Other neuropsychological tests exist for measuring vigilance that do not require multiframe presentations (see Figure 13.1). The most commonly used vigilance tests of this type are *cancellation tests* (e.g., Diller, Ben-Yishay, Gerstman, Goodkin, Gordon, & Wemberg, 1974). *Cancellation tests* require the patient to scan a sheet of paper (single frame) in order to detect a particular stimulus or sequence of stimuli. Several versions of this task have been developed that use stimuli created from different domains (e.g., letters, digits, and geometric shapes). Performance is measured as a function of the time taken to complete the

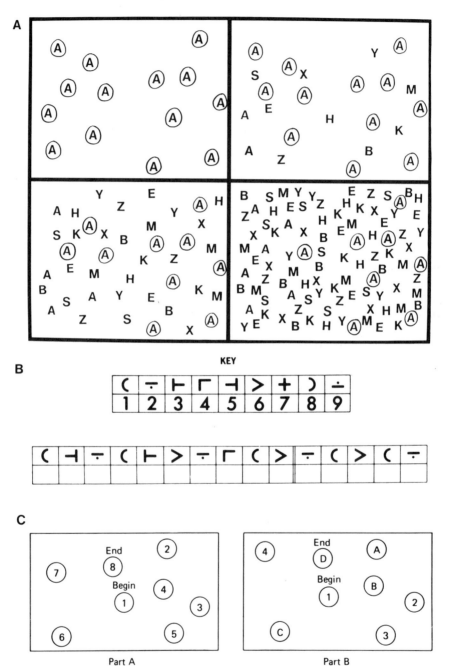

FIGURE 13.1. Examples of several commonly used neuropsychological tests that provide information regarding attentional dysfunction: (A) letter cancellation; (B) Symbol Digit Modality Test (Smith, 1973); (C) sample items from the Trail Making Test.

task and is based on the number of target stimuli that are not detected by cancellation. Failure to detect stimuli is considered an indicator of inattention.

As in the case of the *CPT*, *cancellation tests* assess sustained attentional performance under conditions of limited task demand. The nature of this task is also not likely to induce high levels of interest in subjects. *Cancellation tests* differ from the *CPT* because of the necessity of visual scanning in order to perform cancellations. The visual *CPT* usually uses a single fixation point with a series of stimuli presented at that point. On *cancellation tests*, patients must scan across a page. Deficits related to eye movement, lateral inattention, or other spatial characteristics may be apparent on these tests, but not on the *CPT*. In fact, cancellation tests are a tool for evaluating the presence of hemi-inattention and neglect syndromes.

Another distinction between *cancellation tests* and the *CPT* arises out of the use of a multiframe versus a single-frame methodology. Although *cancellation tests* require sustained attention, the patient is able to scan using his or her own strategy. As the stimuli are stationary, scanning is directed by the patient's own intention. There is no demand to maintain a pace with stimuli that are being presented at a rapid and sustained rate. Therefore, the two types of tasks tap into different aspects of sustained attention and vigilance.

Sustained Attention with Increased Task Demand

Both the *CPT* and *cancellation tests* can be modified in order to enhance task demand. On the *CPT*, this is done by increasing the number of rules to be followed (e.g., respond to *X* when preceded by an *A*), and by adjusting parameters such as memory load, interstimulus time, or the presence of more than one stimulus in a target field on a trial. In concept, each parameter could be varied to determine how attentional performance changes in relationship to these variables. However, this is rarely done in clinical practice, partly because of time constraints and the demands this would place on the patient.

Tests have been developed that have increased demand because of the requirement to perform a cognitive operation over repeated trials. The *serial addition* and *serial subtraction tests* are examples of this method, as patients are asked to add or subtract beginning from a particular number (Smith, 1967). For instance, subtracting serial 7s requires the subject to subtract 7 from 100 and then to continue subtracting 7 from the result of each calculation until instructed to stop. As this task can be difficult even for patients without brain injury, caution must be used when interpreting results. Individuals who are weak in mathematical skills may perform poorly owing to deficiencies that cannot be explained solely as inattention. When using tests of sustained performance that have greater task demands, the clinician must first determine whether the patient is capable of performing the basic operations that are required, before assessing the serial characteristics of performance.

Standard *serial addition* and *subtraction* tasks do not control for the rate of presentation of the stimuli to be processed, as the subjects control their own speed of performance. The *Paced Serial Addition Test* (*PASAT*) controls for the variables of interstimulus interval and computational difficulty (Gronwall & Sampson, 1974; Gronwall & Wrightson, 1974). The *PASAT* is very sensitive to brain disorders. Factors that influence information-processing capacity are likely to affect performance on the *PASAT*. Considerable effort is also necessary to perform this task. Therefore, some patients with severe brain pathology (e.g., Alzheimer's disease) cannot direct themselves well enough to complete the *PASAT* even partially. Although the *PASAT* is sensitive to disturbances in attention, the difficulty of this task may limit its clinical utility.

The *Symbol Digit Modalities Test* (*SDMT*) (Smith, 1968) is another sensitive test requiring sustained attentional performance in the completion of a task involving a more complex cognitive operation. The *SDMT* does not require calculations; instead, it requires the rapid processing of symbolic information and the transcription of numbers that are paired with the symbols on a tracking task. The demands of sustained attention are different on this task than on other sustained attentional measures that we have mentioned, as the length of the *SDMT* is present at 90 sec. The attentional demands of this task are created primarily by the memory requirements of the task (i.e., the need to learn the pairings of symbol and digit), the requirement of visual tracking, the perceptual-motor demands of the task, and the time constraints that are placed on the patient.

The fact that the *SDMT* requires multiple resources for adequate performance makes it a good measure of overall information-processing ability. Some investigators may choose not to include this test as a true measure of attention because of its sensitivity to a range of neuropsychological impairments. However, it is our feeling that this sensitivity to subtle information-processing problems makes the *SDMT* an excellent tool for assessing attentional performance. Often, patients who show relatively intact performance on measures of language, perceptual-motor processing, and memory perform poorly on the *SDMT*. Even though they have the capability of performing the specific cognitive operations necessary for this task, they are unable to allocate these cognitive resources efficiently. As a result, the time they take to complete the task increases. The *SDMT* illustrates the interrelationship of information-processing demands and attention.

Assessment of Executive Functions

Executive functions can be regarded as including those processes involved in the generation of plans and the direction of responding relative to goals. Executive control depends on the ability to inhibit responding to irrelevant stimuli and to facilitate responses that are goal-appropriate. A mechanism for "switching" between response alternatives is necessary for executive control.

Executive control is a critical component of the attentional process. Tests that measure the individual's ability to inhibit irrelevant responses and to switch according to changes in the response requirements provide information that is critical to the analysis of attention. Neuropsychological tests of executive functioning can be separated into tests of four factors: (1) the capacity to inhibit interference and to maintain a pattern of responding; (2) the ability to alternate between response sets; (3) the ability to plan, organize, and derive solutions on tasks requiring hypothesis testing; and (4) a capacity for response generation.

Tests of Response Inhibition

Perhaps the most well-known test of the ability to inhibit distractors is the *Stroop Interference Test* (Stroop, 1935; Nehemkis & Lewinsohn, 1972). The patient is first asked to read 100 words containing the names of colors. Next, the patient names the colors of 100 stimuli. Finally, on an interference trial, the patient names the colors on another set of 100 stimulus words, which are printed so that the actual color of the word differs from the color specified by the meaning of the word. The interference created by this stimulus competition causes slowing relative to the times needed to complete the first two tasks. In patients with impairments that affect their freedom from distraction, the degree of slowing on the interference task is much greater, and often, these individuals are unable to inhibit the competing stimuli effectively.

Other more basic tests of the ability to inhibit motor responding include the *motor impersistence test*, the *go–no-go test*, and the *recurring-figures test* described by Luria 1966). These tasks require the patient to follow a simple repetitive response pattern. Individuals with frontal lobe dysfunction often fail to inhibit their responding effectively. They may perseverate by maintaining an initial response even when there are signals to switch, or they may break from the response set and produce responses that are inconsistent with the original demands. The simple motor actions that are evaluated by these tasks bridge the areas of motor system function and attentional control.

Dichotic listening tests have occasionally been used in divided-attention paradigms to provide information about the ability to attend to two sources of simultaneous input. A greater-than-expected drop in performance may suggest a deficit in the ability to filter relevant from irrelevant input or problems with temporal inhibition. There is disagreement over a number of theoretical issues related to this paradigm, such as the role of serial and parallel processes in divided attention. For this reason, as well as because of the difficulty of conducting dichotic listening measurements, this paradigm is not widely used in the clinical assessment of attention.

Tests of Response Alternation

Several of the tasks described previously (e.g., alternating sequences and go–no-go) require the alternation of response patterns and therefore provide information about this capacity. However, one of the most commonly used tests of response alternation ability is the *Trail-Making Test* (Reitan, 1958). Subjects complete Trail A, which requires them to connect 25 numbers sequentially by placing a line between each number in order. On Trail B, patients must alternate in sequence between numbers and letters. Errors occur when the patient fails to alternate and skips between two letters or numbers, or when there is a break in the sequence and a particular item is omitted. As in the cases of other neuropsychological measures of attentional performance, the time needed for task completion is an indicator of the difficulty encountered when trying to make consistent alternations without breaks in responding.

The sensitivity of the *Trail-Making Test* to brain damage is very strong (Lezak, 1983). Performance on the *Trail-Making Test* has been shown to be related to impairments of executive functioning in patients with damage to anterior regions. This task also requires adequate visual scanning ability, and performance is affected if deficits related to visual processing are evident. Other factors, such as motoric slowness and conceptual problems, can also affect performance on this test, so that it is not a pure test of response alternation. Slowing on Trails A and B has been associated with lateralized damage to both right and left hemispheres.

There are other tests of complex executive processes that assess the ability to switch between response alternatives. For instance, the *Wisconsin Card Sort Test* (*WCST*; Berg, 1948) measures the patient's ability in concept formation and hypothesis testing. The patient is asked to determine where a stimulus card should be placed by using categorical information that can be extracted about different featural dimensions (color, shape, and number). The goal of the task is for the subject to determine the rule being used for the correct categorization of the stimulus card based on binary feedback (correct-incorrect) provided by the examiner. After a series of correct responses, the response criterion is changed by the examiner, so that the patient must now determine a new rule and switch his or her response to a new alternative. Alternatives to the *Wisconsin Card Sort* include the *Modified Card Sorting Test* (Nelson, 1976), and the *Object Sorting Test* (Goldstein & Scheerer, 1941). These tests provide information that is similar to that provided by the *WCST*.

Failure on the *WCST* and other sorting tasks of its type can occur owing to an inability to generate adequate conceptual categories. However, in some cases, subjects may generate many categories but may perform poorly because they cannot easily switch conceptual categories based on the feedback that is provided. Patients with frontal lobe damage affecting the dorsolateral region have particular problems with this test (Milner, 1963, 1964). They obtain fewer conceptual categories than patients with lesions in other cortical areas. They also perseverate in their responses (i.e., they continue to respond by placing the stimulus cards based on a particular conceptual rule, even when the feedback suggests that they should shift to a new alternative).

Performance on the *WCST* may also be affected by attentional factors that are not related to structural brain damage. For instance, Cohen and his colleagues (1984) found that patients exhibiting bipolar affective disorder showed different response characteristics depending on whether they were in a state of mania or depression at the time of the assessment. Manic patients showed a tendency to make disinhibited responses by shifting sets prematurely, even though the feedback suggested that the response they were making was correct. Depressed patients showed a greater problem in generating new conceptual alternatives and tended not to shift even when their response strategy was not working. Therefore, performance on this test reflects the response biases of the patient.

Tests of Response Generation

In order for individuals to choose responses that will yield positive consequences, they must have a capacity to initiate and generate responses. Attention depends on the individual's ability to generate a response and to sustain responding, in accordance with feedback regarding the outcome of the response. Feedback is used to either maintain a consistent direction of response or to modify the response. Therefore, response initiation, generation, and switching are central to executive and attentional control.

Methodological difficulties are encountered in trying to measure capacity to generate responses. As *response generation tests* should reflect the patient's capacity for self-generated behavior, tasks that require the individual to respond to overt stimuli confound the goal of assessing this dimension. Naturalistic observation of individuals in their normal setting may give the best indication of their normal response-generation characteristics. However, naturalistic observation lacks the experimental control of a laboratory assessment, and such data are also difficult to obtain in most clinical contexts. Therefore, to assess this capacity clinically, it is necessary to use tests that require minimal stimulus analysis and that depend on the ability of the patient to produce a train of responses after an initial task requirement has been presented.

Controlled word-list-generation tests meet some of the requirements of the assessment of response generation ability. The patient is given a task of producing as many words as possible that belong to a particular associative class based on phonemic or semantic characteristics (Spreen & Benton, 1969). In the semantic task, subjects are asked to generate as many words that fit a semantic category, such as animals. The phonemic task requires the patient to generate as many words as possible that begin with a particular letter (e.g., *F*, *A*, or *S*). On both types of tasks, the patient is given a limited amount of time to produce as many words as possible (e.g., 60 seconds). Fewer words are usually produced on the phonemic task, presumably because of the restriction of the response or associative set that is necessary when producing words in phonemic categories.

Deficits in word list generation are clearly evident in patients with aphasic disorders. The sensitivity of these tests to language disturbances extends beyond what can be considered attentional phenomena. Yet, there are instances in which reductions in the quantity of word output are noted in patients who have no other language impairments, and who are fluent in normal discourse. For instance, patients with frontal lobe dysfunction often show impaired word-list-generation performance (Benton, 1968), which correlates with other executive control deficits.

Tests of motor functioning, such as the *Grooved Pegboard Test* (Klove, 1963), provide information about the ability to generate primary motor responses at a rapid and sustained rate. Although motor speed and dexterity may be intact in patients who have severe impairments of spontaneous response generation, it is worth noting the impairment on pure motor tasks may correlate in some cases with executive dysfunction, which affects other aspects of response generation. Certainly, motor system deficits need to be considered when one is assessing whether a response generation deficit is related to attentional-executive impairments, and occasionally, problems in the motor domain may be a confounding variable in the interpretation of neuropsychological results. However, deficits in the ability to persist in motor tasks may also reflect secondary problems in executive functioning. For instance, patients suffering from multiple sclerosis show fatigue that extends beyond their motor deficits (Cohen & Fisher, 1988). This fatigue has been shown to be related to attentional deficits in these patients.

Other response generation tests have been developed. For instance, Lezak (1978, 1983) described a constructional test (the *Tinkertoy Test*) in which patients are given an open-ended task of making whatever they want to with a set of materials. The construction of the objects created by the patients is rated for complexity, level of organization, and spatial quality. Also, the persistence of the patient in performing the test is determined by assessing whether the patient has made a construction and also how much of the allotted time has been used. Tasks of this type also hold promise for providing other sources of information about the relationship between response generation ability and other cognitive operations, such as visual-spatial construction.

BEHAVIORAL ASSESSMENT METHODS

We previously described a variety of tests that are used in the assessment of attention. Neuropsychology has traditionally made use of tests as a cornerstone of clinical assessment. Tests provide a level of control in the assessment process that is difficult to achieve through clinical observation alone. Yet, there are excellent behavioral methodologies for assessing attention that are based on careful clinical observation and monitoring of the activity of the patient. These methodologies arose from the field of behavioral psychology that had as its foundation the perspective that the best approach to clinical evaluation is the documentation of overt behavioral responses.

The reader who is interested in a detailed review of behavioral assessment methods is encouraged to examine Bellack & Hersen (1988). We summarize here several of the strategies that have been used in the behavioral assessment of attention. For the most part, these techniques are based on the sampling of behavior and the quantification of occurrences of behavior that are either on- or off-task. The measures used for sampling behavior include (1) recordings of events (i.e., the frequency of occurrence of desirable or undesirable behavior); (2) interval recordings of particular behaviors; and (3) scan sampling.

Event recording is divided into the techniques of frequency recording and trial scoring. These methods are the most common behavioral assessment techniques and involve the recording of each discrete occurrence of a particular behavior. When assessing attention, an event recording of the number of times a child breaks from a task during brief time intervals may prove to be a useful measure. Event recording may be difficult for very high- or low-frequency behaviors.

Interval recording is another common technique in behavioral assessment; it is similar to the scan-sampling method. However, with interval recording, the behavior is sampled in a binary way for very short time periods. It therefore combines some of the characteristics of both event recording and scan sampling. The disadvantage of this procedure is the fact that, in a given interval, the event is scored as a binary occurrence, and events that occur repeatedly in an interval are not counted.

Scan sampling is useful when the duration of a behavior is a more useful indication than frequency. With this technique, the observer periodically samples the behavior of the patient and determines whether the behavior is occurring or not. The sampling may be done at a preset interval or on a random basis. The advantage of this technique is its capacity for longer duration monitoring. The disadvantage is that a binary measure of occurrence or nonoccurrence is provided at each sampling, but not the intensity of responding at the given moment. A second disadvantage is that, with very frequent, but erratic behaviors, the observer may miss the occurrence of an event. This technique has been used extensively in studies of sleep–wake behavior.

Behavioral assessment research has contributed greatly to the study of single-case methodologies (see Hersen & Barlow, 1976). As neuropsychological studies often require the assessment of a unique case, which it is not feasible to include in a group with other patients, single-case methods provide a means of making comparisons of the patient with himself or herself. This method may be particularly useful in the study of toxic effects. For instance, Zaret and Cohen (1986) used a single-case methodology to demonstrate the effect of valproic acid in inducing a reversible dementia. Many single-case methodologies depend on showing a change in behavior secondary to the introduction of a new condition that reverses when the condition reverts back to previous states (ABAB design). In the multiple-baseline methodology, a number of different responses are assessed over time. The change in a particular response with the introduction of an independent variable is assessed by comparing that response to the other behavioral responses that did not change. Unfortunately, these methods are not as useful with disorders that are attributable to the introduction of an external or independent stimulus variable.

A general methodological difficulty of behavioral assessment is the necessity of ensuring interexaminer agreement on what constitutes a behavior. Therefore, much emphasis is placed on ensuring assessment reliability through the control of interrater reliability. Although the problem of reliability can also be a dilemma in standard neuropsychological measurement, often the structure of a test eliminates some of the biases that may exist in behavioral observation.

Despite some limitations of behavioral observation methods, these techniques offer a valuable tool for the assessment of attention. In particular, behavioral assessment offers a way of studying attention and other neuropsychological functions in a natural setting. At this time, these techniques are more commonly used in the study of childhood attention-deficit disorder (Barkley, 1988) than in adult attentional assessment. A reason may be the greater ease of using these techniques in school settings or with parent training. The assessment of adult behavior in natural settings is more difficult to accomplish, except in hospitals or rehabilitation centers, where the environment is more controlled.

EXPERIMENTAL APPROACHES TO ATTENTIONAL MEASUREMENT

The rapid growth of interest in the processes of attention among cognitive researchers and neuroscientists has led to the development of many experimental techniques for quantifying the parameters underlying attention. Many experimental techniques from the cognitive sciences have relevance to neuropsychology. We conclude this chapter with a brief review of some of these experimental approaches.

Although many experimental techniques have relevance to neuropsychological assessment, they have not been widely incorporated into standard clinical methods. One reason may be the difficulties encountered in trying to use in a clinical context cognitive tasks developed for experimental studies. Neurologically impaired patients often have great difficulty performing complex cognitive tasks. Also, before experimental techniques can be used for clinical neuropsychological assessment, they need to be administered to large groups of patients to yield normative data, including measures of reliability and validity. This necessity imposes constraints that slow the clinical development of these techniques.

Equipment limitations often make the universal clinical application of complicated attentional paradigms difficult. For instance, there are still many neuropsychological clinics that do not use, or make only limited use of, computerized stimulus-presentation techniques. Tachistoscopic methods are not widely incorporated into clinical neuropsychological assessment, even though many psychophysical approaches depend on that level of experimental control. The experimental analysis of attention often depends on the extension of methods developed to study other cognitive phenomena. When studying attentional phenomena, cognitive researchers have commonly modified paradigms developed in the field of sensory psychology. Yet, the more rigorous methods of psychophysics and sensory psychology have not been fully incorporated into the field of clinical neuropsychology. The performance of neurologically impaired patients on basic psychophysical and perceptual tasks needs to be established before these techniques can be fully applied to the clinical measurement of attention.

Although the translation of experimental cognitive methodologies into clinical neuropsychological techniques may continue at a slow pace, it should remain an important goal for neuropsychological researchers, particularly those concerned with the measurement and evaluation of attention. At this time, there are several experimental cognitive methods that seem to have relevance to clinical neuropsychology. These include methods that require different operations, including scanning and search, sustained vigilance, cuing, divided attention, and shadowing. Many of these methods were originally developed for the purposes of studying cognitive phenomena other than attention. For example, divided attention has been studied by means of dichotic listening techniques. Dichotic listening was originally used primarily to study cerebral dominance in patients with unilateral brain lesions (Kimura, 1967).

Many of the experimental methods that are useful in the study of attention depend on techniques arising from the theory of signal detection (see Green & Swets, 1966), and from reaction time methods (see Posner, 1978). Signal detection theory enables the researcher to assess response accuracy under different conditions, and reaction time provides an indication of the processing demands placed on the subject. Often, these two variables can be analyzed simultaneously to provide the best indications of attentional performance.

Signal Detection Theory

Most modern experimental studies of attention incorporate signal detection theory, either explicitly or implicitly, in their methodologies. Therefore, a brief review of the methodological features of this theory is provided here to facilitate the discussion of other experimental approaches. A description of signal detection in the context of selective attention theory is contained in Chapter 2. A discussion of some of the theoretical considerations of signal detection and information theory is contained in Chapter 21.

Procedures developed from signal detection theory have great utility in the neuropsychological assessment of attention. The most straightforward is a procedure in which the subject is asked to indicate, by either yes or no, whether a target stimulus has occurred. It is assumed that noise will occur randomly in any environment, and that it will be normally distributed around a mean level based on some featural characteristics (e.g., sound frequency). The introduction of the target stimulus into a field of noise does not change this normal distribution of signals. However, if the signal is strong enough to stand out from the noise, it will produce a distribution with a mean that is shifted away from the mean of the noise. The mean of the distribution of the signal + noise is defined as d' with a standard deviation of 1. The mean of the noise is assumed to be 0, as the random signals average out to no value, though the standard deviation remains as 1. The size of the difference between the means of the distribution of signal + noise and the noise determines the likelihood of detection, which is equal to d'.

In addition to the actual separation between the signal and the noise, the probability of correct detection also depends on the response criterion (β) that is established. If there is a bias to be cautious and to indicate yes only if there is certainty, the likelihood of misses increases, and the likelihood of false alarms decreases. The opposite effect occurs if a liberal criterion is established with a bias never to miss a signal when it is present. In this case, there are likely to be many false alarms. Four outcomes are possible in this framework, based on which of two possible stimulus types has occurred. Either there will be a correct hit or a miss if the target has been presented, or there will be a correct rejection or a false alarm if only the noise has occurred. Figure 13.2 illustrates a theoretical distribution of signal and noise using d' and criterion values that are set.

Signal detection is very analogous to the statistical principles underlying the test of a null hypothesis. If the distributions of signal-noise and noise are nearly identical, d' is very small, and the likelihood of detecting a difference between the distributions is small. If the distributions are very different, there is a high likelihood of correction. A graph of the relationship of the probabilities of correct detections versus false alarms yields different curves depending on the size of d'. If $d' = 0$, there is a linear relation between these probabilities, as there is a 50% (i.e., random) chance of correctly responding. As d' increases, the curve becomes more hyperbolic, with the likelihood of a false alarm being noted when there is a strong bias for making hits rather than missing targets.

As it is often difficult to determine Receiver Operating Characteristics (ROC) curves on an *a priori* basis, there are several nonparametric methods for estimating the sensitivity and response criteria. The response criterion always depends on the sensitivity of the individual in making detections. Methods for calculating sensitivity and response criteria were described by Swets (1964, 1973, 1984).

Signal detection tasks often require a forced choice among a number of alternative stimuli. The ROC curve that is produced is similar to that generated in experiments which require discrimination of signals from noise (yes-no decisions). Therefore, this methodology can be used in various types of tasks. By a comparison of detection rates under different conditions of attentional demand, it is possible to obtain indications of the attentional component in a particular task.

The use of signal detection methods in conjunction with chronometric techniques has yielded a number of interesting findings pertinent to the analysis of attention. Attentional demands typically increase the reaction times noted on signal detection tasks. Often, there is a trade-off between accuracy of detection and reaction time.

Information-Processing Methods

Attention has been studied by means of a number of different experimental methods. These methods usually share the dependent variables of accuracy of signal detection and reaction time. However, they differ with respect to the actual task requirements. We provide a brief review of several of these methods.

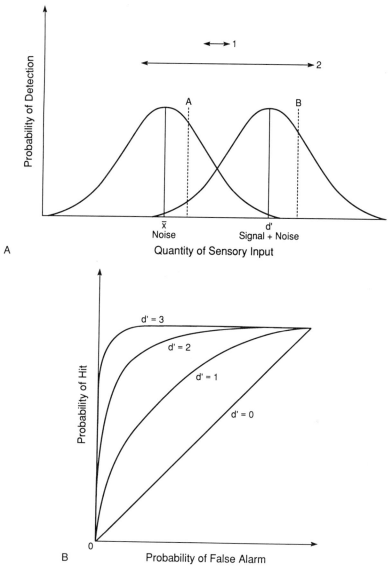

FIGURE 13.2. Signal detection methods. (A) Theoretical distributions that show the relation of noise to signal + noise. As the arrows indicate, these distributions vary as a function of the difficulty of discriminating the signal from the noise. For very intense target stimuli, the distance between the means of two distributions is great. For weak target signals, the two distributions are close together, indicating difficulty in discriminating signal from noise. The beta value associated with the response criterion varies as a function of variables such as the subject's motivational state and incentive to respond in a certain way. In Case A, the response criterion is shifted in the direction of always detecting the target, but making numerous false positive detections. The opposite is true in case B, as the subject will now miss many targets but will rarely respond when there is no signal. (B) Theorectic Receiver Operating Curves (ROC) for different levels of d'. This reflects the relationship between the signal and the noise. When it is difficult to discriminate signal from noise, d' approaches 0, whereas if such a discrimination is easy, d' increases as a hyperbolic function.

Vigilance Tasks

Vigilance tasks measure the ability to sustain attention over long periods. Most vigilance tasks are extensions of the methodologies first described by Mackworth (1950) in studies of radar operators. These tasks usually require the performance of a simple but monotonous task for a long duration. Because arousal and alertness vary in all people across the day, vigilance is likely to fluctuate. The continuous-performance task (CPT) is an example of this experimental technique. From the standpoint of signal detection methods, vigilance tasks involve a modification, as performance is not stable over time during vigilance. To account for this variation, investigators may calculate inconsistency scores that reflect fluctuations in performance over a time series. For example, Cohen and Fisher (1988, 1989) described increased inconsistency in a study of fatigue in multiple sclerosis. Vigilance tasks have been developed that have a rate of stimulus presentation that varies as a function of either reaction time or response accuracy (Buchsbaum & Sostek, 1980). These modified CPT paradigms enable task parameters to be modified in an ongoing manner in accordance with the subject's attentional performance at different times during the task.

Scanning and Search Tasks

When visual fields are studied, it is common to create a map of the distribution of sensory recognition. This is done by indicating whether the individual was able to detect a signal at various coordinates in the field. If a patient makes a certain percentage of correct detections at a particular spatial location, it is assumed that the field is intact at that position. Assessment of the spatial distribution of the visual selective attention relies on a signal detection methodology (see Chapter 19 for further discussion). Psychophysical parameters such as stimulus intensity, duration, spatial frequency, and movement can be varied to influence the recognition rates at different spatial locations.

The spatial distribution of visual attention can be evaluated in a similar way, although modifications in methodology are necessary. Neisser (1969, 1976) studied visual search by measuring the time taken to scan a matrix of items for a particular target. The search times were greatest when there was a high similarity between the targets and the distractors. This finding was interpreted as an indication of feature detection and analysis. Subsequent studies have generally supported Neisser's findings, although other investigators have demonstrated the parametric characteristics of performance with changes in psychophysical dimensions, as well as memory load.

Sperling and Melchner (1978) mapped the spatial distribution of visual search accuracy in a 7 × 7 array. They found that search accuracy is highest above the foveal fixation point, and that extreme points in the vertical dimension are the least likely to be accurately searched.

The accuracy of a visual search depends on the attentional demands of the task. Accurate detection should occur at an almost perfect rate when the location of the target is obvious and not difficult to discriminate. Reduced speed and accuracy occur when the target is shifted in the visual field and its location is uncertain. Cuing the subject to the spatial region to search improves performance, a finding suggesting an attentional effect.

Priming and Cuing Techniques

Priming and cuing techniques enable the investigator to measure the influence of anticipatory processes on performance. Attention is often viewed as a process by which individuals allocate their resources to a certain stimulus or response set. The allocation of resources before a task should enhance performance, as an expectancy is established that allows individuals to generate response alternatives before the actual stimulus onset.

Cues have been used in different ways in attentional research. In studies of visual-spatial attention, a neutral cue is sometimes presented in a spatial location before the onset of a target. The accuracy of detection and reaction times can then be measured as a function of the anticipatory cue to either correct or incorrect spatial position (Hasher & Zacks, 1984; LaBerge, Petersen, & Norden, 1977; LaBerge, Van Gilder, & Yellott, 1971; Posner, 1980, 1986; Posner & Cohen, 1984; Posner, Snyder, & Davidson, 1980; Sperling, 1984). Sperling (1960) used cues to test attention in iconic memory tasks by presenting the cue after a spatial matrix of stimuli. The fact that the subjects showed near-perfect recall of the stimuli that they were cued to indicated that their attention had been effectively directed to a spatial position on the icon.

Cuing has also been used to assess the allocation of attention in other cognitive tasks. Cohen and Waters (1985) used a cue to direct subjects to the appropriate cognitive operation to be performed in a levels-of-processing paradigm. The cue indicated the type of effortful processing that would be required and also served as an anticipatory stimulus. The psychophysiological response to the cue was shown to habituate over the course of successive trials, a finding suggesting that its role had become primarily informational, rather than establishing a strong emotional expectancy.

The use of cues to allocate resources to the required cognitive operation has been frequently studied using reaction time indices (LaBerge, Petersen, & Norden, 1977; LaBerge, Van Gilder, & Yellott, 1971; Posner, 1986). Cuing was shown to produce greatest decreases in reaction time when it signaled information about the upcoming task.

Divided Attention

When individuals are required to perform more than one task at a time, by definition they must divide their attention. Driving a car while listening to the radio and talking is an example of divided attention. Much research effort has been devoted to specifying whether people are capable of performing multiple tasks simultaneously (i.e., parallel processing), or whether their performance actually consists of a serial chain of processing steps. The theoretical issues surrounding this debate have been discussed previously. Most cognitive researchers now agree that people are capable of at least some degree of parallel processing. However, attention to simultaneous tasks depends on the tasks' demands and the type of information to be processed. The quality of performance on simultaneous tasks decreases as a function of the number of tasks to be performed, the degree of similarity of the tasks to be performed, and a host of other factors.

The most common way of measuring divided attention is the dual-task method, which requires the subject to respond on one task while performing a secondary task as well. Instructions are given to attend to only one of the tasks. Performance on measures such as reaction time and detection accuracy on the secondary task can then be contrasted as a function of the different primary tasks. By using this method, it is possible to determine how much attentional processing demand is created by the primary task. If performance on the secondary task decreases to a greater extent in the presence of one of the primary tasks, that primary task is assumed to require more processing capacity. This type of methodology has been used extensively by Posner (1986). It has not been widely incorporated into clinical neuropsychological assessment.

Another approach to the study of divided attention is the use of interference to prevent the optimal performance of a primary task. Interference methodologies do not require simultaneous task performance; rather, they measure performance on one task, while some form of noise is presented to interfere with attention. The Stroop test (1935) is an example of this type of task. It has been used extensively in clinical neuropsychology to provide information about distractibility and filtering capacity. However, the Stroop test, as it is commonly used, does not enable the examiner to control many of the attentional parameters that would be useful when evaluating divided attentional capacity. For instance, the degree of interference during the task cannot be adjusted. In our laboratory, we have recently begun developing computer-generated divided attention tasks that may yield more precise information about the threshold of interference for particular patients.

Dichotic listening tasks have been used extensively in studies of cerebral dominance and asymmetry (Kimura, 1967; Springer, 1986). This technique is also useful in studying divided attention, as the presentation of different stimuli to the ear provides the essential tool necessary for studying simultaneous auditory processing. Dichotic listening has been used in shadowing paradigms which measure the capacity of the subject to repeat immediately the material being presented auditorily in one ear, while processing a competing message in the other ear.

Shadowing was a favored method of early information-processing researchers. Cherry (1953) found that subjects have great difficulty extracting information from the non-shadowed ear during dichotic listening, but that they can detect physical changes in the stimuli to that ear. Subjects also show little memory of the material presented to the nonshadowed ear.

Subsequently, other investigators examined other shadowing conditions, including some tasks requiring more than one sensory modality. Treisman and Davies (1973) found that subjects attended better to the nonshadowed channel when different modalities were used. It is possible to learn to attend to the nonshadowed channel as reported by Underwood (1976), who found that well-rehearsed subjects detected stimuli presented to the nonshadowed channel with high accuracy, whereas naive subjects performed poorly. Shadowing provides a well-controlled methodology for studying divided attention.

Physiological Methods

There is now an extensive experimental literature pertaining to central and peripheral manifestations of the attention processes. Chapter 6 dealt with this body of knowledge, as well as with some of the problems of interpretation. In our view, the field of psychophysiology provides a rich source of information for understanding attention phenomena, although it has yet to be fully integrated into clinical neuropsychology. The use of neuroimaging techniques such as Regional Blood Flow (Risberg, 1990), Magnetic Resonance Imaging (MRI) spectroscopy and Position Emission Tomography (PET) hold promise for the future.

Summary

In this chapter, we have discussed three broad approaches to the assessment of attention:

1. The psychometric approach
2. Specific neuropsychological tests
3. Behavioral methods

The most traditional method of psychologists is the interpretation of psychometric data from intellectual or commonly used tests. Another common approach is to rely on indirect clinical observations. Although this second approach can provide useful insights, it is

TABLE 1. Commonly Used Neuropsychological
Measures of Attention

Attention span	Response intention and planning
Digit Span	Controlled word generation
Corsi Blocks	spontaneous verbal generation
Consonant trigrams	Sustained performance and vigilance
Divided attention	continuous performance
Stroop Test	paced auditory serial addition
dichotic listening	cancellation tests
Switching	Information-processing speed
Trail-Making Test	Symbol Digit Modality Test
motor impersistence task	
go–no-go task	
Wisconsin Card Sort	

subject to obvious confounds. More controlled methods of behavioral observation provide a better methodological avenue. Surprisingly, these methods have not been widely used by neuropsychologists.

The neuropsychological approach uses psychometric theory, but attempts to development tests capable of providing specific measures of attention. Although there are a number excellent neuropsychological tests that are sensitive to attentional disturbances, it is not possible to use a particular measure to characterize all forms of attentional deficit. Therefore, the neuropsychological assessment of attention depends on a multivariate framework. Some tests that are particularly useful in assessing attention in a clinical context are listed in Table 13.1.

We have grouped these tests into attentional components. In doing so, we recognize that these components are not orthogonal, and that most of the tasks that are listed also measure at least some features of the other attentional components. These groupings are primarily meant to provide an organizational scheme on which to build future efforts to characterize attentional performance.

As we described previously, most of the standard neuropsychological tests commonly used to measure attention miss several important dimensions. They tend to be cross-sectional in nature and therefore are not very sensitive to serial variations. Also, they tend not to be very useful for assessing the characteristics of performance variability. Although most tests provide statistical measures of variance, these are used only for purposes of reliability estimation. However, our work has suggested that variance may be an essential characteristic of attentional processing.

Traditionally, neuropsychological methods have not emphasized establishing attentional parameters across various stimulus, task, and response dimensions. For instance, it is not clear how visual attentional performance relates to auditory attention in most brain-damaged populations. This will be an important area for future investigations. In the next chapter and in Part III, we discuss some of these parametric considerations, along with constraints that place limits on attentional processes that should be taken into consideration.

Neuropsychological Models of Attentional Dysfunction

RONALD A. COHEN and BRIAN F. O'DONNELL

Over the last several years, neuropsychological models have been proposed to explain how attention is controlled by the brain. These models have often been based on data obtained from the analysis of specific clinical neuropsychological syndromes. Some investigators have attempted to integrate data from broader clinical populations to establish a taxonomy of attentional dysfunctions (e.g., Mirsky, 1978, 1989). We will review several of these models of attention as a way of summarizing the information derived from the field of clinical neuropsychology.

Two models derived from studies of patients with hemi-inattention syndromes are discussed here (Heilman, Watson, & Valenstein, 1985; Mesulam, 1985). Although based on studies of hemi-inattention and neglect, these models have great relevance to analysis of the neural systems governing normal attention. We follow with a discussion of the theoretical frameworks of Pribram and McGuinness (1975) and Luria (1966), researchers who have made major contributions to the neuropsychology of attention. We conclude with a discussion of a recent attentional taxonomy (Mirskey, 1990) that reflects recent efforts to characterize the forms of attentional disturbance. The models and concepts discussed in this summary chapter have often been based on different populations of brain-damaged patients. The disorders that have generated particular attention deficits and models were characterized in greater depth in the preceding chapters.

MODELS OF ATTENTIONAL DISTURBANCE

The neglect and hemi-inattention syndromes have been the source of many of the recent neuropsychological models of attention. These syndromes usually involve specific lesions that are well localized, and that produce circumscribed behavioral disturbances. We describe here two models of hemi-inattention syndrome: Heilman, Watson, and Valenstein (1985) and Mesulam (1985).

Heilman, Watson, and Valenstein

Attention is regarded as involving two components: sensory attention and motor intention. The sensory attention model has seven points at which impairments may occur

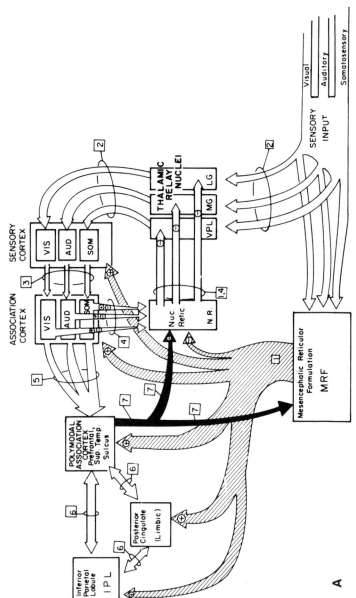

FIGURE 14.1. Schematic representation of the pathways considered important in sensory attention and response intention. From Heilman *et al.* (1985), with permission. (A) Sensory attention is viewed as depending on seven neural system components: (1) arousal; (2) sensory transmission; (3) association cortex; (4) **not defined**; (5) nucleus reticularis projections; (6) inferior parietal and limbic connections; and (7) cortex arousal. AUD = auditory; LG = lateral geniculate; MG = medial geniculate; NR = nucleus reticularis thalami; SOM = somatosensory; Sup. Temp. = superior temporal; VI = visual; VPL = ventralis posterolateralis.

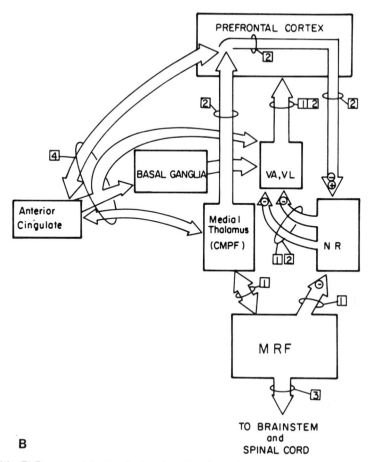

FIGURE 14.1. (B) Response intention is also viewed as depending on several components: (1) arousal from the mesencephalic reticular activating sytem (the MRF); the thalamic–frontal cortical system, including the nucleus reticularis; (3) descending activation from the MRF for the orienting response; and (4) limbic–subcortical interactions. CMPF = centromedial parafascicularis thalamic nucleus; VA = ventral anterior thalamic nuclei; VL = ventrolateral thalamic nuclei.

that will produce hemi-inattention. Figure 14.1A is a schematic representation of the pathways that Heilman, Watson, and Valenstein considered important in the control of sensory attention.

Sensory Inattention

In this model, normal attention is considered dependent on (1) arousal; (2) sensory transmission; (3) intact sensory-association-area projections; (4) projections to the nucleus reticularis of the thalamus; (5) sensory convergence on the heteromodal cortex; and (6) parts of the cortex, such as the inferior parietal lobule with (7) limbic connections. Heilman and his colleagues proposed that sensory neglect is an arousal–attention disorder created by a dysfunction of a corticolimbic-reticular-formation loop.

Arousal is generated by the mesencephalic reticular formation (MRF). Although there are some problems in the concept of arousal as originally proposed, stimulation of the MRF usually produces a desynchronization of cortical activity. Although the exact neurotransmitter systems responsible for the generation of central arousal have not been clearly established, the ascending reticular formation contains several catecholamine pathways that are probably responsible. The MRF seems to project polysynaptically to several thalamic nuclei, some of which relay information to many different cortical areas, including the sensory association cortex. Increased arousal usually produces heightened states of vigilance and sensorimotor preparedness. Arousal mediates the behavioral response to sensory information flowing through cortical regions.

The limbic and frontal areas also provide inputs into the sensory association cortex, which modulate the attentional response of sensory association areas such as the inferior parietal lobules. These inputs inhibit or facilitate attentional response in accordance with information pertaining to stimulus significance, motivational state, and the goal orientation of the animal.

The cortical systems responsible for visual attention include the neurons of the inferior parietal lobe, including projection neurons, fixation neurons, visual tracking neurons, saccadic neurons, enhancement neurons, and light-sensitive neurons. The enhancement neurons are of interest because they produce selective activation to stimuli of particular spatial characteristics based on prior motivational input. The projection, fixation, and tracking neurons facilitate attention by responding to stimuli in behaviorally specific ways. For instance, projection neurons fire in response to an intention to act, such as reaching.

The model of sensory inattention proposed by Heilman *et al.* maintains that neglect may occur owing to lesions at several different neuranatomical sites, including the disruption of critical pathways. Damage to neurons of the inferior parietal lobe can result in a failure to register current spatial information. Damage to other neurons may cause an inability to maintain fixation, to reference attention to movement or to track visually. All of these deficits may produce unilateral inattention. Unilateral damage to the MRF may also give rise to a similar disorder, but for a different reason: failure of the sensory cortex to be adequately aroused and prepared for further processing. Similarly, limbic damage may produce neglect because of a motivational failure. In effect, different brain disorders result in a common presentation.

Intentional Neglect

Response preparation and intention depend on four critical pathways, according to Heilman *et al.*: (1) the mesencephalic reticular formation (MRF) and nucleus reticularis (NR); (2) the medial thalamic frontocortical–nucleus-reticularis system; (3) pathways from the MRF to the brain stem and spinal cord; and (4) limbic subcortical connections. Damage to any of these systems may produce a unilateral intentional disorder (see Figure 14.1B).

Within this model intentional neglect parallels sensory neglect, though it has a different mechanism and also is produced by different task demands. Intentional neglect occurs when an individual cannot respond to stimuli in one hemispatial field, despite the demand of the task to respond to that side.

The phenomenon of intentional neglect was demonstrated by Watson, Miller, and Heilman (1978) after unilateral frontal ablation in primates, as animals were unable to make a unilateral response to one side. Watson *et al.* (1978) suggested that this finding might indicate a unilateral hypokinesia related to a defect of intentional preparation, as a failure to make an appropriate response to one side of space was dissociated from a failure of sensation on one side. This finding was consistent with earlier findings of neglect following unilateral dorsolateral frontal lesions (Welch & Stuteville, 1958) and also with theories that have suggested a dissociation of sensory and response components of attention (Pribram & McGuinness, 1975). The distinction between sensory and response components of attention is evident even within a single task, when the psychophysiological components of attention are examined (Cohen & Waters, 1985). The distinction between hemi-inattention and intentional neglect has been confirmed in other neuropsychological investigations (e.g., Butter, Rapcsak, Watson, & Heilman, 1988; Coslett & Heilman, 1984; Verfaellie, Bowers, & Heilman, 1988; Verfaellie & Heilman, 1987). The task required the production of a unilateral response; however, the animal was unable to respond unilaterally, because of a defect in "intentional" preparation.

Hemi-intentional disorders may occur owing to damage to arousal pathways and therefore may coexist with sensory inattention. However, Heilman *et al.* proposed that other thalamic nuclei are involved in intentional disorders (i.e., the contromedial parafascicularis). Also, the prefrontal cortex, the cingulate gyrus, and the basal ganglia play pronounced roles in this form of neglect.

Mesulam

Mesulam (1981, 1985) described a neuropsychological model from a more general systems approach. He concluded that normal attention depends on the interactions of two functional systems: the attentional matrix and the attentional vector. The attentional *matrix* or state function represents those systems in the brain that regulate overall information-processing capacity, detection efficiency, focusing power, resistance to interference, and signal-to-noise ratio. This set of functions can be related to tonic attention and is influenced by the reticular activating system. The *vector* or channel function regulates the direction and target of attention in any one of the behaviorally relevant areas of the spatial environment. (Mesulam noted that these spaces may be covert representations, for example, memories.) The vector aspect of attention is related to selective attention and is associated with more rostral CNS elements, especially the neocortex. The vector function may be sensory and motoric in character. For example, it may be involved in selecting a stimulus for exploration, or in selecting a behavior.

The Attentional Matrix

The biology of the attentional matrix involves structures at different levels of the nervous system between the brain stem and the cortex (see Figure 14.2). The reticular activating system may provide global regulation of "attentional tone" for the whole forebrain. At one extreme, bilateral lesions of the midbrain reticular core lead to permanent stupor or coma. In terms of normal behavioral activity, the reticular activating system appears to regulate sleep cycles and general alertness. It appears, then, to play a major role in modulating arousal. This global influence may be mediated by cholinergic projections from the upper brain stem, serotonergic pathways from the midline raphe nuclei, and noradrenergic pathways from the locus coeruleus.

The cortex is influenced by the reticular formation and in turn influences the reticular formation, through relay nuclei within the thalamus. This interaction may be best described in terms of the orienting response (OR) described by Sokolov (1960, 1963, 1969), who suggested that the OR requires an interaction of reticular and cortical components. Global responses to pain and gross changes in the physical environment may produce an OR with little cortical

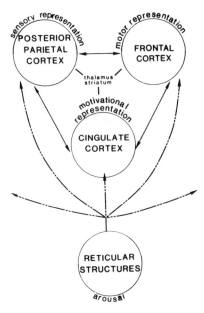

FIGURE 14.2. A simplified attentional matrix. From Mesulam (1985), with permission.

mediation. An OR to a novel word or a complex figure, on the other hand, requires cortical analysis at a semantic or visuospatial level. In this case, the cortex initiates an orienting response through descending impulses to the reticular formation. Similarly, habituation may be mediated by cortical or brain stem structures, depending on stimulus complexity. More complex stimuli require greater cortical involvement for habituation to occur.

Damage to unimodal sensory association areas may result in modality-specific attentional deficits. More complex attentional responses are mediated by the polymodal association cortex. These polymodal association areas include the prefrontal cortex, the posterior parietal cortex, and the ventral temporal cortex. Lesions to these areas may lead to confusional states. The frontal lobe is the most important contributor to the attentional matrix. Frontal lobe damage is often associated with attentional problems, including impersistence, distractibility, perseveration, and difficulty with response inhibition.

Disorders of the Attentional Matrix

Multifocal lesions or functional disturbances of the brain can result in confusional states. Acute confusional states are associated with a variety of attentional disturbances. Clinically, three features are associated with confusional states: disturbance of vigilance or heightened distractibility, inability to maintain a coherent stream of thought, and inability to carry out a sequence of goal-directed movements. The attentional disturbance is not a direct function of global arousal. Arousal can vary markedly: The affected individual can be nearly stuporous, apathetic, or agitated, depending on the etiology of the disturbance. Acute confusional episodes can be brought on by a variety of brain disorders, including toxic-metabolic encephalopathies, multifocal brain lesions, head trauma, epileptic seizures, space-occupying lesions, and focal brain lesions of key attentional areas in the right hemisphere.

Directed Attention and Neglect

Mesulam discussed neglect as a disorder of one aspect of vector attention; directed attention to extrapersonal space. Directed attention to different areas of extrapersonal space is often impaired by lesions to the parietal lobe, the frontal eye fields, the thalamus, the striatum, or the cingulate region. Neglect may have sensory, motor, or motivational components.

In sensory neglect, stimuli in the extrapersonal space contralateral to the lesion have a diminished impact on behavior, whereas stimuli in the space on the same side as the lesion dominate consciousness. It is as if the mental representation of the visual fields has been altered, with suppression of one part of the space and enhancement of the contralateral area. In terms of motoric neglect, visual scanning and motor exploration of the environment are suppressed contralateral to the lesion. Motivation may also be a factor in neglect. Mesulam recounted a case in which monetary incentives to detect targets in the neglected hemifield improved the performance of a patient.

An Anatomical Model for Directed Attention

Based on human and animal studies of neglect, Mesulam proposes an anatomical network that subserves directed attention to extrapersonal space (Figure 8 from Mesulam, 1985). The posterior parietal cortex maintains a sensory representation of extrapersonal space, and the frontal eye fields and associated cortex maintain a motor representation. The activity of these areas is influenced in turn by projections from the cingulate cortex, which mediates motivational input, and from the reticular structures, which modulate arousal. These major structures are also interconnected via the thalamus and the striatum, which may be why unilateral damage to thalamic or striatal nuclei can result in neglect.

Lesions of the right hemisphere are more likely to produce neglect than lesions of the left hemisphere, and typically, right-hemisphere lesions result in more severe and persistent neglect syndromes than left-hemisphere lesions. Mesulam proposed that the right hemisphere is dominant for directed attention to extrapersonal space, arguing that the left hemisphere provides directed attention only to right extrapersonal space, whereas the right hemisphere can direct attention over the whole of extrapersonal space. Moreover, the right hemisphere devotes more "synaptic activity" to all attentional tasks than the left hemisphere. For these reasons, damage to the left-hemisphere attentional mechanisms can be compensated for by right-hemisphere mechanisms, but not vice versa. In addition, damage to the right hemisphere (but not to the left) can result in a confusional state, a finding suggesting that it has a major role in maintaining overall attentional coherence.

Luria's Concept of Attention

Because of the importance of Alexander Luria, a Russian psychologist in the field of neuropsychology, a text on attention would not be complete without reference to his theoretical position. Luria (1986) emphasized the importance of executive functions in the control of behavior and provided an early account of the role of the prefrontal cortex. He also made one of the early distinctions relative to types of attention. Luria and his colleagues gave attentional systems a central place in their models of normal and disturbed brain function. In this section, we review Luria's model of attention (1966) and summarize the clinical as well as the psychophysiological evidence presented in support of it.

Luria defined (1966) attention as the systems that maintain the *selectivity* and *directivity* of mental processes. As in contemporary information-processing models of attention, Luria stressed the importance of selection at several points in the stream of cognitive and behavioral activity: in the selection of *sensory stimuli* to be evaluated; in the selection of movements necessary to generate an appropriate *response* or to real a goal; and the selection of *memory traces* that correspond to current intentions and environmental demands. Out of the vast number of stimuli, responses, and memories available to a person, a small number are selected as being relevant to the current situation, and are synthesized into a coherent model of the world, from which plans are generated and are responses made. These responses are temporally directed as well, to permit intentions to be translated into an adaptive and consistent behavioral sequence. The focus of attention is narrowed to relevant events, and other stimuli, responses, and memories are inhibited.

Luria considered two extreme historical positions with respect to attention. Attention and perception had been distinguished as separate processes by introspective psychologists such as Wundt (1973) and Titchener (1908). They stressed the importance of mental direction in the focus of attention. An opposing view associated with Gestalt psychology stressed the importance of the structure of the environmental field as the major determinant of attentional focus, with a minimal need for the involvement of cognitive processes.

Luria approached the nature of attention from a different perspective, using information regarding attentional processes from developmental psychology, psychophysiology, and the effects of brain lesions on attention. Luria first noted that the orienting reaction to intense, novel, or biologically meaningful stimuli can be observed in the first few months of the child's development. An infant shows the *orienting response* to complex salient stimuli. The reflex consists of motor, electroencephalographic, and autonomic components. The infant turns its eyes toward the stimuli, then turns its head, then focuses on the stimulus if it is visually available, and then shows changes in respiration, heart rate, brain electrical activity, and other physiological indices associated with arousal by external events. This response to salient stimuli is elementary and involuntary and requires very little cognitive development. The orienting response is highly selective in character, rapidly habituating if a stimulus is repeated, and reappearing if the properties of the stimulus change.

Attention directed by cognitive processes, on the other hand, takes much longer to develop. Luria used Vygotsky's work (1962) on the development of language and thought to describe the development of internally directed attention. This type of attention is socially learned and is based on the purposeful discrimination of objects in the environment, initially in conjunction with prompts from an adult. For example, a parent may point to and say the name of an object, directing a child's attention toward it. The child may respond by fixating on the object or manipulating it. The child's attention can later be directed simply by naming the object. The child learns to name the object and can use the name to direct attention. In this way, attention gradually develops from an externally directed to an internally directed process. This development is quite slow. For example, not until age 4 or 5 can the child follow a spoken instruction to attend to a familiar object when other novel objects are in the same area. In earlier years, the orienting response to novel stimuli often overrides linguistic direction of attention.

In the adult, then, two attentional mechanisms operate in parallel: a reflexive and environmentally triggered *orienting response* to novel, biologically meaningful, or conditioned stimuli, and *volitional attention*, directed by a person's cognitive interpretation of the current situation and her or his goals within it. Volitional attention often appears to be mediated by external or internal speech. In a normal adult, these processes operate in conjunction, allowing a person to pursue goals guided by very specific stimuli and intentions, while automatically monitoring the environment for important, often unexpected events that may require an immediate response or some modification of a planned behavioral sequence. Both types of attentional activation are associated with physiological changes indicative of increased arousal.

Luria cited clinical evidence that attentional activation and inhibition may be mediated by limbic and frontal cortex in the human brain. Patients with damage to the limbic region, particularly the hippocampus, show fatiguability, an inability to maintain a goal over time, and distractibility. Physiological measures of the orienting response may be absent or may fail to habituate. Interestingly, such patients can use verbal instructions provided by another person to direct their behavior and to sustain their attention on a task. Patients with severe frontal lobe damage also show an inability to maintain attention and resist distractions. They show impulsive, often socially inappropriate, reactions to irrelevant stimuli, as if the orienting response had taken complete control of their behavior. In support of this interpretation, the orienting response in these patients is often enhanced. In addition, verbal prompting usually does not enable them to direct their attention appropriately.

In summary, Luria proposed two attentional systems: One system, based on the orienting response, is reflexive, appears early in development, is subject to rapid habituation, and does not depend on cognitive processes. The second attentional system develops slowly through social learning, is associated with cognitive and particularly linguistic mediation, is volitional in nature, and permits sustained, intentional behavior. In patients with limbic or frontal lobe damage, the system directing volitional attention is often disrupted, and the orienting response takes control of response generation. The behavior of such patients is often impulsive, lacks goal direction, and is bounded by immediate environmental events.

Pribram and McGuinness

Pribram and McGuinness (1975) proposed that attention is controlled by three physiological systems: arousal, activation, and effort. Based on neurophysiological data from both human and animal investigations, they concluded that arousal and activation can be dissociated and that each form of physiological reactivity is associated with a different component of the brain's response to task demands. The role of the limbic system is emphasized in the control of sensory integration, and activation reflects the readiness to make a response produced by the reticular system. The coordination of arousal and activation produces effort, which is reflected in a third neurophysiological response associated with sensorimotor integration.

This model is important for historical and theoretical reasons. It was one of the first attempts to present a comprehensive neuropsychological model based on evidence from neurophysiological studies. It also delineates the importance of arousal, reinforcement, and other concepts derived from the behavioral sciences to an understanding of attentional processes.

The model emphasizes the role of the limbic system, the frontal cortex, and subcortical structures in the control of attention (see Figure 14.3). Attention is considered a component of behavioral response selection. In this sense, Pribram and McGuinness's model anticipated the need to incorporate intentionality as a component of attentional control. As we have discussed, this perspective has recently received consideration in the neuropsychological literature (e.g., Heilman et al., 1985).

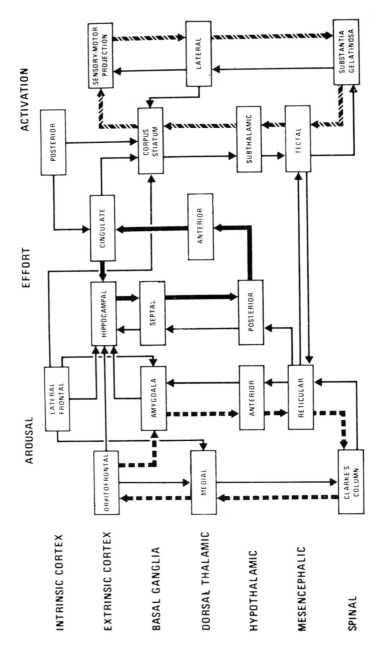

FIGURE 14.3. The neural systems proposed by Pribram and McGuinness (1975, with permission) to underlie arousal, activation, and effort for the control of attention.

Posner

The neuropsychological models described so far were developed by researchers drawing on the fields of behavioral neurology, neuropsychology, and neurophysiology. In contrast, Michael Posner is a cognitive psychologist who has been a leading influence in the emerging field of cognitive neuroscience.

One of Posner's most significant contributions to the neuropsychology of attention is his systematic application of methods from cognitive psychology to the neuropsychological study of attention. In particular, Posner has had a major influence on the development and application of chronometric techniques. His use of response time as an index of the costs and benefits associated with overt and covert shifts of attention provided an important tool for determining the efficiency of attentional selection and detection (Posner, Snyder, & Davidson, 1980). Posner's use of positional cues to direct attention to spatial locations prior to the presentation of a target is a primary paradigm for studying spatial selective attention. Using this paradigm, a cost–benefit analysis can be conducted to determine the effects of valid or invalid positional cuing, which ultimately provides information about the effects of uncertainty on attentional selection.

In addition to his methodological contribution, Posner's neuropsychological research has suggested the existence of two neural systems that contribute to different types of attentional control: (1) a neural system governing spatial selection in the parietal lobes, and (2) an anterior neural system that influences *intensive* attention. The parietal system directs covert shifts of spatial attention according to Posner. The general features of his model do not differ greatly from the models described by Heilman *et al.* (1983) or Mesulan (1981), though it provides a somewhat different explanation for how the parietal lobes direct covert attention.

Posner maintains that the primary deficit associated with parietal damage is an impairment of attentional disengagement. Parietal damage tends to cause difficulty with covert shifts of attention to the area contralateral to the lesioned hemisphere. However, Posner has demonstrated that this impairment is greatest when the patient must disengage their attention focus from a position in the ipsilateral hemispace and direct attention toward the contralateral hemispace. Therefore, Posner proposes that shifts of spatial attention are controlled by the parietal lobes by a *disengagement* mechanism.

Posner has suggested that a second type of attention exerts a primary effect by enhancing the intensity of cognitive operations directed toward particular tasks. Again, Posner's proposal does not differ in general terms from the process of *intention*, which has been described by Heilman *et al.* (1983). However, Posner has suggested a broader application of this anterior brain system and the process of intensive attention to account for attentional effects beyond the clinical syndrome of hemi-inattention and neglect. In particular, Posner and his colleagues have provided evidence through studies of PET scan activation for the role of the cingulate cortex in regulating attentional intensity. Furthermore, Posner has suggested a role for these systems in the direction of attention relative to semantic information.

Mirsky

Mirsky (1989) proposed a model of attention that is built on a taxonomy of attentional functions. He concluded that there are five fundamental attentional functions: focusing, executing, sustaining, encoding, and shifting. Mirsky then analyzed neuropsychological test data from brain-damaged populations using factory-analytic methods. He used the following neuropsychological tests: Trail-Making, letter cancellation, Digit Symbol Substitution Test, Stroop Interference, continuous performance test, Arithmetic Subtest (Wechsler

Adult Intelligence Scale—Revised—WAIS-R), Digit Span, and the Wisconsin Card Sort. He derived four factors that correspond to the dimensions of sustaining, encoding, executing/ focusing, and Shifting. Mirsky then used a deductive method to determine how these four factors are expressed in reference to neuroanatomical systems. This methodology is distinct from the approach of traditional beahvioral neurology, which seeks to define behavioral expression as a funciton of lesion site.

Mirsky constructed a phenomenological taxonomy of attention and then fit this taxonomy to the existing knowledge about the effects of different types of brain dysfunction. In this manner, he localized the four elements of attention that were empirically derived. As described below, this localization is similar to that described by Heilman, Watson, and Valenstein (1985) and by Mesulam (1985).

Reticular Formation

The tectum and the mesopontine regions are important in the maintenance of consciousness and attention.

Thalamic Systems

The medial thalamic region, including the reticular nuclei, is an important relay for the transfer of reticular activation to cortical regions.

Corpus Striatum

The basal ganglia structure of the corpus striatum appears to be important in the gating of information. It has particular relevance to the control of motoric and premotoric impulses.

Limbic System

The hippocampus and other limbic structures influence attention by mediating the affective value attributed to signals that are attended to. It is also critical in memory formation and therefore affects attention by influencing encoding. The medial frontal cortex, including the cingulate gyrus, also is important in normal attention.

Prefrontal Cortex

The prefrontal cortex is essential to executive control, as described elsewhere in this text.

Parietal Cortex

The inferior parietal lobe has been shown to be critical in sensory selective attention. It contains cells that show enhanced response when motivationally directed attention occurs. This region is particularly important in visual attention and is often impaired in neglect syndromes.

Temporal Cortex

The superior temporal sulcus appears to be improtant in heteromodal sensory associative processing. This region may influence attention by integrating converging multisensory inputs.

There are two weaknesses in Mirsky's taxonomy. First, it relies on factors derived from traditional neuropsychological measures. Although these measures adequately assess for the factors that Mirsky derived, these measures do not deal as adequately with other related processes, such as motivation, behavioral timing, and other factors that also seem to be critical in attentional functioning. Second, the four attentional factors that Mirsky specified are said to correspond to specific neuroanatomical systems, though little empirical support is provided.

A TAXONOMY OF ATTENTION

As can be appreciated from the review of neuropsychological tests of attention, the clinical assessment of attention currently lacks a unitary theoretical basis. In this section, we discuss a conceptually organized approach to assessment and suggest tests for behaviors that are typical of different types of deficits. This approach is based on the division of attentional processing into four factors: sensory attention, response selection and executive control, capacity, and sustained attention. In Table 14.1, we describe the components underlying the four attentional factors, as well as the neurobehavioral task variables that should be considered in studying these components.

Sensory Selection

Sensory attention comprises several mechanisms that select specific stimuli for further processing, including integration and filtering, passive shifting (e.g., OR), and active focusing and enhancement. Passive processes are largely driven by stimulus properties (bottom-up) mechanisms, while active processes are driven by task-related (top-down) mechanisms.

Passive Integration

Passive sensory integration operates on the basis of intrinsic properties of the stimulus field. Gestalt mechanisms of stimulus grouping are the classic example of these types of phenomena. The inability of patients to automatically segregate figures from ground, to avoid "collisions" when copying figures, and the tendency to neglect areas or objects in the visual field typically indicate a failure of these fundamental mechanisms, which usually operate effortlessly.

Sensory Filtering

Filtering entails a selection of a stimulus for attention because it possesses a particular feature, usually a simple physical characteristic. The feature which allows selection of a particular stimulus or message might be the spatial location or gender of a voice, or the spatial location of a visual display, such as a television screen. Filtering permits a rapid, automatic, and early selection of relevant stimuli when an identifying feature can be

TABLE 14.1. Neuropsychological Taxonomy of Attention

Attentional component	Task variables
Sensory selective attention	
Filtering	Stimulus complexity
Focusing/selection	Computational demands
Automatic shifting	Orienting-response parameters
Response selection and control	
Intention	Task and information salience
Initiation and inhibition	Multiple response onsets (e.g., go–no-go demands)
Active switching	Alternation of responding
Executive regulation	Categorical switching
	Rule-governed decisions
Attentional capacity	
Energetic factors	
Arousal	Intrinsic biological state
	External stressors
Motivational state	Consequences/payoff
Effort	Task demands/salience
Structural factors	
Memory capacity	Short-term memory (STM) demands, rehearsal, etc.
Processing speed	Individual differences
	Testing different modalities
Temporal dynamics	Serial/multiframe designs
Spatial characteristics	Spatial frame design
Global resources	General cognitive demands
	Complexity of operations
Sustained performance	
Vigilance	Signal/target ratio
	Task duration
	Arousal
Fatiguability	Salience, payoff
	Intrinsic biological state
Reinforcement contingency	Schedule of payoff and costs

recognized. Broadbent contrasts filtering with pigeonholing, or categorization. Pigeon-holing entails the sorting of stimuli which differ by multiple sensory features into categories (or pigeonholes), and is often associated with response selection. If no category is appropriate, then the event is ignored. Since pigeonholing requires the detailed analysis of a stimulus on a number of dimensions, it occurs later in time, may take a longer time to complete, and requires more active processing than filtering. Both processes may be involved in generating a single response. For example, a child may respond only to the sound of his mother's voice in a gathering, but the type of response will depend on interpretation of the message which his mother provides.

The measurement of filtering processes in attention is closely identified with the dichotic listening paradigm. In this paradigm, a subject is required to shadow, or repeat, a spoken message presented from one source and ignore speech from another source. This procedure has been used most often in the assessment of hemispheric processing of language, rather than in the assessment of attention deficits. Brain-damaged patients are usually able to transiently attend to appropriate stimuli on the basis of common physical features in the absence of sensory, perceptual, or agnostic disturbances. This may be a result of the pervasive filtering mechanisms at every level of the nervous system, which isolate and enhance meaningful features in the environment.

Automatic Attentional Shifting

In the natural environment, people tend to orient to unexpected events (e.g., the appearance of an object on a road surface). The orienting response appears to represent an environmentally actuated system that detects unexpected but possibly significant events and shifts attention to them. Unlike other attentional processes, the orienting system requires no effort or conscious awareness to maintain. Traditional neuropsychological testing seldom addresses this system, although the orienting response can be disturbed by both neurologic and psychiatric disorders such as frontal lobe syndromes and schizophrenia.

Focusing-Enhancement

The most active attentional operations conducted during early stages of sensory processing involve focusing and enhancement. Prior to the arrival of new stimuli, processing biases exist that are determined by expectancies and the history of previous information. These biases enhance the allocation of cognitive resources to particular featural characteristics or spatial positions. The bias that is created based on expectancy occurs prior to stimulation and enhances the likelihood of attention being drawn to particular stimuli or environmental features, thereby creating an attentional focus. As information flows through the sensory systems, there is continual modification of the attentional focus, in relationship to the salience of the information that is processed.

The neural mechanisms underlying attentional focusing are just now beginning to be understood. Neurophysiological investigations have demonstrated a neural enhancement mechanism that facilitates response to certain regions of the spatial environment based on expectations from cues (see Chapter 9). Eventually, mechanisms similar to those involved in neural enhancement will probably be shown to be involved in various types of attentional focusing.

Response Selection and Control

The attentional operations that we have just described enable selection of sensory information during the early stages of information processing. However, other attentional operations that are more closely associated with response production also play an important role in attentional control. Under normal conditions, information processing occurs in situations in which some type of response is required. Therefore, attention to sensory stimulation is usually either directly or indirectly influenced by response demands. Our taxonomy contains four primary components of response selection and control that have significant influence over attention: (1) intention, (2) initiation, (3) active switching, and (4) executive control.

Intention

Prior to the response, a response intention usually forms, except in cases where the response is elicited in an automatic reflexive manner (e.g., OR). Intention reflects the activation of response preparation in relation to motivational pressures or reinforcement. Based on the development of intention, humans frequently generate a plan of action or initiate pre-motor programs.

Initiation

Following the formation of intention, humans typically initiate a series of iterative processes, through which they test alternative response outcomes. While these iterative processes may involve actual pre-motor activation, in humans they do not require actual motoric responses, but rather are carried out covertly through feed-forward operations. These operations constitute hypothesis testing, and may occur relative to associative information, even when no overt response is required. The efficient initiation of these iterative processes has a great influence over attentional control. When the capacity to efficiently initiate pre-motor programs or actual motor responses is disrupted, attentional performance is compromised. The attentional performance characteristics of patients with Parkinson's disease illustrates this point.

Active Attentional Switching

In addition to response initiation, response selection and control also depends on active switching processes. Active switching depends on the inhibition of one response tendency and the initiation of another. In order to attend effectively, the individual must be capable of efficient switching among responses, so that a behavioral continuity is maintained. Attention is typically impaired in cases of defective response switching, as failure to disengage an earlier response tendency interferes with attention to information that is currently appropriate. This type of problem occurs with many disorders that affect frontal lobe and subcortical functions.

While normal individuals shift attention fluidly as task demands change, patients sometimes have great difficulty making such transitions. They get "stuck" in a given response set. This phenomenon has been referred to as pathological inertia (Luria, 1974), or perseveration. The inability to shift response sets in spite of feedback can be observed on the Wisconsin Card Sorting Test. Intrusions of earlier responses on new tasks is a striking example of this tendency, particularly on graphemic tasks. Sometimes the patient will be unable to inhibit a perseverative response even after verbally noting its occurrence. Abnormal performance on certain tasks, such as the go–no-go and the Stroop tests, often provides evidence of faulty response inhibition or switching. These tests vary in their response demand, from simple motor control (go–no-go) to a more complex verbal response (Stroop Test). Yet both tests require response inhibition and switching, illustrating that this attentional component is evident at various levels of cognitive operation.

Executive Control

All of the components of response selection and control that we have discussed can be considered as aspects of the domain of executive control. However, executive control connotes an even broader cognitive capacity, one that is responsible for top-down, meta-cognitive control over attention.

Executive functions facilitate higher cognitive operations such as categorization. Pigeonholing deficits and problems with categorization are ubiquitous among patients with brain dysfunction, particularly when high-level neural systems that are necessary for cognitive flexibility are damaged. Notably, lesions of the frontal lobes are known to impair the ability of humans to perform these types of operations, as patients with frontal lobe damage lose their ability to plan, categorize, take perspective, and use abstraction. Ultimately, failure of these higher executive functions affects the ability to control attention.

Attentional Capacity

Attentional capacity can be divided into two realms: capacity as determined by nonspecific energetic factors, such as arousal or effort, and capacity as determined by structural factors, like working-memory capacity or processing speed.

Arousal and Energetic State

Although factors like effort, arousal, and activation can be experimentally distinguished, in the clinic they are usually considered a variable, nonspecific factor that influences performance across tests. In this section, arousal is regarded as encompassing the range of the factors that influence performance by varying the energy applied to it. In the laboratory, arousal is typically measured through psychophysiological techniques, which are impractical in a clinical setting. However, qualitative assessment of the tonic and phasic components of arousal should be part of the whole assessment.

Tonic arousal may be depressed or elevated by disturbances in brain function. Diminished tonic arousal may be characterized by such behavioral signs as decreased alertness, a generalized slowing of speech and responses, lack of spontaneous movement, reduced reactivity to the surroundings, or failure to initiate conversation or activity. Diminished arousal is typically observed in depression and is often a nonspecific concomitant of brain damage, particularly damage to brain stem or frontal structures. Diminished arousal can also be produced by drugs. Hyperarousal is typical of manic disorders, may be observed in schizophrenia, and may be produced by stimulant medication.

Disturbances in phasic arousal are a common result of brain dysfunction. The classical laboratory index of phasic arousal is the effect of readiness on performance. Typically, if performers are given a warning signal just before an event requiring a response, their response time is shortened and their accuracy may be improved. This effect rapidly decays over time. The inability to take advantage of warning signals suggests that a person is unable to sustain arousal. If a person is unable to transiently increase or sustain arousal for a task, performance deficits will be observed on a variety of tasks. Performance shows striking variability from one trial to another and between tests. In extreme cases, a patient may respond correctly to easy items and miss hard items on a test. On tests demanding sustained effort, such as Digit Symbol or word generation, fatigue may cause a rapid decay in performance. Disturbances in phasic arousal can be dissociated from specific cognitive deficits. For example, a disturbance in arousal can be inferred when a patient is not anomic, speaks fluently, and has a good vocabulary but is unable to generate words fluently by letter or category.

Structural Factors

Disturbances in span of apprehension and working memory are commonly assessed by means of the Digit Span tests or its variants. Digit Span Forward provides a measure of span of apprehension. Gross deficits on Digit Span Forward are usually seen only in cases of severe brain damage, such as aphasia or dementia. Performance variability on digit strings of the same length is a more common problem, suggesting difficulty in maintaining concentration over trials. Digit Span Backward makes greater demands on attention, in that a person is required to hold symbols in memory and to perform an operation on them (Craik & Lockhart, 1972).

Processing speed on cognitively demanding tasks, such as the Symbol Digit Modalities Test and the paced serial addition tests, is impaired by many types of brain damage. Choice reaction time is delayed in a variety of syndromes, including schizophrenia, depression, head trauma, mental retardation, and dementia. Processing speed is usually delayed more on complex than on simple tasks. The biological substrates of delayed processing speed are typically unknown. As argued in Chapter 17, it may be reasonable to regard processing speed measures as indices of global capacity for effortful performance, rather than as a direct reflection of slowing of neural transmission.

Other structural factors include the temporal and spatial processing characteristics, the memory, and the overall cognitive resources of the individual.

Sustained Attention

The ability to sustain attention on tasks is quite vulnerable to neurological and psychiatric disturbances. Vigilance performance, even on very simple discriminations, is often impaired in these patients, who have great difficulty sustaining attention on a channel of information with a low event rate. The continuous-performance test provides quantitative information regarding a patient's vigilance performance at different levels of task difficulty. Distractibility is clinically apparent in patients who are pulled off-task by external events, or who impulsively articulate task-irrelevant thoughts during performance. Distractibility may be more apparent outside the quiet and structured testing milieu, and therefore, the patient and the family members should be asked about such difficulties.

The bases for difficulties in sustaining performance levels are quite varied. Deficits in sustained performance may be due to failures of filtering, pigeonholing, arousal, response selection, or lack of effective reinforcement. Effective filtering requires a person to monitor an appropriate channel over time, and to resist distraction that causes the attention to shift to a task-irrelevant channel. Pigeonholing similarly requires that a person maintain an appropriate set of responses to a series of stimuli, and to consistently categorize stimuli into their correct response bins. Deficits in arousal result in a tonic decrement in sensitivity (d'). Patients may be unable to inhibit well-learned but inappropriate responses to a stimulus. Finally, patients may be unresponsive to formerly reinforcing activities and consequences or may lack sensitivity to contingencies. They therefore fail to sustain attention on tasks despite intact cognitive processing, it has been often remarked that patients with frontal lobe syndromes or head trauma show a paucity of deficits on traditional neuropsychological testing but are profoundly impaired in natural-world performance. The experimental neuropsychological literature suggests that measures of vigilance may be a more sensitive measure of brain dysfunction than traditional tests of intellectual performance. With the advent of inexpensive computers, such tests may supplement or replace psychometric tests, which have been the mainstay of neuropsychology. In addition, the examiner should be aware that it is impossible in the clinical environment to duplicate some of the common demands of the natural world, such as planning a work day in the office when multiple tasks must be assigned priorities executed serially, and interruptions must be fielded. Good interviewing and observational techniques remain an irreplaceable component of attentional assessment.

TABLE 14.2.   Disturbances of Attention

Probable level of Impairment (for Tables 14.1a, b, c): ++ = Moderate to severe impairment; + = Mild impairment; +/? = Possible impairment; − = Not significantly impaired; −/? = Probably not impaired, but not enough information known.

14.2A.   Neuroanatomical Lesions

	Parietal	Frontal	Limbic	Reticular	Hypothalamic
I. Sensory attention					
Select/focus	++	+	+/?	+	−
Automatic shift—OR	+	++	++	++	++
Sensory filtering	++	−	−		−
II. Capacity					
Arousal	+	++	++	++	++
Motivation		++	++	+	++
Processing speed	+	+		+	++
Temporal dynamics	?	++	++	+/?	++
Spatial distribution	++	+	+	−	−
Memory	+	+	++	+	+
Global capacity (IQ)	+	+	+	+	+
III. Response selection and control					
Intention	+/?	++	++	−	++
Initiation	+/?	++	++	+	++
Inhibition		++	++	−	+
Active switching	+/?	++	+	+	+
Executive control		++	++	+	+
IV. Sustained attention					
Fatigue	−	++	+	++	++
Persistence	+	++	++	+	++
Vigilance	+	++	+	++	++
Reinforcement	−	++	++	−	++

14.2B.   Neurological Disease[a]

	CHI	MS	AD	PD	MD	NPH
I. Sensory attention						
Select/focus	−	+/?	++	+	−	+/?
Automatic shifts—OR	+	?	++	+/?	+/?	+/?
Sensory filtering	−	−	+/?	−	−	−
II. Capacity						
Arousal	+	++	+	++	++	+
Motivation	+	++	++	+/?	++	+
Processing speed	++	++	++	++	+	++
Temporal dynamics	++	++	++	++	+/?	+/?
Spatial distribution	−	−	+	+/?	−	−
Memory	+	+	++	+	+	+
Global capacity (IQ)	+	+	++	+	+	+
III. Response selection and control						
Intention	++	+/?	++	+	+	+
Initiation	+	+	+	++	+	++
Inhibition	++	−	++	++	+	++
Active switching	++	++	++	++	+	++

(Continued)

TABLE 14.2.   Neurological Disease (*Continued*)

14.2B.   Neurological Disease (*Continued*)[a]

	CHI	MS	AD	PD	MD	NPH
III. Response selection and control (*Continued*)						
Executive control	++	+	++	++	+	+
IV. Sustained attention						
Fatigue	−	++	−	++	+	+
Persistence	++	++	+	++	+	++
Vigilance	++	+	+	++	+	++
Reinforcement	+/?	+/?	+/?	+/?	+/?	−/?

[a]CHI = closed head injury; MS = multiple sclerosis; PD = Parkinson's disease; AD = Alzheimer's disease (early to middle stage); MD = metabolic disorders; NPH = normal-pressure hydrocephalus.

14.2C   Psychiatric Disorders[a]

	ADHD+	ADHD−	SCHIZ	DEP	MANIA	ANX
I. Sensory attention						
Select/focus	−	++	++	+/?	+/?	+/?
Automatic shifts—OR	++	++	++	++		?
Sensory filtering	−	−/?	+/?	−	−	−
II. Capacity						
Arousal	++	+	+	++	++	++
Motivation	++	++	++	++	++	−
Processing speed	+/?	?	+/?	+	+	−
Temporal dynamics	++	+/?	++	++	++	+
Spatial distribution		+	+	−	−	−
Memory		+	+	+	+	−
Global capacity (IQ)	−	+	+	−	−	−
III. Response selection and control						
Intention	+	+/?	+/?	++	+	−
Initiation	−	+/?	+/?	+	−	+
Inhibition	++	+/?	+	−	++	+
Active switching	++	+/?	+	+	++	+/?
Executive control	+	+/?	++	+	++	−
IV. Sustained attention						
Fatigue	+	+	−	++	−	−
Persistence	++	+	+	++	++	−
Vigilance	++	++	+	++	++	++
Reinforcement	++	+/?	+/?	++	++	−

[a]ADHD+ = Attention deficit disorder with hyperactivity; ADHD− = attention deficit disorder without hyperactivity; SCHIZ = schizophrenia; DEP = major depression; ANX = anxiety disorder.

Clinical Manifestations

Attentional disturbances are a frequent concomitant of both psychiatric disturbance and brain damage. Although many tests are sensitive to attentional deficits, the specific type of attentional deficit cannot be defined by a single test. The clinician is required to integrate information from interview, observational, and formal tests within a conceptual framework in order to define an attentional disturbance. A comprehensive attentional assessment should consider the ability of the patient to modulate arousal, to select stimuli and responses, to sustain attention over time, and to shift attention.

The neuropsychological taxonomy that has been described was derived from a multivariate analysis of the neuropsychological performance of both normal control subjects and patients with different clinical diagnoses. Attentional performance does not vary homogeneously across clinical populations. Different patterns of attentional dysfunction are evident across patient groups when a large number of attention measures are analyzed. In Table 14.2, we summarize patterns of attentional deficit found across several different patient groups that have been described by neurobehavioral studies.

The results that emerge show that subtypes of attentional disturbance exist. Although severe brain damage may interfere with many different attentional components, a predominant area of attention dysfunction is often apparent. With localized brain lesions, there may be greater specificity of the attention impairment. It should be emphasized that our studies of subtypes of attention disturbance are in a preliminary phase. Yet, these early results are promising and suggest that additional research is needed to fully characterize the components of attention associated with different brain and psychiatric disorders.

Toward an Integrated Attentional Framework

Consciousness and Self-Directed Attention

The distinction between outside reality and our experience of it has been a fundamental concern of philosophers throughout history. Some have seen subjective experience and the "mind" as separate from physical reality, and others have considered them extensions of one another. The mission underlying these philosophical quests has been to understand the nature of human "consciousness."

Scientists have reacted with ambivalence and occasionally outrage to the concept of consciousness. Although they have acknowledged this subjective experience, most have argued that consciousness is a metaphysical phenomenon that is not within the realm of scientific inquiry. Yet, perspectives regarding the relationship between consciousness and reality are often either explicitly or implicitly evident in scientific theory. For instance, the nature of consciousness has not been a central topic of study within physics. Yet differences in theoretical perspectives regarding the relationship between external reality and the human observer led to radically different interpretations of universal structure. This point is illustrated by the theoretical divergence between Heisenberg and Einstein over the issue of certainty in the observation of the outside world. These theoretical perspectives reflect fundamentally different philosophies regarding the relationship between subjective experience and external reality. Ultimately at issue is whether there is a limitation to human awareness. Therefore, while it is not defined as a topic within the field of physics, the nature of consciousness may have great significance in explaining the capacity of science to explain physical reality. These theoretical perspectives reflect fundamentally different philosophies regarding the relationship of subjective experience and outside reality.

Consciousness and awareness have always held a precarious position in psychology. Although an understanding of consciousness has often been an implicit desire of psychological theorists, psychological scientists, more often than not, have rejected the position that consciousness can or should be studied. Wundt and many of the early psychologists considered consciousness and awareness central topics for psychology. To them, apperception, the process by which external reality interfaces with the individual's internal state, is a primary psychological process. William James was also concerned about the nature of consciousness and the relationship of brain to awareness. His theory of emotions proposed that emotional experiences and meaning resulted from the perception of physical or behavioral reactions to events; that is, perceptions of reality gained meaning as a result of the context in which they were experienced. James considered attention the "taking posses-sion of the mind." Attention was considered an indication of clarity or "clearness" of consciousness by structuralists like Titchener.

Subsequently, psychological science largely rejected the study of consciousness in favor of empirical behavior. The reasons are largely the same as those for rejecting the need for an attentional construct. Objections to consciousness were even stronger because it was a "mental experience" that was even less accessible to empirical science. Even with the advent of cognitive psychology, there has generally been a reluctance to consider constructs like consciousness and awareness.

An inescapable characteristic of human experience is the capacity for self-awareness. Furthermore, when we experience "consciousness," the whole seems to be greater than the sum of its parts. Self-awareness is not easily explained by traditional behavioral or cognitive theories. As a result, consciousness has slowly reemerged as a viable neurobehavioral construct over the past few years. Some neuroscientists have gone so far as to conclude that a "concept of consciousness is necessary . . . for a scientific understanding of man's psycho-logical processes" (Pribram, 1976, p. 46).

As we discuss subsequently in chapter 21, there is now considerable philosophical debate over the relevance of recent efforts in the cognitive neurosciences to more clearly understand mental experience (Churchland & Churchland, 1990; Daugman, 1990; Pyly-shyn, 1973; Serle, 1990). For these philosophers, accounting for the nature of consciousness and self-awareness is central to the meaningfulness of cognitive neuroscientific efforts. Some neuroscientists have also recognized the need to consider the nature of consciousness (e.g., Sperry, 1969).

SELF-AWARENESS CAPACITY

If consciousness is a by-product of self-regulating systems, the capacity for conscious-ness should depend on the extent to which people are self-aware. It is clear that humans are not always aware of all their neurobehavioral and physiological processes. Some cognitive experiences remain unconscious until attention is directed to them. For instance, as I type this page, I do not consciously recognize my kinesthetic and somatosensory signals. Yet, if I direct my attention to these sensations, I become aware of them.

The ability of healthy people to bring unconscious "automatic" processes to aware-ness is quite strong for many types of information. Most people are able to report the experience of self-awareness, and to identify with a feeling of "consciousness." However, humans exhibit a mixed capacity for self-awareness, as their awareness may not always be accurate. This capacity depends on the type of awareness that is considered.

Studies of visceral self-perception and awareness suggest that there are marked differ-ences in the ability of human subjects to accurately detect physical responses such as heart rate (Katkin, 1985; Drescher, Heiman, & Blackwell, 1977; Williamson & Blanchard, 1979). Although people are generally able to report the sensation of their heartbeat, their accu-racy in determining the rate is quite variable. Interestingly, the accuracy of heart rate detection increases under conditions of stress and emotional arousal.

There are also marked differences in the ability of humans to report or recognize emotional experiences. Studies of patients with "psychogenic" illnesses suggest that a significant percentage have difficulty labeling these experiences (Nemiah & Sifneos, 1970; Sifneos, 1973). This condition has been called *alexithymia*. These patients lack insight into their self-experiences. Although they describe physical ailments like pain, they are unable to provide a qualitatively rich description of this experience. Furthermore, they seem to lack awareness of other aspects of their internal state. Whether alexithymia is due to abnormalities of verbal self-report, affective registration or labeling, or some other process has not yet been established. Yet, it appears that the subjective quality of these patients' self-consciousness is different from that of other individuals.

Even in people without alexithymia, there is considerable variation in awareness of or attention to internal state. Some individuals are highly introspective and very aware of their "mental" activities, and others show a limited inclination for such activity. Although individual differences in these and other experiential tendencies have been demonstrated by psychological investigators, at this point little is known about the relationship of these tendencies to attention or neurobehavioral control processes.

MODELS OF CONSCIOUSNESS AND AWARENESS

Cognitive and neuroscientific theories regarding the nature of consciousness and self-awareness fall into five general classes, based on the suppositions that consciousness and self-awareness are (1) by-products of cognitive self-regulation; (2) an emergent property of the total activity of the brain; (3) the product of a supervisory system in the brain; (4) by-products of states arising from other processes, for example, short-term memory (STM); or (5) do not exist and should be ignored. For the purposes of this discussion, we consider the first three possibilities.

The first hypothesis that self-consciousness and awareness are the result of cognitive self-regulation, has much appeal. A metacognitive process is implicated that provides supervisory control over cognition. Such a process would depend on an intricate feedback arrangement that would enable the brain to have information regarding its cognitive operations. This feedback could then be labeled in accordance with previous experience. Therefore, as a memory of past life events is evoked, the brain recognizes that it is having this experience and then labels it as an "old" memory. This model is an offshoot of the Jamesian theory of emotion, as it suggests that these experiences result from multiple sequential processes. The idea that self-regulatory mechanisms underlie these metacognitive phenomena has several lines of support, which we will address later.

The second hypothesis, that consciousness is an emergent property, suggests a somewhat different possibility—that self-awareness and the experience of consciousness are not the same thing. Although the brain may be capable of self-monitoring through feedback mechanisms, the quality of consciousness is a result of the sum of all neural activity, which then compounds the results in the completely integrated experience that we call consciousness. Models that consider consciousness an emergent property are more difficult to test, as they are based on the gestalt principle that the whole is greater than the sum of its parts.

The possibility that a supervisory system generates consciousness stems from the idea that awareness is associated with attentional control over action. Without supervisory control, a state of pandemonium would exist, so that no single process would have priority. As attentional selection usually occurs relative to response demands, some theorists (e.g., Shallice, 1972) have maintained that a supervisory system must exist that establishes the dominance of certain actions. Consciousness is the by-product of this supervisory control.

These three theoretical perspectives are not mutually exclusive and, in fact, may be quite compatible. A neural system that contains multiple feedback arrangements could provide for the recursive reprocessing of information about its own responses. Self-awareness of this recursive quality of processing would then provide the basis of the human experience of consciousness. Consciousness would be an emergent property of this self-regulatory characteristic, which would also serve to provide supervisory control over behavior. Furthermore, supervisory control could be established by a "prepremotor" neural arrangement that modulates feedback from the preparation of response alternatives. This concept was discussed in chapters 3 and 10 and has some neuropsychological support.

Attention and Consciousness

Early cognitive theories of attention occasionally come close to using the construct of consciousness. The early bottleneck theories maintained that one reason for attention was that it reduced information load, as only one item could be handled at a time. This was made evident by the fact that we can be aware of only one thing at a time within our frame of awareness. Furthermore, tasks with intense attentional demands are often perceived as effortful, a perception suggesting a subjective quality to attentional processes. In fact, the distinction between automatic and controlled attentional processes has been made partly on the basis that automatic processes can be performed effortlessly and without awareness. Therefore, self-awareness seemed to be intertwined with attention.

Humans seem to be capable of voluntary attention. They can decide to direct themselves to a particular task even when there are no immediate stimuli to elicit this response. When we exercise voluntary attention, conscious awareness usually results. Other attentional processing seems to occur without conscious awareness. For instance, the reflexive act of shifting our attention to a new stimulus (the orienting response) usually occurs with little conscious awareness. Yet, we may be aware of our orienting response (OR) after it occurs, as we recognize that we have turned our head to a distant sound. Therefore, attention and consciousness are not synonymous.

Pribram (1976, 1980) distinguished between attention and consciousness on the grounds that attention is a process, whereas the term *consciousness* refers to a state, which contains informational content: "Attention refers to processes that organize these contents into one or another conscious state" (p.48). For Pribram, different states of consciousness exist, exemplified by the distinction between perceptual awareness and self-consciousness. Perceptual awareness reflects attention to the external environment and actions relative to that environment; self-consciousness reflects attention to internal state. Both states of consciousness and attention are intricately related to attentional processes through feedback or "feedforward" systems.

Shallice (1972) postulated that consciousness is a by-product of supervisory control, as the neural system ensures that "one action or control process has control" over behavioral actions (p. 48). He suggested that neural "action-systems" compete for dominance. Although feedback is involved at multiple levels, there must be a selection or control process that "creates dominance" of certain actions, perceptions, or cognitions. This occurs as a result of amplifying systems that, through positive feedback, accentuate the difference between competing processes. Amplification would result from a self-exciting neural assembly (Hebb, 1949) that strengthens the priority of one action over others. The sequential variations in action and in cognitive and perceptual dominance create a "stream" of consciousness.

In Shallice's model, the relationship between states of consciousness and attention arises from supervisory functions that establish a dominance of potential actions. Particular neural systems are thought to provide this control (e.g., frontal and subcortical structures). Other models of consciousness and attention have implied a "bottom-up" attentional process, in which consciousness is the by-product of other basic processes. For instance, Atkinson and Shiffren (1971) suggested that consciousness is synonymous with short-term memory. Other authors have taken the position that consciousness is not the result of a single process like STM, but the result of constructive processes that create models from traces of sensory information (Turvey, 1977). Obviously, the exact relationship between consciousness, attention, and the underlying neural processes is not yet well established, though neuropsychological studies of brain function have suggested a role for multiple neural systems.

NEUROPSYCHOLOGICAL EVIDENCE REGARDING SELF-CONSCIOUSNESS

Neuropsychological studies have indicated that disorders of self-awareness and consciousness are commonly associated with two factors: the total extent of the brain damage and the disruption of particular neural systems. In neuropsychology, a distinction is often made between specific (localizing) and nonspecific (nonlocalizing) deficits. After generalized brain damage, patients exhibit conceptual impairments, slowness of ideational process, reduced scope of attention, and reduced memory efficiency, which vary as a function of how much damage has occurred (Goodglass & Kaplan, 1979). This corresponds to the principles of mass effect described by Lashley (1929).

With massive brain damage, such as is evident in Alzheimer's disease, patients lose their general cognitive capacity and therefore their capacity for attention, self-regulation, and self-awareness. Although it is difficult to assess self-consciousness in a patient in the end stage of a progressive dementia, it is common for family members to report that the patient no longer seems to be the same person. Typically, a regression to primitive states occurs, with a disintegration of personality characteristics.It can be assumed that at this point, the patient's self-consciousness and awareness have deteriorated. Parametric analyses of self-consciousness, attention, and brain damage have rarely been conducted. Therefore, the exact relationship between extent of brain damage and capacity for self-consciousness is not well established.

Focal brain damage can also produce specific disturbances of consciousness (Plum, 1972). This in fact is important, as it supports the position that consciousness is not simply an emergent property of total brain activity. Specific neural structures influence self-consciousness. Disorders of consciousness arise from damage to several different brain systems: (1) the prefrontal cortex; (2) the nondominant hemisphere; (3) the corpus callosum; and (4) the limbic system.

Anosognosia refers to a denial of illness or lack of concern for obvious impairments in patients with brain damage. While clinicians have observed anosognosia in neurological patients since the early 1900s, only recently have these disorders been investigated. Heilman (1991) has proposed that anosognosia may result from the failure of four processes: (1) self-monitoring, (2) absence of feedback, (3) false feedback, or (4) improper setting of the monitoring system. Anosognosia is commonly observed in cases of neglect and is associated with other symptoms, like extinction (Hier, Mondlock, & Caplan, 1983). Hemineglect is common following damage to structures of the nondominant hemisphere. The neglect syndromes were discussed in Chapter 9. In addition to inattention to one side of space, patients with this disorder often exhibit a lack of awareness of their own bodies. Though patients may move or feel sensations in one arm, they may deny that it is their arm, arguing that it belongs to someone else. This body schema disturbance suggests that the right parietal region is involved in normal self-experience, and that it may contain a topographical representation of body schemata.

Patients with damage to more anterior regions of the right hemisphere, including the frontal, the anterior parietal opercula, and the basal ganglia, may also exhibit anosognosia secondary to aprosodia and disorders in affective expression. The disturbance in affective processing associated with such damage suggest that the integration of affective and motivational information is also necessary for normal self-consciousness. Limbic system disturbances that alter affective and motivational influences on behavior also influence qualitative self-experience. Although patients with amygdaloid or septal damage may be self-aware, the character of this awareness markedly changes. The value, meaningfulness or emotional labels attached to their experience is affected. Although these changes have not been systematically studied with respect to the question of self-consciousness, it is clear that attentional capacity is disturbed after limbic damage.

Damage to the prefrontal cortex produces qualitatively different impairments of consciousness and self-directed attention. The importance of the prefrontal cortex in attentional processes is obvious if one considers the "frontal lobe syndromes" (Chapter 10). The impairments in planning, behavioral control, and directed and sustained attention that occur with prefrontal damage illustrate the "supervisory" role of this region.

The prefrontal cortex seems to have a regulatory capacity over other cognitive functions. Recursive feedback and feedforward processes seem to be controlled by selective activational and inhibitory influences of the prefrontal cortex. The prefrontal regions modulate affective signals from the limbic system that provide for the salience of information. This arrangement is illustrated by the effects of cingulotomy, which produces a disruption of signals between the limbic and prefrontal systems. After cingulate lesions, patients still experience affective signals, including pain, but do not seem to care as much about it (Cohen *et al.*, 1990). In effect, they experience a background pain that may occasionally be obvious to them, though they are not aware of it or as attentive to the pain most of the time. This effect illustrates the intricate relationship among feedback arrangements in the prefrontal cortex, attention, and self-awareness.

CONSCIOUSNESS, SELF-AWARENESS, AND ATTENTION

The extent to which consciousness, awareness, and attention are interdependent has much relevance to the analysis of attention. If attention is a reflection of only those cognitive processes that have gained access to conscious awareness, then attentional selection will be greatly constrained. As only one unit of information can be the focus of awareness at any point in time, then the attention must be governed by a serial bottleneck arrangement that gates the entry of information into awareness.

The perceived close relationship between conscious awareness and attention clearly influenced the development of the bottleneck theories of selective attention (e.g., Broadbent, 1958; Treisman, 1964). Other theorists (e.g., Neisser, 1967; Hochberg, 1970) explicitly addressed the relationship of consciousness and attention. Neisser equated perceptual analysis with focal attention and ultimately with consciousness. Hochberg proposed a somewhat different relationship, by separating awareness and perceptual analysis. According to Hochberg, perception is viewed as the confirmation of changing expectations about future events, while awareness results from the generation of expectations. Both models of attention suggest that attention and awareness are intimately connected.

As we discussed previously, there is a fundamental problem with considering attention and awareness as synonymous, as there are many instances of behaviors to which humans attend, but have little conscious awareness. Furthermore, the latency for conscious awareness often approaches the latency required to make a response, such as a reaction time (Kahneman, 1973), precluding the possibility that awareness must precede attention. Demonstrations of automatic forms of attention (Schneider & Shiffrin, 1977; Hasher & Zacks, 1979) provide strong evidence that attention without awareness is possible. Furthermore, parallel distributed models provide a means by which information processing can be explained without the constraints of serial processing arrangements.

While attention occurs without the requirement of awareness, attention and awareness are interdependent. The intensity of attentional focus seems to govern whether information processing enters awareness. The degree of effort required for adequate task performance provides a good indication of whether awareness is evoked. Therefore, awareness may be a byproduct of the overall extent or intensity of processing resources allocated to attention. Whether awareness is a requirement or a facilitator of effortful attention is yet to be known.

Consciousness, awareness, and attention are interdependent. Some attentional operations may occur outside normal awareness. However, as task demands intensify, there is a press for effortful controlled processing, which is usually subject to awareness. Consciousness is a state that reflects the pinnacle of the ongoing cognitive processing of the individual.

The distinction between consciousness as a state and attention as a process is necessary, as consciousness emerges as a result of attentional direction against the backdrop of cognitive organization. The temporal-spatial organization of experience is mapped relative to neural coordinate systems. We have discussed several brain systems that provide this organization. For instance, the parietal cortex contains spatial representations, including a body schema on which humans establish a physical sense of the self. The organization of experience relative to this map creates an important aspect of consciousness. Modifications in this organization may occur as a function of environmental influences, which affect the self-experience of consciousness.

The temporal-spatial organization of experience by itself is not sufficient for consciousness. Humans have an active selection system that provides for the supervisory control of experience. We modulate information intake relative to our existing state of consciousness. This modulation is accomplished by self-regulation systems of the prefrontal cortex, in conjunction with salience provided by the limbic system. The attentional control mechanisms provided by these systems creates regulatory control over the state of consciousness. Norman and Shallice (1984) have suggested, it may do so by influencing "dominance" relative to "action systems."

In summary, consciousness is the by-product of attentional processes that act in reference to temporal-spatial organizational systems in the brain. This organization exists with respect to both the external environment and the internal schemata of body and memory. The recursive nature of this attentional control process may create the quality of "metacognition" that characterizes the human experience of consciousness. With damage to the systems that control temporal-spatial organization, we often see a disturbance in body schemata or inattention to part of the environment. In such cases, the specific contents of consciousness are altered. With damage to the systems that regulate and attach significance to this organization, a loss of "depth" and "richness" of conscious experience is often evident. Disturbances in the "stream of consciousness" and the capacity for self-directed experience result.

Just as attention is a process determined by multiple factors, consciousness is a multidetermined state. The characteristics of attention influence consciousness, and conversely, the nature of consciousness has implications for attention. They create mutual constraints that require neuropsychological address.

Neural Constraints on Attention

Cognitive scientists are occasionally criticized for not ensuring that their models are feasible in light of what is known about how the brain works. The neuroanatomy and physiology of the brain constrain the types of mechanisms that can be the neural substrates of attention. Cognitive models that contain processes that are incompatible with neurobiological constraints do not reflect the way cognition is represented in the brain.

Can a model of cognition that does not fit with the natural constraints of the human nervous system be meaningful? For the investigator who is interested in artificial intelligence, the answer may be yes. The success of a computational model may depend only on whether it enables a machine to perform a particular cognitive operation. However, this criterion is not acceptable to scientists interested in the analysis of human cognition. Machines do not have biological pressures to respond. Their operation is totally dependent on the intentional action of the human operator. Models of attention that are based on a machine metaphor have difficulty accounting for this capacity of living organisms to initiate action. Some computational models of behavior have incorporated stochastic properties that enable them to have generative qualities. However, these models do not fully capture the impact of organismic factors on the generation, selection, and control of behavior.

Attention depends on a system that generates self-directed and self-organizing activity. If there were always a complete linear relationship between a stimulus event and the occurrence of a response, there would be little need for an attentional construct. Responses would always occur reflexively to particular stimuli. This obviously is not the case in humans and other higher animal species. Although very predictable relationships can be demonstrated in controlled experimental paradigms, in natural environments responses often depend on selection among various stimulus and response alternatives. This selection process is at least partly driven by intrinsic biological factors. For instance, when the animal's body indicates through physiological signals that it is hungry, it looks for food. The need to eat catalyzes a wide range of behaviors and therefore is often labeled as a *drive*. The study of attention requires that these organismic factors be considered.

The validity of a particular cognitive model of attention depends not only on its fit with existing neural constraints, but also on whether it is compatible with the basic biobehavioral characteristics of the animal. A model that is inconsistent with the structure and functions of neural systems, and that therefore does not meet the conditions of neural and biobehavioral compatibility, is of questionable value, if the goal is to understand natural human cognition. In this chapter, we identify some of the neural constraints that must be addressed in studying processes of attention. These constraints are discussed with respect to the development of cognitive models of attention. We also address how these constraints affect the neuropsychological analysis of attention.

CELL TYPES INFLUENCE AND PROCESSING CHARACTERISTICS

The characteristics of neural cells vary across different brain regions. Therefore, it seems reasonable that the differences in cells noted across brain regions relate in some manner to their functional properties. Cell types are generally classified according to their morphological or synaptic characteristics. The broadest characterization is the distinction between pyramidal and nonpyramidal cells. Pyramidal neurons often contain axons that project outside the cortex. These neurons have dendrites with multiple spines, and with a wide range of different patterns of branching.

Nonpyramidal cells are characterized by distinctions in their shape as compared to that of pyramidal cells. They have many different features and therefore are more difficult to categorize. Their projections are often very diffuse. Morphological distinctions have been made between different types of nonpyramidal neurons, including neurons with and without spines, neurons with different types of synapses, and neurons with unique structural features. Unique cell types include the bipolar, basket, and chandelier cells. These different cell types seem to have unique functional characteristics. For instance, some neurons have a potential for the excitation or inhibition of other groups of neurons. Others seem to have their primary influence through interconnections with other neurons in associative networks. Neural cells can be functionally distinguished on the basis of their firing rate, the type of signals they respond to, and how they interact in groups of neurons (see Kandel & Schwartz, 1983, for a detailed review).

Although the exact role of each type of neuron is not known, it is likely that many neural cells are connected in groups to perform operations in a computational network. However, the neuroanatomical data pertaining to this issue are confusing, as cells in the neocortex typically do not interconnect directly with cells of a similar type. Instead, neurons usually interconnect with neurons of other cell types, often in a different cortical layer (Crick & Hsanuma, 1986). For instance, cells have been detected in the visual system that respond to specific featural characteristics (Hubel & Wiesel, 1963, 1968, 1977) and spatial frequencies (Pollen & Ronner, 1975; Pollen, Gaska, & Jacobson, 1990; Pollen, Jacobson, & Gaska, 1988). Yet, it is not clear how the interaction of groups of these cells influences perception.

The presence of cells that may respond to particular spatial orientations, directional movements, or featural qualities indicates that the brain is tuned to respond to the inherent properties of the stimuli. Many of these cells are part of secondary or tertiary cortex and therefore respond to signals from other primary neural firings. Desimone and his colleagues (Desimone, Albright, Gross, & Bruce, 1980; Desimone, Schein, Moran, & Ungerleider, 1985) have produced results suggesting that some of the higher order responses of temporal visual cells have attentional properties. They direct visual orientation in anticipation of an impending stimulus. Furthermore, these cells seem to fire in response to the aggregate input of groups of neurons, rather than to a single neuron's output.

Some theorists have proposed that specialized "grandmother" cells may exist in the brain and that these cells are tuned to respond to salient complex stimuli. These cells received their name because they are presumably sensitive to very specific and idiosyncratic information, such as the face of one's own grandmother (Feldman, 1982). Although there is not much empirical evidence for this type of cell at this time, the concept of grandmother cells raises an important theoretical issue in the study of attention. The extent to which individual cells are capable of responding to very specific types of stimuli is likely to determine the constraints placed on attention. If grandmother cells are responsible for the representation of important information, like familiar faces, then major efforts should be directed to a search for these cells. Information representation would be very dependent on the functional characteristics of these cells.

Empirical data refuting the grandmother cell theory would support the view that it is the interaction of neurons in networks that is essential for cognition. Such a finding would lessen the importance of the neurobiological characteristics of individual neurons in the cognitive neurosciences. Of course, in the long run, this information is still necessary if we are to understand the response characteristics of cells, as well as the rules governing their interactions.

There is now beginning to be some resolution of these questions pertaining to the selectivity and specialization of individual neural cells. Although it has been well known for some time that cells of the visual cortex are capable of responding to specific types of spatial frequency information, recently the specific response characteristics of neural cells at different levels of the visual cortex to complex stimuli have been demonstrated. Investigators have isolated cells in the V4 region of the monkey that seem to respond selectively to faces or hands (Bruce, Desimone, & Gross, 1981; Desimone *et al.*, 1980). The pattern of neural firing from individual cells in the primate visual cortex, when computationally analyzed, may yield a visual representation that approximates the original stimulus (Pollen, Gaska, & Jacobson, 1990). The neural firing pattern has a high degree of correspondence to the featural characteristics of the original stimulus. These findings suggest that individual cells may be capable of very complex computations, providing a high degree of specificity to their functional properties.

PATTERNS OF ACTIVATION

The activation of networks of neurons provides one possible mechanism for information processing and representation in the brain. Patterns of neural cells acting as networks presumably respond in a unique form of activation, which holds the informational value of the stimulus. The fact that neural cells may be tuned to accept different types of stimulus information accounts for one basis for activation. Clusters of cells that are predetermined to be sensitive to certain stimulus features may provide for an inherent stereotypy of sensory experience. However, it is hard to imagine that there are enough different cells tuned to specific features to account for all of the different stimulus combinations that exist.

The firing patterns of neural cells provide important information about the types of processes that are possible for individual cells. If the pattern of activation reflects an on-off occurrence, most of the information being transmitted must be a by-product of the network of groups of cells. However, it is possible that the pattern of neural firing acts as a code that provides information besides whether the cell has turned on.

How do individual cells that are relatively similar to each other activate in different ways to result in a heterogeneity of experience. Neural cells that transmit signals over distances of more than 1 mm do so through the production of an action potential that occurs as a binary on-off response lasting approximately 1 msec. Most neural cells have spike discharge rates that vary from 50 spikes per second to as many as several hundred spikes per second for brief intervals during stimulation. They have resting levels that may be on the order of several spikes per second. Therefore, the coded information contained in single-cell firing must occur within the constraints of these cell-firing parameters.

Most perceptual processes occur in lengths of time that are less than 200 msec in response to stimulation. As a result, there is a limit in the number of spikes that can occur before initial perception. This limit imposes a constraint on the amount of information that can be provided by the firing pattern of neurons during perception. So far, these constraints have not been well delineated. However, there are only a limited number of different patterns that a particular neural cell can produce, given even the most liberal time constraints.

NEURAL SPEED AND INFORMATION FLOW

Neural speed imposes constraints on cognitive processing by influencing the flow of information in the brain. For instance, if a model proposes a transcallosal mechanism for attention, then it is constrained by the amount of time required for the passage of information across the corpus callosum. If such a crossing takes 10 msec, and it can be shown that attention occurs in a shorter time, then a transcallosal model can be discounted. This methodological approach enables a test of the feasibility of hypothetical cognitive mechanisms.

Hypothetically, it should be possible to determine the neural speed of every pathway, neural circuit, and system of the brain. Neural speed reflects the time taken for an informational impulse to travel along a particular neural pathway, or to be processed by a particular system. It may also be possible to derive an index of the overall neural speed throughout the brain (John, 1967, 1972). The determination of neural speed is, in fact, a complicated matter, and one that is open to much debate. It is much easier to determine the speed of impulses along a single neural unit (e.g., the squid axon). The speed of even the fast axons is relatively slow compared to the speed of electrical impulses along a wire. Therefore, it is easy to see that the flow of billions of impulses across regions of the brain is temporally constrained.

Even though neural transmissions are much slower than the speed of electrical impulses over a wire, the brain is capable of much greater cognitive flexibility than a computer. Humans are able to perform tasks that are well beyond the capability of even the most advanced machines. In its own right, this fact is not difficult to accept. Obviously, neural speed is not the only factor that defines the brain's resources. However, with respect to our discussion of attention, it raises a more interesting problem. A computer requires thousands of sequential steps and much processing time to perform many tasks that humans can perform in little time. Given how much slower the human brain is, one would predict that it would take people much longer to solve similar problems if they were doing so sequentially. The fact that we are able to outperform the computer on many tasks suggests that we do so without following the serial algorithms that constrain computers. Humans are often able to derive solutions based on incomplete data, and through the use of heuristics.

A system operating in parallel would deal with the neural speed problem by selective information from the environment on the basis of heuristics. The neural system would select a stimulus and make a response, if the majority of the criteria for a particular solution were met. By settling on a solution that fit with the minimal allowable criteria for a particular task, the system would essentially make an "educated guess." A response would be made if a target stimulus fit the broadest features of the category appropriate for the particular task. A more precise and narrow selection would be pursued only if a task required a higher level of resolution. In such cases, the task demands would create a pressure to engage in more time-consuming sequential operations. If the neural system were not capable of this type of search, it would become trapped in endless "do-loops," without the flexibility to shift to other response alternatives until the completion of the entire search.

As there are limits on the number of serial operations that can be performed, individual neurons or groups of neurons must be capable of performing complicated operations simultaneously. The neurophysiological characteristics of neurons make it unlikely that an individual neuron is capable of performing very complicated operations. It is more likely that cooperative groups of neurons are the basis for complex parallel processes. Networks are generated by the interactions of groups of individual neurons, which respond in on-off patterns of activation. Neural networks must organize these patterns of activation to produce a more complex operation. Recently, cognitive theorists have developed computational models to account for the attentional control of simultaneous parallel operations (see Chapter 21). These models have incorporated processes like "competitive learning" to describe how a neural system could compensate for the computational limitations of serial processing.

Although parallel processing networks solve a time constraint problem, they also make it more difficult to use neural speed as a direct index of the sequence of events occurring during a cognitive process. It is difficult to account for how multiple operations occurring in parallel translate into temporal organization. Models of brain function that address parallel processes are forced to deal with the nonlinearities in their systems. The presence of nonlinearities makes it difficult to assume that the time required for each operation to be performed will add up to yield a total processing time.

TIMING PROPERTIES

Attention provides a temporal organization for cognition and behavior. Synchronization of behavior and sequencing of information from the environment require a neural system that can switch the direction of responding and sensory analysis to the information necessary for task performance. As this is often accomplished in a series of steps, attention would be facilitated by a neural time-keeping system. In fact, neural systems seem to be tuned to respond optimally to information occurring in certain temporal patterns, as opposed to signals that lack temporal coherence. The "attunement" of neural systems seems to influence their attentional characteristics.

As we have previously described, a common feature of attentional disturbance is a breakdown in the consistency of responding. Response consistency may occur either as a direct function of an internal clock or indirectly, as a result of the temporal characteristics of physiological processes that have the properties of a timekeeper, but that, in their own right, are not true biological clocks. For instance, heart rate has a rhythmic quality that hypothetically could serve as a timekeeper for behavioral processes. Besides relying on biological clocks, animals may establish a temporal organization in their behavior through the use of cues from the external environment. The sequence of events in a chain of responses may enable the individual to estimate the time needed for the successful completion of tasks.

The isolation of the suprachiasmic nucleus (SCN) as a biological clock that controls circadian timing was a major breakthrough (Lydic, Albers, Teper, & Moore-Ede, 1982). The discovery of the SCN provided the first strong evidence of an internal timekeeper that is capable of synchronizing complex behaviors. Although the SCN exerts great influence over long-term timing, the relationship of this clock to the timing of shorter term activity is less evident. Although investigators have shown a disregulation of attention and short-term timing capability when there is damage to the SCN (Cohen & Albers, 1991), it is unlikely that this structures serves as a primary clock for short time frames.

Discovery of the properties of the SCN led some investigators to search for other neural structures that may function as internal clocks. Recently, the hippocampus and the cerebellum have been shown to have rhythmic characteristics that qualify them as potential timekeepers (Ivry, Keele, & Diener, 1988). Cells from the dentate region of the cerebellum pulsate rhythmically, in a synchronized manner with motor responding. This response characteristic suggests that this region may have a timing function, making it a candidate for a second internal clock.

Although there is increasing evidence that biological clocks within the brain play a role in many behavioral functions, there are also many cases of cognitive operations that do not seem to require timing with a clock. For instance, the auditory system is able to extract important sound-localizing information based primarily on the order in which impulses arrive at each ear. Many cognitive analyses are highly dependent on the sequential nature of the information being processed. Other behavioral phenomena, such as learning, may depend on timing without the aid of an internal clock. For instance, differential rate of low-level responding (DRL) conditioning paradigms require that the animal wait a certain period of time before responding in order to receive a reward. Animals can learn to delay responding reasonably well. Although a clock mechanism has been proposed to account for this performance (Meck, 1984), it also appears that animals rely on cues to facilitate their timing. There are many other examples of nontemporal control of timing, suggesting that the representation of time in the brain is very complicated (see Chapter 20).

Neurophysiological models have been proposed to describe mechanisms for timing that do not depend on a clock. Certain brain regions have pulsative properties suggesting that they may act as pacemakers, even though they are not actual clocks. For instance, Crick (1984) proposed that the interaction of bursts of reticular and thalamic activation at 50-msec intervals may cause a natural window for the shifting of attention. According to Crick's proposal, these 50-msec activational bursts cause a transient short-term alteration in the synaptic strengths of neurons in the cortex. The sequential nature of these bursts of activation may produce a temporal organization that is strongly linked to the changing associative strengths that result from synaptic alterations. The binding of synaptic alterations with a temporal sequence of activations is critical in processes of attention. Attention requires a system that is "plastic" in its response to stimulus variations and synchronized in its organization of information processing over time. Therefore, it will be important to further characterize the temporal properties of various neural systems.

NEURAL NETWORKS THAT FACILITATE ATTENTION

In order for networks of neurons to be effective, they must be capable of a large number of interactions with other neurons and neural systems in the brain. The brain has an extremely large number of neurons (estimated to be over 10 billion), which obviously enables an astronomical number of possible interactions between neurons. It has been determined that neurons synapse with as many as a 100,000 dendrites on other neurons (Crick & Asanuma, 1986). The large number of neurons also creates an organization in which no neuron is more than several connections away from another neuron of the brain. The brain's capacity for simultaneous processes is obviously enhanced by its large number of interconnections.

One might think that the tremendously large number of neurons and interconnections in the brain would create an impossible state of chaos, so that it would be difficult to have any behavioral stereotypy across people. The brain's complexity suggests that there is an astronomical number of permutations of how the brain may be organized. This should cause such variability across individuals that there would be few behavioral similarities. Of course, this actually is not the case. Although there is great diversity across people, humans are remarkably similar in the way they function. Even though there is an incredible complexity in the brain, there also seems to be an underlying organization that creates functional consistency.

The neurons of the brain are organized topographically in systems. As neurons in one region are likely to interact most intimately with nearby neurons, the nature of neural interactions is somewhat constrained. Communication between distal neurons occurs when there is a pathway that traverses regions. Cortical organization is also built around sensory and motor systems. For vision and audition, as well as motor function, there are primary cortical regions that enable a primary level of processing. Secondary and tertiary cortex is organized around the primary regions, enabling other levels of processing.

Within given regions, the cortex is organized in fields. This fact has been known for some time and is clearly illustrated in the case of vision. The visual cortex is arranged in spatially distributed fields that correspond to the spatial positions of the environment. Neurons across these fields exert excitatory and inhibitory influences on each other, which provide for temporal-spatial integration. It is likely that, as other brain regions are mapped, they will show similar arrangements, largely the number of neural fields that interact. An understanding of the structural arrangement of these regions will further define the processing characteristics of the neural system. The architecture of the brain sets the parameters for the interaction of neurons, provides constraints on the processes that are possible, and enables animals to have a behavioral stereotypy.

REDUNDANCY AND STEREOTYPY

The brain also seems to have functional and structural redundancy. Some neural systems are very localized and specialized for function. For instance, the calcarine cortex is very specialized for vision, and damage to selective regions is likely to cause specific changes in the visual field. However, it is also apparent that many brain areas contribute to most cognitive processes. Although damage to isolated brain areas may impair performance, individuals are often able to maintain functional capacities even after significant amounts of tissue damage. Therefore, brain functions seem to be distributed across cortical regions, and associative functions are likely the result of parallel distributed processes (Rumelhart, Hinton, & McLelland, 1986).

The functional redundancy of the brain may reflect the way in which outside reality is organized. The idea that cognitive experience is organized according to the structural characteristics of the environment is not new. For instance, Gibson (1950, 1979) developed a theoretical framework to explain human perception that is rooted in a similar concept. He proposed that the environment contains "invariances" that determine the perceptual form that we experience. According to Gibson, perception is largely governed by the spatial structure of the external world acting on a perceptual analyzing system that is relatively consistent across people. The fact that the world contains many invariances creates a predictable order by which experiences can be cataloged. When engaging in a perceptual search, the neural system "settles" on the solution that best approximates these invariant templates. If a stimulus is relatively close in form to a particular environmental invariant, the system registers that it belongs to that particular class of objects.

Several recent computational models have suggested hypothetical mechanisms to account for how a neural system is able to settle on a solution during task performance. The constructs of "relaxation search" (Hinton & Sejnowski, 1986) and "competitive learning" (Grossberg, 1980; Rumelhart & Zipser, 1986) have been formulated as two possible mechanisms. An assumption underlying both constructs is that the neural system is most comfortable with conditions of environmental stability. Environments containing high levels of redundancy offer greater stability, as it is then easier to detect relevant features in the surrounding field. Under such conditions, the system responds actively when there is an inconsistency or a mismatch with the existing schemata. A system that operates in this fashion would be tuned to the redundant patterns of external stimuli and would seek to resolve discrepancies in these patterns. The detection of discrepancies produces an initial orienting response, which quickly habituates. Pressures to continue searching occur only if the observed inconsistencies suggest that the new stimulus is salient.

The internal architecture of the brain also seems to have considerable structural redundancy. Although the functional reasons for a redundant organization are not well understood, it is possible that such an arrangement provides consistency in the way information is represented across the brain. Structural redundancy probably has adaptive value, as it serves to prevent total system failure if damage occurs. Redundancy may also reflect the architectural realities of biological systems. An examination of the coding of DNA reveals considerable redundancy in the pattern of bases along a given strand of genetic material. Although the reasons are not fully understood, one explanation is that redundant codes serve to ensure consistency in the information that is stored across the system.

From the standpoint of attentional processes, redundancy may facilitate the organism's selection of stimuli and responses, so as to ensure a correspondence with the external environmental order. Systemic redundancy provides a constraint on cognition, as it sets the organizational possibilities for the individual. The recursive nature of brain organization may facilitate the formation of templates with which new stimuli can be compared for the "best fit." However, the ramifications of this type of arrangement are far from being well understood.

MEMORY CONSTRAINTS IN NEURAL SYSTEMS

Memory emerges as a critical factor in specifying the influences on attentional processes. In Chapter 17 we delineated the interrelationship between the processes of attention and memory. Although these two cognitive processes have important functional interdependence, memory also places neurophysiological constraints on the processes of attention. When a memory trace decays, there is not only a functional loss of information, but also presumably a physical change in some neural state.

The memory constraints that have particular relevance to attentional processes include (1) limits on the nature of memory storage; (2) the characteristics of plasticity; (3) the nature of the interaction of short-term working memory with entry into long-term memory (LTM); (4) the way in which associative memory interacts with incoming perceptual information; and (5) the anatomical localization of different types of memory processes.

Limits on short-term memory (STM) storage exert a major influence on attentional capacity, timing, and the flow of information through the system. These limits are undoubtedly set by the neurophysiological constraints of the brain. For instance, the ability of most humans to handle approximately seven chunks of information at a time must be a function of a property of the system. However, why the system is able to hold only this amount of information in STM is not yet known. The most important limits on memory storage that affect attention are the rate of trace decay, the capacity of STM, and the rate at which information can be encoded into LTM (Atkinson & Shiffrin, 1968).

PLASTICITY OF NEURAL SYSTEMS

Neural plasticity is probably critical to both memory and attention. In order for a memory to be encoded, the brain must be capable of making some type of structural or neurochemical change. It is likely that some brain systems are much more plastic than others. For instance, some areas of the visual system are relatively stable in response characteristics, and other areas of the brain seem capable of changing the criteria under which activation occurs. Some of the neurophysiological mechanisms that are thought to underly neural plasticity were discussed in Chapter 7. Despite much research directed to delineating the mechanisms of neural plasticity, relatively little is known about the functional impact of neural plasticity.

In principle, brain regions that are capable of greater plasticity are able to form new associative networks and therefore have a capacity for adaptation. Brain systems that lack plasticity are more invariant in their response patterns, which provides a consistent structure on which information from the external world can be organized. There are advantages in having a system with both types of neural characteristics. Animals need to have some reference system that they can rely on to provide an invariant temporal-spatial framework, but they also need to be able to change their responses to incoming information under certain conditions.

The brain seems to take care of both these needs. There are primary sensory and motor areas that are designed with less plasticity, as well as secondary cortical areas with integrative capability that have greater plasticity. This allows the stimulus–response (S-R) part of the learning process to be more reflexive, and the intermediate processes of integration of the new information with existing memory to be more flexible.

Recent studies have suggested that certain sensory regions that have traditionally been thought to be unchanging in function may actually be relatively plastic. Merzenich, Kaas, Wall, Sur, Nelson, and Feldman (1983) found that the spatial map of the surface of the hand changes its neural representation after damage to the nerves that innervate it. After damage to the nerves of the hand, the region of the monkey's somatosensory cortex that had previously responded to stimulation of the hand failed to do so. Instead, the somatosensory region reorganized and became responsive to the somatic stimulation of other related anatomical areas.

Plasticity has been detected across many brain regions, including subcortical structures such as the reticular system and the thalamus (Singer, 1979, 1982). The hippocampus seems to have plasticity-modulated catecholamines, such as norepinephrine (Hopkins & Johnston, 1984). The locus coeruleus has also been shown to exhibit plasticity, a finding suggesting that the production of catecholamines within this nucleus can be modified by behavioral factors (Kasamatsu, Pettigrew, & Ary, 1979). Plasticity seems to occur in varying degrees across a broad range of neural structures. How plasticity is distributed in the brain is not yet well established.

CONSTRAINTS ON INFORMATION FLOW

Cognitive scientists have long debated how memory is represented in the brain and what is the arrangement of storage systems. Early cognitive models postulated compartmentalized memory stores and stages of processing with discrete functions (e.g., STM and LTM). It was thought that information passes through a "pipeline" of serially arranged operations. Investigators working from this perspective are likely to place STM at an earlier processing stage than LTM. Other models have discounted such a sequential arrangement of functional compartments and have suggested other types of memory organization. In some of these models, STM is considered not an information store, but an index of cognitive processing. The idea that STM reflects a comparison process between incoming information and memories from LTM leads to a different expectation regarding the flow of information in the brain.

A comprehensive model of memory should also describe the flow of information through the brain as it is transformed into various types of storage. Models of this type could be validated by tracking the flow of information from sensory areas to other brain regions during information processing. Unfortunately, it is extremely difficult to establish methodologies for accomplishing this goal. One approach that has been used in the past involves recording electrophysiological activation from multiple sites during different stages of information processing. Examples of the investigations that have attempted to show the interactions between different cortical regions during attention and learning were described in Chapter 4. We also discussed investigations into the neural bases of learning and attention (Chapter 7). There is an obvious need for additional research in this area.

Study of the neuroanatomical basis of memory is still in its infancy. Although progress is being made in understanding how memory is encoded in certain neural structures like the hippocampus, there is still much to be learned about how structures of the limbic system interact with association areas of the cortex. How LTM is represented in the cortex is not yet well established. Although sophisticated computational models have been proposed to account for distributed memory representation, neurophysiological evidence supporting a particular model is still sparse. Therefore, our understanding of the relationship between memory and attention is constrained by the limits of our knowledge of the neural representation of memory and information flow.

MODALITY-SPECIFIC CONSTRAINTS

The characteristics of attention vary as a function of sensory modality. The pattern of neural connectivity influences the way attention operates in each modality (see chapter 7). All sensory modalities have very specific cortical pathways and neural systems that perform modality-specific processing of stimuli based on primary features. For most sensory modalities, higher-level analysis is performed in secondary- or tertiary-association cortical areas. In the case of the visual system, spatial selective attention appears to be governed by such a cortical system (e.g., the inferior parietal lobule). Attentional systems for auditory and somatosensory information have not yet been well-documented, though presumably they also exist. Ultimately, it will be important to characterize the relationship between cortical systems that govern primary sensory registration and analysis and systems that govern attentional focusing relative to sensory information for each sensory system. The parameters underlying this relationship will undoubtedly enable investigators to better specify neural constraints on attention.

Most sensory systems also contain subcortical components that facilitate detection of stimuli prior to subsequent higher-level analysis. These subcortical systems play an important role in attention, as they enable an initial rapid response based on gross stimulus features. This response frequently facilitates a shift of attention, which in turn facilitates subsequent cortical processing. The relationship between subcortical and cortical systems illustrates that attentional operations occur at different stages of information processing. While much is now known about these subcortical systems, there is still relatively little data regarding the interaction of subcortical and cortical attentional systems. Parametric characterization of these interactions is extremely important for specification of the temporal dynamics of attention.

The pattern of connectivity between the sensory cortex and the system also is an important determinant of attention for each sensory modality. The olfactory system has direct access to the limbic system, which greatly influences the characteristics of olfactory attention and contributes to the strong appetitive nature of this modality. Other modalities, such as the visual system, have an extremely complex pattern of limbic connectivity, which enables great specificity of response to stimulus features. This pattern of connectivity represents another neural constraint that influences the characteristics of attention. Ultimately, it will be necessary to specify the unique features of each sensory modality as it relates to the processes of attention as we attempt to sepcify the neural constraints on attention.

FEEDBACK AND FEEDFORWARD ARRANGEMENTS

Many of the original information processing theories maintained that cognition depended on a serial processing arrangement comprised of sequential stages of cognitive operations (e.g., Sternberg, 1966). Most serial processing models contain some provision for feedback, so that information from the later stages of processing can be used to influence subsequent early information operations. However, researchers studying selective attention (e.g., Treisman, 1964) have provided strong evidence for selective attention at an early stage of information processing, without the benefit of feedback from response outcome. As there are limits to the number of feedback loops that can be executed in the brief duration of many cognitive operations, automatic attentional operations provide a mechanism for selection at these early stages of processing. Automatic attention does not depend on recursive serial processes, as many aspects of automatic attentional selection can be explained within a parallel processing framework. Attentional selection is governed by the predetermined salience of incoming information.

Still, there are many tasks for which feedback is a necessary component of attentional control. Some tasks cannot be performed using rapid automatic selection. For instance, the type of focused attention required to analyze potential moves in the game of chess depends on feedback from recursive cognitive operations. Generally, feedback from early (automatic) stages of information processing is necessary to maintain the sequential character of sustained attention. In order to perform a sustained attentional task, the individual must be able to make multiple recursive searches. A feedback component must be assumed to be part of such a process, as feedback would enable information derived form previous attentional operations to be used for later sequential comparisons.

In order to accommodate sequential attentional operations, a memory store must be present that will hold the information for repeated comparisons. There must also be a mechanism by which repeated searches are generated. The concept of executive control has obvious relevance to this generation process. Finally, there must be a feedback mechanism, that takes the information resulting from a comparison of new stimulus input and existing schemata and redirects it to these executive mechanisms for further processing. These requirements for serial attentional processing were delineated in computational terms in the early models of manual tracking (see Chapter 21). The compensatory tracking models of Licklider (1960) and others specified feedback networks that take information about the subject's attempt to hit a target and relay it back to a subtractor system that determine the difference between the response and the actual target position. This information is then used to approximate the next response.

Feedback is thought to be generated within the brain by the comparisons of incoming stimuli with existing memory. The characteristics of the information resulting from such comparisons are not known. It appears likely that activation by reticular, hypothalamic, and limbic stimulation facilitates attentional processing during sequential operations by providing an energetic catalyst. It is also well known that the various cortical association areas have descending pathways to limbic and other subcortical structures. These pathways seem to provide feedback from cognitive operations that influences further sequential attention processing. This influence would be accomplished through selective excitation or inhibition.

There are many cognitive operations that could produce a modulation of activational response. One likely basis of this effect is the hypothetical comparison process that we previously alluded to, by which incoming stimuli are compared to existing templates. Earlier in this book, models of the orienting response were reviewed that suggested this type of comparison process. For instance, Sokolov's model (1963) of habituation proposes that the result of this type of comparison determines whether the animal will continue to respond to the stimulus or will habituate. Subsequent, neurophysiological models of habituation have also been proposed. The neural systems that are necessary in providing feedback for habituation will indicate how this atttentional response is modulated.

Feedback appears to be critical in most cognitive and behavioral functions. For instance, motor control is very dependent on feedback from the body regarding position, trajectory, and speed. Studies of the extrapyramidal control of movements like reaching suggest that there are processes that allow for a fine level of approximation as a movement is executed. Often, there is initially a very gross movement. As the trajectory of the movement is established, feedback from the limb that is moving enables small adjustments so that the individual is able to approach the target accurately.

The feedback to be effective in controlling the broad range of attentional behavior, there must be a large number of pathways that are highly flexible (plastic) and that have considerable specificity in their ability to resond to certain types of cortical output. Neuroanatomical researchers have devoted much effort to delineating the feedback arrangements that exist between limbic structures, the hypothalamus, the reticular system, and cortical regions. Although significant strides have been made, little is known about the functional specificity of the pathways between these structures.

The type of feedback that has been described for sustained attention enables the integration of sensory information with response production. As a result, a series of processing "steps" can occur as the system responds to sensory information, adjusts its response, and then establishes feedback for the next selection. This series of steps is the basis for controlled attention.

We suggested earlier that feedback may not be required for automatic attention. An example is the orienting response (OR). The OR is associated with an attentional redirection that occurs in an automatic, reflexive manner. Yet, a different type of feedback may be an essential part of some automatic attentional processes. From the standpoint of the neural network models that we have discussed previously, the term *feedback* refers to the pattern of connectivity between activational units. When stimulus elements interact with each other, they may produce excitatory or inhibitory effects that influence the relative strength of an associative connection. If the neural system is actually multilayered, as some network models suggest, there is also feedback between different levels of associative organization. This feedback differs from that involved in directed or effortful attention because, in a parallel network, feedback does not imply an executive action. Instead, it reflects those interactions among associative elements that result in a change in attentional bias. Feedback of this type would be highly related to the plasticity of the neural elements in different brain regions. Outside those studies that have investigated the interaction of the neural cells contained in cortical fields, little is known about the neurobehavioral basis of this type of feedback.

Attention may also depend on feedforward arrangements that enable the system to generate a response program when certain conditions are met. In the case of feedback, information regarding a response outcome is used to adjust future sensory selection criteria (i.e., selection that occurs during earlier stages of processing). With a feedforward arrangement, the attentional system can adjust the criteria for executing a particular response sequence based on the effects of information that has been selected. Feedforward mechanisms account for recursive (iterative) operations that influence many executive functions that require a self-generated search, such as problem solving and categorization. Feedforward mechanisms may also play a role in self-awareness, as self-directed attention probably requires a self-generated search for internal cues. Feed forward loops may facilitate the shift of attentional focus from perception to action (McLeod & Posner, 1984).

SUMMARY

The structural and physiological properties of the brain influence the types of operations it can perform. Although this statement seems obvious, psychological researchers did not always view the physical properties of the neural system as relevant. From the perspective of cognitive neuroscience, brain structure and function are intricately related, and the properties of the neural system determine whether particular cognitive models are feasible.

There are many ways in which the functional characteristics of neural systems constrain how information is processed. Some of the constraints discussed in this chapter that seem to influence attentional processing include:

1. Neural speed
2. Neuronal response properties
3. Activational characteristics
4. Temporal attunements
5. Memory dynamics
6. Plasticity
7. Information flow dynamics
8. Feedback arrangements
9. Neural network organization

The parameters underlying these factors have not been specified across all neural systems of the brain. Therefore, it is difficult to estimate the relative contribution of each constraint in determining the capacity or limitations of attentional performance. In some cases, these limitations have been specified in experimentally controlled situations. For instance, the limits of STM pose constraints on attention that are very robust; however, the neural basis for STM is still not clear.

In most cases, there are relatively little data from the neurosciences so that it is difficult to delineate the physical bases for each constraint. Therefore, it is not easy to specify the parametric relationship of these factors to the control of attention.

Processing Speed and Attentional Resources

BRIAN F. O'DONNELL and RONALD A. COHEN

Does the speed of information processing within the CNS influence the quantity of information that can be evaluated and, consequently, attentional capacity? Processing speed, as measured by reaction time, was studied intermittently as an indicator of individual differences in mental function in the late nineteenth century, but this line of investigation was essentially abandoned until the 1970s (Vernon, 1987).

One reason why this line of work was abandoned might be the implausibility of its premise, that studies of reaction times on simple discrimination tasks might predict performance on far more complex tasks, such as verbal reasoning. Given the richness and complexity of human intellectual behavior, such a hypothesis seems absurdly reductionistic. The resurrection of reaction time—or more generally, processing speed—as a candidate predictor of more abstract measures of intelligence probably has more to do with the emergence of models of mental capacity in which mental speed plays a central role than with the persuasive power of sporadic studies of reaction time and "IQ." Such a relationship is implicit in constructs such as channel capacity or attentional capacity, which reflect the speed at which mental operations can be performed.

ATTENTIONAL CAPACITY AND INTELLIGENCE

Attentional capacity and the limits it places on performance have a central role in information-processing psychology. Attentional capacity is required to carry out effortful or novel tasks whose performance has not been automatized. Attentional capacity is frequently said to be limited by the availability of cognitive or processing resources, which are frequently referred to as the *resource pool*. Performance of more than one effortful task at a time is difficult from both an experimental and an introspective perspective. Therefore, dual-task performance has been one of the primary tools for the investigation of attentional capacity.

Although cognitive resources are frequently invoked as an explanatory principle in theories of attentional capacity, the neuroanatomical or mental elements that compose resources have been little discussed. Cognitive resources can be thought of as composing a single pool that all volitionally organized tasks draw on, or as consisting of multiple independent resource pools that can be tapped independently for performance on a given task. Hirst (1986) noted that cognitive resources are described in at least two ways, in terms of structures, like working memory, or of fuel, like arousal or effort. Shiffrin and Schneider (1977) stressed the importance of the limitations of working memory as a structural constraint on attentional capacity. Kahneman (1973) stressed the role of arousal and effort in modulating performance. Wickens (1984) discussed evidence for a variety of structural resources, or pools, that constrain performance, such as spatial versus verbal encoding.

Attentional capacity has several attributes in common with intellectual capacity as described by psychometric theory (Table 17.1). Like attention, intelligence has been described in terms of single or multiple factors; has been determined by structural and fuel-like components; and is best measured by tasks that demand effortful processing. Attentional capacity is said to be determined by an aggregate of cognitive resources, which have been described as a single pool, or as consisting of separable resource pools. Intelligence has also been described as a single entity that is drawn on by many types of tasks or as a complex aggregate of many factors. Attentional capacity has been described as being determined by cognitive structures and fuels, such as effort or arousal. Intellectual performance has been posited to be jointly determined by abstract-thinking capacity and personality factors, such as motivation or persistence. Attentional capacity is used up by controlled processes but is unaffected by automatic processes. Consequently, attentional capacity is usually tested in relation to performance on two effortful tasks. Similarly, intelligence is typically measured by performance on tasks that demand controlled or effortful processing. If these analogies are correct, then individual differences on measures of intelligence ought to correlate with measures of attentional capacity.

ATTENTIONAL CAPACITY AND PROCESSING SPEED

From the standpoint of classical information-processing theory, a system's information-processing capacity is directly related to the rate of processing within the system: faster rates of processing are characteristic of larger capacity systems (Broadbent, 1958; Shannon & Weaver, 1949). If the human mind can be conceptualized as a serial, single-channel processor at the level of consciously directed performance, even a simple task could provide an index of processing rate that would have more general significance in determining intellectual performance.

Processing rate might be especially critical on tasks that require the manipulation of information within working memory. Because the contents of working memory rapidly decay, encoding of information in "chunks" and storage in long-term memory are required before further information can be accepted into working memory. If new information is

TABLE 17.1.   Attributes of Attentional Capacity and Intelligence

Attribute	Capacity	Intelligence
Types	Single vs. multiple pools	Single vs. multiple factors
Components	Cognitive structures	Factors
Energy	Effort and arousal	Motivation
Measurement	Tests of controlled or effortful performance	Tests of controlled or effortful performance

acquired before working-memory space is available, either the new or the old information will be lost. As the perceiver usually does not control the rate at which information is presented in the environment, this loss is not an uncommon occurrence.

Most people have had the experience of finding a classroom lecture going too quickly for note taking (shadowing) or assimilation in a classroom. Or after asking for directions of a local person, we receive a rapidly paced description of distances, turns, and landmarks that become irretrievably jumbled by the time we take to the road again. In both cases, the rate of information presentation has exceeded working-memory capacity and rate of processing; the result is degradation of the information. Performance failures due to inadequate processing speed were called *divided-attention deficits* by Shiffrin and Schneider (1977).

The relationship of reaction time to capacity demands was further specified by Norman and Bobrow (1975). Although attentional capacity is typically characterized through a dual-task paradigm, Norman and Bobrow hypothesized that demands on attentional capacity by a task may be directly reflected in reaction time measures. Moreover, the relationship of error rate and reaction time may be determined by the nature of the task, rather than solely by the response criteria adopted by the performer. Norman and Bobrow distinguished between data-limited tasks and resource-limited tasks. In data-limited tasks, performance is limited by environmental properties, like signal-to-noise ratio in a signal detection experiment. In resource-limited tasks, performance is limited by the resources of the performer.

Accuracy and reaction time have different relationships on data-limited tasks and on resource-limited tasks. On data-limited tasks, reaction time is inversely related to accuracy. Shorter reaction times are typically related to better performance, particularly when the task involves a brief signal presentation. On data-limited tasks, easy discriminations are associated with short, accurate reaction times, and hard discriminations are associated with long, less accurate reaction times. There is no speed–accuracy trade-off. In resource-limited tasks, on the other hand, there is a speed–accuracy trade-off. Accurate responses take more time, as accurate decisions require cognitive operations that may go on long after the end of a stimulus event. On resource-limited tasks, rapid decisions are often made at the expense of accuracy.

Although Norman and Bobrow (1975) did not consider the implications of these proposed relationships in the study of individual differences, it is probable that a person with more resources to deploy on a task will complete it more quickly. If cognitive resources can be described as a single pool or channel called *attentional capacity*, reaction time on a resource-limited task may provide a direct index of the resources within a system. If cognitive resources are related to intelligence, then individual differences in reaction time would be correlated with measures of intelligence as well. This hypothesis has received substantial empirical support over the past two decades.

PROCESSING SPEED AND INTELLECTUAL PERFORMANCE

Several recent theories of intelligence stress the critical importance of mental speed in a system that operates as a single-channel processor with a short-term memory of very limited capacity and rapid decay (see Eysenk, 1987, for a historical review of this work). Motivated by these theories, a series of empirical studies have shown that choice reaction time, reaction time variability, and, less consistently, the slope of reaction time on the number of response alternatives in bits correlate with measures of intellectual performance (Jensen, 1982; Vernon, 1987). Shorter reaction times, less reaction-time variability, and more shallow reaction-time slopes are associated with better performance on psychometric tests of intelligence. The correlation between IQ-type measures and reaction time (RT) averages about .30 across studies, but coefficient magnitudes range widely in value. As different studies have used different samples, different RT paradigms, and different psychometric tests, this variability is not unexpected.

Some investigators have reported remarkably high RT-IQ correlation coefficients. For example, Brand (1981) summarized a series of studies that correlated a RT task requiring the discrimination of line length with measures of IQ. The correlation between RT and tests of verbal intelligence was in the range of .60 and .90, depending on the sample characteristics and the type of IQ test used. Counterintuitively, this spatial RT task did not correlate with visuospatial IQ.

Jensen and Vernon (1986) argued that choice RT is primarily reflective of mental speed, because the task makes no demands on higher cognitive processes. Taking issue with the characterization of choice RT as a simple task, Detterman (1987) cogently argued that it may be influenced by a number of cognitive or personological factors, such as the comprehension and interpretation of the task instructions, motivation, sensory acuity, response selection strategies, memory, and attention. The importance of RT variability, in particular, argues for the influence of attentional factors on task performance. For these reasons, it is impossible to draw the conclusion that mental speed or neural speed directly modulates intellectual performance. From the perspective of channel-capacity or attentional-capacity predictions, this is not a major issue, as these models posit that processing speed is modulated by an aggregate of cognitive resources.

PROCESSING SPEED AND BRAIN DYSFUNCTION

If processing speed is a function of the capacity of the brain to carry out conscious, attentionally demanding tasks, then brain dysfunction associated with a reduction in intellectual performance will be also associated with a slowing in processing speed on effortful tasks. Indeed, choice reaction time is slowed in a wide variety of brain disturbances, including schizophrenia, head trauma, Alzheimer's disease, mental retardation, and multiple sclerosis. As these diseases are associated with varied clinical and neuropathological findings, the slowing of processing speed appears to provide a relatively nonspecific index of mental capacity. Investigators have provided evidence that changes in intellectual function in the course of aging are best characterized by a slowing in processing speed (e.g., Birren, Woods, & Williams, 1980; Salthouse, 1982).

Reaction time measures cannot directly isolate the specific contributions of sensory, cognitive, response-selection, and response-execution speed to performance. Evoked-potential measures offer the possibility of obtaining premotor measures of processing speed. The P3, or P300, response, an electrophysiological measure whose latency reflects the time required to evaluate a stimulus, has been investigated in both normal and brain-damaged individuals. Prolongation of the P3 response of the auditory event-related potential has been repeatedly associated with changes in brain function related to aging and dementia. P3 slowing over the adult life span was first reported by Goodin, Squires, Henderson, & Starr (1978). Even more dramatic P3 slowing has been observed in patients with dementia (Goodin, Squires, and Starr, 1978, 1983). P3 latency prolongation was subsequently reported in a variety of adult-onset neurological disorders associated with impaired intellectual or memory performance, including heterogeneous groups of demented patients (Pfefferbaum, et al., 1984; Polich, Ehlers, Otis, Mandell, & Bloom, 1986; Syndulko et al., 1982), Parkinson's disease (Goodin & Aminoff, 1984; Hansch et al., 1982; O'Donnell et al., 1987), and Huntington's disease (Homberg, Hefter, Granseyer, Strauss, Lange, & Hennerici, 1986).

If P3 prolongation reflects a disturbance in a specific mental process (e.g., span of apprehension or auditory working memory), then P3 prolongation would be expected to correlate most strongly with experimental, psychometric, or clinical measures of such deficits. If P3 prolongation reflects reduction of the overall processing capacity of the brain, it would tend to correlate with a broad spectrum of clinical and psychological measures of mental function.

In studies to date, variations in P3 latency have been reported to correlate with a wide variety of psychometric measures, a report suggesting that, like choice RT, it reflects changes in overall capacity rather than specific stages in information processing. Polich *et al.* (1986) reported that P3 latency showed a curvilinear relationship to the severity of qualitative estimates of global cognitive impairment in dementia. Although the relationship between P3 latency and severity was monotonic, the most significant change in P3 latency occurred in patients with severe cognitive impairment. Kraiuhin *et al.* (1986) found that, after accounting for the effect of age, 57% of the variation in P3 latency among elderly subjects could be related to psychometric performance. The strongest predictors of P3 latency were a test of word learning, and Block Design from the Wechsler Adult Intelligence Scale–Revised (WAIS-R). O'Donnell *et al.* (1990) found that measures of P3 latency correlated with psychometric performance in elderly adults and in patients with dementing disorders. In a pooled group of persons at risk for Huntington's disease and patients with Huntington's disease, Homberg *et al.* (1986) reported that P3 latency correlated with verbal and performance subtests of the WAIS-R, as well as with other tests of memory and intellectual function. P3 latency was most strongly related to tests requiring concentration, immediate recall, and speeded processing of visual material. P3 latency was not influenced by depression or psychotic symptomatology. In Parkinson's disease, Hansch, Syndulko, Cohen, Goldberg, Potvin, and Tourtellotte (1982) found that P3 latency was most strongly related to the Symbol-Digit Modalities test, although other psychometric measures and a clinical disability score were also related to P3 latency. O'Donnell *et al.* (1987) replicated the strong relationship between P3 latency and Symbol-Digit performance in Parkinson's disease patients. They also found that P3 latency was correlated with tests requiring the learning or the mental manipulation of information, but not with measures of verbal performance, digit span, motor disturbance, or depression.

P3 latency, therefore, shows a consistent relationship to measures of intellectual function in disorders associated with dementia. P3 latency appears to be most reliably associated with performance on tests of speeded visual processing, concentration, and learning. P3 latency seems less associated with noncognitive aspects of brain dysfunction, such as depression, psychosis, and motor disturbance. In none of the above studies was N1 latency a reliable correlate of intellectual performance. As P3 latency is influenced by cognitive variables, whereas N1 latency in this paradigm is primarily responsive to stimulus properties, this dissociation suggests that a measure of processing speed provides more information about mental capacity when it reflects the performance of a cognitive process.

SUMMARY

Measures of processing speed obtained in the context of discrimination paradigms have been consistently correlated with psychometric tests of intellectual performance. Choice RT, RT variability, and P3 latency are all associated with cognitive performance in normal individuals and in patients with brain dysfunction. These findings provide strong empirical support for the notion that attentional capacity, or the capacity of the system to carry out conscious, effortful processing, can be characterized as a serial processor whose performance is roughly proportional to processing speed. The strength of this relationship has varied among studies, however. In various studies, the correlation between measures of processing speed and intellectual performance has varied in magnitude from .10 to .90. The sources of this variation are not clear. The number and variability of the subjects in the study, the nature and difficulty of the processing-speed task, and the psychometric properties of the intellectual tests used clearly have an impact on coefficient magnitude, but these relationships have yet to be adequately described. From a theoretical perspective, the correlation of measures of attentional capacity from classic dual-task paradigms with psychometric and RT measures of performance may provide empirical support for the hypothesis that attentional capacity and intelligence (as measured by intelligence tests) expresses the same underlying factors.

The psychobiological basis of the relationship between processing speed and intellectual performance remains unknown. It is unlikely that processing speed directly reflects neural conduction times, or that mental speed is an innate property of the mind. Rather, processing speed for consciously motivated performance probably represents a complex interaction of biological substrates, conscious strategies, and learned skills.

The Mutual Constraint of Memory and Attention

Throughout this text, we have emphasized that the processes of attention and memory are interrelated. In fact, all of Chapter 4 was devoted to a discussion of how attention was accounted for in behavioral learning theories. Even though most of the original models of conditioning did not specify an attentional process, much emphasis was placed on describing how the response tendencies of an animal vary as a function of changes in the field of stimuli during conditioning. Furthermore, the factors governing stimulus and response selection were a central focus of the conditioning studies, which often described phenomena that we might now label as *attentional* when attempting to specify the rules governing learning. Therefore, for learning theorists, learning, memory, and attention were conceptually linked.

With the emergence of cognitive psychology, there has been a tendency among some theorists to view memory and attention as separate faculties in the sequential flow of information processing. Much debate has been focused on whether attention and memory are distinct processes that need to be studied separately or are nested properties of each other. The distinction between memory phenomena and attention is not always clear-cut. The early information-processing models proposed that memory was organized in storage systems that varied in accordance with their durability (Atkinson & Shiffrin, 1968). Subsequently, a concept of *working memory* emerged that broke from theories that considered memory a passive storage system. The levels-of-processing framework is an example of a theoretical perspective that rejected memory as a passive form of storage (Craik & Lockhart, 1972). Memory was viewed as a by-product of the active processing of the individual relative to the salience and associative properties of the information being presented (Baddeley, 1966a,b). Investigators advocating a working memory were likely to consider attention a direct correlate of the processes of memory encoding.

There are compelling reasons for considering the constraints placed by the characteristics of memory encoding and storage on attention. Learning and memory have a direct impact on the processes of attention and vice versa. Specification of memory parameters better enables prediction of attentional charcteristics. Conversely, determination of the influences of attentional processes on memory operations is also important. Therefore, in this chapter we consider the mutual constraints of memory and attention.

SYSTEMIC MEMORY CONSTRAINTS ON ATTENTION

The influence of memory on attention seems to depend on the type of memory that is considered. Models of memory vary considerably with regard to proposed underlying neural mechanisms. Therefore, it is important to first consider the hypothetical processes suggested by different models. Since the neurobiological foundations of memory storage are still not well understood, the validation of specific models of memory based on physiological evidence has not been possible. The relationship between attention and memory first must be established by analyzing how attention is affected by certian behavioral or phenomenological characteristcs of memory. Then, a proposed memory constraint on attention can be tested for fit with existing neurophysiological evidence.

The early information-processing theories tended to view attention and memory as two discrete phenomena. For instance, Broadbent (1958) suggested the presence of sensory, short-term, and long-term memory storages that were serially arranged in an information-processing sequence. The concept of multiple memory storages was elaborated by Atkinson and Shiffrin (1968). *Attention* referred to processes that controlled the selection of information passing into and out of short-term (STM) and long-term memory (LTM). Within these frameworks, the processes of attention occurred at different stages of processing.

The sequential nature of the multistore stage models was heavily scrutinized. The early processing stages (e.g., perceptual recognition) depend on the analysis of information contained in LTM. Therefore, the later stage of entry into LTM must affect the earlier stages in the processing sequence. Models that proposed stages of processing had difficulty accounting for how late-stage processes could affect processes at earlier stages. Bower and Hilgard (1981) argued that if multiple memory storage systems exist, there must be considerable interaction among them.

Norman (1968) proposed an alternative to the two-stage memory models. He suggested that the distinction between LTM and STM is not as fixed as originally proposed. Instead, STM storage reflects the state of activation of elements from LTM storage. Activation can be induced by incoming stimuli. Therefore, STM would reflect the active processes of attention and learning, while LTM would refer to the broader domain of all information stored by the individual. Estes (1950) anticipated this distinction in his statistical learning theory, when he proposed that both the conditioning and availability of information must be accounted for during learning.

There is an advantage to considering STM a very different form of storage from LTM. By viewing STM as a passive buffer that holds information for short periods prior to entry into LTM, one must accept the presence of separate storage areas that are arranged serially, like the components of a computer prototype. The problems suggested by Bower and Hilgard then become quite evident. On the other hand, if STM is the by-product of activation induced by incoming information interacting with existing LTM information, then separate storage areas do not have to be present. In this case, STM can be viewed as a transient form of storage with durability determined by the system's processing characteristics, and the rate at which information fades from active processing.

The distinction between LTM and STM has been supported by the fact that during some types of tasks, information is held for brief time periods but not stored permanently. For example, subjects are typically able to recall seven digits or words in sequence after short time periods. However, the items are not recalled after long durations unless the information is salient or the subjects are instructed to learn the items for later recall. The apparent universality of STM capacity at approximately seven bits of information indicates that there must be limits to the size of STM, again distinguishing it from the limitless LTM. Many other distinctions have been suggested, some based on how the content of these memories differ.

ON THE NATURE OF STM

While it is beyond the scope this chapter to review all of the proposed differences between STM and LTM, it should be noted that this functional dichotomy has held up for many years. Yet there continue to be disagreements over the processes underlying STM. The most traditional view is that STM is a short-duration buffer comprised of some transient form of "memory trace," with characteristics similiar to a sensory trace. Alternatively, some memory researchers have considered STM to be a by-product of "working memory." From this perspective, STM results from a process, such as an articulatory loop, through which recently presented information is covertly handled in a recursive feedfoward manner. According to both these views, the duration of STM is constrained by some charcteristic of the proposed underlying mechanism.

Some theorists maintain that STM and LTM may not actually be separate froms of memory. For instance, in Anderson's (1983) adaptive control of thought (ACT) model of semantic memory, STM is conceptualized to be the activated region of the semantic network. This view of STM substitutes *activation* for an actual memory buffer system. Interestingly, this type of model may actually provide the most direct link between memory and attention, since the activated state that produces STM would also reflect the current attentional focus. While this view of STM is intriguing, the characteristics of the "activational state" and the parameters that would underlie such a state have not been fully resolved. Therefore, while there is widespread agreement regarding the functional distinction of STM, there continues to be many unresolved issues surrounding the nature of the processes that result in STM.

Very-Short-Term Memory

Distinctions between STM and even shorter duration memories have also been shown. Sperling (1960) developed a paradigm that demonstrated that subjects could store very large amounts of information for several hundred milliseconds following presentation when partial recall was required. This finding suggested the presence of a very-short-term iconic memory that decayed quickly. Studies of auditory memory have suggested an analogous form of sensory registration (Massaro, 1972, 1975). The possibility that both short-term and very-short-term memory may be forms of sensory storage has been suggested (Cowan, 1984). The fact that both forms of short-term storage decay over relatively brief periods, when entry into LTM is prevented, is a basis for considering that they are forms of sensory storage. However, Cowan argued that there are two forms of STM: one that is sensory and one that is nonsensory.

Support for the idea that STM contains a form of sensory memory comes from studies of spatial effects on recall. Spatial location of visually presented information affects the decay rate of the stimulus template. This was shown on tasks that required a subject to match a second new stimulus with a previously presented template to make a same-different judgment (Phillips, 1974; Walker, 1978). When the target was in an identical location, STM span was longer than when the location was varied.

SPECIFIC MEMORY CONSTRAINTS ON ATTENTION

Storage capacity and the rate of memory trace decay are particularly important constraints on attention. Unfortunately, determining the rate of memory decay and the capacity for storage is not a simple task. Memory storage characteristics vary as a function of the sensory modality and of the characteristics of the information to be processed. Many cognitive researchers now believe that memory is not a unitary entity; rather, there are multiple forms of memory storage. If so, it may be difficult to establish one univeral set of parameters for decay rate and the amount of information that can be stored.

Decay Rates

Regardless of whether one accepts that STM exists in two forms (sensory and non-sensory), it is obvious that the decay rates for different types of sensory memory have a bearing on the influence of STM on attentional processes. Decay rates vary as a function of the sensory modality and of the amount of interference blocking attention to the stimuli. There is now considerable neurophysiological evidence for multiple types of memory, each with specific time-dependent characteristics (e.g., McGaugh, 1966).

The presence of a very-short-term sensory storage, with a durability of several hundred milliseconds, and a longer term sensory storage that has a durability of multiple seconds (Cowan, 1988) has been demonstrated. The first type of sensory memory seems to contain a literal template of the original stimuli. One can disrupt the durability of the very-short-term sensory trace by introducing a masking stimulus. The mask causes an erasure of the original trace. This type of sensory memory was originally thought to be a component of visual processing since auditory information seems to have a longer echoic trace. Shorter-duration auditory traces that lasted approximately 200 msec have also been described (Cowan, 1988).

The longer-term sensory memory has been shown to have a duration of between 10 and 20 sec. The durability of longer-term sensory storage can be reduced by the introduction of interference, though the mechanism seems to be different from that in the case of the very-short-term store. This memory may not contain a literal sensory representation of the original stimulus; instead, it may be the result of higher level information processing.

Although STM may have a sensory component, there are also indications of a nonsensory type, which can be established by studies in which the storage of sensory memory is prevented while the durability of nonsensory storage is assessed. The Consonant Trigram task developed by Peterson and Peterson (1959) provides one means of testing nonsensory STM. Subjects typically show a dramatic decline in performance over the course of 18 sec when an interfering task is introduced during the time delay. Studies have been designed to discriminate between the contributions of sensory and nonsensory interference, by having the subject perform the interfering task either in the same sensory modality or in a different modality from the memory component of the task. Generally, greater interference is noted when the two tasks are in the same modality.

LIMITED CAPACITY AND SHORT-TERM STORAGES

The capacity of STM was established many years ago in studies by G. Miller (1956). The fact that individuals can hold approximately seven units of information in short-term storage indicates that this form of memory is of quite limited capacity. Subsequent studies have suggested that this capacity is actually more robust, as the seven units can range from simple, unidimensional sensory elements to complex chunks of information. Although seven words and seven phonemes have an identical number of units, the words ultimately provide more than seven bits of information. Nonetheless, STM is relatively limited in its capacity.

The capacity of very-short-term sensory memory is not as limited as that of short-term memory. Studies of iconic memory illustrate that vast fields of information may be accessible in sensory memory for short periods. However, the capacity of this form of memory is restricted by its rapid rate of decay. As iconic memory lasts for only several hundred milliseconds, only a small part of a large stimulus field can actually be retrieved.

SHORT-TERM STORAGE AND ATTENTION

With respect to our consideration of attention, it is worth noting that, during interference, the redirection of attention to a new task seems to reduce the durability of both sensory and nonsensory STM. This reduction is a function of the degree of effort required for the distracting task. A task that requires a subject to perform serial addition by 3's is likely to cause greater decrements than a simple counting task. The durability of STM also has a direct effect on attentional processes. This relationship was discussed in Chapter 2, where we considered Schneider and Shiffrin's distinction (1977) of effortful and automatic processes in the control of attention. However, for an attentional process to become automatic, presumably it must handle information or a procedure that is already in LTM.

The relationship between STM and attention is more complicated. As STM may be composed of a sensory storage, the durability of this memory should facilitate attentional performance on tasks that fall within the time limits of this sensory trace. It is difficult to establish exactly how very-short-duration sensory memory influences spontaneous attention. In the early studies of iconic memory, the relationship between storage and attention was determined by the characteristics of the experimental paradigm. When the subject was cued to scan at a certain spatial position after the original stimulus array was removed, very accurate memory recall was possible (partial report). Performance declines when recall of the entire list is required, since the time frame of iconic storage is surpassed.

In the original partial report paradigm (Sperling, 1960), attention is directed by the examiner. In natural situations, the direction of attention to elements of the stimulus field must occur as a function of the task requirements, or as the result of an internally mediated process. As the duration of iconic storage is extremely short, its effect on attention can occur only as the result of a rapid selection of salient elements from the stimulus field. Attentional selection of this sort must be automatic, as effortful serial processing would not be possible within this time. Very-short-term sensory memory may constrain the parallel processing that occurs during the early stages of attention. However, the impact of this type of storage on selective attention is not well established.

LONG-TERM STORAGE: CAPACITY AND DURABILITY

In contrast to the shorter term memory storages, LTM is generally thought to be of limitless capacity. Humans are capable of recalling a tremendous quantity of remote information. The retrieval of information on popular board games such as Trivial Pursuit reflects this fact. Yet, there may be some constraints on the capacity of LTM, which arise from the manner in which information is represented in this type of memory. How information is organized in LTM associative memory is a major field of cognitive study and well beyond the scope of this book. For the purposes of our discussion, the important point for consideration is that the concept of capacity that holds for STM does not seem to have the same meaning in connection with LTM.

A potential indicator of the breadth of LTM is the quantity of information knowledge that individuals have. Information knowledge is an index of stored semantic information that is available to the individual and that may provide an indication of the current holdings in the LTM of a given individual. However information knowledge cannot be used as a measure of LTM capacity, as the current knowledge is a function of previous exposure. An individual with limited information knowledge may have a limitless capacity but may not have received the information at the same rate as other people with greater funds of knowledge. Furthermore, LTM contains more than discrete units of information, such as the name of the current president. It also seems to contain networks of associative information that may be highly integrated and non-specific or, conversely, very exact in associative reference (Wickelgren, 1975, 1979). For these reasons, evaluating LTM memory capacity is a difficult proposition.

The concept of a limitless LTM must be considered in light of the differences between information storage in LTM and in STM. Information in LTM may not be stored as a direct representation of the initial sensory features of the stimulus; rather, it may exist in a more integrated or consolidated form. It may be a reconstruction of past information or a representation based on the collective activation of a network of associative characteristics. Long-term storage is typically activated in response to internal or external demands. The process by which the individual selectively retrieves information from LTM can be considered attention. In this sense, attention reflects the selective activation of LTM. In the next section, we will discuss the relationship between attention, context, and the semantic networks that many theorists believe constitute LTM.

SEMANTIC AND CONTEXTUAL CONSTRAINTS

Given that attention involves the selective focusing and directing of cognitive operations, it should be no surprise that the semantic and contextual factors greatly influence how attention is allocated. Attention directs cognitive processing toward information that is salient, meaningful, or contextually relevant, enabling one to ignore or disengage from information that is irrelevant or meaningless.

The relationship between attention and semantic associative memory as considerable relevance for cognitive science. Ultimately, "thinking" may be viewed as the interaction between our attentional focus and the semantic organization of associative information derived from previous learning. From this perspective, the interaction of attention and semantic memory should be a central topic of cognitive psychology. Semantics and context influence how information or knowledge is represented in memory. While the existence of some types of human memory with minimal semantic underpinnings appears likely (e.g., procedural memory), there is overwhelming evidence that much of knowledge is organized in memory on the basis of semantic and contextual properties, which reflect the significance or "meaning" of information. Therefore, consideration of the mutual constaints of memory and attention requires determination of how semantic and contextual factors influence attention.

At issue is a larger question: How does knowledge from already existing memory representations influence our efforts to derive meaning from ongoing experience and thereby govern our attentional focus? There has been little research directed specifically at the nature of this relationship. Cognitive theorists who are interested in the nature of associate representation usually assume that attention is simply either a by-product or an emergent property of the current state of activation within the associative network. Conversely, attentional researchers have frequently focused on topics such as spatial selection or the parameters underlying attentional capacity, avoiding the murkier issues surrounding the relationship between attention and semantic memory. Despite the lack of research directly related to these issues, there have been attempts to link the processes of attention and semantic memory. Knowledge about this relationship has also emerged from investigations of other cognitive phenomena.

The relationship of semantic and contextual factors to the allocation of attention has been discussed indirectly in the context of earlier topics of this book. For instance, in our consideration of the orienting response we described how researchers have demonstrated a relationship between the OR and the conditioning of the semantic information of verbal stimuli (Maltzman, 1968, 1979). In his consideration of the neuropsychological bases of attention, Posner and colleagues (1988) suggested that certain brain systems, such as the anterior cingulate cortex, may influence the intensity of attentional focus on the basis of semantic relevance. Given the relevance of these issues to determining the focus of attention and to understanding the mutual interaction of attention and memory, we will now briefly consider some of the ways by which semantic and contextual factors constrain attention.

Stimulus Salience and Attention

One of the most fundamental principles derived from the early classical and operant learning theories is that behavior is influenced by the salience of the presented stimulus. During Pavlovian conditioning, an unconditioned stimulus (UCS) is almost certain to elicit a reponse, while the likelihood of a response diminishes based on the strength of the conditioined stimulus (CS). Furthermore, certain CSs gain maximum strength when presented in the context of other stimuli. Similiarly, operant conditioning is greatly influenced by the salience of the stimulus that is provided as reinforcement for a particular response. In both cases, the behavioral repsonse is a direct by-product of the organismic value of a salient stimulus.

The orienting response (OR), which is a direct outgrowth of classical conditioning research, provides an obvious example of how the salience of stimuli influences attention. Both the amplitude of the initial OR and subsequent habituation rate vary in proportion to the salience of the eliciting stimulus. While a response can be considered a true OR, only if the eliciting stimulus is not an UCS or already conditioned (CS), stimuli differ in their instrinsic salience (e.g., amplitude, novelty, etc.). As a result, it is relatively easy to demonstrate not only the effect of specific stimulus parameters on the overt attentional response, but also the underlying neurophysiological mechanisms that influence orienting. For instance, the P300 evoked brain potential response that is elicited during auditory "oddball" paradigms provides a direct measure of how stimulus uniqueness produces a specific attentional response.

Salience, Semantics, and Attention

Orienting response variations that occur relative to the degree of intrinsic stimulus salience reflects a more primitive level of attention than can be reasonably attributed to *semantics*. Yet, moving from the level of salience charcterized by stimulus features to semantic properties does not require a major conceptual leap of faith. Semantics reflect the relationship between signs, symbols, and referential meaning, and semantic value is a by-product of the associative properties of these signs and symbols relative to the underlying objects or concepts that they represent.

The idea that a relationship may exist between the development of the associative–symbolic representations and basic attentional responsses such as the OR is not new. Maltzman (1968, 1979) maintained that "changes in the direction of thinking" depend on shifts of attention rather than simply the evocation of associations. Maltzman went on to demonstate that distinctions could be made between ORs based on the semantic characteristics of a task and that conditioning, extinction, and generalization of autonomic response to semantic presentations (i.e., words) took place even when no prior conditioning occurred. In one study, Maltzman, Langdon, and Feeney (1970) instructed subjects to make a motor response whenever the word *light* was presented. However, the word *light* never occurred, but instead a series of irrelevant words were presented until the subject habituated. Subsequently, test words were presented that had some associative relationship to the word *light*, along with irrelevant words. Subjects exhibited greater autonomic response (galvanic skin response) to the test words that were semantically related to *light* than to irrelevant words. This finding of semantic generalization without conditioning was interpreted by Maltzman to be an indication that semantic activation leads to a"dominant focus" of attention. This attentional focus increases activational strength of semantically related information within the associative set, without the need for conditioning.

As we discussed previously, the magnitude and characteristics of psychophysiological and attentional responses elicited during cognitive processing depend on the type of semantic operations required during the task (e.g., Cohen & Waters, 1985). Tasks that demand more complex semantic processing elicit greater activation and attentional allocation. Therefore, both the semantic properties of stimuli (salience) and the demands for semantic processing directly affect attentional allocation. If we take this line of evidence one step further, there is at least some theoretical basis for believing that semantic associative memory is a by-product of the interaction of smaller units of activational states resulting from the essential features of input. Theories that assume such an underpinning for associative memory provide a conceptual link for bridging phenomena such as the OR, physiological activation during semantic processing, and underlying semantic networks.

Semantic Memory Organization

Many cognitive theorists now believe that human memory is best thought of as distributed associative networks (McClelland & Rumelhart, 1986), or as a semantic–episodic network such as described by Anderson (1983). From the human associative memory perspective, symbols achieve their semantic value through association with a cluster of more basic properties or input units that together constitute the essence of the particular object. When activated, the associational network that represents a particular object influences the entire state of the processing system at the particular time. For instance, when we conjure up a mental image of a dog, a host of basic features are likely to arise that we associate with dogs, such as barking, fur, and other aspects of its phycial appearance. Together these features form an associative cluster for our concept of a dog. Therefore, semantic value depends on the associative integration of the most salient features that constitute the particular object. If, as discussed previously, the salience of primary stimulus characteristics affects the OR, then semantics should also differentially affect attention, if semantic value is a by-product of the associative relationship among primary stimulus features.

A number of different models of semantic memory have been developed to account for the factors that govern the search for semantic information in associative memeory, including hierarchical models (Collins & Quillian, 1969), feature comparison models (Smith, Shoben, & Rips, 1974), and spreading activation models (Collin & Loftus, 1975). Within all of these models, semantic information is represented as a network based on some semantic characteristic such as the "semantic relatedness" or the underlying features of the semantic item. Therefore, each model proposes a specific organizational structure for how information is represented in the network. For instance, the hierarchical models propose that semantic information is organized on the basis of subordinate and superordinate categories, so that memory search requires moving up or down a hierarchy of semantic categories. In contrast, the feature comparison models propose that memory organization is based on basic featural similarities among the objects in memory. The spreading activation models maintain that it is simply the overall level of semantic relatedness based on the number of associative links between objects in memory that governs search. While these models differ in very fundamental ways, each predicts that the speed, efficiency, and result of associative memory search depends on the region of the semantic network that is activated. If particular semantic representations are primed initial trials, then subsequent search for related semantic information will be facilitated. The efficiency of decisions relative to information in the network depends on the intersection of associative paths that link "close neighbors" (i.e., semantic information that shares common characteristics).

Memory Probes

The use of cues to activate memory and to facilitate retrieval has bearing on the relationship between memory and attention. Cues that are used to facilitate retrieval presumably activate relevant associative memory networks. In this capacity the cue serves as a link between external factors that create demand for the attentional and the memory representational systems of the individual. However, the extent to which attention plays an active role in accessing semantic information from the memory associative network depends largely on the particular theory of semantic memory that is examined.

Encoding, Retrieval, and Context

Perhaps one of the best illustrations of the relationship among attention, memory, and context comes from the work of Tulving and his colleagues on the *encoding specificity effect* (Tulving & Thomson, 1973). The essence of this effect is that memory retrieval depends on matching the specific encoding. If a word is encoded in a particular semantic context during initial learning trials, then it will be more easily retrieved if retrieval cues trigger the original semantic context. For instance, the encoding specificity effect maintains that if the word *bark* is originally presented in a context to mean part of a tree, semantic cues presented later during retrieval related to this concept will increase the likelihood of retrieval, whereas a cue such as *dog*, which relates to another meaning of bark, will be less effective.

While the encoding specificity effect was originally developed to account for memory phenomena, the use of a cue to activate retrieval incorporates an attentional device. By cuing the subject to a particular semantic category, the experimenter essentially directs the attention of the subject in an implicit manner.

Semantics and Automaticity

As discussed earlier, one of the main topics of cognitive research on attention over the past decade has been the distinction between automatic and controlled attentional processing (Schneider & Shiffrin, 1977). Why is it that some tasks can be performed rather effortlessly and with considerable automaticity while other tasks require effortful, controlled attentional processing? While most of the early studies of this question investigated response to simple stimuli based on low-level visual features, it is noteworthy that automaticity for semantic information has been reported. Schneider and Fisk (1984) used a set of words that were examples of one semantic category (e.g., robin and canary as types of birds) to test whether training for detection of words from another semantic category facilitated detection of other words from the same category. They found evidence to support such semantic transfer and that the search for new stimuli that belonged to the old semantic category (e.g., bluejay) was rapid. This finding illustrates that attention may become increasingly automatic based on prior activation of a semantic network. Information that is a well-integrated part of the semantic associative network (LTM) will generally be easier to attend to than new information that is only available in STM. Furthermore, when information in LTM is consistently activated, there will be greater capacity for automatic processing. Accordingly, automaticity is governed by the strength of associative memory and the certainty that this information will occur.

Determinants of Attention to Semantic Associative Memory

Automatic semantic associative search can be accounted for without the requirement of an independent and discrete attentional or *executive* process. As described previously, in most models of semantic associative memory, the parameters underlying search, detection, and semantic decisions can be accounted for on the basis of the properties or organization of the semantic network. By activating a particular region of the semantic network, we can predict search characteristics. Search efficiency is a function of how activation spreads throughout the network across the links that connect associative nodes. Search of the network may be driven largely by what region of the network is activated by the stimulus probe. Of course, outside of the experimental situation, stimuli that activate the semantic network are not probes per se, but rather the new incoming information to which the individual is exposed. Therefore, this type of automatic attentional selection of semantic information may occur during an earlier parallel stage of processing. The interaction of newly arriving stimuli with existing information represented in the semantic associative network would result in continual variation in the allocation of attentional resources. Discrepancy between existing schemata in LTM and new information creates a potential catalyst for attentional redirection. Changes in the direction of attention could be induced by minimal discrepancies between the new stimuli and existing templates. Shifts in associative strength resulting from the interaciton of new inputs with the existing network can be accounted for by such computational approaches as the parallel distributed processing (PDP) model (see Chapter 20). While a semantic search may occur automatically without the requirement of a discrete attentional or executive mechanism, can we conclude that there is little relationship between semantic memory and controlled attention?

It would be a mistake to reach such a conclusion for several reasons. First, it is apparent that the effects of automatic processing may have direct impact on future action and attentional selections. When semantic information is selected through an automatic search, the semantic region associated with this information is presumably activated, creating the *semantic-relatedness effect*. As a result, information that is semantically related to the activated information becomes more available and the semantic network is then biased relative to this semantic set. Therefore, the automatic activation of semantic information serves to direct future attending. The activated attentional state may create an increased drive and/or executive decision to direct additional controlled attention to the semantic information.

Furthermore, while semantic selection may occur automatically based on a spread of activation through the network, in many cases attention is driven based on anticipation of future action (Allport, 1987). In fact, as we have discussed earlier in this book, there is strong neuropsychological evidence supporting the existence of neural systems that govern response execution. These systems play a role in low-level motor response control as well as the shifting of categorical set and decisions that relate to what logical path is chosen during problem solving. Given that these systems seem to play a role in high-level cognitive functions, where shifts in set are required, there is a compelling basis for considering how these executive functions influence the direction of attention relative to semantic associative information. As the individual exerts executive control, the frame of attention is shifted, which will then influence the information that is available to future automatic processing.

Given the probable influence of both automatic and controlled attention relative to semantic associative memory, it is likely that two processing sequences may occur:

1. With the arrival of new information, automatic featural and semantic processing is activated. Based on the salience of this information and prevailing tasks demands, additional attention may be allocated. With effortful controlled attention, the processing of the new information can be enhanced, resulting in a more complete encoding of the new information. Furthermore, directed attentional allocation of this type may result in forcing a search through a semantic pathway that was not initially selected. Such a search could result in the development of new associative relationships. This type of semantic search requires much greater effort than automatic selection and probably involves the executive system.

2. The second sequence differs in the origin of the semantic memeory search. In most semantic models, activation of the relevant region of the associative network occurs as a result of the introduction of an external stimulus probe. In natural contexts, semantic search often may be self-generated. In such instances, semantic activation may occur with minimal executive constraints (i.e., free association). However, self-generated semantic search usually is governed by some *intention* or, as Allport (1987) has suggested, selection-for-action. The resulting sequence would be driven by controlled attentional (executive) processes, such that an automatic semantic spread of activation would follow directed attention to a region of the semantic network.

Effort during this type of controlled attentional search may result when individual is required to respond in a manner that is contrary to the easiest associative pathway available in the network. a number of recent computational models have suggested that the neural system normally seeks the easiest solution during processing (e.g., harmony theory). This may be accomplished by the neural system choosing a selection that fits some minmal constraints. In order for effortful processing to occur, the system must bypass these weak constraints and opt for alternative attentional selections. This could only occur through a sequence of serial operations, during which the system pushes beyond the initial attentional selections.

SUMMARY

Memory and attention share many overlapping features and operate together in the performance of many cognitive operations. Thus attention and memory are highly interdependent. Some aspects of memory can be analyzed without consideration of attentional operations. For instance, factors such as the strength of associative connectivity, the reate of trace decay, and the characteristics of long-term potentiation reflect basic neurobiological properties of memory and do not require an attentional component. In fact, memory investigators often choose to eliminate attentional factions from experimental paradigms in order to control for confounds that may affect the analysis of memory. By minimizing attentional effects, the investigator hopes to establish how memory works in isolation of other factors.

Yet, it is unlikely that an understanding of memory independent of attention will explain most complex cognitive phenomena. The processes of memory formation and degradation do not account for how the animal selects a particular stimulus or how it will behave at any given moment. In this chapter, we have discussed how different cognitive models of memory explain encoding and storage. Some models considered attention and memory as separate compartments in a flow of information-processing steps while others considered attention to be the by-product of operations that result in memory.

We have taken the position that attention and memory should be considered as separate but interdependent processes. There are compelling reasons not to consider attention as a completely independent compartment in a "pipeline" model. Attention is the by-product of the processing of multiple neural systems. To designate separate attentional and memory compartments in a box model leads to the suggestion that a single locus of attention can be isolated. This possibility appears to be unlikely. Instead, attention seems to comprise different processes that interact with memory. Paradoxically, memory may be considered to be one component of attentional phenomena while attention may be viewed as a by-product of memory. This paradox may be explained as follows. Since attention depends on the comparison of new information with existing templates in memory, attention may be considered to be a superordinate process, of which memory is a critical component. However, as memory is formed through the intentional or incidental processing of new information, it naturally creates pressures (through associative weighting) that will influence the future direction of attention. This paradoxical relationship between memory and attention is apparent in other theoretical dichotomies that have emerged in the study of attention. The distinction between automatic and controlled processes provides an illustration of this point.

Some attentional processes are rather automatic with apparently little executive top-down control. Other attentional processes are much more effortful and seem to involve an executive control mechanism in which the response production tendencies of the individual are a determinant. Automatic and effortful attentional mechanism may interface with the different forms of memory in different ways. The long-term storages may interact in a direct way with incoming perceptual information to produce automatic attentional selections. Long-term memory may also direct the production of an executive program, which will direct the attention of the individual in a more effortful manner. The short-term storage of information interacts with attention by establishing parameters for the flow of information through the system. It determines how much information can be handled at a given stage of processing as well as how long information can be held before it must be either encoded in a more durable form or further processed in an active manner.

The study of attention requires a careful consideration of the memory characteristics of the system. Attentional research must control for or at least consider memory parameters when designing experiments or assessment techniques. This issue becomes paramount when studying patients with brain damage. A patient with an amnesia may experience altered attentional performance as a result of failure to encode or access information in memory. Similarly, memory disorders can often result from failures of attentional control. When considering the effects of memory on attention, factors that effect the rate of memory formation, the rate of decay of short-term memory, and capacity will have direct bearing on the attentional characteristics. Delineation of these memory parameters also helps to establish the constraints on the related process of attention. While significant strides have been made in this regard, much more research is necessary to specify the parametric relationships between memory and attentional processes based on knowledge of the neural properties of the brain. A number of questions still exist. How do automatic and effortful attentional processes mutually interact in the generation of a working memory? How do the neural substrates of basic attentional processes, such as habituation and sensitization, relate to more complex forms of attention, learning, and memory? The relationship among attentional control, awareness, and memory is also far from understood. Continued research on the constraints that memory and attentional processes place on each other appears to be a necessary and logical step toward better understanding the factors influencing attention.

Spatial Determinants of Attention

When an animal engages in a directed course of action, it organizes its behavior with reference to the position of its body, using the spatial coordinates of the surrounding environment. All natural environments have a spatial organization that can be mapped in a Cartesian coordinate system. Although this fact seems intuitive today, the question of how space is represented within the observer has been one of the enduring problems for philosophers and scientists throughout the ages. Kant (1931) argued that humans have an intrinsic spatial grid that provides an internal representation of external Cartesian space. According to Kant, this spatial grid provides an *a priori* framework on which all external reality is organized.

The idea that people have an intrinsic spatial organization is not universally accepted. Historically, some philosophers argued that spatial awareness is not innate but learned as a function of the individual's interactions with the environment. This perspective assumes that humans are born without an *a priori* spatial framework for mapping experience; they begin life with a *tabula rasa*, on which all organization is imprinted from the environment. Modern neuroscientists would generally agree that the external environment provides input that is necessary for establishing spatial awareness. Without sensory experience, the animal would not have a spatial frame of reference. The importance of sensory input into spatial organization is evident from studies of sensory deprivation. Under conditions of prolonged sensory deprivation, subjects lose both their spatial and their temporal orientation.

Although sensory input is necessary for normal spatial awareness, the conclusion that spatial experience is derived solely from the structure of environmental information appears incorrect. There is also compelling evidence that spatial awareness and spatially directed behavior are influenced and constrained by the characteristics of the brain's structure and function. If spatial behavior were determined solely by environmental variables, people from different experiential backgrounds and environments should have difficulty relating to the same spatial framework. The fact that all people relate to the same spatial coordinate system supports the idea that our neural system places important constraints on the way we organize spatial experience. Therefore, the spatial organization of behavior depends both on a continuous flow of multimodal sensory information and on an intact nervous system capable of integrating this sensory input according to a relatively spatially invariant template.

If there is an intrinsic spatial frame of reference for behavior, it is important to specify the constraints that it places on behavior, cognition, and, for our purposes, attentional processes. Attention is strongly influenced by the spatial characteristics of the individual relative to the environment. This point is illustrated by the peculiar neglect found in patients with hemi-inattention syndromes, who fail to attend to part of their spatial field. The neuropsychological models of neglect discussed earlier in the text differ with respect to the proposed underlying mechanisms. Yet, these models are almost universal in positing that the neglect syndromes involve a fundamental disturbance of attentional distribution relative to either the internal or the external spatial representation. A central feature of these syndromes is their hemispatial character. Therefore, the analysis of attention requires a consideration of the way in which space is represented both cognitively and within the neural system.

PHENOMENOLOGICAL CONSIDERATIONS

There is now considerable evidence that the brain has an intrinsic capacity for organizing and mapping spatial representations. Yet, the neuropsychological characteristics of this spatial organization and its impact on attention are still not well established. Spatial behavior is difficult to study because there are multiple spatial frames that affect the individual at any given time. In a given situation, spatial orientation can have reference both to the broad distinction of figure–ground relationships and to the finer spatial distinctions between objects in the visual field. Furthermore, spatial representations are influenced by the response tendencies of the individual. This fact was demonstrated in neurophysiological studies that we described earlier (Mountcastle, 1978; Mountcastle, Anderson, & Motter, 1981; Mountcastle, Lynch, Georgopoulos, Sarata, & Acuna, 1975; Mountcastle, Motter, Steinmetz, & Duffy, 1984). Given the complexity of spatial experience, it is important that the investigator clearly specify the level of spatial organization of interest when studying spatial phenomena. Spatial experience does not appear to be a unitary representation.

Grusser (1983) provided one of the most comprehensive phenomenologies of spatial experience. He postulated that there are four levels of extrapersonal space that can be delineated on the basis of the proximity of the spatial frame to the individual's actions: grasping space, near-distant action space, far-distant action space, and visual background. The distinction among these levels is the degree to which direct contact with objects in the spatial frame is possible.

Grasping space is the most proximal level of spatial organization and therefore involves the greatest degree of multimodal integration. Objects contained within this spatial frame are likely to have strong tactile and proprioceptive qualities. As one moves farther from the individual to near- and far-distant action space, there is greater reliance on nontactile signals and particularly on visual input. The most distal level of the visual background creates a field that is necessary for figure–ground relationships.

Grusser's taxonomy is interesting because it postulates that spatial representations are organized around the characteristic actions of the individual. The more distal spatial representations based on figure–ground relationships are highly dependent on the visual modality. However, somatosensory feedback is also important in determining figure–ground relationships, and probably contributes to the ability of humans to make correct determinations regarding spatial position and orientation (Hein & Diamond, 1983; Held & Hein, 1963; Wilkin, 1959). Some people show a preference for cues from body position, and others show a visual preference. As one moves toward more proximal objects in space, it is obvious that spatial behavior depends on the integration of multiple modalities. Furthermore, in proximal space, motor acts of responding seem to be highly integrated with visual processing.

SPATIAL CHARACTERISTICS OF ATTENTION

Attentional selection requires a search for salient stimuli within the spatial field. Spatial position is determined by several factors, including the position of an image on the retina, the position of the eyes relative to the head, the position of the head on the body, and the general orientation of the body in space (Miles & Evarts, 1979). In addition, auditory signals regarding localization, vestibular signals, and proprioceptive inputs yield signals that may be integrated to provide information about spatial position (Gottschalk, Grusser, & Lindau, 1978). In sum, spatial organization seems to occur as the result of information from several sources.

Spatial behavior is often thought of as primarily sensory. However, studies of oculomotor activity illustrate that the motor activations of saccadic tracking produce spatial rather than retinal patterns. Spatial organization seems to evolve from the interaction of motor activity in response to sensory input (Hallet & Lightstone, 1976). In fact, humans are able to generate accurate eye movements even when they do not register the visual stimulus that they are tracking (Jeannerod, 1983; Perenin & Jeannerod, 1978).

The well-known studies of Held and Hein (1963) illustrate that coordination of visual feedback with motor feedback is necessary for the development of visually guided locomotion. When cats were reared under conditions in which they did not have access to visual cues during the learning of locomotive skills, they failed to develop the ability to direct their movements in space. In another study, the movement of limbs toward a target was shown to depend on visual feedback about the movement of the limbs. Cats that were provided information about the movement of their limbs without information from actual locomotion also failed to develop guided reaching (Hein & Diamond, 1972). These studies demonstrate the mutual interactions between body awareness and visual information about spatial position in the learning of directed actions. Other studies by these researchers (Hein & Diamond, 1983) demonstrated through surgical immobilization of specific neural systems that eye movements and proprioceptive feedback from eye muscles are the critical components in the formation of spatial representation.

SPATIAL DISTRIBUTION OF VISUAL SELECTIVE ATTENTION

When the visual fields are studied, it is common to create a map of the distribution of sensory recognition by indicating whether the individual is able to detect a signal at various coordinates in the field. If a patient makes a certain percentage of correct detections at a particular spatial location, it is assumed that the field is intact at that position. Assessment of the distribution of visual fields relies on a signal detection methodology (see Chapter 13 for further discussion). Psychophysical parameters such as stimulus intensity, duration, spatial frequency, and movement can be varied to influence the recognition rates for detection at different spatial locations.

The spatial distribution for visual attention can be evaluated in a similar way, though modifications in methodology are necessary. Neisser (1969) studied visual search by measuring the time taken to scan a matrix of items for a particular target. Search times were greatest when there was high similarity between targets and distractors. This finding was interpreted as an indication of feature detection and analysis. Subsequent studies have generally supported Neisser's findings, although other investigators have demonstrated the parametric characteristics of performance with changes in psychophysical dimensions, as well as memory load.

Sperling and Melchner (1978) mapped the spatial distribution of visual search accuracy in a 7×7 array. They found that search accuracy was highest above the foveal fixation point, and that extreme points in the vertical dimension were the least likely to be accurately searched (see Figure 19.1).

The accuracy of visual search depends on the attentional demands of the task. Accurate detection should occur at an almost perfect rate when the location of the target is obvious and not difficult to discriminate. Reduced speed and accuracy occur when the target is shifted in the visual field and its location is uncertain. Cuing the subject as to the spatial region to search improves performance, a finding suggesting an attentional effect.

Signal detection methods have been used extensively to characterize the distribution of visual attention. By specifying the hits, misses, correct rejections, and false alarm errors of the subject during attentional tasks with varying memory load, stimulus set size, and response demand, it is possible to characterize the spatial distribution of attention. This distribution reflects the likelihood of the two error types across various positions of the spatial field.

Sperling and his colleagues conducted many experiments using their partial report methods to establish attentional parameters for search tasks having either "concurrent" or "compound" demands. Concurrent tasks require performing two or more tasks simultaneously. Invariably, this is more difficult than performing a task in isolation. Compound tasks require performing more than one task over a series of trials, but only one task at any given time. Compound tasks have intrinsic uncertainty, as the subject does not know ahead of time which target or task will be called for on a given trial.

The compound-concurrent distinction reflects the difference between tasks performed in series or in parallel. Sperling (1984) attributed the difference between these tasks to the "resources" required for adequate performance. As the subject cannot determine the resources necessary for an upcoming compound task, optimal resources will be necessary at all times if the subject is to be prepared for all possible task alternatives. Sperling concluded that the speed and accuracy of target detections on spatial search tasks vary as a function of the task structure of spatial search and detection tasks.

Variations in the response time needed to detect visual stimuli presented at various distances and positions relative to the focus of attention provide even more dramatic evidence that attention is spatially distributed. Hughes and Zimba (1987) presented precues to different coordinates of the visual spatial field that served to orient their subjects' attention to those positions. The probe stimulus that followed often occurred in an unexpected location, which typically increased the response time (RT) for detection. The diminished performance (RT) was then studied as a function of the degree of spatial discrepancy between the two stimuli. A three-dimensional map was generated that reflected the variations in RT based on stimulus discrepancy and spatial position as seen in Figure 19.2. This methodology provides an important tool for studying spatial constraints on attention and also demonstrates the normal boundaries of the spatial spread of attention.

Rizzolatti and his colleagues conducted a series of related experiments to evaluate the characteristics of attention as a function of other spatial variables. Several of their findings that pertain to the spatial distribution of attention are described below.

Attention in 3-D

The distribution of three-dimensional spatial attention follows many of the rules noted for attention in two dimensions (Gawryszewski *et al.*, 1987). Rizzolatti and his collaborators demonstrated that attention can be directed to spatial depth without the necessity of eye movements (Rizzolatti, Riggio, Dascola, & Umilta, 1987). Interestingly, they noted that subjects respond faster to spatial points between the attentional fixation point and the

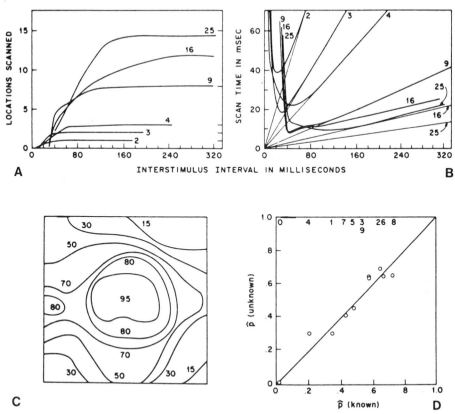

FIGURE 19.1. The relationship among spatial position, task variables, and search characteristics is illustrated in this series of graphs. (From Sperling, 1984, with permission.) (A) The likelihood that a spatial location will be scanned is a function of the interstimulus interval and the number of stimuli to be processed. (B) As a result, there is also a trade-off among the scan time, the interstimulus interval, and the number of stimuli in the visual array. (C) The likelihood that a particular spatial location will be scanned can be plotted as in this figure. Central locations are the most likely to be scanned. (D) Search accuracy varies as a function of how familiar the stimuli are to the subject.

observer, than to points deeper than the attentional fixation point. This type of effect was not noted in the two-dimensional frontal plane, as the reaction time to points between the foveal fixation point and the spatial point of attention was not enhanced.

Attention Without Spatial Expectancy

In a second series of experiments, Gawryszewski et al. (1987) demonstrated that, during a neutral condition in which attention is not directed to a spatial position before target onset, response times reflect a diffuse, nonfocused attention. Posner (1978) had proposed that, when subjects do not expect a stimulus at a particular location, their attention should remain fixated at a neutral position (i.e., near the foveal center). The findings of Gawryszew-

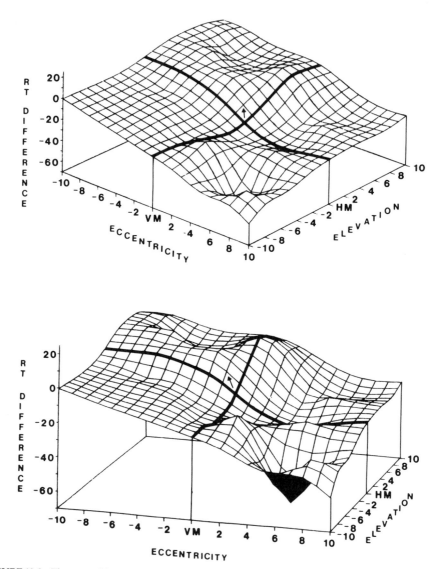

FIGURE 19.2. The natural boundaries of the spatial distribution of visual attention can be represented by plotting the reaction time (RT) differences between uncued or probed stimuli in different spatial locations. By plotting these reaction time differences as a function of spatial position, Hughes and Zimba produced a three-dimensional graphic representation that depicts the effect of valid and invalid attentional expectancies across the spatial field averaged across four subjects. The costs and benefits of being cued to either correct or incorrect spatial position is a function of the reaction time differences relative to the difference between the anticipated spatial position to which attention was directed and the position at which the stimulus actually occurred. From Hughes and Zimba (1987), with permission.

ski *et al.* suggest a different possibility, that attention is diffusely and equally distributed across space when there is no spatial expectancy.

Attention Across Midline

Rizzolatti and his colleagues (1987) demonstrated that the reorientation of attention across the horizontal and vertical dimensions occurs with some costs. They conducted studies in which attention was incorrectly cued on a proportion of trials (30%), and they found that correct orienting of attention yielded slight benefits, whereas incorrect orienting produced significant costs, as reflected by slowed reaction time. The cost of the incorrect orientation of attention varied as a function of the spatial distance from the point of incorrect orientation and the actual target.

The cost of incorrect orientation was greatest when attention had to be redirected across the vertical or horizontal midline. Rizzolatti *et al.* concluded that this effect could not be explained by hemifield inhibition or a gradient of attention but must be due to the increased time necessary to execute two different motor programs (see Chapter 3 for a discussion of premotor mechanisms of attention).

Tassinari, Aglioti, Chelazzi, Marzi, and Berlucci (1987) investigated the aftereffects of orienting attention to a spatial position. They had subjects fixate centrally while deliberately allocating covert attention to other spatial positions. The reaction time of the subjects to targets presented after a short duration improved when in the same spatial location but increased for targets in other positions. Following orientation to a spatial location, aftereffects were noted for subsequent presentations of the cue and target stimuli. Reaction time to the target increased when it was repeated in the same position, and no cost was noted for stimuli in the opposite hemifield. These findings suggested hemispatial effects of premotor readiness.

Habituation of Spatial Selective Attention

Maylor and Hockey (1987) demonstrated that when subjects were required to orient repeatedly to a specific spatial location, their response time to a subsequent target depended on the time interval between the cue and the target stimuli. With short durations between stimuli (e.g., 100 msec), there was no change in reaction times over a series of trials. However, with longer interstimulus durations, the reaction time increased as a function of the run of cues before the target occurred. The investigators interpreted this finding as indicating habituation to the anticipatory cue when the interval was long. When there was a short interstimulus interval, repetition of the cue facilitated response to the target.

NEURAL DETERMINANTS OF SPATIAL ATTENTION

Spatially directed behavior depends on the coordination of visual input into the retina with spatial information derived from eye movements. The nucleus of the optic tract of the pretectum has been identified as a likely structure for such integration (Hoffmann & Schoppmann, 1975, 1981; Precht & Strata, 1980). This structure seems to be particularly sensitive to directional movements. Cells of the right nucleus respond to movement from left to right, whereas the left nucleus prefers movement in the opposite direction. The movement specificity of this nucleus establishes a basis for spatial directionality of eye movements in response to movements across the retina.

Other nuclei have also been implicated as points of integration of visual target and positional information. For instance, researchers have identified a thalamic region (the internal medullary lamina) that responds to the target goal to be reached by the eyes, rather than the current position of the target (Schlag & Schlag-Rey, 1983; Schlag-Rey & Schlag, 1981). This thalamic nucleus acts as an anticipatory generator for eye tracking. Interestingly, it receives inputs from the superior colliculus (Harting, Huerta, Frankfurter, Strominger, & Royce, 1980) and projects to the basal ganglia, the frontal eye fields, and the parietal lobes. As a result, it is well situated to direct the sensorimotor integration of spatial information.

The superior colliculus appears to be a center for the control of saccadic eye movements (see Figure 19.3). Lesions of this nucleus disrupt the spontaneous production of saccades. When these lesions are coupled with damage to the frontal eye fields, these movements are eliminated. Studies by Sparks and Mays (1980) have suggested that the superior colliculus encodes for errors in mismatch between eye position and retinal image.

CORTICAL INFLUENCES ON SPATIAL ORGANIZATION

In addition to thalamic and subcortical structures, cortical areas play significant roles in spatial organization. The most important areas are the frontal eye fields and the parietal lobes. As the role of these structures has been discussed in Chapters 9 and 10 we will only briefly review the contributions of these cortical areas to spatial organization. The frontal eye fields have a critical influence on the visual scanning of the environment. Lesions to this area result in a failure of visual search of the entire field during attentional tasks. The specific characteristics of the impaired visual search can be summarized as a failure of intentional scanning. Disorders of this system produce a gaze inertia, as patients fail to maintain a course of directed action during scanning.

Damage to the parietal lobes can impair spatial organization through several possible mechanisms. Cortical region ? serves as a higher order visual processing system for sensory information arriving from V1. Neural cells of this region respond to stimulus characteristics such as movement and even spatial orientation. Therefore, part of the parietal lobe seems to be tuned to the spatial characteristics of the target that is being processed.

The superior parietal regions process somatosensory information from the postcentral gyrus. This information is integrated to produce a body schema. Spatial sense can be derived from kinesthetic and proprioceptive signals without the necessity of visual input.

Unilateral lesions of the inferior parietal lobule (particularly area PG) are known to produce neglect syndromes. As we have discussed in Chapter 9, there are several models for why hemispatial inattention results from this type of damage. In their model of hemineglect syndrome, Heilman, Watson, and Valenstein (1985) proposed that hemi-inattention is interrelated with spatial directionality.

Damage to the parietal lobes may cause syndromes such as right–left disorientation, problems with spatial mapping, constructional difficulties, and a host of other problems that result from a failure to organize spatial information effectively. It is widely accepted that the parietal lobes integrate information from different modalities to produce a spatial schema.

THE CHARACTERISTICS OF PARIETAL SPATIAL DISTRIBUTION

The fact that visual input is distributed in a spatial grid is now well established. The pioneering studies of Hubel and Wiesel (1963, 1968, 1977) on the mapping of visual input on cells of V1 demonstrated a direct correspondence between retinal and cortical regions for

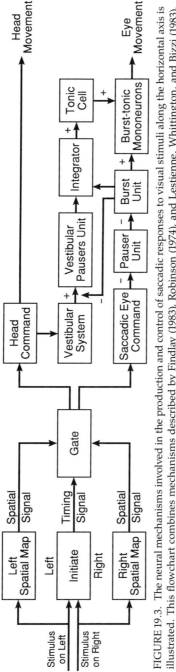

FIGURE 19.3. The neural mechanisms involved in the production and control of saccadic responses to visual stimuli along the horizontal axis is illustrated. This flowchart combines mechanisms described by Findlay (1983), Robinson (1974), and Lestienne, Whittington, and Bizzi (1983). Stimuli to either the right or left visual field activate parallel saccadic initiation processes which generate a timing signal. The initiation of the saccade is referenced to a spatial signal produced by comparing of the visual stimulus with a spatial map. The spatial and temporal signals interact at a gating mechanism. The output from this saccadic initiation process causes the generation of two response sequences: occular and head position. The size of the occular saccade is influenced by burst motorneurons that produce the movement and burst-tonic motorneurons that respond to this saccadic burst and feedback about the movement. A second process under the influence of the vestibular system influences the direction of head movement. Occular and head movement information is integrated so that control of the saccade is possible, and visual searching is directed to the correct spatial position.

visual perception. An image that is imprinted on the retina has a direct mapping to certain cortical cells, so that the image produces a template in the pattern of cortical activation.

Since Hubel and Weisel's initial demonstration of this phenomenon, there have been a large number of investigations of the mapping of visual input in other cortical regions. The high degree of correspondence between retinal image and cortical activation that is found in V1 is not as apparent when one moves to visual centers of the parietal lobes. Yet, there is evidence the activation of neural cells in the parietal regions evokes differential responses according to the spatial distribution of stimuli in the spatial field.

The posterior inferior parietal lobe of the cortex appears to be a major center for spatial representation. It receives input from the striate cortex, and from the superior colliculus through the dorsal thalamus. This region is important in object localization in space. It has less relevance to object recognition, as demonstrated by the studies of Ungerleider and Mishkin (1982). The dissociation of object recognition from spatial localization is theoretically important, as it demonstrates that the brain is indeed sensitive to the spatial characteristics in the visual modality.

Mountcastle, Anderson, and Motter (1981) conducted elaborate experiments to delineate the response properties of parietal visual neurons in different spatial patterns of stimulation. Stationary stimuli were flashed to monkeys that maintained fixation on a target. The receptive field of the parietal visual neurons was shown to be very large, often encompassing both halves of the visual field. These neurons also tended to respond maximally to rapidly presented stimuli in half of the visual field, rather than to a stationary central stimulus. Finally, these neurons did not respond specifically to stimuli or different featural characteristics. When all of these findings are considered together, it would appear that the cells of this region are sensitive to the spatial characteristics of stimuli.

The presence of movement sensitivity in cells of the parietal region (Motter & Mountcastle, 1981) provides a further indication of the spatial character of this cortical region. The receptive field of some parietal cells seems to be sensitive to specific spatial orientations of movement. In fact, these authors determined that over 90% of neurons in this region respond to the direction of movement from different spatial orientations. Interestingly, the directional response properties of parietal neurons are often not distributed uniformly, as certain orientations seem to be favored over others. This finding suggests that there are inherent preferences for particular spatial orientations among these neural cells.

The spatial characteristics of parietal visual neurons may depend on the organization of these neurons in networks to form a spatial map, as well as on the response characteristics of individual neurons. Some of the functional properties of the parietal visual neurons involved in spatial analysis that were described by Mountcastle *et al.* (1981) are

1. Large bilateral receptive fields.
2. Sparing of fovea response, with greater response to peripheral stimuli.
3. High sensitivity to high-velocity movement.
4. Strong directional sensitivity for most parietal visual neurons.
5. Less sensitivity to static spatial localization.

The limited sensitivity of these parietal visual neurons to static spatial information is intriguing, since nondominant parietal lobe damage produces attentional neglect, even for stationary objects. This finding may reflect the fact that the parietal lobes contain multiple neuronal systems, some involved in movement perception, and others involved in attentional processing. However, there may be other explanations as well. Attentional neglect occurs when there is a breakdown of information regarding the person's spatial position relative to the environment. Movement perception requires that neurons be tuned to sequential changes in spatial position. Therefore, it is possible that attentional neglect is influenced by a disintegration of sequential feedback from movement-sensitive areas that govern visual tracking to the spatial analysis systems of the parietal lobe.

RESPONDING IN A SPATIAL ENVIRONMENT

The relationship between motor responding and the visual processing of spatial information has been demonstrated in recent neurophysiological studies of the interaction between looking and grasping (Goldberg & Bushnell, 1981; Goldberg & Robinson, 1977, 1980). In a series of experiments, Goldberg and his colleagues demonstrated that the superior colliculus responds to the attentional act of directed eye movements to an area of the visual fields. Monkeys trained to look at a stimulus in the visual field had enhanced activity of the superior colliculus when they saccaded to that region of the visual field. This activity preceded the saccade, suggesting that it was related to anticipatory attentional response. When the stimulus was removed from the visual field, the anticipatory activation of the superior colliculus diminished. Therefore, the increased activation in the presence of the stimulus was not due either to the solo effects of the saccades or to the visual analysis of the stimuli, but to the integration of the sensory and motor acts in an anticipatory response.

Heilman, Watson, Valenstein, and Goldberg (1988) suggested that the enhancement of the sensory response is a neural analogue of sensory selective attention. In addition to the superior colliculus, the frontal eye fields and the striate cortex have also been shown to produce attentional enhancement of sensory information through interaction with saccadic movement (Wurtz, Goldberg, & Robinson, 1982; Wurtz, Richmond, & Newsome, 1984). Attentional selection is directly related to the integration of the act of looking (i.e., the saccade) with the preparation and activation of spatial analysis systems of the inferior parietal lobule.

Parietal lobe neural cells have been shown to produce an attentional enhancement of spatially selective information that does not depend on a specific form of movement (e.g., Bushnell et al. 1981). These cells can respond to attentional activation independent of a motor component. A similar pattern of activation is seen in this area regardless of whether a saccade is made or not. Therefore, a dissociation seems to exist between selective attention with and without motoric response requirements. This dissociation has bearing on the distinction made between sensory and motor aspects of attention that we discussed earlier.

From the standpoint of our discussion of the spatial distribution of attention, it is important to note that the spatial orientation of the stimulus is a primary determinant of the attentional characteristics of different neural regions. Attentional activation of the superior colliculus depends on behavioral factor different from those that influence the activation of parietal neurons. Yet, in both cases, activation is sensitive to specific spatial characteristics of the stimulus. When an animal is trained to respond to a specific spatial orientation, it shows decreased responsivity to stimuli in other regions, thus demonstrating attentional specificity with respect to spatial distribution.

The basis for the spatial distribution of attention may not be the same for different cortical regions. The spatial response characteristics of posterior parietal neurons may be determined to a greater extent by the tuning properties of cells in this region, whereas the response of other cortical regions may have a less specific spatial map. For instance, factors related to the conditioning of a stimulus to a particular spatial region may have greater bearing on the response of cells in certain cortical regions. The parameters underlying the spatial mapping of cells in different cortical regions and the relative influence of conditioning on these parameters have not yet been exactly determined.

SPATIAL PROPERTIES OF VISUAL ATTENTION

The demonstration of a spatial organization of the visual system represented a significant step in establishing a conceptual foundation for selective visual attention. If neural cells of the parietal lobe are sensitive to specific spatial factors such as directionality, so that certain cells show a bias for particular orientations, then it is easier to envision a mechanism by which selective attention can be derived.

Neural cells of the parietal lobes have been shown to respond differentially in accordance with changes in behavioral state. For instance, cells of the inferior parietal lobe in monkeys respond more intensely to stimuli that have greater behavior relevance (e.g., food vs. nonfood). The presence of a behavioral goal seems to be a triggering mechanism for the response of these neurons. Mountcastle and his colleagues (1984) and several other groups have conducted experiments that illustrate the role of the inferior parietal cortex in directing attention to parts of the visual spatial field. When monkeys were presented visual stimuli to one region of the visual field on repeated trials, neural cells in the parietal cortex did not respond to the initial appearance of the target light. The response of these cells was enhanced when they had to respond to specific task demands, such as detection of dimming of the light, as the monkey fixated for a particular time interval over repeated trials. A reward was given for correct performance. The response of the monkey's parietal cells was also measured during an intertrial period. Interestingly, the response of the cells during the intertrial interval varied, as some cells continued to respond over the course of this interval, and other cells actually increased in responsiveness. When the response of the cells to relevant stimuli was compared with their response to nonrelevant stimuli in the same spatial positions, a clear distinction could be made (Mountcastle *et al.*, 1981, 1984). These findings illustrate the interrelationship between spatial attention and the salience of the stimuli to be processed. The importance of task demand in determining the responsiveness of neural cells of the parietal lobe to spatial tasks is also apparent.

There is also evidence that activation of a specific visual spatial region of the field is not necessary for attentional activation to occur. Studies by Mountcastle's group have suggested that the parietal visual neurons of the monkey become activated even when attention is directed away from the fixation point of the original target position. Therefore, the spatial region of previous activation may not be a critical determinant of the activation of parietal neurons. Furthermore, the activation of these parietal neurons during attentional fixation seems to represent a different phenomenon from the neural "enhancement" noted in cortical cells associated with saccades to a target (Mountcastle *et al.*, 1981, 1984). Yet, both responses can be classified as determinants of spatial selective attention.

As we previously noted, Heilman and his colleagues have distinguished between selective attention with and without intention movements. A central issue in their distinction was the absence of a relationship between saccadic movements and attentional activation in cells of the parietal lobe. At first glance, this distinction may seem discrepant from the results of these other studies of behavioral influences on parietal activation. Cells of the parietal lobe are responsive to motivational variables when directing spatial attention, thereby indicating an intentional influence on the selective attentional response of this cortical region. However, a more careful examination of the concept of *intention* reveals that these conclusions are not in conflict. Heilman *et al.* (1985) specified intention narrowly, to refer to the preparation and selection of motoric responses. By means of this criterion, a distinction can be made between the preparation to initiate an action (intention) and the activation of selective attention based on behavioral changes and motivational consequences. Parietal neural activation may be associated with selective spatial attention in a manner that is behaviorally influenced by motivational variables, but that does not depend on the actual preparation for a motoric act.

CONSTRAINTS ON AUTOMATICITY OF SPATIAL SELECTION

Considerable research over the past decade has been devoted to specifying factors that influence whether attentional selection can be accomplished with automaticity. An assumption underlying these efforts is that automaticity occurs when multiple units of information can be processed simultaneously in parallel. When automaticity is not possible, an alternative for selection occurs, which involves effortful controlled attention. Controlled attentional selection requires serial processing, such that only a limited quantity of information is processed at each time point.

Schneider and Shiffrin (1977) demonstrated that by controlling three variables (frome size, memory set size, and mapping characteristics) it is possible to dissociate controlled from automatic processing. Memory set size referred to the number of potential targets that the subject had to hold in memory for future detection. Frame size referred to the number of items presented simultaneously with the target. The greater the frame size, the more difficult is the detection of the target, since more distracting stimuli would be present to compete with the target for attention. The third variable—mapping characteristics—had two conditions: variable and consistent mapping. When subjects performed under the condition of consistent mapping, the target stimulus was never presented as a distractor across other trails, whereas under the variable mapping condition, the target stimulus could occur as a distractor on other trials. Therefore, with the variable mapping task, the subject could not memorize the targets across trials to facilitate detection, but with consistent mapping task, memorization would facilitate detection.

Using reaction time as a dependent measure, Schneider and Shiffrin (1977) found a general increase in reaction time as a function of increasing frame size and memory set size only during the condition of variable mapping. Increasing memory set size from two to four slowed reaction time considerably, as did increasing frame size. With consistent mapping, there was not a major increase in reaction time as a function of memory set size. Furthermore, when distractor items that had been consistently mapped to a particular spatial position were subsequently presented along with the target stimulus, there was a 22% decline in rate of correct detection of the target.

These findings demonstrated that spatial selective detection depends on the relationship of the target to distractors, since increasing frame size slowed response time. However, it was primarily the consistency of mapping of items and spatial position in memory that affected automaticity. That response time did not increase much as a function of frame or memory set size when consistent mapping was allowed suggested that automaticity was possible. However, when consistent memory mapping was prevented, automaticity was not possible, resulting in slower serial processing.

Spatial Focus and Interference

While a major determinant of automaticity during spatial selection is the consistency of the information to be detected and its relationship to the present memory set, the automaticity of attentional selection of targets in the spatial field also depends on how the stimuli are spatially distributed. It is extremely difficult and perhaps impossible to simultaneously direct attention to multiple spatial positions when these positions have large spatial separations. This observation has led to the concept of spatial attention as spotlight. Theories of spatial selection that incorporate this spotlight metaphor predict that time is needed to redirect attention among spatially separated positions. However, it also appears that with greater spatial separation, there is less interference between targets and distractors (Johnson & Dark, 1986). When the distance between targets and distractors decreases, interference increases, which then may hamper automaticity.

Feature Integration Theory

The relationship between spatial position and automaticity becomes apparent when detection characteristics are analyzed as a function of the featural relationship targets and distractors. Treisman and Gelade (1980) developed a feature integration theory that attempted to characterize the limitations associated with perceptual encoding. They studied target detection under two featural conditions: conjunctive and disjunctive. Conjunction exists when features of the target stimulus share characteristics with the background distractor stimulus, whereas disjunction exists when the targets and distractors do not have overlapping features. Detection of stimuli under conditions of featural conjunction is much more difficult than under disjunctive conditions. For instance, detection of blue circles from a set of blue circles and red triangles is relatively easy and can be performed automatically. In contrast, detection of blue circles from a set of blue squares and yellow circles is not easy, since the underlying features overlap with multiple distractors. Treisman and Gelade (1980) found that detection of objects with conjunctive features of this type requires serial controlled attentional processing.

The findings of Treisman and Gelade demonstrate that attentional detection depends on the difficulty of featural analysis that is required to make a selection. Furthermore, they found that when subjects had poor information about where a stimulus would occur in the spatial field, their detection rates for stimuli with conjunctive features was near chance. This was not true for targets with disjunctive features, since detection of these stimuli was possible even when spatial position was not certain. Therefore, spatial position is a determining factor in specifying the increased demand for controlled attentional processing associated with the segregation of overlapping perceptual features.

Demands for Action: A Determinant of Spatial Selectivity

Most of the constraints on spatial selective attention that we have discussed arise from the characteristics of spatial representation or the way attention is directed relative to the spatial frame. While spatial selective attention can be accounted for largely on basis of these factors in laboratory situations, there is reason to believe that spatial constraints are dependent on the prevailing demands for response or, in a broader sense, action. This fact led to the development of theories that proposed that attentional selection occurs at a late stage of processing (e.g., Deutsch and Deutsch, 1963). While these theories were partially refuted, there is still strong evidence suggesting the influence of response-related (premotor) factors in the control of attention (See Chapter 3).

Some attentional theorists have suggested that spatial selective attention also depends on a need to generate organized and controlled action (e.g., Allport, 1987; Neumann, 1987; Shallice, 1972). For instance, Allport has maintained that since goal-directed action requires the specification of a unique set of execution parameters, if motor acts were always driven unidirectionally by sensory spatial selective attention, an inefficient situation would result. There would be no way to use feedback regarding the results of movement to guide sensory selection, since crosstalk between spatial selection and the motor response would create interference. Allport proposed that a selection process must exist to map information from spatial selection, with control parameters governing the particular action (e.g., reaching and grasping the object in space). The selection process for this type of mapping would require spatial and temporal segmentation of the spatial field relative to response parameters. There is considerable complexity associated with the integration of visual–spatial and motor processes. Therefore, the mechanisms that might underlie the type of mapping that Allport has proposed are not yet well established.

Temporal Constraints on Attention

Attention is temporally distributed. The inability of humans to perform optimally at all times is often an indication of attentional variation. Momentary performance variations are commonly labeled as *lapses in attention*. The construct of attention would be unnecessary if humans performed optimally at all times, by always selecting the most relevant information from the environment. The temporal inconsistency of behavioral performance is a core feature of attention.

Attention varies as a function of the temporal characteristics of both the situation and the organismic state. Under stable environmental conditions, attention varies in accordance with changes in neurobiological state over time. Under changing environmental conditions, attention is influenced by information-processing demands relative to existing time constraints. When individuals have large amounts of time to search their environment for information, they perform better than when their response time is limited. As time is a determinant of attentional performance, it is natural to question how it is represented in the neural system, and how this representation influences attentional processing.

Attention provides for the sequential selection of stimulus and responses, and for the shifting of processing allocation over time. Although it is possible to characterize sensory and response selection at isolated points in time, attention normally reflects the variability of selection over multiple trials or over spans of time. This was a central consideration of the early cognitive models of attention (e.g., Treisman, 1960, 1964, 1967), which proposed that attention was the result of a bottleneck. As people can perform only a limited number of behaviors at a time, the attentional bottleneck provided a hypothetical mechanism for information reduction. It was assumed that humans could better handle information serially. Attention provided for the sequencing of information over time. Although it is no longer assumed that serial processing is the basis for all attentional operations, it is clear that attention is related to the production of behavioral sequences. Attention is a process that provides for the allocation of cognitive resources over both time and spatial position.

PSYCHOLOGICAL TIME

The study of human time experience is made difficult by the fact that we cannot directly see or feel time. Although humans are able to report the subjective experience of time, this awareness is not a direct result of primary sensory experience. Yet, the sensation of time's passage is something that all humans experience. Time is a fundamental component of all human behaviors, as almost all cognitive processes have a time reference. For instance, the encoding of episodic information is tagged to some estimate of duration. Our auditory processing is also strongly based in time. Speech always has a syntax that reflects a sequential flow. Syntax provides a representation of temporal organization in our language. Therefore, time is paradoxical; it is intangible (unlike the spatial dimensions), but it is a fundamental characteristic of our experience.

When Immanuel Kant postulated that humans have an intrinsic spatial organization on which experience is mapped, he also emphasized that there must also be an intrinsic temporal framework. He proposed that people have an internal capacity for separating object representations in "relation to time." The logical extension of this view is that the human brain possesses a temporal-spatial coordinate system providing an organizational grid for mapping new experiences. Of course, epistemologists like Kant never speculated on the physical characteristics of such a brain system. Although the relationship between time and space has been a central focus of theoretical physics over the past century, there has been relatively little research regarding the cognitive characteristics of "time representation" or the mechanisms that may account for a temporal organization of behavior. Yet, many cognitive processes reflect an underlying relationship between behavior and time. For instance, an intrinsic determinant of "memory" is its durability (i.e., its stability over time). Therefore, how time is represented in behavior and cognition has implications for neuro-psychological inquiry.

Within the behavioral sciences, time is often used as a dependent variable. For instance, reaction time and time to criterion are two dependent variables that have been incorporated into many behavioral paradigms. In both cases, time is used as an indication of behavioral or cognitive processing characteristics. For instance, when measuring rate of learning, an investigator may use a temporal criterion (e.g., the time until some performance level is reached). As, more commonly, the number of trials to criterion is used to measure learning rate, there has been much historical debate over whether trials reflect time. Reaction time, a dependent measure used by even the earliest behavioral researchers, provides a more direct temporal marker of the speed of cognitive processes. In this sense, reaction time may reflect the temporal characteristics of the neural system and the constraints of processing speed on attention.

Time can also be an independent variable, if the central question is how performance varies as a function of duration. The most common use of time as an independent variable is in memory paradigms that use a time delay to test recall from storage. Time is an essential parameter for defining the strength and durability of memory. Memory durability is one important temporal characteristic of the neural system, which clearly constrains attention. Furthermore, memory provides a representation of time.

Although time has been an important variable in behavioral research, the characteristics of behavioral timing and time awareness are not usually the central focus of these investigations. The capacity for time awareness and estimation may reflect how time is represented in cognitive processes. The capacity of humans to estimate time may reveal the extent to which time constrains their behavior. There has been a recent upsurge of interest in the topics of time awareness and estimation. Another temporal constraint comes from the capacity of animals to time their behavioral responses. Behavioral timing may be facilitated by the capacity for time estimation. However, behavioral timing may also be influenced by intrinsic organismic characteristics and external factors that are largely unrelated to the capacity for time awareness or time estimation.

The mechanisms underlying temporal representations in cognition and behavioral timing are relevant to the study of attention. Attentional control depends on the precise timing of stimuli, responses, and duration. The regulation of attention over time may be associated with either intrinsic attributes of the neural system or nontemporal factors associated with task demand, arousal, affective state, or other components of information processing. In this chapter, we will consider how time is represented in the brain, as well as the constraints that time places on attentional processes.

TEMPORAL AND NONTEMPORAL CONTROL MECHANISMS

Time may be represented in human behavior and cognition in two very different ways. The experience of time and the timing of behaviors may result from intrinsic timekeeping mechanisms in the brain (i.e., a biological clock). However, it is also possible that contextual factors such as the sequential nature of behavior provide critical cues that may be sufficient to enable the timing of behavioral responses. In this chapter, we use the term *nontemporal* to refer to behavioral timing control that may occur without a biological clock. While the idea of nontemporal control of timing may sound like a contradiction in terms, the time denotes the concept of timekeeping without an actual clock mechanism.

Many cognitive scientists have taken the position that a clock mechanism is not necessary to explain most aspects of behavioral timing and time experience (e.g., Michon & Jackson, 1984). The need for a clock mechanism is minimized if the "psychological" time is an outgrowth of the sequential character of behavior. In the context of learning theory, behavioral responding is the by-product of the history of prior conditioning relative to the available discriminative stimuli in the environment. Therefore, behavioral timing may result from the sequential chaining of behavioral responses, without the need for a clock. A temporal reference would be established based on the order of steps in a behavioral sequence, rather than by time itself. Therefore, a clock may not be essential to make behavioral estimates of time.

How might the sequential character of behavior be used for timing without a clock? Timing may be accomplished without a clock by relying on a relative duration of certain behavioral events relative to others. An animal's behavior is comprised of a large number of responses of different durations. By establishing the "basal duration" associated with the response of shortest duration, the animal may learn to estimate other responses of longer durations. The resulting "scaling" process would enable the animal to estimate duration without knowing the exact time associated with its responses. A "quantal" time unit would be established that is referenced in an indirect way to real time, but that actually reflects the shortest duration response of the animal. Given that all behavioral events occur within the same temporal frame of reference, it would be possible to time behaviors relative to this shortest duration response (i.e., the quantal unit). Within this framework, timing results from the scaling of behaviors relative to one another.

If the minimum "real" time necessary to perform a particular simple behavioral operation is known, it would provide the building block for time estimations of more complex behaviors. For instance, if scanning a visual spatial field takes 50 msec, this duration represents a basal time unit for any operations requiring visual scanning. This interval could also serve as a time index for other behaviors that require such scanning. Therefore, the minimum duration necessary for simple responses provides a temporal constraint on any task that requires this response. Chronometric analyses assume this premise when accounting for cognitive processes on the basis of reaction time measures.

As attempts to show a relationship between biological rhythmicities and the estimation of time intervals have generally met with only limited success, some cognitive investigators have concluded that an invariant biological clock is not necessary for time estimation. They have discounted the role of biological rhythmicity in regulating short-duration timing for cognitive and behavioral operations. Support for their position has come from studies that showed that behavioral timing is influenced by a host of nontemporal factors. For instance, the estimation of the temporal duration of behavior varies as a function of the behaviors that fill the particular time interval (Jones & Boltz, 1989; Ornstein, 1969). Equivalent time intervals are often judged as having different durations, depending on the task that is performed during the interval.

Despite some findings from cognitive studies of time estimation that minimize the need for an invariant timekeeping mechanism for short-duration behaviors, there continues to be much appeal in the idea that neurobiological clock mechanisms facilitate the behavioral timing of sequential responses and the scheduling of behaviors. Biologists have long been interested in factors governing certain rhythmic activities, ranging from hibernation and sleep to endocrine cycles. The existence of biological rhythmicity suggested that behavior may be influenced by biological systems that have the properties of a clock. This has led to intensive investigations in search of neural systems that may serve as timekeepers for behavior (Aschoff, 1981, 1984).

Is a neurobiological clock a prerequisite for the production of sequential behavior and time estimation? Perhaps a neural clock mechanism is not required if nontemporal control of timing is possible. Yet, behavioral timing would certainly be facilitated by such a timekeeper. A neural system with precise timekeeping properties would be able to handle larger quantities of information—and, therefore, attentional operations—more efficiently. In the following section, we discuss evidence for the role of biological clocks used for behavioral regulation.

CLOCKS, PACEMAKERS, AND QUANTAL DURATIONS

Until recently, the need for an internal biological clock for behavioral timing was largely a matter of theoretical conjecture, as a biological clock had never actually been demonstrated. This stance changed dramatically with the discovery that the suprachiasmatic nucleus (SCN) of the hypothalamus has a circadian timekeeping capacity (Aschoff, 1981; Lydic, Albers, Tepper, & Moore–Ede, 1982) (see Figure 20.1). For a neural structure to serve as a potential biological clock, three criteria must be met: (1) it must possess a relatively invariant timing interval; (2) it must maintain its pacemaker function, even when isolated from other neural systems; and (3) it must have influence on other behavioral or biological functions. The SCN meets these criteria and thereby provides strong evidence that there is an endogenous biological clock with important influences on the timing of biological and behavioral events in a daily rhythm.

The temporal properties of the SCN are now reasonably well understood. The degree of variance of this clock has been established with reasonable accuracy, as it has a relatively invariant period, approximately equal to 1 day. The SCN acts with circadian rhythmicity, even when it is isolated from other brain systems, and it therefore meets the second criterion. Its role in the temporal measurement and regulation of other physiological systems and behavioral responses has also been well demonstrated.

There are other physiological systems that meet some of these criteria, but that do not have all of the properties of a clock. For instance, the heart beats at a fairly consistent rhythm over short time periods, and its beat serves to influence other systems and physiological responses. However, cardiac rhythm is highly irregular over longer periods of time and

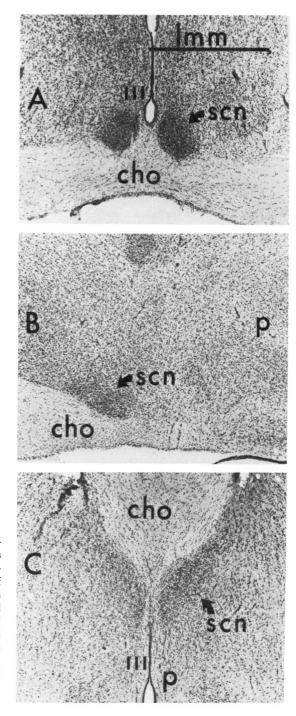

FIGURE 20.1. The suprachiasmatic nucleus (SCN) as seen in brain sections taken from a rat and a monkey. (A) Coronal section from photomicrograph of cresyl-violet-stained rat SCN (0.4 mm from the rostal SCN pole). (B) Sagittal section (0.5 mm from midline) of SCN in a squirrel monkey. (C) Horizontal section (0.2 mm from the ventral surface) of the SCN in the squirrel monkey. p is posterior, III is third ventricle, and cho is underlying optic chiasm. From Lydic *et al.* (1982), with permission.

therefore would not be a very accurate clock. More important, there is little evidence at this point that the heart is used by the brain to time behavioral responses. This is not to say that the heart has no timing capacity. If the heart's pacemaking action also serves as a clock, the mechanisms underlying this function have not been defined.

An important point is raised by this example of cardiac rhythm: There is a distinction between clock and pacemaker functions. Pacemakers are similar to clocks in that they pulsate in a rhythmic manner, which produces a periodic physiological effect. However, pacemakers do not necessarily act as timekeepers for temporal regulation. The heart is a pacemaker, as it contracts in a rhythm that supplies blood to the body in a periodic way. Yet, it has not been shown to serve as a clock for temporal control.

If there are multiple biological clocks, each should have a different fundamental unit of time to which it is tuned. The possibility that there are also neural clocks capable of timing shorter term behaviors has been suggested by some cognitive researchers (e.g., Kristofferson, 1980). If the capacity for timing short durations is controlled by a clock mechanism, it should be possible to delineate a small "quantal" time unit. The quantal unit would be the finest level of temporal discriminability and resolution that is possible for a particular functional system. Much effort has been devoted to determining whether there is a quantal time unit used for determining short durations during behavioral timing, as well as for time awareness.

NEURAL CLOCKS FOR BEHAVIORAL REGULATION

All living species have physiological and behavioral periodicities that can be specified across varying time frames of a day, a month, or a year. Often, these periods are synchronized with external periods, such as day and night, the lunar phases, or the seasons of the year. There is now evidence that organisms have internal clocks that act as self-sustaining pacemakers synchronized with these periods (Aschoff, 1981, 1984). Like manufactured clocks, internal pacemakers have a synchronized, regular character in their movements, leading to their description as circaclocks (e.g., circadian, circannual). Although these clocks run without the need of external input, it is also true that they synchronize their timing with cues from the environment (*Zeitgebers*), so as to maintain consistency with environmental periods (Pittendrigh, 1981).

The circadian clocks are the most well-documented and best understood of the internal biological clocks. They provide a daily rhythm that synchronizes various functions such as endocrine release, sleep, and various appetitive behaviors. One of the most invariant circadian rhythms is core body temperature. Circadian rhythmicity has been demonstrated in species ranging from simple one-celled organisms to primates. The demonstration of circadian periodicity in primates by Albers and his colleagues (1991) provided evidence that a clock is present even in animals that are very similar to humans. Furthermore, the demonstration of circadian variation in basic cellular processes, such as messenger RNA levels, in the SCN (Albers, Liou, Ferris, Stopa, & Zoeller, 1991; Schwartz, Davidsen, & Smith, 1984) suggest that these rhythms may be controlled by genetically mediated processes.

It has been known for some time that circadian periodicity influences cognitive performance. The performance of individuals on demanding cognitive tasks varies over the course of the day in a manner that roughly corresponds with the circadian phase. Kleitman and Jackson (1951) found that auditory and visual reaction times varied in a manner that correlated with circadian temperature period. Interestingly, time estimation for even short durations of several seconds has been found to vary in a circadian period. This finding suggests that circadian factors influence short-duration timing. There are many other experimental studies of performance variability as a function of circadian period (Folkard, 1979a,b; Hockey & Colquhoun, 1972).

The role of the SCN in the maintenance of circadian rhythmicity has been well established in laboratory animals, including primates. Demonstrating the role of the SCN in humans is much more difficult because of obvious methodological limitations. Although it is clear that humans have circadian rhythms for a variety of physiological functions (e.g., temperature and cortisol levels), how strongly the SCN influences these rhythms has not been fully established, partly because of the capacity of humans to override the biological pressures created by their appetitive states. For instance, people often prevent themselves from sleeping, thereby overriding this urge. Yet, the presence of circadian rhythmicity goes without question, and there is good reason to believe that the SCN provides an important influence on the temporal organization of human behavior.

The analysis of clinical neuropsychological cases provides one means of showing a potential role for the SCN in temporal behavioral control in humans (e.g., Cohen & Albers, 1991). Cohen and Albers studied a patient with damage to the hypothalamic region containing the SCN resulting from craniopharyngioma. They observed numerous behavioral and cognitive disruptions that reflected temporal disregulation, presumably because of the disruption of a clock mechanism.

Patients with seasonal affective disorders have provided another source of clinical data regarding biological rhythmicity in humans. Investigations into the behavioral characteristics of these patients over the course of the day, at various times of the year, suggest that alterations in the light–dark cycle occurring with seasonal variation create a disregulation of normal periodicity, which may disrupt neuroendocrine patterns (Rosenthal & Blehar, 1989). Disregulation of the periodicity of neuroendocrine release may produce asynchronies between environmental signals of light onset and the circadian clock.

Unfortunately, behavioral findings regarding the relationship of circadian periodicity, light–dark cycles, and cognitive performance are not always clear-cut. Some contradictory evidence has been found. Results often depend on the exact parameters of the tasks used. For instance, Folkard and his colleagues conducted experiments using memory measures as well as attentional tasks such as a letter cancellation task and measured the relationship between performance and biological rhythm (Folkard, 1981a,b; Folkard & Nank, 1980). They found that performance was highly correlated and in phase with circadian variations in body temperature when subjects had to detect two-letter stimuli, but was out of phase with circadian variations in temperature when the task required the detection of six-letter targets. This finding is difficult to explain.

The relationships among light–dark conditions, human behavioral performance, and circadian rhythm have been studied extensively (Aschoff, 1981, 1984). Human subjects were kept in an isolation chamber for long durations (several weeks). Light–dark cycles were maintained by the experimenter. By the use of cues signaling various time periods, the human circadian period could be entrained to other time periods (e.g., 26.67 hr). Therefore, the circadian period can be altered by environmental manipulations. In a related study, Aschoff (1984) found that the light–dark cycle is not the primary determinant of variations in motor response over the course of the circadian period. When different light–dark schedules were maintained for long periods, most performance characteristics did not vary as a function of schedule. Instead, performance (e.g., finger tapping) varied as a function of the intrinsic circadian period (Aschoff, 1984).

Several factors besides light–dark cycle affect the entrainment of circadian rhythms. Anticipatory activity has a particular influence on behavioral rhythms, a finding suggesting the role of motivational influences on the circadian clock. Changes in the pattern of presentation of social cues, food, and sleep allocation influence circadian periodicity. These factors may directly affect timing and time estimation. Although factors such as motivational state may affect circadian rhythm, the inverse is not necessarily true. Lesions to the SCN that produce circadian disturbances may not disrupt motivational state. For instance, the anticipatory behavior in restricted-feeding paradigms has been shown to be unimpaired following these lesions (Terman, 1983). Therefore, the relationship between behavioral variables like motivation and circadian timing is very complex. Systems governing these interactions may not always respond in a reciprocal manner. Efforts to manipulate or to control for the interaction of circadian periodicity and performance have raised many new questions. Some studies have supported the role of external stimuli in influencing circadian variations in behavior, and others have suggested that performance varies in a circadian pattern regardless of what *Zeitgebers* (i.e., periodic environmental signals) are entraining the circadian period.

The analysis of circadian variations in the accuracy of time perception contains similar complexities. In general, it has been shown that subjects tend to underestimate moderate durations of time (e.g., 1-hr intervals) when they are very alert, and to overestimate these durations when they are tired. Their estimates follow a circadian pattern. However, the relationship between time estimation and circadian period varies as a function of the duration to be estimated. Aschoff (1984) reported that estimates of short durations (10 sec) are not highly correlated with circadian phase in subjects kept in isolation, whereas their 1-hr estimates are highly linked. Furthermore, the short-duration estimates have considerable between- and within-subject variability estimates, whereas long-duration estimates show much less variability.

These findings have led some investigators to postulate either that additional circadian oscillators are operating (Wever, 1979), or that an entirely different, noncircadian process is responsible for performance differences. Unfortunately, the possibility that there are multiple interacting internal clocks with different rhythmicities raises many complications for current models of the temporal regulation of behavior that advocate an underlying time base or clock. Also, the SCN is the only neural structure that has been established as a true biological clock.

Short Duration Timing

As discussed earlier, circadian periodicity influences behavioral performance over the course of each day. Attentional performance is likely to be much different in the morning from what it is late at night. Circadian neural systems produce a daily rhythm. The influence of circadian phase on performance is greatest for long duration tasks and becomes less critical when estimation of the shorter durations is required. Variations in neurobiological state over the circadian period are the basis for performance differences. Normally, there is less variability within short intervals of the daily period. Therefore, short-duration time estimates to the circadian rhythm are relatively insensitive.

It is unreasonable to assume that a circadian clock is responsible for all forms of behavioral timing. Two other possibilities are more likely: (1) other neural clocks enable the consistent measurement of short durations, or (2) neural clocks are not essential for the behavioral timing of short durations. The existence of a circadian clock does not eliminate the possibility that nontemporal factors influence short-duration timing. In fact, there continues to be much debate among some cognitive theorists over this issue. Later in this chapter, we reconsider arguments for the nontemporal control of short-duration behavioral timing. There is also growing evidence that other neural systems have clock or pacemaker functions in behavioral timing. Therefore, we explore here how a short-duration clock may operate to provide a short-duration temporal organization for behavior.

Models of Short-Duration Clocks

Michael Treisman (1963) proposed one of the first cognitive models to account for a short-term clock. His model contains a pacemaker that keeps time. The pacemaker interacts with a counter, which enables the neural system to count the number of time intervals occurring during a particular period. Treisman suggested that the speed of the pacemaker is influenced by central nervous system arousal. He gave three hypotheses regarding the relationship between generalized arousal and the pacemaker function: (1) generalized arousal differs from specific arousal, which influences the pacemaker, but these two forms of arousal interact; (2) the generalized arousal acts nonspecifically on a pacemaker system; and (3) the various rhythms associated with arousal (e.g., alpha activity) create a pattern of activity with frequencies that create a pacemaking function.

In order to test these hypotheses, Treisman studied the spectral power characteristics of the EEG of subjects engaged in time estimation tasks during different states of generalized arousal. Spectral power analysis provides an indication of the dominant frequency of electrical brain activity over time. Faster activity reflects higher levels of alertness, and slower activity reflects decreased vigilance or increasing drowsiness. Treisman found that the hypothesis of a common pacemaker for timing and generalized arousal was not supported. The stability of the arousal pattern, as indicated by alpha activity, was much greater then the stability of the timing function. He also found that the temporal pacemaker was not just a specific expression of generalized arousal. The frequency characteristics of the temporal pacemaker and the arousal function differed. This finding led Treisman to the conclusion that there must be separate oscillators controlling temporal regulation and generalized arousal. Although these oscillators may interact, they do not vary in a consistent relationship.

The properties that would be necessary for an internal clock to be capable of short-duration timing were summarized in a recent by Church (1984) (see Figure 20.2). Such a clock must be a temporal pacemaker that has a pulse rate that is modifiable, as duration judgments for short durations often vary. The clock must be sensitive to a host of factors, such as stress and biochemical, metabolic, and motivational state. It must have a switching mechanism that allows it to start, stop, and reset. The clock must act as an accumulator that sequentially, summates quantal time units. The quantal unit is the smallest fundamental unit of time that the system is capable of using for purposes of behavioral timing.

According to Church, the temporal accumulator must be able to transform its time count to another form of information, and to relate the derived duration to events in an episodic memory at a later stage of processing. This transformation should be under the influence of external factors such as new input into the system. The memory that is generated from information from the accumulator must be capable of being reset (i.e., so that old memory is dumped, and new memory space is allocated). Church went on to argue that there must be more than one pacemaker module capable of performing these processes, as humans are capable of carrying on simultaneous temporal processes.

Despite the inherent complexity in a system with multiple clocks, it seems at least plausible that there is more than one neural center with "clock" properties. If there are multiple clocks, it would be important to determine how a common time standard is maintained among them, as each would have a different periodicity. For multiple clocks to work efficiently, they must be nested within each other, with some form of master control. It is not at all clear how the brain would coordinate multiple clocks in a uniform reference system. A system with multiple clocks is possible only if there is a way of synchronizing the short-duration clocks with the circadian clock.

If there is a short-duration clock that is separate from the circadian system, a fundamental question remains: Where is this pacemaker located? Recent findings have provided some

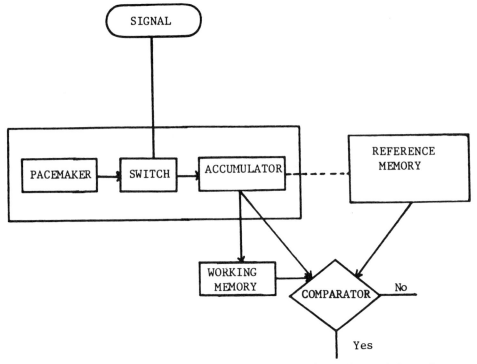

FIGURE 20.2. Model proposed for a neuronal clock for the control of short-duration behavioral timing. From Church (1984), with permission.

clues to the answer, as several other neural structures have been shown to have pacemaker characteristics that may influence behavioral timing, including regions of the cerebellum, the basal ganglia, and the hippocampus. For instance, the cerebellum has been shown to produce oscillatory rhythms that provide a temporal base for motor timing (Ivry, Keele, & Diener, 1988). The hippocampus has also been implicated as a source of timing that may influence the temporal characteristics of episodic encoding. The hippocampus generates an activational rhythm that may influence its temporal capacity. Interestingly, lesions to parts of the fornix create a signal gap that may cause the resetting of temporal memory. Although this type of finding has yielded new avenues of experimental pursuit, there is still much to be learned about the neurophysiological underpinnings of these potential pacemakers.

TEMPORAL FACTORS UNDERLYING ATTENTIONAL TIMING

How does the temporal organization of behavior influence attention? Conversely, how does attention influence the way we experience time? Previous experimental work has focused on two areas that may have relevance to these questions: (1) time perception and duration estimation, and (2) the timing of behavior and cognitive operations. While these two topics are conceptually related, they have a slightly different focus.

The topic of time perception is concerned with the nature of the human time experience and the capacity of humans to perceive and estimate time. The goal of these efforts is often to define the psychophysical parameters underlying time perception. In contrast, the study of behavioral timing often has been directed at determining how temporal factors are used to facilitate behavioral or cognitive performance. Both topics are of theoretical relevance to attention, as most attentional tasks require sustained performance over time. Some tasks make an explicit demand for time estimation or precise timing of responses. For such tasks, the nature of temporal processing may be central to an understanding of how attention is controlled. Other attentional operations may not require behavioral timing, yet are implicitly dependent on the temporal parameters underlying the task to be performed. Because of the relevance of temporal factors to attention, we will consider some of the factors that influence time perception and estimation, and then subsequently behavioral timing.

Time Perception and Duration Estimation

Although time is intrinsic in the structure of behavior, some cognitive processes can be explained without a process for temporal measurement. For instance, auditory processing requires the registration and encoding of sounds that are sequenced in time. Yet, time perception is probably not critical in the perceptual synthesis of information from sound. Speech recognition is a by-product of the temporal relationship between sounds, but not necessarily of the estimation of the duration of sounds. Modifying the timing of speech output interferes with reception because of limitations of the quantity of information that can be accurately processed in a given time interval, not because of problems with time duration estimation. The capacity to measure time seems to have little bearing on this temporally based operation.

Other behavioral processes depend more directly on the estimation of time. For instance, certain conditioning paradigms require the animal to wait a certain duration before responding in order to receive a reward [differential rate of low-level responding (DRL)]. Animals can learn to make very accurate duration judgments. There are many examples of time judgments in human behavior as well. For instance, musicians require a precise sense of timing in order to maintain rhythms while they play. The perception of time is, in fact, essential to the ability of humans to organize their activities over the course of a day. This necessity is illustrated by the fact that humans invented mechanical clocks to facilitate timekeeping. Although these clocks may have decreased our reliance on internal time perception, people still perform reasonably well in estimating time without the aid of a clock.

Temporal Psychophysics

Some investigators have postulated that temporal discrimination and generalization may follow psychophysical rules similar to Fechner's law (Heinemann, 1984). However, the role of temporal perception in information processing is still not well established. Psychophysical studies have demonstrated that, after practicing, humans are capable of making reasonably accurate duration discriminations of times as short as 200 msec. The duration judgments of subjects about repeated time intervals is, in fact, remarkably consistent. They show relatively little variability in their time estimates when state and dispositional factors are held constant. Several investigators have postulated that this temporal invariance reflects the existence of a "quantal time unit" associated with a clock that provides a metric for short-duration time perception (Hopkins & Kristofferson, 1980; Kristofferson, 1977; Wing & Kristofferson, 1973).

The proposed quantal time unit acts as a primary unit of time measurement (see Figure

20.3). When subjects are asked to discriminate between tones of different duration, there is a smallest duration for which a discrimination is possible. At these short durations, the subject's resolution when making judgments occurs with reference to a basal time unit, which is called a *quantum*. The duration of the quantal time unit relates to the variance of the time estimation for various intervals, which is relatively consistent across people in the making of duration discriminations and judgments.

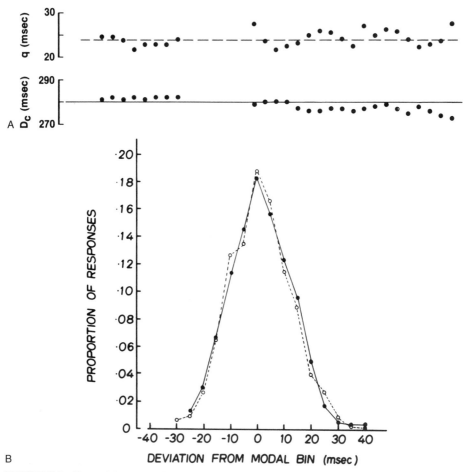

FIGURE 20.3. Quantal time units for duration estimation and motor control have been demonstrated through an analysis of response variance over repeated trials. The subject's task in a study by Kristofferson (1984) was to maintain motor sequences with a particular interbeat interval. (A) The variability in interval duration estimation is distributed around a base duration (D_c), with a quantal time (q) of 48 msec. The variance around the base duration is extremely small. (B) In fact, when interbeat duration is relatively short, low variance is usually found. Distributions of response latencies for two different estimated temporal intervals (307 and 547 msec) are shown. While the estimated intervals differ greatly in magnitude, the variance around these intervals are the same (S.D. = 12), illustrating the temporal invariance in estimation and motor timing for this task. From Kristofferson (1984), with permission.

Kristofferson (1980) estimated quantal unit sizes of approximately 12, 25, and 50 msec, as a function of different base durations that were being judged. The fact that the quantal unit doubled in a rather precise manner suggested that the quantal times of 25, 50, 100, and longer units were built on a fundamental quantum of about 12 msec. This estimate was based on the consistency in the latencies of the subjects' responses to stimulus onsets when making duration judgments. Hopkins (1984) developed a model to account for the role of these quantal temporal units for the synchronization of stimuli and responses. The model was based on the fact these quantal time units are relatively invariant under controlled experimental conditions of short-duration time estimation.

Experiments on the psychophysics of temporal duration estimation illustrate that the nervous system is capable of timekeeping with a high degree of invariance. This temporal invariance provides support for the possible role of an internal clock, as it would be difficult to produce precise time estimates without a consistent pacemaker. However, not all evidence supports the invariance of timekeeping.

When estimates of longer time intervals are required, models that propose that time measurements are accomplished through a quantal metric have greater difficulty. Under these conditions, there is greater variability in duration judgments. Also, differences in duration judgments have been noted across different modalities (e.g., visual versus auditory signals), although fairly accurate judgments can be made in both modalities (Stubbs, 1968, 1979). Other findings suggest that, although there is relatively little variance in the quantal units underlying temporal duration discriminations in human adults, this is not the case in other species or even in human children. They show greater variability (Eisler, 1984). Variability of duration estimates is greatest as durations become long, which may be why children and other animal species have difficulty with activities that have long durations or that involve delay of gratification. As they have a bias for greater temporal accuracy during shorter duration estimates, they have a tendency to underestimate time as durations become long, which ultimately may result in a failure of staying on-task.

There are several fundamental problems in models that argue for the role of an intrinsic metric like the quantal unit. Timing variability may also be due to factors that are not directly related to the quantal unit or the characteristics of an internal clock. For instance, Gibbon, Church, and Meck (1984) postulated that time estimation variability arises from the interaction of the internal pacemaker with memory. It may be that there is pacemaker invariance, but that the memory for the count of quantal intervals has variability. Also, as there has been a suggestion of more than one quantal interval, can it be assumed that all temporal intervals are built on the metric of a single clock? If not, more than one clock may be needed (Kristofferson, 1984). Whether neurophysiological data will support a system with multiple clocks is still to be seen.

Duration Discrimination without a Clock

Some cognitive theorists have correctly noted that there is considerable ambiguity regarding the metric interval that may underlie timing durations of various lengths. They argue that the ability to make accurate time-duration estimations varies considerably across experimental conditions. The investigator can cause subjects either to overestimate or to underestimate time intervals by modifying either the task or the dispositional factors in the paradigm. Task demand can be altered by manipulating factors like memory load and stimulus set size. Dispositional factors such as motivational and emotional state, as well as arousal level, have also been shown to influence duration estimates.

The time order of events or behavioral processes has been shown to produce distortions in timing and duration estimation (Allan, 1977, 1984; Jamieson, 1977; Jamieson &

Petrusic, 1976). For instance, when subjects are required to estimate the duration of auditory vocal sounds, their performance varies as a function of the order of the sounds. This effect was demonstrated in experiments (Allan, 1984) in which subjects were required to judge the duration of two tones. The two tones differed in duration, so that, in some conditions, the shorter tone preceded the longer tone and vice versa. The task was to choose the longer duration tone. Subjects performed better when the longer tone preceded the shorter tone. This finding suggests that the order of the stimuli was critical, perhaps because of a subjective preference for primacy, or because the first stimulus interferes with analysis of the second (Jamieson, 1977; Jamieson & Petrusic, 1976; Jamieson, Slawinska, Cheesman, & Spinoza-Vargas, 1984).

Allan (1977, 1984) studied temporal variances in the duration estimation of both auditory frequencies and durations. She found that changes in one of these psychophysical dimensions resulted in a parallel change in judgment of the other dimension. For example, estimating increased durations resulted in the subjects' also making estimates of higher pitched sounds. This effect was considered a contingent aftereffect of one psychophysical property's influencing judgment of the other. In these experiments, the effects were also noted to be order-sensitive, as the order of presentation of the sounds influenced the perceived duration and pitch. The presence of *contingent aftereffects* illustrates that duration estimation is subject to considerable variability based on the interactions of fundamental psychophysical characteristics, as well as on the sequence of events.

Sequential factors have been found to influence temporal discriminations in lower species. For instance, Wasserman, DeLong, and Larew (1984) studied duration and order discrimination in pigeons by using operant-conditioning paradigms. They found that, when making discriminations, pigeons rely on information obtained from the temporal order of stimuli. The accuracy of their temporal discriminations is sensitive to the order of the stimuli. In summary, these findings illustrate that variances due to the order of events, as well as to the interaction of the stimulus factors, pose significant problems for the concept of a quantal unit or an invariant clock that marks time. This gives support to the notion that temporal judgment probably depends on factors in addition to a clock mechanism. The fact that estimations of duration vary considerably across experimental conditions has also led to a consideration of timing mechanisms that do not depend on a clock.

Nontemporal Models of Duration Estimation

Several alternative nontemporal models have been proposed to account for time duration estimation. In general these models suggest that temporal information is extracted by the individual based on the type of processing that is being performed. The sequential nature of information processing is thought to provide cues or relative temporal markers enabling duration estimation. The information that fills the time interval is ultimately considered critical in the time estimates that are generated. This effect has been described as the *filled-interval effect*.

The filled-interval effect specifically refers to the fact that two equivalent intervals are often judged to be different as a result of the type of information that fills them. Ornstein (1969) accounted for this effect by postulating that variances in time estimation are primarily a result of the complexity of the information being encoded into memory and the amount of memory storage required to handle this information. Although this model has some appeal, its predictions are difficult to demonstrate.

Subsequently, other models were developed to explain temporal estimation that considered intervening processes besides memory storage. Michon and Jackson (1984) proposed that attentional factors are important in explaining temporal estimation. Block (1978) attributed capacity for time estimation to cognitive operations that evaluate changes in situational context. Emphasis on active cognitive processing versus the size of the memory distinguishes these models from Ornstein's proposal. All of these models have some difficulty accounting for the full range of behaviors in which temporal estimations occur.

More recently, Jones and Boltz (1989) proposed an alternative explanation that is of considerable interest in light of our focus on attention. They suggested that temporal duration estimations are essential to attending, as they place constraints on the act of attending. Starting with the assumption that all time periods occur relative to other periods, Jones and Boltz argued that the coherence of these time intervals depends on their relationship to events in the spatial environment of the given individual. They also made the point that some natural events have much underlying coherence in their temporal structure, whereas others are less predictable and thus less temporally coherent. Some processes, such as motor action and melodic production, normally have considerable temporal coherence. Other processes, such as speech, fail to meet the criteria for temporally coherent information, as most of the information conveyed in speech is not determined by a temporal structure. In fact, the unique temporal patterns conveyed in speech often serve to convey meaning.

Jones and Boltz suggested that the temporal structure implicit in information's being processed by the system influences the attentional allocation that is necessary, as well as the tendency to shift attention. Conversely, the individual's goals in a situation influence her or his "attunement" to particular temporal rhythms. The concept of *attunement* is used to refer to the sensitivity of the attentional system to particular environmental rhythms. As attention to speech, body actions, and other environmental events depends on sensitivity to these rhythms Jones and Boltz concluded that attention involves an interactive setting of attunements with regard to patterns of activity in the environment. Attention is considered an active process of tuning the neural system to a dynamic environment. Shifts of attention involve the shifting the attunement to a different temporal pattern. Presumably, a similar attunement can be postulated on the basis of spatial pattern.

According to this model, inexact time estimations occur when there is a failure of attunement. This can happen when a cognitive process or an environmental event is very complex and has weaker temporal coherence or temporal patterns that are more difficult to resolve. Failed attunement can also occur as the result of attending based on an orientation to future events. Although anticipatory state predicts a particular temporal pattern, confusion results when the expected temporal pattern is not present. Accordingly, estimations of temporal duration are influenced with regard to the mode of attending.

Behavioral and Cognitive Timing

A number of other temporal factors besides time estimation may also influence attention. As we mentioned previously, the parameters that influence the timing of specific cognitive and behavioral processes are also potentially important determinants of attentional control.

When studying behavioral timing, it is not always clear whether time should be treated like other experimental variables, such as stimulus intensity and reinforcement type, or whether it should be considered fundamentally different. It may be that, although time is inherent in all behavioral phenomena, it is of less importance than physical stimuli like food. If this is the case, too much emphasis on the variable of time would be a mistake. The sequence of the events that are occurring at different time points would be of greater relevance. Time may be a valid attribute of behavior, but one that does not influence performance directly. On the other hand, time may directly influence cognitive processes, and other cognitive and behavioral processes may affect timing mechanisms. Time may be viewed either as a passive characteristic of information or as an attribute that is actively processed by the system. Investigations of the role of timing in behavior have focused on different processes, including motor responding, conditioning, and cognitive operations. We briefly discuss findings regarding the timing of these processes and how it influences attentional control.

Timing of Motoric Responses

The production of motor responses depends on the synchronization of a large number of responses over time. There are several possible relationships between timing and motor production processes. The production of a motor act may be generated according to a pre-established response schema or motor program that is adjusted as necessary after the initiation of the response. Accordingly, there is a predetermined timing characteristic for the motor response, and adjustments in timing are based on new information over the course of the response. Feedback from muscles may provide the information necessary for the timing of a "force–time" pattern (Keele, 1981). Force–time patterns coordinate the appropriate muscular force at each moment in time for a particular action.

Another aspect of the relationship between motor responding and timing is that motor responding has a natural temporal character that is determined by the temporal-spatial parameters of the task. For instance, a motor task which requires that a person tap their index finger at a particular rate has inherent temporal and spatial characteristics that govern the range of responses that are possible. The range of possible responses is further limited by characteristics of the motor system and preexisting motor programs for a particular type of movement. The net effect of all of these factors is that there is relative invariance to the way most humans execute skilled motor responses (Rosenbaum, 1991). Therefore, motor timing may be governed by the nature of the motor response that is required for a particular task. Evidence for this position has come from analyses of the stereotypy of handwriting (Viviani & Terzulo, 1980). For tasks requiring more precise timing, animals seem to have the capacity to direct their motor timing to the proper level of temporal resolution (Stelmach, Mullins, & Teulings, 1984). When there is a need for gross movements with minimal dexterity, less temporal resolution may be generated than for skilled high-dexterity movements.

The possibility that a pacemaker influences the timing of motor acts has been suggested by studies in which the subject is required to maintain a consistent motor rhythm (e.g., tapping). Wing and Kristofferson (1973) demonstrated variances in motor production that they attributed to two interacting processes. Variability in response pattern may be produced by imprecisions in a hypothetical pacemaker, or by interference created by the generation of responses that are triggered by this pacemaker. Within this model of motor timing, the pacemaker is given an important role. Wing and Kristofferson (1973) conducted studies to test the role of pacemaker function in repetitive movements. Support was found for a two-process model, in which the pacemaker shows greater invariance than the motor system itself. Wing, Keele, and Margolin (1984) provided evidence that the timing deficits noted in Parkinson's disease may be related more to pacemaker dysfunction than to delays in the motor system.

Motor timing is probably controlled by both a central pacemaker function and cues obtained from force–time feedback from the actual motor response. By manipulating the experimental paradigm, it can be shown that either the pacemaker function or the motoric feedback information gains greater relative importance (Semjen, Garcia-Colera, & Requin, 1984). However, the extent to which motor acts are typically under the control of serial processes is not entirely clear.

A theoretical alternative can be derived from the parallel-processing approach. Although motor acts are sequential by nature, they may be controlled in a parallel fashion. Rumelhart and Norman (1982) suggested a model of motor control in typing, which postulates that a schema is generated when the typist determines what word to type, so that after initiation of the response, a whole pattern is generated for the production of the entire word. This raises problems in understanding the neural basis of timing during motor responding. It is possible that the timing of the execution of schemata is sequential, whereas the production of motor responses within a schema is more automatized and under the control of a central pacemaker. Schweickert (1984) reviewed the complexities involved in timing dual tasks.

Verbal Learning

There has been some debate regarding the role of timing in cognitive processes. Temporal variables have been studied in the context of verbal learning, memory encoding, perpetual identification, and other cognitive operations. For instance, the temporal spacing of stimulus presentation during verbal learning paradigms influences the rate of learning. During paired-associates learning, distinctions between massed and spaced practice have been demonstrated (e.g., Izawa, 1971). Spaced practice has advantages that may be related to the time necessary to consolidate the material in memory. Although this temporal parameter clearly influences performance, it can be argued that it is not actually a timing effect. The intertrial interval simply provides time for processing.

However, some investigators consider timing important in verbal learning. Tzeng, Lee, and Wetzel (1979) argued for the importance of sequence in the derivation of temporal information in the processing of verbal material. Subjects who are presented with words to study for latter recall rely on old memories of these words for rehearsal in working memory. The comparison of new material with old memories is an indication of sequential processing according to Tzeng et al., and therefore, temporal information may be a by-product of this type of rehearsal.

Cognitive Processing

The influence of temporal factors on information processing is apparent across a wide range of cognitive functions, including perceptual judgments of duration, motor responding, and learning and memory. In all of these process, the sequential nature of information processing places constraints on performance. According to Heinemann (1984), stored temporal information has psychophysical properties that are similar to other variables such as stimulus intensity. The temporal characteristics of memory should be very predictable for factors such as duration. The extent to which the temporal dynamics of the memory trace influence variables such as interstimulus interval may ultimately determine how memory influences timing.

The duration of events provides information about the identity of the event that is being processed. The time course of perceptual processes may have great relevance to the meaning of the information that is being transmitted. For instance, speech sounds of different durations may convey very different information. Massaro (1972, 1975, 1984) demonstrated that the perception and processing of auditory information depend on information provided by temporal cues.

Temporal order effects have also been demonstrated for verbally processed material, as subjects show a preference for word pairs presented in logical order (Michon & Jackson, 1984). These findings suggest that the temporal information given by sequence influences the quality of both auditory and visual perceptual processing.

The accuracy of perceptual analysis depends on the temporal order of the stimuli to be processed. Collard and Leeuwenberg (1981) demonstrated that the perceptual analysis of shapes depends on the order of presentation. Subjects performed recall better when a difficult shape was followed by a shape that was easy to analyze, than when the shapes were presented in the opposite order.

Some cognitive scientists have disputed the notion that temporal information is critical to normal information processing. Michon and Jackson (1984) argued that temporal information is not easily encoded unless meaning can be derived from that information. A variety of nontemporal factors, such as the level of processing, the context, the instructional set, and the sequential characteristics of the stimuli, influence the temporal characteristics of cognitive performance. Michon and Jackson concluded that timing is relatively unimportant.

Animal Conditioning

As we have discussed previously, conditioning is influenced by many temporal variables, such as the contiguity between the unconditioned stimulus and the conditioned stimulus. Temporal factors have a bearing on the rate of learning, extinction, and a host of other performance factors. Furthermore, memory is a function of temporal factors such as the rate of trace formation and decay.

Although temporal contiguity alone does not account for conditioning (Rescorla & Wagner, 1972) temporal parameters influence conditioning in many paradigms (Gibbon, 1981; Jenkins, 1984). Delayed nonmatching to sample and delayed alternation are two of the paradigms most commonly used in studying memory formation in primates. Performance on conditioning tasks depends on the size of the delay between the acquisition and recall trials. The animal must often remember a sequence of operations and then learn to modify its response accordingly. The ability to make accurate responses may be related to subtle factors such as the recency of the stimuli and the spacing between the trials. The temporal demands of these types of conditioning tasks is quite apparent.

Both delayed nonmatching to sample and delayed alternation depend on both temporal discrimination and event memory (Staddon, 1984). The temporal variables affecting delayed nonmatching to sample have been studied extensively. Four variables that have a particular influence on this task are the length of the sample stimulus presentation, the latency between the sample and the comparison stimulus, the interval between the successive sample-stimulus presentations, and the interval between the successive trials. Roberts and Kramer (1982) argued that the influence of these temporal variables can be explained in terms of the parameters of trace decay. Therefore, temporal discriminations on this task may be secondary to the characteristics of memory.

Meck (1984) conducted a series of investigations of the temporal parameters underlying animal conditioning. These investigations provide the most comprehensive treatment of the relationship among timing, conditioning, and attention that is currently available from the field of animal learning. Meck (1984) demonstrated that it is possible to create an attentional bias in animals during the course of conditioning. According to Meck, this attentional bias influences memory by altering the parameters underlying temporal discriminations. Meck used two temporal discrimination procedures in which rats were required to wait a specified period of time before making a bar-press response. He then created unbalanced probabilities of reinforcement in one procedure, so that the likelihood that the rat would respond in a particular way was influenced. In another procedure, the rats were cued by means of a prior-entry method. Regardless of the method, an attentional expectancy was established. This expectancy affected the timing of durations of future trials in different modalities (e.g., visual versus auditory). Differences were noted depending on whether the animals were to switch from the visual to the auditory modality or vice versa. Meck, Komeily, and Church demonstrated that the interaction of timing associated with stimulus processing may be subject to interference from response timing, suggesting a complex interaction of stimulus and response factors in timing.

Meck's results illustrate how attentional allocation may effect temporal judgments during operant responding when the task requires duration estimates (see Figure 20.4). He concluded that variance in the capacity of animals to time their behavior is due to the influence of attention on internal clock speed. Presumably, the time required to switch attention to another modality causes a reduction in clock speed, which was extrapolated to be a function of the number of pulses of the pacemaker system. However, the clock mechanism used for timing these intervals is inferred from the behavioral characteristics of responding and is not specified in physiological terms. Meck proposed that some type of physiological clock is necessary for timing these behaviors.

If animals actually have neural pacemakers that provide relatively invariant intervals for short-duration discriminations, how could attention influence the variability of behavioral timekeeping. The speed of internal clocks may be modifiable through motivational influences (Killeen, 1984; Killeen & Fetterman, 1988). By influencing the strength of reinforcement associated with particular response alternatives, it is possible to change the timing of behavioral responses during conditioning. Killeen argued that the speed of the neural clock

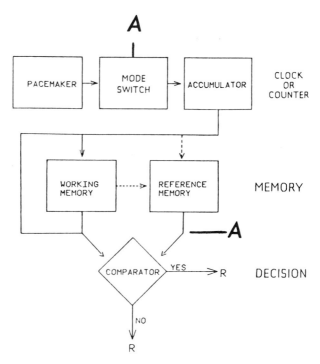

FIGURE 20.4. Model of a hypothetical neural clock for temporal discriminations in laboratory animals. Meck (1984) demonstrated that attentional biases associated with particular tasks influenced temporal discrimination performance. Attentional biases toward particular stimuli mediate the latency to onset of timing for duration estimation and response decision rules. Meck proposed that attentional biases influence the start of an internal clock mechanism. In this diagram, A is attentional process and R is response. From Meck (1984), with permission.

involved in this type of timing is a function of the rate of reinforcement. Platt (1984) demonstrated that rats show a preference for short-duration timing during temporal differentiation paradigms, a finding suggesting that the immediacy of reinforcement influences the timing of responses.

TEMPORAL INFLUENCES ON ATTENTION

Relatively few studies have directly evaluated the role of timing in attentional control, and temporal processing has not generally been considered a primary determinant of attention processes. Yet, there has been much interest in the temporal constraints that influence attention. Often, time has been included as a variable in studies of attention, since only a limited quantity of information can be processed within a particular time frame. In terms of information theory, this phenomenon can be described in terms of the bits of information that a channel can transmit per unit of time. If too much information is presented in a short duration, attention acts to limit the stimuli that should receive further processing.

Serial Processes

The early information-processing theorists recognized that time places constraints on attention. They devoted much energy to characterizing the attentional processes that reduce information from multiple sources to a serial arrangement so that only a limited amount needs to be processed at each time point.

Sternberg's analysis (1966, 1969) of the processing stages during digit-naming tasks is an example of this approach. He developed a chronometric model of information-processing performance that assumes that each cognitive operation requires specified amounts of time. As serial processing is necessary to take information from sensory registration to an eventual response, processing time depends on the number of individual operations to be performed. The model predicts that the time needed to complete various processes may be summed to give a total time for task completion. This additive-factor model attempts to specify the relationships among time, information load, and information-processing characteristics.

The shift away from traditional serial-processing theory that has been apparent since the early 1980s raises the question of whether temporal considerations are still relevant. If cognitive operations are performed in parallel, timing may not be as critical, as there would be less need of sequence information. Although the advent of parallel-processing approaches has added many complexities to the analysis of attention, these approaches do not do away with the necessity for sequential operations. Furthermore, several recent theorists have addressed the temporal constraints underlying network models that assume parallel processing. For instance, Schweickert (1984) proposed a model that modifies the temporal-additive-factor model proposed by Sternberg to accommodate more complex parallel-processing tasks.

Vigilance

Temporal factors become most obvious in studies of sustained performance and vigilance (see Chapter 3). When attention is required over long durations, performance is influenced by a number of intrinsic and extrinsic variables. Task variables such as base

rates of stimulus occurrence, information load, stimulus complexity, and response requirements influence performance. Organismic factors such as motivational state and natural
variations in neurobiological state are also significant. For instance, vigilance under conditions of long duration is likely to be influenced by circadian factors. When vigilance is
required for long durations, temporal constraints arise primarily because these organismic
and task demands are more likely to exert influence.

Automatic and Controlled Processing

The paradigms proposed by Schneider and Shiffrin (1977) to differentiate controlled
and automatic processes illustrate the influence on performance of temporal variables
such as the number of trials, the intertrial interval, and the duration of stimulus presentation.
These variables interact with memory parameters to account for differences in attentional
performance across tasks. The distinctions between automatic and effortful processing are
based on the attentional task demands created by the informational load and the need for
effortful processing during controlled attention.

Some investigators have suggested that temporal information is automatically encoded
during information processing, as time is an intrinsic component of the task. Hasher and
Zacks (1979) suggested that the encoding of temporal information is important to the
distinction between the two types of processes (automatic and controlled).

Other investigators have argued that this may not be the case. For instance, Michon and
Jackson (1984) presented evidence that temporal information is not normally conveyed
through automatic attentional processing. They demonstrated that temporal information
is not easily encoded, and that people do not always process this information unless
meaning can be derived from it. They reached this conclusion because a large number of
factors, such as the level of processing, the context, the instructional set, and the sequential
characteristics of stimuli influence the capacity of subjects to access temporal information.

When subjects have to make sequential judgments about temporal order, speed and
accuracy can be shown to vary with the randomness of the intervals of stimulus presentation
(Jackson, Michon, & Vermeeren, 1984). However, as we mentioned before, this approach
emphasizes order rather than time.

A novel approach to this issue is seen in a study by Skelly, Rizzuto, and Wilson (1984).
They presented moving stimuli on a computer screen that changed position at either a
random or a fixed time interval. On some trials, the stimuli appeared in the same movement
path, and on other trials, the position shifted. It was found that the latency of the N2
response of the visual evoked response varied as a function of the attentional demand,
as well as of the timing pattern. Irregular patterns produced longer latencies. This study
provides an interesting approach to studying the effects of timing on attention, though the
authors did not provide a detailed review of their methodology for analyzing the electrophysiological results.

Cohen and Fisher (1989) demonstrated that temporal variability on tasks with attentional demands is a key indicator of the fatigue associated with multiple sclerosis. Although
patients with this disease could perform many tasks at near-optimal levels for short
durations, their ability to perform consistently diminished over time. This performance
characteristic was noted across a variety of different tasks having both high and low motoric
demands. These findings led the authors to the conclusion that analyses of the temporal
characteristics of performance should be a critical part of the assessment of attentional
processes. Yet, temporal variability is often not emphasized in the development of tasks
that measure attention.

The extent to which temporal variability in attention relates to variances in central clock mechanisms still needs to be established. Cohen and Albers's study of A.H. (1991), a patient with hypothalamic damage involving the SCN, suggests that this nucleus may play a role in regulating the temporal flow of behavior. A.H. showed extreme variability in behavioral state that was characterized by sleep–wake disregulation, as well as lability of cognitive and affective functions.

ATTENTION AS A FUNCTION OF SENSORY MODALITY

The temporal characteristics of attention vary as a function of sensory modality. Visual attention typically involves the processing of multiple channels of information in a single time frame. While attention to visual information may require sustained vigilance over time, it is relatively easy to specify conditions for which considerable information is derived from the spatial array that is present at a particular point in time. Therefore, visual attention requires parallel processing systems capable of simultaneously extracting more than one unit of information.

In contrast, auditory attention almost always involves serial processing across multiple points in time. Situations exist for which auditory attention can be characterized as an attentional response at one point in time. For instance, a fire alarm is likely to elicit an orienting or startle response at its onset. Yet for this type of event, all of the information conveyed at that one moment is uniform. Attention to other sounds occurring at the time of the alarm, requires further processing at subsequent points in time. There are many instances of multiple units of simultaneous auditory information (e.g., an orchestral arrangement). However, people generally cannot attend to all of the different sounds that they hear at one particular instant. Instead, the different sounds of an orchestra create a complex arrangement of sounds that at each moment combine to produce a different musical quality. The overall musical experience requires the integration of sounds over a period of time.

Similarly, auditory attention to linguistic information is time-dependent. As demonstrated by cognitive studies involving techniques such as dichotic listening and shadowing, humans are only capable of dividing attention among competing auditory stimuli to a very limited degree. Language has an inherent temporal structure which is conveyed through syntax. This temporal structure creates an obvious demand for serial processing, since all the information in a verbal communication is not conveyed at a single point in time. While language represents a special form of auditory information, its temporal structure reflects a fundamental character of most auditory information. Obviously, attention to information that is transmitted through the auditory system will be influenced by this temporal character. Auditory attention is governed by a host of factors, such as the amplitude, pitch, and signal value of the auditory stimuli, that are present each moment. However, in humans language is dominant, to the extent that semantic content of speech may be the most powerful influence over degree of attention that is allocated to incoming auditory information. Regardless of the factors that govern what is "listened" to, our auditory attention is highly constrained by serial processing requirements.

If attention to information is other sensory modalities is considered, the unique temporal characteristics of the different forms of sensory information become apparent. We will not review each sensory system to characterize its temporal dynamics. In fact, there is very little empirical data that directly address the issue of the temporal dynamics of attention as a function of the various sensory modalities. Yet, when addressing the temporal parameters of attention, care must be taken to not generalize across all sensory modalities.

SUMMARY

The variability of behavior over time is an important marker of attention. The fact that optimal performance levels are not noted in people at all times indicates that their attentional state is not consistently directed. Individuals who cannot sustain directed activity or stay focused on tasks are said to have an attentional disturbance. Since performance varies over time, it seems intuitive that the processes of attention are greatly influenced by temporal factors. Regardless of whether temporal constraints on attention arise from the intrinsic properties of a biological clock or result from the sequential nature of behavioral events, it would seem that attentional processes are constrained by the temporal character of the situation and the information to be processed.

It is somewhat surprising that more effort has not been directed to establishing the temporal parameters underlying attentional processes. In their review of cognitive aspects of temporal information processing, Michon and Jackson (1984) state that "the construction of a time base . . . for timing of a particular behavior sequence is a highly idiosyncratic activity from which few general insights can be derived" (p. 305). They went on to emphasize the importance of determining the temporal attributes of "sequential stimuli configurations" and concluded that temporal information may be largely a by-product of the content of the associative context. In this is true, then much of the information that is used to establish a subjective flow of time is actually a function of a large number of cognitive and motivational variables. Furthermore, if cognitive, motivational, or contextual factors govern how humans experience time, then trying to understand the neural mechanisms underlying timing may have little relevance to conscious time experience.

Cognitive scientists, who believe that a neural timekeeper is an unnecessary construct for explaining behavioral timing, are likely to emphasize the importance of sequential factors in the determination of timing. The extent to which a time period can be broken down into a series of discrete events is likely to influence timing. Other factors, such as the signal–noise ratio of the stimuli being processed, the discriminability of the stimuli, the rate of information flow, the structural characteristics of the information, the level of effort, the motivational state, the anticipatory state, and the processing time, may also influence behavioral timing. If all these factors influence behavioral timing, one can truly question the relevance of a central timekeeper to attentional control.

There seems to be a strong need for additional research on the temporal characteristics of behavioral performance. Relatively few clinical tests of attention incorporate a temporal component. The continuous performance task (Rosvold, Mirsky, Sarandon, Bransame, & Beck, 1956) is probably the best example of a test designed to investigate performance across the temporal dimension (see Chapter 13). However, in its original form, no provisions were made for scoring performance as a function of time on-task. Recently, this paradigm has been expanded by several investigators to provide measures of performance variability (Cohen & Fisher, 1988). Previously, clinicians often made judgments about temporal variability from their observations of the performance of their patients during assessment.

There are several possible reasons for temporal variability, most of which do not depend on a central nervous system clock. There may be an increased likelihood of interference as time progresses because of the natural probability that a salient event will occur to distract the individual. There may also be physiological fatigue effects that are not related to timing, but that increase in likelihood over lengthy tasks. Attentional variability may occur as a function of difficulties in sequencing operations when task demands increase owing to task length, information load, or other factors of this sort. While multi-step sequential operations are likely to vary as a function of temporal parameters, an actual clock mechanism may not be required to explain the increased variability.

Even if a central mechanism is proposed to account for attentional variability, factors other than clock variance may be responsible. For instance, variations in arousal mechanisms may occur independently of the direct influence of a "pacemaker" that is responsible for timing. Treisman's description (1984) of three hypothetical bases for temporal variances illustrates this point. He went on to make a strong case that external influences affect a pacemaker function through both general and specific arousal influences. Assuming that the rate of a central pacemaker can be influenced by task-related factors, it would still be necessary to establish how the pacemaker rate biases attentional performance.

In many models of attention, the important temporal unit is the "trial" rather than time itself. Although intertrial change provides a valid index of sequential effects, it is not synonymous with duration. The investigator of attention must address both trial and duration effects when assessing temporal effects. To discount the relevance of a real time base to cognitive processes such as attention would, in our view, be premature. The study of attention requires a careful consideration of timing and the way in which events are mapped in a temporal dimension. This is as important to our goal of understanding attention as an understanding of spatial parameters. It is safe to say that temporal factors place significant constraints on attention that need to be further specified in future studies.

Computational Models for the Analysis of Attention

The resurgence of interest in the cognitive sciences since the early 1970s has been accompanied by a dramatic acceleration in the development of theoretical models. Cognitive scientists develop models in order to characterize the formal properties of the processes that they are studying. Efforts to model cognition led to a recent focus on "neural networks," computer-based computational systems that simulate the characteristics of actual neural brain processes. Neural networks are designed by means of computational modeling, which is a direct result of advances in the fields of mathematical psychology and computer science. Computational models are created with the hope that they will provide a formal mathematical basis for understanding cognitive and behavioral processes. These models seek to specify the parameters underlying information processing and therefore are of considerable interest to investigators of attentional phenomena. Although at times these models seem to do little more than provide a mathematical description of processes that are typically characterized less formally, they may be useful for identifying the constraints and parameters underlying attentional operations.

PHILOSOPHICAL ISSUES

In a recent paper, John Daugman (1990) gave a philosophical analysis of the recent surge in interest in computational models that are designed to explain behavioral and neural phenomena. He equated this development with the rise of other metaphors in science over the past century and cautioned cognitive scientists not to become too enamored of a particular metaphor. He argued that, as in the case of other metaphors, the computational approach may be logically consistent with a particular paradigm, yet may not help to explain the behavioral phenomena.

Daugman described several dominant scientific metaphors that have had been used to explain mechanisms underlying behavior and cognition: the mechanical-hydraulic, electronic-optical, network, and computational frameworks. These metaphors parallel a major development in the study of physics, and each has had a significant influence on all other sciences, including psychology and the information sciences. Daugman argued that it may be inappropriate to apply constructs derived from one scientific discipline (physics) to phenomena observed within a very different theoretical framework (cognitive science). He concluded that to do so leads to haphazard, incomplete, and "sporadic reformulations in terms of the technological experience of the day" (p. 9). Furthermore, there may be a tendency to "rephrase every assertion about the mind or brain in computational terms" (p. 17). The result is likely to be a weak fit between the formal properties of the model and the actual characteristics of the cognitive process.

These are valid concerns. It would be a mistake to view the neural networks developed from computational modeling as synonymous with the underlying cognitive phenomena that they are designed to explain. Yet, there is also danger in throwing away a "scientific metaphor or paradigm" when it does not provide a complete theoretical account or a method for understanding all aspects of cognition. If one starts with the assumption that only one of Daugman's metaphors is correct, it is easy to reach his conclusion that the underlying theoretical framework is inadequate. However, these metaphors need not be mutually exclusive or orthogonal. The hydraulic metaphor may be appropriate for explaining mechanisms underlying some aspects of behavior, and computational models may provide a better approach to characterizing other phenomena. Therefore, applying a theoretical framework from one branch of science to the characterization of phenomena in another scientific domain seems both necessary and meaningful.

Searle (1990) addressed an even more basic philosophical issue in a critique of computational modeling approaches. He suggested that efforts to develop computational models capable of functioning like the human brain inevitably result in failure. He argued that researchers who believe that thinking is the equivalent of the symbol manipulations performed by a computer are mistaken. Searle went on to state, "You cannot get semantically loaded thought contents from formal computations alone, whether they are done in serial or parallel" (p. 28). The gist of his position is that a fundamental distinction exists between the quality of thinking from which meaningfulness is derived and the mechanical operations of symbol manipulation: "Syntax by itself is neither constitutive of nor sufficient for semantics" (p. 27).

Developing computers that "think" as humans may be an impossible challenge. Unless it becomes possible to create a machine that has biological drives, it will be hard for computational models to capture the essence of thinking. Although work in computational modeling is often propelled by the hope of developing computer systems that mimic human brain activity, it may be more likely that a machine will be developed that has emergent properties that have many of the qualities of thinking. Some philosophers take the position that these emergent properties may be a basis for thinking in both humans and computers (Churchland & Churchland, 1990). Philosophical debate over this issue may not be easily resolved, as it reflects basic attitudes about what it means to be human.

Regardless of one's philosophical viewpoint, computational modeling seems to provide a valuable method of studying cognition. Models provide a means of testing the adequacy of hypotheses about the processes underlying cognition. Computational models may ultimately provide "a literal description of mental activity," as Pylyshyn (1973, p. 111) suggested, or they may simply act as a heuristic for forming and testing hypotheses about cognition. Ultimately, the resolution of this issue may be less important than the fact that computational models provide another tool for studying processes like attention.

As many volumes have been devoted to an analysis of current computational models of behavior, a comprehensive review of the entire field of mathematical psychology is not attempted here. Instead, some of the major developments in this field are highlighted, with an emphasis on how these theoretical approaches handle the processes of attention. We review several recent theoretical advances in computational modeling that have dealt with attention in intriguing ways. Although at times these computational models seem to do little more than provide a mathematical description of processes that may be effectively characterized less formally, computational models may help to clarify what constraints and parameters need to be analyzed in studying attentional processes.

MATHEMATICAL MODELS AND ATTENTION: A HISTORICAL PERSPECTIVE

Given the recent upsurge of interest in the computational neurosciences, it is easy to lose sight of the origins of current computational approaches. Yet, consideration of early mathematical theories of behavior illustrates current computational theories evolved from two major theoretical perspectives, learning theory and information theory. While the mathematical models associated with these perspectives are conceptually related, they have different theoretical roots. As we have discussed previously, both learning theory and information theory directly influenced current thinking regarding the nature of attention. Therefore, it is useful to initially consider the mathematical models that developed from these two theoretical perspectives.

With these goals in mind, we review several of the early mathematical approaches to modeling behavior, including a description of Hull's hypothetico-deductive theory. This was one of the first attempts at a comprehensive mathematical model of behavior. Next, some of the constructs originating from statistical learning theory and information theory are reviewed, with a consideration of how attention is accounted for in models developed from these frameworks. We conclude with a brief discussion of how attentional processes have been incorporated into current computational and network models. The review characterizes the computational characteristics of these models.

Hypothetico-Deductive Method

The formulation of the hypothetico-deductive method and theory (Hull, 1943) marked a significant milestone in the development of a mathematical psychology. Hull's purpose was to produce a unified and mathematically consistent theory that would relate various psychological processes, such as drives, learning, and inhibition (see Chapter 4 for a more general review). Although Hull's theory has been criticized for being too ambitious (i.e., attempting to describe too many behavioral processes simultaneously through a set of unified equations), it is evident that this work served as a foundation for the development of mathematical psychology.

Hull advocated the development of formal systems for psychological phenomena such as learning. A formal system is a theoretical description of a phenomenon that expresses the relationship between its underlying components through mathematical or logical statements. Hull's formal system contains 16 postulates and 5 corollaries, which he meant to provide an exact relationship among the factors influencing the behaviors associated with learning. He developed postulates based on several experimental observations: (1) the determination of an upper limit for the galvanic skin response to reinforcement after a series of trials; (2) an exponential decrease in reaction times for verbal responses during successive trials of reinforcement during learning; (3) the increase in an animal's "resistance to extinction" secondary to the number of preceding reinforcements until it reaches an asymptote; and (4) in learning situations involving a choice between response alternatives, the increase in the percentage of correct choices as a function of the strength of reinforcement. Hull felt that he could account for the general occurrence of these observations in the following equation:

$$_sH_r = m(1 - e^{-iN})$$

H is habit strength, relative to a specific stimulus (S) and response (R). The number of reinforcements is specified as N, while m and i are constants. Hull postulated that the rate of change in habit strength is exponentially determined (e), so that H varies as a function of the number of reinforced trials and the constants.

The value of the constant m is then established to be a function of the amount of reward (w), and m defines the upper limit of habit strength that is possible for the animal:

$$m = m'(1 - e^{-kw})$$

Other constants (m' and j) are specified as contributing to the determination of the amount of reward. To establish the value of m', Hull again made use of an exponential function (e), which specifies the rate of change from maximum habit strength (m) over time (t).

$$m' = m''e^{-jt}$$

Experimental analysis indicated that maximum habit strength should also decrease as a function of the time between conditioned stimulus (CS) and the unconditioned stimulus (UCS). Therefore, another equation was derived to formalize this phenomenon:

$$m'' = Me^{-ut'}$$

In this new equation, t' is the time between the CS and the UCS, and two other constants (M and u) are used to specify a more exact relationship between these variables. Hull later combined these equations into one formal statement:

$$_sH_r = M(1 - e^{-kw})(e^{-jt})(e^{-ut'})(1 - e^{-iN})$$

The eighth postulate of Hull's model predicts that the likelihood of behavior is a function of a reaction potential ($_sE_r$), which is determined by habit strength, as well as by drive (D), the dynamism of the stimulus trace in producing a habit (V), and the incentive reinforcement (K). The resulting equation is a grand determinant of behavioral response tendency:

$$_sE_r = D*V*K*_sH_r$$

Hull defined drive as the product of the interaction of a primary drive (D') and a monotonic accelerating function (e), which decreases from 1 to 0. D' increases as the time of deprivation of a particular UCS such as food increases, and e decreases as a natural function of time. Drive state (D') was determined primarily by the time of deprivation:

$$D' = 37.824 \times 1/h + 4.001$$

The decay function is assumed to provide a balance with the drive-inducing effect of deprivation and is specified as

$$e = 1 - .0000104h^{2.48}$$

In both equations, h = time. Hull provided a remarkable degree of precision in this equation. A homeostatic balance was proposed, in which drive is maintained by opposition forces created by the deprivation of a biologically necessary substance and a natural state of drive decay. Within this framework, deprivation plays a critical role in generating an internal energetic state that catalyzes responding. The strength of incentive is also shown to be an important influence on drive strength, and behavioral responding has the effect of reducing drive strength.

Despite his noble attempt to integrate experimental data into a cohesive formal theory, Hull's equations have significant problems. Although many of the theory's predictions about behavior have held up, the specific formulations of the models received much criticism. For instance, with respect to the concept of drive, D' can be operationalized by the use of time of deprivation as an index. Yet, deprivation time clearly departs from the notion of some that it is an internal energetic state that catalyzes action. Intuitively, drive seems to suggest a force, push, or pressure that stimulates or prevents action. However, defining drive as an intrinsic state independent of a variable such as time of deprivation does not permit easy empirical validation of the construct.

Other problems were encountered by researchers who tried to test Hull's model. The assumption that learning occurs as a function of the number of reinforcements came under fire by theorists who demonstrated one-trial learning. A problem more relevant to the system's utility as a mathematical model of behavior is its reliance on many complex equations, which are based on a very limited number of specified variables. For instance, in determining habit strength ($_sH_r$), five constants have to be estimated in order to make the equations meaningful. There are four experimental variables (w, t, t', N) that can be manipulated more directly, though the w (amount of reward) is difficult to specify exactly. Therefore, Hull's system was criticized for not being mathematically rigorous.

The hypothetico-deductive theory was followed by a theoretical shift to neobehaviorism, characterized by the work of Spence (1951). Advocates of neobehaviorism held onto many of the fundamental principles of behaviorism but sought to expand the horizons of topics that were within the realm of behavioral study. Spence provided many theoretical and experimental insights that have bearing on behavioral analysis (see Chapter 4), but his work did not advance the field of mathematical modeling far beyond Hull's model. Subsequently, several theorists working from the neobehavioral perspective developed models that attempt to account for attentional phenomena. Kendler's cue dominance theory (1971) and Wagner's continuity theory (1972) are examples of these attempts.

Kendler and Kendler (1962) attributed the transfer of learning in their paradigms to the occurrence of excitatory (E) and inhibitory (I) tendencies that can be mathematically specified (see Chapter 4).

Excitatory tendency (E_t) was specified by Kendler (1972) to be a function of the strength of the excitatory stimulus cue during the current learning trial, relative to the maximum excitatory stimulus cue strength (M_E) for all the cues that have occurred in the individual's reinforcement history. The maximum cue strength can vary from zero to some maximum value depending on its excitatory potential as a reinforcer. The effect of reinforcement on any learning trial is to increase the excitatory strength of the stimulus cues that are present. The increase in excitatory strength can be specified as a function of the trial number ($N + 1$) and a parameter (θ) that specifies the learning rate for the individual:

$$E_{r_{n+1}} = E_{R_n} + \theta(M_E - E_{R_n}) \text{ and } E_{C_{n+1}} = E_{C_n} + \theta(M_E - E_{C_n})$$

Where (R) and (C) are the two stimuli to be discriminated. A similar equation can be specified for each stimulus cue that has been reinforced. The net effect of all of the stimulus cues that have been conditioned can be specified as an interaction of simultaneous equations of this type.

Similarly, a hypothetical inhibitory tendency has been postulated that is a function of a generalized effect of all the inhibitory stimulus cues (I_t) that provide incorrect information regarding reinforcement payoff. Like the excitatory tendency, the inhibitory tendency varies as a function of the inhibitory strength of the incorrect cue on a given trial (m+1), a maximum inhibitory tendency (M_I), and individual differences (ϕ). The increase in excitatory strength on any reinforced trial can be specified by the equation:

$$I_{G_{m+1}} = I_{G_m} + \phi(M_I - I_{G_m}) \text{ and } I_{T_{m+1}} = I_{T_m} + \phi(M_I - I_{T_m})$$

Kendler proposed that the effective excitatory strength (E) of a given stimulus cue varies as a function of the difference between the excitatory and inhibitory tendencies of all the stimulus cues that contribute to the overall cue strength. A particular stimulus can have an excitatory strength comprised of the net interaction of multiple excitatory stimulus tendencies and multiple inhibitory tendencies that are a function of prior reinforcement history. Therefore, the tendency to select one cue over another (d_t) on a trial (n), where (R) and (G) are again the two stimuli to be discriminated, can be represented as:

$$d_{RG_{n,m}} = \overline{R}_{R_{n,m}} - \overline{R}_{G_{n,m}} = (E_{R_n} - E_{G_n}) + (I_{G_m}) - I_{R_m})$$

When discriminations across more than one stimulus dimension are required [e.g., shape (S) and color (C)], a compound stimulus situation arises. The tendency to discriminate on a particular stimulus dimension is a function of the difference between the effective excitatory strengths of the two stimulus dimensions (E_C and $\overline{R}_S$):

$$\overline{R}_{C_{n,m}} - \overline{R}_{S_{n,m}} = (E_{R_n} - E_{R_n} - E_{G_n}) + I_{G_m} - I_{R_m}) + E_{D_n} - E_{T_n}) + (I_{T_m} - I_{D_m}) = d_{C_{n,m}} + d_{S_{n,m}}$$

where red (R), green (G), diamond (D) and triangle (T) are different stimuli across two stimulus dimensions, size (S) and color (C) to be discriminated.

Estimating the characteristics of the compound stimulus obviously becomes an extremely complex problem when one moves beyond the level of two stimulus dimensions. Nonetheless, Kendler demonstrated that for simple experimental contexts, this method can be used to estimate the salience of new stimuli that are to be discriminated, as well as the individual's initial tendencies for making certain discriminations.

The process of "stimulus compounding" that was postulated by Kendler (1971) accounts for the formation of a smooth gradient of excitatory strengths as a function of the broad range of stimuli that actually exist in most situations. The concept of intrinsic cue dominance provided an explanation of why certain stimuli with inherent salience are responded to in preference to stimuli with weaker cue strength. The resulting model specifies many of the behavioral factors needed to account for stimulus selection and is therefore a behavioral description of attention.

Intrinsic cue dominance occurs as a result of the natural characteristics of stimuli in relation to the organism. Kendler (1971) demonstrated an intrinsic dominance of color cues over shape cues in rats. The intrinsic dominance of brightness cues over orientation cues has also been shown in rats (Basden, 1969). However, the dominance of certain cues can be manipulated by varying the difficulty of discrimination in a particular psychophysical dimension. Ultimately, the presence of an intrinsic dominance of cues points to the interrelationship between the inherent organismic qualities of stimuli and the process of learning.

Perhaps the aspect of the neurobehavioral approaches used by Hull, Spence, and later theorists that had the greatest impact on subsequent efforts to develop mathematical psychology was their use of "stochastic" methods to predict the probability of particular responses. The term *stochastic* comes from the Greek word meaning "to shoot at," but in modern usage, it means "to guess." Considering behaviors probabilistic phenomena had a significant influence on later mathematical models. Stochastic modeling can be seen as a direct correlate of concurrent developments in the field of physics, which established the constraints of uncertainty in the observation of atomic events.

The mathematical approaches that followed Hull's made a more direct effort to establish models that were formal, testable, and more rigorous. Two different theoretical directions were taken, which resulted in a statistical learning theory and an information theory. These theoretical approaches shared many features but initially had very different emphases. The goal of statistical learning theory was to formalize the components of conditioning and verbal learning. Information theory was concerned with formalizing the parameters underlying the transmission and selection of information. As these two approaches had great impact on current computational models, as well as the study of attention, we summarize some of their relevant features.

Statistical Learning Theory

Estes (1950, 1959) presented a formal model to describe the mathematical parameters underlying conditioning, which led to a statistical learning theory. A fundamental premise of this theory is that learning occurs in a fashion that can be specified statistically, as long as the experimenter is able to determine several key rate-setting variables. Estes postulated that learning involves two independent processes: the selection of a stimulus from an available pool and the conditioning of individual stimulus items into permanent storage. The selection of stimulus elements is considered a fundamental component of learning within this model because, if a stimulus is not available to the animal for conditioning, it will not be learned. According to Estes, the subject samples from a set of stimuli on each trial of learning. On a given trial, stimuli from the sampled set may be conditioned to responses. Accordingly, the probability of a response is equal to the number of sampled stimulus elements that are conditioned divided by the total number of the elements that were sampled:

$$\Delta_x = s_c \frac{S_c - x}{S_c}$$

where x is the number of elements conditioned on a given trial, S_c is the total number of stimuli in the set, and (s_c) is the mean number of the stimuli that are available to be conditioned on a trial (T). One can predict the rate of acquisition at any time during acquisition by the equation:

$$\frac{dx}{dT} = s_c \frac{S_c - x}{S_c}$$

This leads through integration to:

$$x = S_c - (S_c - x_0)e^{-qT}$$

where q is the ratio of s/S. This equation sets the upper bounds for learning on a given trial to an amount that is, of course, less than S_c. Expressed as a probability, the likelihood of a response (R) after any number of trials is a function of the number of reinforced trials and the probability of R at the initiation of learning (p_0):

$$p = 1 - (1 - p_0)e^{-qt}$$

As Estes was studying conditioning paradigms in which rate of learning was measured as a function of trials to criterion, it was important to account for the time required for learning on each trial. A curvilinear decline in the average time per trial (L) was predicted so that:

$$L = \frac{h}{1 - (L_0 - h)e^{-qT/L_0}} = \frac{Sh}{S - (S - x_0)e^{-qT}}$$

where h = an asymptotic minimum time per trials after a series of learning trials. Through this equation, Estes estimated the upper and lower limits of the time of a learning trial, as a function of the number of previously reinforced trials. The probability of a response (r) is a function of the rate of responses (R) and the time spent in acquisition (t), which can be shown to result in the following equation, where $w = 1/h$ and $B = s/Sh$:

$$r = \frac{dR}{dt} = \frac{dT}{dt} = \frac{wx}{S} = \frac{w}{1 + (S - x_0/x_0)e^{-Bt}}$$

By knowing the initial rate of conditioning at the onset of a learning task $(x0)$, one can predict a whole set of different learning curves.

Estes and Burke (1953) generalized this original model to account for the fact that, in normal situations, the environment of the stimuli (S) is not constant. The presence of variability in the stimulus set requires that models account for the probability that a stimulus will occur or will be available at a given time (T). To investigate this condition, Estes and Burke limited the number of possible environmental alternatives to two states (a and b), as well as the probability of stimulus elements being selected (θ_a and θ_b). When both states are simultaneously present, the probability of stimulus selection (θ) is:

$$\theta = \theta_a + \theta_b - \theta_a\theta_b$$

Across a series of trials, the probability of a particular response's occurring $(p(T))$ is a function of the initial probability of a stimulus's being selected, the number of elements in the set, the trial number, and the degree of variability in the available stimuli:

$$p(n) = \frac{1}{N}\theta\Sigma\,\theta[1 - (\theta_i)^n] = 1 - \frac{1}{N\theta}\Sigma\,\theta_i(1 - \theta_i)^n$$

Using this framework, one can compute a mean and a standard deviation for the probability of a response in any given trial, if the initial parameters, such as the initial number of stimuli, are known. Through this generalized model, Estes and Burke (1953) provided a mechanism for establishing the parameters that are necessary to predict patterns of behavior. Their initial condition of a two-alternative stimulus pool is very restricted so as to allow a simplified account of variability in stimulus availability. Under normal conditions, there may be a much larger set of stimulus alternatives, a condition that complicates the estimations of these equations. Nonetheless, this model of learning represents significant advance, as it offers hypotheses that can be tested. It specifies, in mathematical terms, some of the critical variables underlying conditioning.

Within this model, the probability of conditioning depends on the probability that a stimulus will be sampled. Stimulus variability is assumed to be a critical determinant of the probability of future responding. The statistical learning model was intended to explain factors that determine the rate of conditioning (Atkinson & Estes, 1963). However, because it specifies the importance of stimulus sampling on each trial, another factor separate from the act of conditioning is postulated. Estes may have anticipated the need for an attentional factor, which he defined behaviorally as stimulus sampling. In the context of current concepts regarding information processing, Estes's concept of stimulus sampling implies a process of selective attention.

Other Models of Statistical Learning

Several other investigators have made significant contributions to the development of statistical learning theory. Bush and Mosteller (1951) combined aspects of statistical learning and signal detection in their models of behavior. Bush and Mosteller emphasized the operator characteristics of the subject relative to her or his response tendency. They established a linear assumption indicting that, on a given trial, there are two probabilities, p and $(1 - p)$, associated with the probabilities that a response will either occur or not occur (two response alternatives). The probability of a response on a given trial (n), where λ is an asymptote of performance and a_i is the sampling rate, is interpreted to be:

$$p_{n+1} = a_i P_n + (1 - a_i)\lambda_i$$

This equation can be extended in normal situations in which more than two alternatives exist by a linear operator (T_i) that characterizes a transitional step between successive trials, so that:

$$\vec{p}_{n+1} = T_i \vec{p}_n$$

Bush and Mosteller later suggested that this linear operator is stochastic by nature and can be derived from Estes's stimulus-sampling theory. The major distinction between these two models arises from the way in which the response term (R) is handled (i.e., whether it is considered a variable to be studied independently of the stimulus).

Psychological Implications

Statistical learning theory has been expanded by other investigators to account for a variety of phenomena associated with conditioning and verbal learning. The application of a modified version of the stimulus variation model to paired-associates verbal learning is seen in the work of G. Bower (1961). He proposed that the conditioning of a stimulus word with a paired response can be explained as an all-or-nothing event. However, before conditioning of the stimulus–response pair, the subject guesses at random from the available sample of unlearned items. Bower predicted that the rate of learning would be a function of both the rate of conditioning and the selection of possible word choices. His models are based on stochastic equations in which the probabilities of conditioning and of stimulus selection are covaried to produce a probability of learning verbal associations across trials.

Statistical learning theory has been applied to a range of learning phenomena, including partial reinforcement, avoidance training, experimental extinction, stimulus-and-response generalization, punishment-escape learning, and discrimination learning. The modeling of stimulus-and-response generalization has relevance to the study of attention, as generalization enables previous conditioning to affect future response tendencies. This has obvious implications for the direction of attention (see Chapter 4 for a detailed review of the relationship of generalization to attention).

Stimulus discrimination is also particularly relevant to our discussion of attention, as this process enables the animal to select among the stimulus alternatives according to previous learning. Restle (1955) proposed a model to account for discrimination learning that makes use of two factors (conditioning and cue type) with two states (conditioned-unconditioned) and two cue types (relevant-irrelevant). According to this model, cues that are irrelevant cannot be conditioned, whereas cues that are relevant may or may not be conditioned. A second condition is then placed in the model: When an irrelevant cue occurs, it may be adapted to, which means that in the future it will not be perceived or attended to. Based on the assumptions of this two-state model, a set of stochastic equations were generated that provide for the probability of a correct response given the occurrence of cues that are either relevant or irrelevant, adapted or not adapted, and conditioned or unconditioned.

Even though statistical learning theory represented a major advance in attempts to establish a mathematical foundation for behavioral study it was not without problems. As its name suggests, models generated from this theoretical framework consider learning a probabilistic event, which can be formalized through stochastic statistics. Statistical learning theory requires the investigator to establish certain initial parameters, such as the initial size of the stimulus set, in order to predict future learning curves. Even though precise, these models have difficulty accounting for mechanisms of learning on a given trial. Furthermore, this approach is strongly behavioral in perspective.

Cognitive processes such as attention are not directly addressed by this theoretical framework. However, investigators studying statistical learning can argue that the process of stimulus sampling accounts for attentional effects. These models provide a framework for studying cognitive processes from the perspective of conditioning.

Some researchers have extended the methods of statistical learning to test for attentional effects during learning. For instance, Lane (1980) used a statistical learning methodology to demonstrate that attentional capacity rather than attentional selectivity accounts for age-related differences in performance for two types of learning (incidental and central). However, this type of study extends beyond the original limits of statistical learning theory and employs constructs arising out of the other major theoretical perspective, information theory.

Information Theory

Information theory has had a direct impact on the development of modern theories of attention. As described previously in this text, information theory has influenced researchers studying perceptual processes and has resulted in the creation of signal detection methods for analyzing attentional performance. Two approaches to the study of information can be traced to the period after World War II. The first is concerned with how transmitted signals accurately reflect the actual information being generated. This approach characterized by the work of Cherry (1953) and MacKay (1951) focuses on characteristics of information, to ensure its integrity and its coherence with the original environment. Research has been devoted to quantifying the featural aspects of information.

A second approach, characterized by the work of Wiener (1948) and Shannon and Weaver (1949), is concerned with a slightly different problem: how information is transmitted, and what constraints there are during communication that limit the information that can be received. Both approaches have obvious relevance to the study of attention, as a fundamental aspect of information theories is the selection and discrimination of information from noise. It is noteworthy that, within this approach to information theory, the statistical principles again emerge as an important theme. The detection of information does not occur with certainty and therefore must be viewed as an event with a specified probability. As attention can be thought of as a process that affects the probability of stimulus detection or selection, mathematical models developed in the context of information theory have much relevance to our current analysis.

Information theory is often concerned with the characteristics of signal transmission. Three primary factors influence how information will flow in a particular system: the nature of the transmitter, the operator, and the transmission environment. Much effort has been directed at specifying the parameters underlying these three factors.

Information Parameters

Information can be studied in an ideal environment (noiseless) or in real (noisy) environments. Noiseless environments are easier to analyze but are not natural. In contrast, noisy environments are natural but have complexities that impede mathematical analysis. In a noiseless environment, there can never be confusion about the source of a message, as there is only one source. In noisy systems, there may be multiple messages, some relevant and others irrelevant (noise). The noiseless system is easier to deal with initially, as one source of variance is eliminated by the constraint of being noiseless. If one assumes that the information being transmitted in such a system is compatible with both the transmitter and the receiver, and that it occurs as units of information in time units, then one can determine the capacity of the system to communicate information (Luce, 1960). This can be called the channel capacity of the system (C), where for each unit of time (T),

$$C(T) = \log_2 \frac{N(T)}{T}$$

which states that the capacity of a channel for an interval of time is a log function of the number of signals per unit time and the overall time of the signal. This determines the bits per signal per unit time. If this equation is taken to its limit, the overall capacity of the channel independent of units of time can be determined:

$$C = \lim_{T \to \infty} C(T) = \lim_{T \to \infty} \log_2 \frac{N(T)}{T}$$

The key to determining the transmission capacity of a noiseless system is therefore to determine $N(T)$ the number of signals per unit time that can be transmitted in the system. However, this model assumes that there is an equal likelihood that any particular message will occur (as equal weights are given to each signal). Of course, this is not the case in real environments, as different signals usually have different probabilities of occurrence. Nonetheless, this idealized model establishes a basis for analyzing information transmission. Shannon (1948) demonstrated that, for information that occurs in binary form, channel capacity can be determined:

$$C = \log_2 W_0$$

if one is able to calculate W_0, which can be derived by knowing the possible states for each unit of time. In the case of a binary string of information (e.g., the Morse code), one can compute an exact value for W_0, which results in $C = 0.539$ bits of information per unit time.

The next step in information theory was to determine the capacity of systems for which equal probabilities for each signal could not be assumed (e.g., the transmission of a language). In this case, each symbol of a message that is transmitted has a probability of occurrence. If one assumes that the selection of one symbol is independent of that selection of other symbols (another idealized assumption), the entire message can be defined as having a probability (P), which is equal to the probability of the individual symbols being transmitted. Shannon demonstrated that one can determine the total information contained in a message by knowing the number of different symbol alternatives. As the probability of a given symbol's being selected (p_n) when there are N possible binary signals, the total information in the particular system can be calculated to be $N = \log_2 n$. When the amount of information (N) is assessed in terms of the different probabilities that are possible for a given symbol, this equation results in the following transformation:

$$\log_2 n = \log_{2n} \left(\frac{1}{p}\right) = -\log_2 p$$

Therefore, the information that is contained in a message is negatively related to the probability of the occurrence of the particular unit of information that is being sent. This leads to the interesting conclusion that rare messages transmit more information than common messages (Luce, 1960). If a message is certain, it does not provide any information. Based on this formulation, one can determine the average amount of information that is transmitted in a message (H) by determining the value of a single signal from the source of the message:

$$H = \lim_{r \to \infty} H_r = -\sum_{i=1}^{n} p(i)\log_2 p(i)$$

which is equal to bits per selection.

This is one of the most significant formulations from information theory, as it predicts the amount of certainty and uncertainty relative to the information that is being processed. Shannon interpreted that H represents the "entropy" of a particular system, as the relationship of uncertainty to certainty in a system provides for the degree of chaos or redundancy. Relative to our current understanding of attentional processes, the concepts of uncertainty and redundancy are evident and are closely related to other aspects of attention, such as expectancy and novelty. For instance, the neuronal model, developed by Sokolov (1963) to explain the orienting response and habituation, has a central premise that the degree of mismatch between a new stimulus and existing models determines the nature of the orienting response (OR) that will be generated. As we have previously discussed, the OR is often viewed as a physiological correlate of attention.

After formulating a theory of information for selections whose probabilities of occurrence are independent of one another, it was necessary to account for the more realistic environment. Normally, the selection of one stimulus affects the selection of others. There is a "nonlinear" relationship between stimuli when they are presented in isolation and when they are presented together. If one considers just two stimuli (a,b), $p(a,b)$ does not equal $p(a)p(b)$ in nonindependent systems. Therefore, in the selection of signals in this type of system:

$$H(a,b) = -\sum_{a,b} p(a,b) \log_2 p(a,b)$$

By determining the entropy for the two nonindependent signals $[H(a,b) = H(a) + H_a(b)]$, it was demonstrated that the entropy of the two signals interactively is less than the sum of the two entropies when they are considered independently:

$$H(a,b) < H(a) + H(b)$$

This indicates that, as more information is introduced into the system, the amount of redundancy increases, and this increase reduces the total amount of new information that is gained. In psychological terms, information redundancy may provide an index of behavioral stereotypy as described by Miller and Frick (1949). Stereotypy is relevant to attentional processes, as it reduces the amount of information that must be processed for the message to be understood. When messages lack redundancy, attentional demands are increased, as every bit of information becomes vital to the correct reception of the message.

Besides specifying the amount of information that can be transmitted in a noiseless system, information theory also specifies a relationship between channel size (C = bits per unit time) and entropy (H = bits per symbol). Entropy, a concept taken from thermodynamics, refers to the degree of chaos and uncertainty in a particular system. Increasing the number of bits of information for each symbol increases uncertainty, as a particular symbol holds more than one piece of information. The maximum rate of information transmission (R) on a given channel is a function of channel size and entropy:

$$R = \frac{C}{H}$$

Therefore, the rate of information transmission limits the maximum channel capacity, and vice versa:

$$C = \max(H^*R)$$

We previously discussed some of the neurophysiological constraints on human information processing. Factors like neural speed or working memory capacity may limit the amount of information that can be handled in a given period of time. Information theory provides theoretical guidelines for establishing the constraints on information processing in ideal systems, which in turn may have utility for defining the processing boundaries for humans.

Noisy Systems

Thus far, we have discussed ideal information systems, in which the entire message that is communicated comes from one source. The only limitations on information in this system are the degree of redundancy and the likelihood that a unit of information will occur. However, in real environments, not all input coming to a receiver is relevant. As some input may be irrelevant, it is necessary to generalize from an ideal "noiseless" system to "noisy" environments. In many respects, the characteristics of a noisy system are similar to those described for nonindependent information. In a noisy environment, the information from one source has competition from a second source that is producing nonrelevant signals (noise). The second, noisy signal reduces the entropy (H) associated with the primary signal. Therefore, noise effectively reduces the information that can be transmitted in a particular system. This is derived from a formulation that is similar to the equations that were described in the case of two nonindependent signals (Luce, 1960). If, in a noisy system, a is considered a primary signal, and b is a second signal that is noisy with respect to a, the rate of transmission in the system (R) is limited by the amount of noise. The total entropy associated with the primary signal $H(a)$ is reduced by the amount of entropy associated with the noise $H_b(a)$:

$$R = H(a) - H_b(a) = H(a) + H(b) - H(a,b)$$

By knowing the entropy associated with both the signal and the noise, as well as the variance shared by both signal and noise, one can compute the average rate of information flow through the system. Channel capacity can be defined as a function of the primary signal minus the effect of noise that affects the reception of the primary signal:

$$C = \max [H(a) - H_b(a)]$$

Therefore, in a noisy environment, one can compute the amount of information that can be communicated at a given time by defining the characteristics of the various signals that are in the environment.

Psychological Applications

Information theory and signal detection theory provided a philosophical framework for researchers studying cognitive processes. It has also helped to define the parameters of human information processing. For instance, through the use of the entropy concept, Shannon (1951) was able to set an upper limit on the amount of information contained in letter combinations of varying length (Fn 3.0 bits/letter). Cherry (1953) estimated the entropy of spoken language, and Shannon and Weaver (1949) estimated the redundancy of the English language, through these equations and then showed that significant portions of messages can be deleted without loss of information.

The determination of informational capacity and the determination of the maximum rates of information transmission in humans are two goals of cognitive scientists trying to extend information theory. Information theory established the upper and lower boundaries of information processing and communication in controlled, idealized systems. Although these boundaries may not directly apply to natural situations, the parameters generated from these models provide theoretical guidelines for the empirical study of information in biological-behavioral systems.

Information theory has been used to establish limits for the range of psychological response including reaction time, psychophysical judgments, memory encoding and recall, and concept formation (Luce, 1960). For instance, the parameters underlying reaction time (*RT*) have been evaluated. Hick (1951a,b) and Hyman (1953) suggested that reaction time should be proportional to the amount of information transmitted by a stimulus. Therefore, as the number of stimulus alternatives is increased, reaction time increments would be expected to follow:

$$RT = k \log (n + 1)$$

Hicks established $(n + 1)$ as a rate limiting amount, as using n in the equation would result in $RT = 0$, when $n = 1$. This assumption was later criticized, and other methods for computing the limits for reaction time were attempted. Information theory has been shown to be useful in explaining reaction time within controlled experimental situations involving simple signal processing, but not with respect to more complex processing tasks (Posner, 1986)

Information Theory and Attention

We previously alluded to some of the ways that information theory is relevant to attentional processes. Two factors limit its utility. Information theory makes estimates of information capacity at given points in time, given certain assumptions about the relationship among stimuli. However, during information processing, the individual is actually making selections over time, and one selection is often contingent on the previous selection. Not only are signals not independent, but they are often very dependent. Therefore, the weights assigned when determining the probabilities for future selection must reflect a changing set of stimulus saliences. Luce (1960) suggested that one can apply Bayes's theorem to determine these weights based on prior data.

A second factor that must be dealt with is the multivariant framework that often exists in real-world situations. Instead of considering only one signal and one source of noise, the investigator is forced to consider the interactions of a large set of signals that must be dealt with in parallel. The original information theory dealt with information being handled serially. For a sequential flow of information, variables such as information rate, entropy, channel capacity, and noise can be characterized at each time point in a dichotomous fashion. Each stimulus is either a signal or noise. However, such a dichotomy does not hold up as well when there are multiple signals, with nonlinear interactions, producing even more complex forms of information. Furthermore, a parallel processing system may enable multiple channels of capacity. It is easy to see that the computational requirements of information theory may become excessive when applied to complex multivariant systems.

If we take these limitations into account, information theory still has utility for the study of attention. For instance, Swets (1964, 1973, 1984) focused considerable effort on extending mathematical models derived from formal information theory to the study of attention. They specified four classes of models that have application to the study of attention: (1) selective; (2) divided; (3) visual-spatial; and (4) sustained.

An Early Model of Manual Tracking

Mathematical models designed to account for specific behavioral phenomena were initially the result of efforts to develop machine systems that could replicate human processes. This was particularly true of manual tracking, as the ability to track objects in space is critical to aerospace, military, and other engineering applications. The relationship of manual tracking to attention is obvious, as the manual tracking depends on vigilance, and on directed search and response in reference to a target. All of these factors are considered fundamental components of attention.

Two problems emerged when researchers tried to develop models of manual tracking: (1) Manual tracking cannot be accounted for by only one or two processes and therefore refers to a series of processes, and (2) that the human operator acts as a linear time-independent system cannot be assumed. Nonetheless, manual tracking provides an illustration of how a model for a complex behavior may first be determined for a simple system that can be relatively well understood and then expanded to account for the real conditions of the system. Such a method was used in the case of information theory and statistical learning, though neither of these approaches was overly concerned with defining the underlying processes involved in the phenomena of information transmission or learning. Estes's model of learning (1950, 1959) suggests two processes involved in learning (conditioning and the availability of stimuli), though no mechanism for these processes is defined.

Manual tracking is fundamentally dependent on a temporal sequence of behavior (time dependence) and the integration of signal input with response output. The adequacy of a particular tracking system depends on the degree of correspondence that can be achieved between the temporal-spatial characteristics of the signal that is processed and the response that follows. Two types of tracking have been previously described: pursuit and compensatory. The main distinction between these types of tracking is whether the individual who is tracking is given information regarding his or her own relative position, as well as that of the target (pursuit), or only the relative difference in position between him- or herself and the target (compensatory). Pursuit tracking is inherently more difficult to model as there are more variables to account for.

Licklider (1960) described one of the first mathematical descriptions of compensatory tracking (see Figure 21.1). In his simplest model, tracking depends on a signal's being transmitted to an operator, who makes a determination of whether her or his previous response was an error based on a signal sent back from the target. This simple system requires a feedback loop that allows the operator to determine her or his next response. The presence of feedback greatly complicates the computational demands of the system, as the feedback signal inherently serves to change the value of the information to be derived from future stimuli.

From the standpoint of information theory, the difficulty in creating a model to account for compensatory tracking stems from the nonlinearity that occurs when feedback is introduced. In human systems, delays in reaction time produce variability in temporal-spatial coordination. Licklider (1960) dealt with this problem by first describing tracking in a linear system, and then extending this model to account for the nonlinear demands. To accomplish this, he described tracking performance as a function of error propagation (ϵ) in a system that detects a movement of a target between two states:

$$\frac{d\epsilon(t)}{dt} = -k\epsilon(t)$$

where (t) = time, e = error size, and k = constant. This equation predicts that, for each tracking attempt, the size of the error decreases at a rate proportional to its initial size. One can extend this simple model to account for error rates in the tracking of more complex state changes, such as a waveform.

As we previously discussed, if the nonlinearities in this system are minimized, the accuracy of the model increases, but the computational complexity that is required may become overwhelming. Models of tracking propose many hypothetical mechanisms for

A

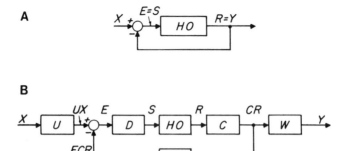

B

FIGURE 21.1. Simplified models of compensatory tracking as proposed by Licklider (1960). (A) The simplest system for tracking requires an input (*X*), which is responded to (*R* = *Y*) by a human operator (*HO*) based on feedback and error analysis. (B) A slightly more complex and generalized system is illustrated in which an input network (*U*) recognizes the signal (*X*) and then compares it with information from a feedback network (*F*), which then creates an error determination. This comparison results in a differential function, which is represented by the circle. The human operator responds to the resulting display (*D*) of the mismatch between target and error to initiate control mechanisms (*C*) for response correction. When an optimal correction is achieved, the output network (*W*) initiates a response. (E = error, S = stimulus, FCR = Feedback loop output). From Licklider (1960), with permission of the publisher.

reducing the error of temporal-spatial approximation. Early efforts to model manual tracking have been fraught with many computational complexities that are well beyond the scope of this chapter. Yet, it is noteworthy that the fundamental mechanisms postulated in these early models remain a cornerstone of recent approaches to this problems. Most models of tracking include processes that enable the system to perform sensory selection and directed responding, and they include a mechanism for adjusting responses based on error. All of these models must compensate for the variability associated the human operator's response tendency. To accomplish this, many contain filters that subtract for feedback that falls outside a particular range. Filters enable the system to correct for the fact that humans do not respond in direct linear correspondence to the stimuli that they receive.

Models of manual tracking were among the first computational attempts to describe attentional operations. They tried to account for a variety of operator and task characteristics that affect tracking performance.

COMPUTATIONAL MODELS AND NEURAL NETWORKS

The primary goal of recent computational neural models is to create a formal description of cognitive processes that closely resembles the features of actual neural events. As in other mathematical models that we have discussed, an attempt is made to ensure mathematical-logical rigor and consistency. This goal is not unique to current mathematical approaches. As we have noted, previous theorists were also concerned about these issues. However, previous mathematical approaches were often less focused on creating models that replicated the natural characteristics of neural phenomena. Those theorists who were concerned about both the neural and the functional aspects of particular cognitive processes lacked the computational power (computers) and knowledge about the nervous system that are now available.

Self-Organizing Systems

The problem of creating a neural network that could learn was central in the early investigations of artificial intelligence. Learning theory had suggested that a strengthening of the associative connection between elements of the network could explain conditioning. However, until recently, there has been little empirical neurophysiological information to suggest what mechanism may produce associative connection. For the investigators of artificial intelligence, the mechanism of memory formation was more clear-cut, as storage characteristics were determined by the constraints of the machine and the algorithms that were used for information processing. However, a different problem emerged: how to create a machine that would learn spontaneously, from information derived from previous processing, rather than as a result of rules supplied by the programmer.

An initial solution to this problem occurred somewhat serendipitously in Rosenblatt's studies (1962) of the perceptron. Rosenblatt invented a simple learning network, which he called a *perceptron*. A characteristic of this network was that, if a sequence of stimuli was presented, it could separate the stimulus units into classes (0,1) based on the weights of the stimulus value. This process would continue until, eventually, all of the stimuli would become grouped into one class. Regardless of how the stimuli were weighted, the result was an all-or-nothing grouping into one or the other class. The machine favored a state in which there was always one end state that was determined by which stimulus class was initially in the majority When the two classes were evenly distributed, the classification preference was determined by random fluctuations in machine state.

This problem was eventually handled by creating a modification, by which the perceptron network would change the weights of the stimulus units before classifying on the basis of a particular feature. The result was that the machine could adjust so as to maintain a stable steady state of classification based on features of the stimuli. Rosenblatt (1962) felt that this reflected the development of a new type of machine that was capable of thinking according to statistical classification rules. This conclusion was strongly criticized by many in the field of artificial intelligence. For instance, Minsky and Papert (1969) argued that perceptrons are vulnerable to the same problems of other computer-based information processing systems. The perceptron is incapable of acting in a way that is inconsistent with its computational properties and the nature of the elements that are used to create its structure. The perceptron was developed with one layer of processing between the stimulus and the output device. Therefore, there is no capacity for feedback arrangements in this system, which limits its ability to perform self-directed learning. Also, symbolic processing approaches had already been shown to be capable of performing many tasks. This led Minsky and others in the field of artificial intelligence to question the usefulness of the perceptron.

Even though the field of study shifted away from the perceptron model that Rosenblatt had originally advocated, it is now evident that his goals had much merit. The capacity for self-directed organization and learning is fundamental to whether a machine is capable of simulating human cognition. Also, self-directed activity defines the attentional characteristics of the system. As we have suggested elsewhere in this text, attentional processes reflect the selective allocation of cognitive resources to a task.

The concepts of parallel processes and human associative organization that arose out of research on information processing have had a particular impact on current computational approaches. Parallel processes have enabled cognitive researchers to avoid some of the problems that plagued previous models. For example, the temporal constraints of a serial processing framework are not as great a problem for neural systems that operate in parallel. Study of the organization of human associative memory has led to new ideas about how learned experience is represented, including the view that memory may be distributed across the cortex. As cognitive phenomena seem to consist of more than the activity of single neurons, it has been important to develop models that can account for the interaction of distributed neurons throughout the brain, acting as networks for either parallel or serial processing.

The computational approaches that exemplify current directions in mathematical modeling include Grossberg's neural network models (1980, 1988), connectionist modeling (Feldman & Ballard, 1982) and the parallel-distributed-processing (PDP) models (Rumelhart, Hinton, & McClelland, 1986). The PDP models are characterized by the thermodynamic models of Smolensky (1986) and Ballard, Hinton, and Sejnowski (1983). All of these models have common features: each provides a formal system for analysis; each is mathematically rigorous; and each accounts for complex cognitive phenomena. The conceptual underpinnings of several of these models come from traditional learning theory, computer science, and cognitive neuroscience. We review some of the features of these models here and discuss the utility of these approaches in the study of attention.

Parallel-Distributed-Processing Models

PDP models are a class of models that was developed by Rumelhart, McClelland, Norman, and their collaborators to extend the principles or parallel processing into a formal theoretical system. These models characterize the relationship among eight components that are thought to be fundamental to cognitive processes:

1. Processing units, u_i
2. States of activation, $a_i(t)$
3. Output values $o_i(t)$
4. A pattern of connectivity, W_i
5. Rules of propagation, net_i
6. Rules of activation,

   $Fa(t + 1) = Wo(t) = \text{net}(t)$

7. Rules of learning, Δw_{ij}
8. Environmental characteristics, p_i

In PDP models, the processing unit is a conceptual object such as a visual, phonemic, or semantic feature. These units are characterized as input, output, or hidden and are organized in a set with the number of units (N). At any given time (t), some elements from the set of units may be in a state of being actively processed; those units are in a state of activation: $a_i(t)$. The possible values that this state of activation can hold depends on the characteristics of the particular model that one chooses to study. Activation may be restricted to binary values ($-1,1$) or to a range of analogue values. When a set of units interact, they are said to produce an output value ($o_i(t)$). This output value may be equal to the state of activation of the unit or may be reduced based on a threshold that is pre-established. The system's overall activational state varies as a function of the activational rules, which are determined by the interaction of all activational influences and patterns of connectivity. Therefore.

$$a(t + 1) = F[a(t), \text{net}(t)_1, \text{net}(t)_2, \ldots$$

Ultimately, the set of processing units interact to form a pattern of connectivity that reflects the strength, or weight (W), of all of the associated units.

The pattern of connectivity is fundamental to the PDP models, as it reflects the nonlinear relationship between a pattern of inputs and the effects of inhibitory and excitatory influences generated by the individual units. The pattern of connectivity is determined by a set of matrices, which are the weighted sums of the strengths of various associative connections. Rules of propagation are necessary to determine the net input ($net_i(t)$), which reflects the interaction of the connectivity matrices (W_i) and the output vectors that are generated, where

$$net_e = W_e o(t) \text{ and } net_i = W_i o(t)$$

where net_e is the net excitatory effect and net_i is the net inhibitory effect. Activation rules define how new inputs into a neural system interact with existing units and with each other to produce a new state of activation. The state of activation is a function (F) of the previous state of activation and the pattern of connectivity as defined by the propagation rules:

$$a_i(t + 1) = F(net_i(t)) = F(\sum_j w_{ij} o_j)$$

Accordingly, changes in activation occur over time as a function of the net ($_t$). In a natural neural system, the pattern of connectivity is always changing as a function of new experience. To account for these changes, PDP models used the rule of learning suggested by Hebb (1949), that the individual weights (w_{ij}) will vary as a function of the state of activation and rate of conditioning (η), where

$$\Delta w_{ij} = \eta a_i o_j$$

As conditioning depends on the specific environmental state at any given time, it is necessary to account for these environmental effects on the neural system. These are represented in PDP models as a set of probabilities that certain stimuli will occur (Rumelhart *et al.*, 1986).

Activational States

One of the most intriguing characteristics of PDP and other models is their incorporation of variables to specify activational states. This provides greater consistency with current neuropsychological and electrophysiological constructs regarding neural function. As we have described previously, the constructs of activation and arousal are central to most current theories of attention that integrate cognitive and psychophysiological evidence for an attentional process. The PDP models direct much effort to delineating the computational requirements of the state of activation. As was the case in previous mathematical models that we discussed, investigators studying PDP models start with simple linear models to explain the relationship between the existing state of activation and the pattern of connectivity. Simple phenomena can be modeled with some accuracy by means of the assumption of linearity. For instance, the example of learning that is given by the equation

$$\Delta w_{ij} = \eta a_i o_j$$

specifies the change in the pattern of weighted connections as a linear function of activation state. However, as we discussed earlier in this chapter, linearity cannot be assumed in real systems.

Current computational models deal with the need for nonlinearity in various ways. In most of these models, nonlinearities are particularly evident when one tries to establish the activational values acting on stimulus units. The early computational models dealt with nonlinearities by assuming a threshold of activation. If activation exceeded a certain value, an activation value of 1 was assigned, and if the value was less than the activation threshold, a value of 0 was given to the processing unit. Based on an analysis of this threshold framework, Minsky and Papert (1969) concluded that a single-step system of this sort could not account for learning. Anderson (1977) described a brain state in a box model that is similar to the linear threshold approach, but in which a feedback arrangement is incorporated so that previous activation can be recycled to influence the current state of activation.

A more recent approach to the problem of activation is seen in the "thermodynamic models" of harmony theory (Smolensky, 1986) and the Boltzmann machine (Hinton & Sejnowski et al., 1986) are based on a stochastic function of inputs. The probability of a given activational state is determined by many of the variables described in the general PDP model, as well as a variable called temperature (T). Temperature sets the probability that a unit will activate when it is close to a threshold value. It also determines the degree of nonlinearity that a set of input units will have over a range of conditions. The higher the value of T, the greater the uncertainty of activation at different values of the input. When $T = 0$, the system will behave as a linear threshold device, with little uncertainty, as there will be a clear-cut pattern of activation or no activation, depending on whether a threshold of the unit was passed. The rules that define the probability of activation are given by the following equation:

$$p(a_1(t) = 1) = \frac{1}{1 + \eta^{-(\Sigma_j w_{ij} a_j + \eta_i - \theta_i)/T}}$$

where n is the input from outside the system, θ_i is the threshold for the unit, and T is the temperature. Both harmony theory and the concept of relaxation search share a core set of principles that characterize thermodynamic theories.

Relaxation Searches, Harmony, and Attention

Smolensky (1986) proposed harmony theory to provide a mechanism whereby a system could make inferences based on uncertainty in the information that it receives (see Figure 21.2). According to this theory, when input is inconsistent with existing schemata, or when it is incomplete, the system settles for the most self-consistent state that is also consistent with the characteristics of the stimuli. Self-consistency can be determined by a harmony function (h). In simplest terms, h is the difference between the number of matches and mismatches between a stimulus and an existing schema. As, in normal cognition, there

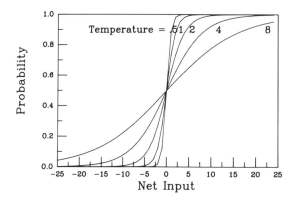

FIGURE 21.2. Harmony theory, as described by Smolensky (1986), is based on a thermodynamic framework. Behavioral change and adaptation are a function of the "temperature" of the system in relation to the net input into the system. New inputs influence the system's stability and essentially disrupt "harmony" which might otherwise remain at steady state. From Rumelhart et al. (1986), with permission.

may be many simultaneous activations of schemata, the most probable state of the environment is determined through a computational analysis of the interactions of these schemata. Harmony theory goes on to use the thermodynamic concept of temperature (T), which is the tendency of a system to settle on a stable, complete solution. With high computational temperatures, the completion of schemata will occur randomly.

Harmony theory uses stochastic assumptions that the machine will generate a series of probabilistic alternatives directed toward a goal. This stochastic characteristic creates the direction of the task, thus serving as an artificial drive. Within harmony theory, the drive is toward self-consistency, which will produce a state of maximal harmony. This model is a direct extension of thermodynamics and Shannon's information theory. Activation associated with the computational temperature and the drive toward harmony serves as a catalyst, by which changes in the pattern of connectivity will occur.

The thermodynamic perspective has been incorporated into the development of machines that learn by principles of "relaxation search" (Hinton & Sejnowski, 1986; Hinton, Sejnowski, & Ackley, 1984). This term refers to a model for learning in which the network settles for the easiest solution at the least cost. According to this approach, during many types of learning (especially visual analysis), the most efficient search occurs when the system settles for a solution or a template match that meets very "weak constraints." Once a state of relaxation is achieved, the system either settles or again searches to the next level of minimum constraint, if a greater degree of precision is necessary.

The advantage of a relaxation search is that the system is not forced to perform a high-precision analysis of every feature at the first step of analysis. By responding to a weak constraint, the neural system may perform a reduced level of processing until more processing is needed. This has obvious computational benefits and also fits the requirements of a thermodynamically driven system. As in the case of harmony theory, stochastic decision rules enable the system to jump to a higher level of analysis. These rules are generated in accordance with the environmental demands of the situation, so that the system's learning is closely integrated with natural characteristics of the context. Hinton and Sejnowski (1986) suggested that this model of learning tends to produce memory representations that resist change after minor system damage.

Relaxation search procedures may account for shifts of attention. Inhibition rules may explain how the system settles at a particular featural level or shifts to other stimulus characteristics.

Computational Models of Attention

Computational modeling has been largely directed at the primary sensory and motor processes, as well as learning and memory. The processes of attention and executive control tend not to be incorporated directly into these models. For instance, Rumelhart, Hinton, and McClelland (1986) stated, "it is certainly true that certain PDP models lack explicit attentional mechanisms" (p. 114). They went on to argue that these models are not incapable of exhibiting attentional phenomena. The fact that artificial intelligence machines generally have great difficulty directing their processing based on the relevance of the material they are processing illustrates the difficulty of creating models for attentional processes. Besides the many theoretical issues that relate to what factors should serve to direct attention, there is a problem in getting a model to self-initiate action. Some models avoid this problem by assuming a stochastic framework, in which attentional direction can be produced by a thermodynamic pressure that serves to generate a series of probabilistic alternatives.

In PDP models, attention may be considered an implicit phenomenon that is the by-product of other specified processes, but that is not specified in its own right. Grossberg

(1988) gave attention a more centralized role in his models. Attention is considered a subsystem in his adaptive resonance theory (1976a). Concepts such as competitive learning, relaxation searches, and harmony, which have been incorporated into different computational systems, provide theoretical mechanisms by which attentional processes can occur.

Competitive Learning

Competitive learning paradigms were developed in order to account for spontaneous learning on tasks that require the categorical determination of a set of stimuli. In certain situations, individuals must learn to determine a salient featural characteristic from a set of stimuli, when there is no *a priori* basis for making a classification. The individual must develop a representation of the stimuli that will allow for future classification. However, the lack of any *a priori* rules for such a classification makes this task difficult to explain in terms of simple associative learning theory. The adequate categorical classification of stimulus input depends on separating stimuli into well-defined groupings with categorical boundaries that are easily distinguished. Competitive learning is a theoretical process that links learning and attention.

Several investigators have proposed computational models to account for competitive learning (e.g., Grossberg, 1976, 1988; Rumelhart & Zipser, 1985). In most competitive learning models, stimulus input patterns pass through layers of filters that allow the dominant features of the stimuli to win over nondominant features. The effect of this competition is the resetting of the filter in correspondence with the changes induced by the new stimuli. Rumelhart and Zipser (1985) accounted for filtering by proposing that stimulus input passes through a series of hierarchically arranged inhibitory layers. At each layer, input units are organized into associative clusters. In each cluster, one element is dominant and inhibits the strength of the other stimulus elements.

Learning occurs in this model through competition between the elements in a given cluster. If a unit is strengthened to the point of having a dominant weighting relative to the other elements of the cluster, that unit becomes active. The activation caused by new competitive learning results in a different pattern of activation at the next layer of the system. This activation is distributed across all elements of the cluster according to the relative weights of all of the elements in the cluster.

The activation of multiple layers of processing clusters within competitive learning enables the system to respond to different levels of featural information. The higher levels may have a different resolution than the lower levels. The filtering of noise is possible because only information that passes through all layers of processing is consistent with the featural characteristics of the original stimulus to be recognized.

Hinton (1981) proposed that such a system can be used to account for both attentional focusing and stimulus equivalence during the recognition of stimulus features. To accomplish recognition, Hinton argued the neural system must be capable of "variable mapping" so that features presented in different orientations can be translated back to some pattern template for comparison. Mapping units are postulated that correct for shifts in orientation of the stimulus to be processed. Once this shift in orientation is learned, it is possible to direct the attention of the system to the correct orientation before the occurrence of the stimulus, based on previous presentations that change the unit strengths of the mapping units. This type of mechanism for mapping was described in great detail by Kohonen (1984) in a model of self-organizing maps.

Within a neural system that performs competitive learning, attentional focusing is determined by the setting of the mapping units that direct processing to a particular spatial orientation. The orientation of mapping units is under the control of previous learning, as repeated presentations of past stimuli tune these units to the proper orientation. This tuning is accomplished by shifts in the weights of particular elements contained in clusters of neural units at the layer of the system concerned with mapping. The rules of competitive learning suggest the basis for the changes in weights associated with featural elements of the stimulus, which influences attentional orientation in this model.

Grossberg (1976a,b) and, more recently, Rumelhart and Zipser (1986) have indicated that competitive learning occurs as a function of the characteristics of the stimuli that are to be processed. If stimuli are highly structured in well-organized clusters, there is a tendency for the system to be very stable. However, if the stimuli to be processed are not well structured, the classification and weightings of associative clusters is more variable and the result is greater instability in the system. This characteristic is particularly relevant to our consideration of attention. The instability of a system creates a pull for further processing. Attentional direction may be a by-product of this instability.

This theoretical interpretation has interesting similarities to the neuronal model for the OR and attention that was proposed by Sokolov (1963) (see Chapter 4). The neuronal model suggests that the OR is a by-product of the degree of mismatch between a new stimulus and existing templates for relevant stimuli in the neural system. The greater the novelty, uncertainty, or discrepancy of the new stimulus, the greater the size of the OR. This may be a reflection of the degree of attentional registration. Cue dominance and stimulus compounding, neobehavioral (Kendler, 1972) are extended in competitive learning models (see Chapter 4).

As competitive learning is dependent on a thermodynamic concept of a system's reaching a steady, stable state, the term *equilibrium* has been used to refer to this state. According to Rumelhart and Zipser (1986), equilibrium is defined as a state in which the average change in the weights of the elements of the clusters that make up the neural system is zero. They specified this state as:

$$0 = g\sum_k \left(\frac{c_{ik}}{n_k}\right) p_k v_{jk} - g\sum_k w_{ij} p_k v_{jk},$$

or at equilibrium:

$$W_{ij}\sum_k p_k v_{jk} = \sum_k \left(\frac{p_k c_{ik} v_{jk}}{n_k}\right)$$

where w = weights of units; v = the probability that a unit (j) will win in competition with other units when a stimulus (k) is presented; and p = the probability of a stimulus (k) occurring. As the competitive learning paradigm allows a unit to assume only two values (0,1), it can be shown that the response of a unit (j) to a new stimulus (Sx) is equal to:

$$\alpha_{j,l} = \frac{\sum_i p_i r_{li} v_{jl}}{\sum_i p_i v_{ji}}$$

where r_{xi} = the overlap of the new stimulus pattern with the previous pattern, when the system is at equilibrium. The stability of the equilibrium state depends on the characteristic of the stimuli that it must process. Stability is estimated to be a value (T) that is a function of the average response of units to new stimuli that create activation (unit = 1) relative to all other units of the system:

$$T = \sum_k p_k \sum_{i,j} v_{jk}(\alpha_{jk} - \alpha_{ik})$$

The size of T determines the stability of a system, so that a large value of T indicates that the system is stable and that there is a reasonable degree of overlap between the patterns being processed by a group of units. This condition would usually be met when each stimulus is well defined, with little ambiguity relative to other stimuli.

Attention in a Computational Network Model

Grossberg (1976a) proposed a model system that is capable of competitive learning and the self-organization of pattern input. This model is one of the few neural network models developed from a computational perspective that incorporates an attentional subsystem. Grossberg used his adaptive resonance theory (ART) as a foundation for this model. Although a discussion of all of the features of ART is beyond the scope of this book, it should be noted that attention is handled by Grossberg's system through processes that involve the self-organization and stabilization of the neural system. These processes are similar to those described relative to competitive learning. Grossberg (1988) argued that self-stabilization allows the system to incorporate old information in such a way that new input does not erase previous learning. Furthermore, he stated that this type of learning system does not run into capacity problems. Unlike in traditional associative learning models, in ART and competitive learning systems, new material is dealt with only relative to existing information. Therefore, information that exceeds the limits of existing knowledge is rejected.

The architecture of this system is shown in Figure 21.3. According to Grossberg (1980), filtering through competitive processes (i.e., adjustments in the weights of stimulus units) occurs during a stage of information processing before long-term memory formation. This processing step is necessary so that long-term traces do not change except when appropriate, based on the salience of new input. In the ART model, attentional control is established through interactions of long-term memory and short-term memory activation in two stages (F_1 and F_2). By including two stages, Grossberg suggested a system that can make comparisons between stimulus units and templates. The system also has the capacity to control the activation associated with the stimulus units, as the system conducts comparisons and amplifies stimulus strength with information from STM.

Grossberg's neural network model (1980, 1988) shares features with the PDP models and theoretical systems we have reviewed. Activation rules govern changes in associative relationship between stimulus units. Although units can have any value, a certain threshold needs to be reached before a unit will affect the strength of another unit. An interesting aspect of Grossberg's formulation is the inclusion of both excitatory and inhibitory effects. As in the PDP models, a multilayer system is proposed, one capable of both top-down and bottom-up activational influences. Activation is determined to be a function of decay rate (A), the maximum level of excitation of the unit (B), and the maximum inhibition (C) that may occur below the resting state of 0. Accordingly, activational state is predicted to be

$$a_j(t + 1) = a_j(t)(1 - A) + (B - a_j)(t) - (a_j(t) + C)\,\mathrm{net}_{ij}(t)$$

which accounts for the effects of both inhibitory and excitatory influences when deriving activational state.

Simulations of Visual Attention

Recently, Sandon (1990) developed a neural network, based on a connectionist model, to simulate selective visual attention. The model is hierarchical, as it contains multiple processing layers that enable features to be extracted, focused, and then extracted again

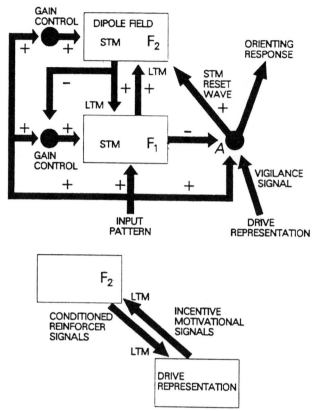

FIGURE 21.3. The adaptive network model (Grossberg, 1988, with permission) is among the first neural-network–computational frameworks to incorporate attentional considerations. (A) Two subsystems are proposed that interact: attentional and orienting subsystems. Input produces bottom-up changes in short-term memory (STM) at a first level (F_1) based on matching with top-down influences such as learned expectations from STM at a second level (F_2). The degree of mismatch activates the second orienting subsystem, which causes STM to be reset, which in turn triggers further attentional search. This activation may also elicit an orienting response. Drive representations produce incentive motivational signals that enhance the sensitivity of the orienting subsystem, thus increasing the likelihood that STM will reset and also interacting with STM at F_2 to strengthen long-term memory (LTM) development (Arrows with a positive value ($+$) are excitatory, while arrows with a negative value ($-$) are inhibitory.). (B) The relationship of these attentional components to operant and competitive learning (CD = drive representation; CS1 and CS2 are conditioned stimuli; SCS1 and SCS2 are sensory representations).

at higher levels of resolution. Furthermore, the model contains processing units tuned to different featural scales, which enable the system to handle feature types. An attention module is included, which gates information that has been activated based on characteristics that have been assigned information value and that are deemed "interesting." According to what featural information is attended to, the system directs focusing to the local spatial region of interest. In effect, the system location is used to mediate the attentional focus.

One of the central problems for models of attention relates to how the unattended-to

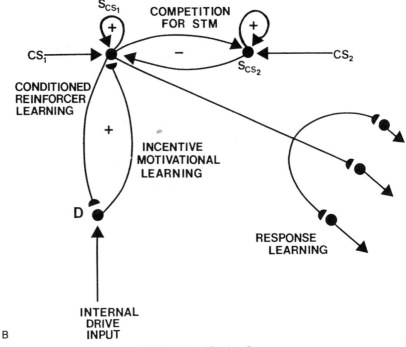

S_{CS_1} COMPETITION
FOR STM

CS$_1$

Scs$_2$

CS$_2$

CONDITIONED
REINFORCER
LEARNING

INCENTIVE
MOTIVATIONAL
LEARNING

D

RESPONSE
LEARNING

INTERNAL
DRIVE
B   INPUT

FIGURE 21.3. (*Continued*)

information is handled by the system. Some recent models assume that unattended-to information is processed on occasion as a function of some probability (Mozer, 1988). Sandon's model allows for some unattended-to information to be passed through to subsequent attentional layers, so that, at times, it may still influence selection. Sandon proposed that a relaxation search procedure enables the system to shift and settle, thereby focusing attention based on inhibitory processes according to the following rule that was proposed by Koch and Ullman (1985).

$$\frac{dy_i}{dt} = y_i(s_i - \Sigma x_j y_j)$$

where x_i represents attentional layer activation, and y_i represents the activation of auxiliary nodes based on the overall information that is available. The level of y_i is determined by the amount of noise and the number of iterations of the relaxation procedure, where

$$y_i(0) = \frac{1}{N} + \eta \ (\eta = \text{noise})$$

before attentional processing. Using this procedure, Sandon was able to show differences in attentional search time and accuracy based on the similarity of stimuli. This model illustrates the direction being taken in recent neural network approaches to attention.

Toward an Integrated Neuropsychological Framework of Attention

This final chapter contains a synthesis of the material presented earlier. Conclusions can now be drawn regarding the cognitive, behavioral, and neural bases of attention. The constructs, models, and theories of attention that have been described are supported by the large quantity of empirical and factual evidence that has been presented earlier. In this chapter, I attempt to pull together this evidence, and to formalize current thinking about what attention is and how it is controlled by the brain.

I describe a theoretical framework that may help to organize the plethora of information regarding the neuropsychology of attention. Within this framework, two types of models are described, based on both cognitive and neural perspectives. The cohesiveness of this theoretical framework still needs to be tested. As the interrelationship among the various cognitive processes and neural mechanisms is extremely complex, the nature of this interrelationship cannot be examined in an isolated experiment. Verification of this theoretical framework depends on determining the fit of its components with data derived from studies using multiple methodologies. Although I believe that this framework accurately reflects the processes underlying attention, perhaps its greatest utility will be as a foundation on which new research can be built.

Before considering the details of this theoretical framework, we should first examine certain premises and observations on which its tenets are based. Hopefully, we have demonstrated that the way one defines attention determines the paradigms and, ultimately, the processes that are found to underlie it. As attention has been studied by researchers from very different scientific perspectives, it is not hard to see why a variety of attentional models have emerged. One common strategy for scientific model development is to assume that there is a correct paradigm for a particular behavioral analysis and to reject models arising from other paradigms. Unfortunately, this approach does not work well for attentional phenomena. As models derived from different scientific approaches are typically concerned with separate aspects of attentional phenomena, it is unrealistic to completely reject one approach in favor of another. A comprehensive neuropsychological model of attention should be inclusive rather than exclusive and, therefore, must seek to incorporate the salient features of all approaches that have utility.

Because of the diversity of scientific perspectives from which attention has been studied, there is not a universal language or set of constructs to facilitate the study of attentional phenomena. The similarities and differences among models of attention are often obscured by distinctions in language and philosophical assumptions associated with particular scientific disciplines. One goal of this book is to unify the language, constructs, and empirical data regarding the neuropsychology of attention, so that it is easier to assess how well particular models fit with reality. Now, at the completion of this project, I am impressed by the fact that certain conceptual themes seem to recur in many of the attentional theories developed since the late 19th century. Although the particular language used to describe attentional processes varies across scientific disciplines, there is often a remarkable consistency in the underlying concepts originating from these different approaches, as each attempts to characterize attention. This is not to say that there is complete redundancy across modern theories of attention. Conceptions of the exact mechanisms underlying attention differ depending on the theoretical perspective that one chooses to consider. Yet, these differences are frequently minimal.

Our theoretical framework reflects the commonalities evident across most modern attentional theories, as well as the unique contributions of the more dominant approaches (e.g., behavioral and cognitive). Whenever possible, an effort has been made to incorporate concepts that seem to be universal across different theories of attention, along with those characteristics of particular theories that explain some unique aspect of attentional phenomena. This theoretical framework is composed of certain underlying cognitive-behavioral principles. These principles are outlined here, in an order that is roughly based on the extent to which they are universally accepted.

1. Attention enables *information reduction*. It is universally accepted that humans cannot simultaneously process and respond to the infinite quantity of information that reaches the sensory systems each moment. Therefore, there must be a means by which large quantities of incoming information are reduced to accommodate cognitive processing. This means is attention. Although researchers have disagreed on the basis of information reduction, most agree that such a phenomenon must occur.

2. Attention provides for *information selection*. This principle is closely related to the principle of information reduction but emphasizes a somewhat different point. Attending not only reduces the quantity of information but also establishes a priority of particular information for further processing. Although widely accepted, this principle is the subject to somewhat greater debate, as some behavioral theorists object to the notion of an active "selection" process. However, if we bypass the issue of active versus passive selection, there is almost universal agreement that in normal behavior situations, certain stimuli are responded to and others are not. This phenomenon can be referred to as *attentional selection*.

3. Attention is the *interface* between perceptual input and higher order cognition and behavioral action. This principle has its roots in the psychological theories of James and Wundt. Among these early psychologists, there was a recognition that sensory input is not analogous to the substance of attentional experience. For instance, a distinction between external reality and internal experience was made by Wundt, who referred to the interface between the two as the apperceptive focus. In the context of current concepts of attention, it is widely accepted that sensory registration is not synonymous with attention. As in the case of hemispatial neglect, individuals capable of normal sensation and perception may fail to respond to certain incoming information as a result of attentional dysfunction after brain damage.

4. Attention provides for the *interaction of incoming information with existing memory*. When one examines the nature of learning and memory formation, it becomes clear that attention influences the encoding of new information. Furthermore, the nature of existing memory representations influences the characteristics of attention. Memory and attention interact reciprocally.

5. Attention is *spatially distributed*. The spatial characteristics of the environment influence the attentional parameters underlying the particular situation. Conversely, attentional behavior influences the spatial orientation of the individual. The spatial reference of attention is underscored, as this principle characterizes an important aspect of attentional behavior: Attention selection often depends on one's relationship to a spatial environment. Attention requires several spatially oriented activities, such as (a) a search of the environment for salient stimuli; (b) a focusing of cognitive processing on a particular spatial location when a relevant stimulus has been detected; and (c) a rejection or inhibition of responses to other locations. Humans also seem capable of diffusing their spatial attention so as to increase the likelihood of detection from all spatial locations. A number of spatial parameters affect attentional performance. For instance, attentional performance varies depending on where a stimulus is presented and whether the animal is oriented to the particular spatial location. Many spatial effects have been demonstrated by researchers studying spatial selective attention. For example, attentional responses to stimuli presented to the fovea differ from those presented to the peripheral visual field. Other spatial factors, such as depth and vertical and horizontal orientation, are also extremely important in specifying the parameters of attention.

6. Attention is also *temporally distributed and variable*. This principle is also very important, as it specifies that attention reflects the selection of information over time. This concept was central to early theories of attention, as it suggests that attentional control is governed by the *serial processing* of human information. Even though not all attentional operations occur serially, the sequence of incoming information has important influences on attention. In certain instances attention may be momentarily pulled by a stimulus (e.g., an orienting response), with the animal showing no subsequent response to that stimulus. Therefore, it can also be argued that attention need not always be temporally distributed. However, this situation is special, as failure to maintain an attentional response is influenced by the occurrence of competing stimuli that have greater priority. Attention produces a tendency toward a temporal continuity of response to a stimulus, but this continuity is subject to competing influences, which produce variations in attention.

7. *Anticipation, preparation*, and *delay* of response are determinants of attention. This principle specifies that the relationship between attention and impending action is contingent on the animal's response to time parameters. Anticipatory, preparatory, and delay responses are temporally based, as they are transitional behaviors that occur before an overt goal-directed response. These responses determine the temporal character of attention. The term *anticipation* refers to a process of sensitization and general activation before a response demand that will happen at a later time. Preparation is the behavioral response to the anticipation of impending demands and is generated to facilitate subsequent performance. *Response delay* refers to the important action of inhibiting immediate responding despite the presence of anticipatory or other pressures to respond. Without the capacity for response delay, sustained attention is impossible, as attention is pulled by any immediate strong stimulus. All three of these processes depend on the animal's time horizon.

8. Attentional selection and focus are governed by *motivational factors*. Although considerable debate has centered on the validity of the psychological constructs of drive and motivation, it is widely accepted that stimuli vary in their salience and reinforcement strength. Not all stimuli have the same attentional value. Some stimuli have intrinsic

qualities that create "cue strength," and others develop value as a function of learning. Attention is influenced by a host of factors that have a bearing on stimulus value, such as stimulus novelty, complexity, and strength. Furthermore, the momentary state of the animal dictates the relative strength of a particular stimulus at each given point in time. The stimuli that have attentional value for a hungry animal may fail to have that value after satiation. Behaviorists have tended to emphasize the importance of the principle of reinforcement when explaining attentional phenomena, while cognitive psychologists working from an information-processing framework have often minimized this factor. Although motivational variables are not the sole determinants of attentional direction, they clearly are an important underlying factor.

9. *Attentional capacity* varies as a function of internal organismic factors. Energetic state, motivational factors, and natural differences across individuals influence attentional capacity. We will reiterate the factors affecting attentional capacity later, as they are cornerstones of modern cognitive theories of attention. For now, the principle of attentional capacity can be summarized as follows: The extent to which humans are able to divide their attention among multiple stimuli, to handle large loads of information, and to sustain attention for long time periods varies both within the individual and across different people.

10. Humans have only a limited capacity for *divided attention* among multiple sources of information. Early attentional researchers generally felt that attention was severely limited and could not be divided among multiple channels of information. Later demonstrations of parallel processing indicated that people have a greater capacity for divided attention than was originally believed. However, even under the best of conditions, the number of simultaneous attentional acts that can be performed is limited. Human capacity for divided attention is determined by the degree to which the information to be processed or the behavior to be performed is already well integrated in long-term memory. Integration in long-term memory produces attentional *automaticity* for well rehearsed information.

11. A distinction can be made between *automatic and controlled* attentional operations, which influence the effortful demands that a task places on the individual. As a general rule, tasks that can be performed automatically require less attentional effort, though this depends on momentary task demands (Shiffrin & Schneider, 1977; Hasher & Zacks, 1984). For instance, the automaticity of attending while driving a car may become effortful and may require controlled attention if road conditions worsen. The attentional demands created by a particular task influence not only momentary performance characteristics, but also the capacity for sustained attention and the subjective experience of effort. Attention to effortful tasks for long time periods is likely to produce subjective *fatigue*. However, the relationships among subjective, behavioral, and physical fatigue are a more complicated issue.

12. As a task requires greater levels of controlled attention it is more likely to produce *conscious awareness*. Although the neuropsychological bases of consciousness and awareness are still largely not understood, the phenomenological relationship between attention and awareness has been the subject of cognitive inquiry. There continues to be debate over whether conscious awareness is a precondition for attention. As people are able to attend to tasks (e.g., driving a car) without being aware of their actions at all times, it would appear that attention does not depend on conscious awareness. This issue is closely related to the distinction between controlled and automatic attention. Without venturing further into this debate, it is safe to say that attention and conscious awareness are interrelated.

13. Attention is the by-product of *multiple interactive processes*. Throughout this text, the argument has been presented that attention is not a unitary process. Hopefully, readers are convinced that the term *attention* actually refers to a set of cognitive-behavioral processes involved in the selection of information and in behavioral response control. Furthermore, attention is determined by multiple factors, and most likely by a network of neural systems.

Therefore, the neuropsychological analysis of attentional phenomena requires a multifactorial perspective.

This principle is not accepted by all psychological researchers, as illustrated by the explanations for attention offered by different theoretical perspectives. On one hand, behaviorists frequently take the position that attention is not a process at all, but only a label used to describe more basic behavioral phenomena, such as extinction and stimulus control. Behaviorists largely reject the need for an attentional construct on the grounds that attentional phenomena are adequately explained within the confines of learning theory. In contrast, many cognitive scientists have postulated the existence of a specific attentional process located at a particular stage of information processing. On one extreme are scientists who reject the existence of attentional processes, and on the other extreme are scientists who maintain that attention represents a single process.

14. Attention is simultaneously governed in both a *bottom-up* and a *top-down* manner. Although this statement seems paradoxical, these two perspectives are not irreconcilable. Attention emerges as a "bottom-up" manifestation of the response to conditioning. An animal's history of previous learning in relation to the reinforcement strength of new stimuli produces attentional direction. From this perspective, attention is not an entity in its own right but a result of the conditioning process. In contrast, cognitive models of attention with "top-down" organization consider attention an independent cognitive function that provides for information selection. Attention is generally thought to exist either as a single process, or as a set of processes, with a supervisory role over other behaviors.

Without rehashing the strengths and weaknesses of each of these theoretical positions as we did earlier in text, it is fair to say that both positions have merit, and that both are correct and useful for explaining certain aspects of attention. There can be little doubt that the direction of our sensory intake and behavior is often governed by external stimulus events. Environmental stimuli are capable of "pulling" our perceptual focus. The reinforcement value of a particular stimulus dictates the duration and stability of that focus. Therefore, it is possible to account for many "attentional" experiences by using a "bottom-up" model in which there is no specific attentional process.

There are other situations in which attention is a by-product of a seemingly higher order plan of action. For instance, when we "look" or engage in other forms of environmental search, our sensory intake is directed by an incentive to locate and act relative to a particular stimulus. Learning theories may also account for such behavior in a "bottom-up" fashion by advocating the importance of schedules of reinforcement and discriminative learning. Yet, it is also clear that the act of looking may be driven by organismic urges before the presentation of a stimulus. At such times, attention is associated with the supervisory control of behavior.

Even in cases of the first type, when attention is pulled by environmental events, additional focusing often occurs subsequently. After an initial response to a stimulus, we may either tune our attention to a finer level of featural resolution or draw our attention to a less specific level of detail. To accomplish such attentional tuning, neural systems must exist that are capable of exerting supervisory control over other neural systems that are responsible for more basic sensory processes.

These brief examples demonstrate that two seemingly incompatible views of attention can coexist and explain different aspects of attentional phenomena. Furthermore, they illustrate why attention should not be viewed as a unitary process but must be considered the by-product of a network of processes that interact to govern responses to an ever-changing stimulus environment.

15. Attentional processes are *adaptive*, as they are most sensitive to changes in environmental state. Generally, attention is enhanced when there are variations in the stimulus set,

whereas attention attenuates under conditions of environmental redundancy. This can be demonstrated both behaviorally and with regard to physiological response characteristics.

NEURAL PRINCIPLES OF ATTENTION

In addition to these cognitive and behavioral principles, our current theoretical framework is based on several principles regarding the neural mechanisms underlying attention.

1. Attention is not localized at one brain site. Instead, attention is the by-product of a *network* of neural systems. This follows from the earlier principle that attention is not a unitary process but a set of related processes. Although the exact nature of this network is still far from being understood, it appears that several major neuroanatomical systems are implicated in attentional control.

2. The neuroanatomical systems involved in attentional control reflect the *functional organization* of the brain. The architecture of brain systems is such that higher order cognitive functions are organized around neural systems that control more basic sensory, motor, or regulatory functions. For instance, visual registration occurs in the primary visual cortex. Yet, higher order visual analysis, featural and object recognition, integration, and abstraction occur in secondary and tertiary cortical areas that surround this primary cortex. Similar arrangements exist for other sensory functions. The relationship of the prefrontal cortex to the motor cortex illustrates such a relationship for motor responding, as the prefrontal cortex facilitates the planning and execution of motor responding. These higher order functions associated with each sensory and motor system seem to play fundamental roles in the control of attention.

3. The neuroanatomical systems involved in attentional control are most broadly divided into two cortical divisions corresponding to the distinction between *sensory* and *motor* functions. Posterior brain systems associated with sensory functions are implicated in *sensory selection*, and anterior brain systems associated with motor functions are implicated in preparation and response *intention*. However, the division between these functional systems is not sharp, particularly with respect to attention, as attention depends on sensorimotor integration.

4. The neural systems involved in attention are *hierarchically* arranged. Besides having a functional organization around basic sensory and motor systems, the brain is organized in a cortical-subcortical axis. This arrangement has an implicit logic and utility for attentional control. Subcortical systems such as the reticular system and the hypothalamus produce activational states that direct the animal to respond. Subcortical systems may control specific biological functions such as the regulation of physiological state or even appetitive behaviors such as eating and sleep. However, these activational states are rather nonspecific with respect to salient features of the environment or previous experience.

At the apex of the subcortex are the limbic system and the basal ganglia. These two systems are similar insomuch as they modulate impulses from both lower subcortical areas and higher cortical sites. These systems have excitatory and inhibitory capabilities and therefore are able to tune less modulated subcortical impulses. Furthermore, these systems seem to be highly flexible in their behavioral repertoire, as they respond to and integrate multimodal sources of information and facilitate the encoding of this information in a distributed cortical system. At the top of the hierarchy, the cortex provides for multimodal mixing and the associative elaboration of new information with previously encoded representations. Communication among different systems in this hierarchy enables an interface between biological pressures that govern behavior and associative processes that shape these pressures in correspondence with experience. This interface creates attentional control.

5. The extent to which the cells of particular brain systems exhibit *neural plasticity* dictates their attentional role. Cortical regions that have cells with highly crystallized architecture seem to be "hardwired," so that their function is very specific and more invariant. Tertiary cortical regions seem to have less specificity of function and greater neural plasticity Mesocortical areas, such as the cingulate gyrus and the parahippocampal and entorhinal areas, are less differentiated and have greater neural plasticity. The limbic system seems to be capable of a high degree of plasticity. Attention seems to depend on the interaction of neural systems with less plasticity that can provide an invariant template on which to map experience, and plastic neural systems that can be modified in accordance with behavioral adaptation. The modification of neural cells in accordance with sensory input is a mechanism by which attentional enhancement may occur.

6. Habituation, sensitization, and *classical conditioning* are among the most basic behavioral processes that underlie attentional response. Habituation and sensitization explain the facilitation and attenuation of the orienting response to new stimuli. In controlled situations, the relationship between stimulus presentation and these responses can be specified with reasonable precision. That the attentional response to simple stimuli with little informational value can be predicted in humans is important, as it provides a starting point from which to examine attention to more complex information. Habituation and sensitization also provide the foundation for classical conditioning, thus creating a link between attention and memory formation. Habituation and sensitization are robust phenomena that can be demonstrated in organisms with many levels of complexity. Furthermore, the neurophysiological and neurochemical mechanisms for these responses are reasonably well understood in some simple organisms. The fact that habituation, sensitization, and classical conditioning appear to be neurally linked establishes a logical consistency between the behavioral and neural bases of attention.

7. Attentional control is established by the interaction of *inhibitory* and *excitatory* processes. Inhibitory and excitatory arrangements are evident at many different levels of the nervous system, from the interactions of large brain systems to events occurring within or between individual cells. These arrangements are critical for normal attentional operations as they provide mechanisms that stop, delay, or maintain responding relative to a particular stimulus. Several of the relevant inhibitory-excitatory arrangements for attention are (a) cortical modulation of subcortical impulses; (b) inhibitory functions of the prefrontal cortex; (c) the reciprocal relationship between amygdaloid and septal influences during limbic system responses to reinforcing stimuli; and (d) lateral inhibition across cells of the visual system that provide tuning to specific spatial frequencies. There are numerous other inhibitory-excitatory neural arrangements that influence attentional response.

8. *Neurochemical mediation* influences attentional response. The actions of neurotransmitters, as well as a number of neuropeptides, provide a means by which neuronal response can be modulated. Neurochemical variation is generally slower than bioelectrical activation, which expands the time horizon of attentional response. Stimuli that produce direct neuronal activation are likely to produce a rapid attentional response, and factors affecting neurochemical state produce more gradual change in attentional tone. Circadian variations in attentional capacity illustrate these gradual changes resulting from a host of neurochemical variations over the course of the day.

Although the relationship between brain neurochemical response and attention is not yet well understood, it is clear that there are both generalized and specific effects on attention. For instance, CNS stimulants like coffee may produce a generalized increase in vigilance. Other drugs, such as LSD, disrupt the selectivity of attention. Dopaminergic agonists change the ability of neural systems to gate information. The administration of peptides to particular brain nuclei may actually induce or block specific behavioral repertoires in laboratory animals, as in the case of flank marking resulting from stimulation of the preoptic nuclei of the hypothalamus. Such a finding demonstrates that a specific attentional focus can be induced by the chemical activation of a particular brain site. Therefore, it seems likely that the distribution of neurochemicals across brain systems plays a key role in attentional response.

9. Neural *processing speed* influences attentional capacity. In general, individuals who exhibit a long latency of neurophysiological response (e.g., P3 paradigms) also exhibit reduced performance on attentional tasks. In certain subcortical brain disorders, such as multiple sclerosis (MS) a breakdown of communication along white matter pathways correlates with reduced attentional capability. Even though MS patients are often able to store information in memory, they have great difficulty with information processing. Their difficulty seems to correspond to psychomotor slowing. Although the evidence is not in yet, one explanation for this impairment is a breakdown in the synchronization of cognitive processes with external events, along with a loss of temporal continuity. The metaphor of a telephone line helps to illustrate this point. If the signal rate along the line falls below a certain speed, the transmitted message will become garbled as a result of interference from other signals. A minimal neural processing speed is necessary for incoming information to maintain its integrity. When there is a slowing beyond this level, input loses its informational integrity, processing becomes effortful, and attentional failures result.

10. Certain neural cells have *special attentional functions*. In addition to the interaction of a network of brain systems for attentional control, there also seem to be certain brain sites that contain neurons with specific attentional functions. Two examples are the cells of the frontal eye fields and the inferior parietal lobule. The frontal eye fields influence saccadic movements and the act of looking. The inferior parietal lobules contain cells that seem to enhance response to spatial location prior to an actual stimulus. Enhancement provides a neural explanation for attentional focusing. As we have discussed these systems previously, we will not review them at this point, except to say that they illustrate that the brain undoubtedly contains cells that perform very unique functions that we do not fully understand yet.

NEUROPSYCHOLOGICAL TAXONOMY OF ATTENTION

Earlier, a neuropsychologically based taxonomy of attention was presented. This taxonomy is based on an analysis of the principle factors derived from experimental and clinical assessments of both patients and normal subjects. The taxonomy incorporates four primary attentional factors: (1) sensory selection; (2) response selection and control; (3) attentional capacity; and (4) sustained performance (see Table 22.1). As these factors have been discussed in considerable detail previously, I will now only summarize them by describing the components of each factor.

The term *sensory selection* refers to attentional processes that operate in association with or soon after the initial sensory registration and perception of a stimulus. Attention provides a vehicle by which animals can select certain stimuli over others. It is now clear that such selection occurs early in the information-processing sequence, before a response intention. Three sensory selection components were discussed: (1) sensory filtering; (2) focusing and selection; (3) automatic shifting. Sensory filtering occurs early in information processing and is closely associated with perceptual analysis. In fact, many sensory physiologists would argue that sensory filtering is actually a perceptual event. Yet it appears that attentional factors may influence what information filters through the system. Filtering

TABLE 22.1.   Neuropsychological Taxonomy of Attention

Attentional factors	Components
Sensory selective attention	Filtering
	Selection
	Focusing
	Automatic shifting
Response selection and control	Intention
	Initiation
	Inhibition
	Active switching
	Executive control
Attentional capacity	
Energetic factors	Arousal
	Motivation
	Effort
Structural factors	Memory capacity
	Processing speed
	Temporal dynamics
	Spatial constraints
	Global resources
Sustained performance	Vigilance
	Fatiguability
	Reinforcement contingency

has been confirmed experimentally by studies that demonstrate that primary sensory cortical systems contain neurons tuned to certain stimulus and spatial features. The attentional processes associated with filtering have a high degree of automaticity.

Sensory attentional focusing seems to be less closely associated with primary perception; rather it is influenced by the input of other neural systems. The phenomenon of *sensory enhancement* demonstrated in experimental studies of primates is probably the neurophysiological correlate of focusing, as the response of parietal cortical neurons to upcoming stimuli is either enhanced or attenuated based on prior attentional priming. *Automatic shifts* of attention occur in conjunction with the orienting response (OR). The mechanisms underlying the elicitation, habituation, and sensitization of the OR have been discussed previously.

Response selection and control are a critical factor underlying attentional processing because the direction of attentional response is often governed by the task requirements at hand, the animal's propensity to explore the environment, or its anticipation of a need to act. Response selection is influenced by four related components: (1) response intention; (2) response initiation and inhibition; (3) active switching; and (4) executive regulation. These components determine the ability to become mobilized to attend, to start and stop attentional responses, and to switch between attentional response alternatives. As these components are hierarchically arranged, they are interdependent. Attentional response selection and control may actually precede sensory selection, in cases in which the animal prepares and orients its body to facilitate attention.

Attentional capacity has been divided into two subfactors: *energetic* and *structural* capacity. This dichotomy reflects the fact that attention is influenced by both stable and transient behavioral and neural characteristics. Stable characteristics are relatively invariant in a particular species or in the individual human being, whereas transient energetic characteristics vary with the individual as a function of momentary energetics, or motivational or biological state. An example of a structural capacity is the human digit span of 7 ± 2. Although structural capacity may be influenced by energetic state, a minimal level of performance can be specified below which normal performance will not fall. The components of structural capacity that influence attention are (1) memory capacity; (2) processing speed; (3) temporal-spatial dynamics; and (4) global cognitive resources. The temporal-spatial organization within the animal influences structural capacity by setting, for a particular animal, the coordinates in time and space to which its attention will be responsive. As we discussed previously, the term *global cognitive resources* roughly corresponds to the construct of intelligence and is therefore a very controversial concept. Yet, it is clear that attention varies as a positive function of the overall cognitive capability of the given person. Situations with excessive cognitive complexity are likely to result in inattention.

Energetic capacity is influenced largely by interrelated components: (1) arousal; (2) motivational state; and (3) task-induced effort. Although the constructs of arousal and motivation are admittedly controversial, these broad terms are used in this taxonomy simply to refer to both nonspecific (arousal) and behavior-specific (motivational) physiological activation. Arousal and motivation provide an energetic catalyst that creates an attentional direction. Reticular activation seems to be central to generalized CNS arousal. Motivation is largely a by-product of the interaction of biological state and the reinforcement received from the environment. Arousal and motivation are also governed by the nature of the task at hand. By modifying situational salience, it is possible to influence those motivational factors that determine attentional capacity.

Sustained attention, the fourth attentional factor, is actually a by-product of the other three factors: Sustained attention is influenced by variables that affect sensory selection, response selection and control, and attentional capacity. Sustained attention is included as a separate factor because it reflects an important and unique aspect of attention. One of the primary characteristics of behavior that creates the need for an attentional construct is that performance varies as a function of temporal task dynamics. The other factors that have been mentioned also influence the sequential nature of behavioral performance, but by themselves they do not capture the fundamental nature of sustained attention. Sustained attention is determined by three components: vigilance, fatigue characteristics, and reinforcement contingencies. The characteristics and influences of these components were discussed earlier.

The factors and components described above are the basis for the current neuropsychological framework. They are not new constructs; rather, they originate from the large body of empirical and theoretical literature on attention developed over the past 25 years. The current framework is an attempt to organize and synthesize these constructs in a manner that is consistent with our present knowledge of the neuropsychology of attention. It is my view that these factors and components must be accounted for if one hopes to account for attention. Furthermore, a comprehensive neuropsychological assessment of attention requires a consideration of these attentional components. The degree to which these factors and components are orthogonal to one another and are independently observable still needs to be determined. The difficulty for neuropsychological researchers will undoubtedly be the overlap of these components. Variables that influence one component are likely to have secondary effects on other components. This makes the empirical dissociation of attentional components difficult. As we described earlier, there are a number of different task variables that, when manipulated, yield information about particular attentional components (see Table 14.1).

STRUCTURAL CONSTRAINTS ON ATTENTION

In the preceding chapters of Part III, we discussed factors that place behavioral and neural constraints on attention. To a large extent, these attentional constraints are a function of the principles of attention and the attentional factors and components outlined above. Many of the behavioral principles have neural correlates, and conversely, most of the neural principles have behavioral manifestations. The primary factors that constrain attention in humans are (1) properties of the neural system; (2) memory properties of the system; (3) spatial representations of attention; (4) the temporal distribution and dynamics of attention; (5) the nature of perceptual representations; and (6) processing speed. These factors are important because they influence what attentional parameters are possible and also set limits for attentional capacity. Variations in attention relative to these six factors typically reflect either the structural or the transient energetic capacity of the system.

One might argue that memory encoding and representation, temporal-spatial organization, and processing speed are not true aspects of attention. However, these factors have both direct and indirect influences on attention. Furthermore, it is difficult to define the neuropsychological parameters of attention without using these factors. Although there is some risk of increasing the complexity of attention beyond a manageable level when considering all of these factors, complexity is unavoidable if one hopes to establish neuropsychological parameters for attentional processes. As attention is not a unitary process but a "matrix" of processes, a multifactorial framework is necessary to characterize its interacting parameters. Ultimately, attention is constrained by all factors that influence the interface of incoming signals, existing memories, and responses to those signals. The factors that were outlined earlier in Part III are only the broadest categorization of the constraints that influence attention.

Most of these constraints influence either structural or energetic capacity. For instance, processing speed may set a limit on the number of signals that can be handled in a given period. Memory also influences attentional capacity by influencing the quantity of new information that requires active, effortful processing. The temporal and spatial characteristics of the external environment, the information to be processed, and the attentional processing system also create capacity limitations.

Attentional capacity is also ultimately affected by constraints established by the nature of the neural system. The way in which memory, temporal-spatial organization, and processing speed come under neural control sets the natural boundaries of attention. Furthermore, attention depends on the interaction of multiple brain systems, which must communicate effectively for optimal attentional capacity. Of course, the brain's architecture and physiological response characteristics also influence the other primary attention factors: sensory selection, response control, and sustained performance. Yet, the influence of these constraints is most evident with respect to attentional capacity, perhaps because attentional capacity reflects the interface among incoming signals, cognitive operations, and pressures to respond. Ultimately, an individual's ability to attend to particular tasks is limited by differences in the components of attentional capacity.

INFORMATION FLOW DURING ATTENTION: COGNITIVE AND NEURAL MODELS

The taxonomy that has been described in this chapter specifies the essential components of attention. However, by itself, a taxonomy does not capture the dynamic nature of attention as a fundamental component of information processing. In this section of the chapter, the flow of information through the cognitive and neural systems believed to be responsible for attention is considered. Models are presented based on the attentional principles that have been discussed earlier. These models incorporate the four primary attention factors and their components and are constructed so that they fit reasonably well with known cognitive and neural constraints on attention. A series of flowcharts are presented that illustrate attentional operations from several levels of consideration.

The first flowchart (Figure 22.1) incorporates the four primary attentional factors that are necessary to account for attention in humans. In this highly simplified model, it is assumed that attention is directed by an external stimulus event. After initial sensory registration, early *sensory selection* and *focusing* occur. However, these attentional processes are influenced by ongoing structural and energetic properties of the system. To maintain consistency with earlier cognitive models (e.g., Kahneman, 1973), we refer to this stage as attentional *capacity*. In a broad sense, this capacity reflects the operational demands on the system by particular tasks, as well as the constraints imposed by the characteristics of the neural systems involved in attention. Capacity is directly influenced by momentary response demands, which influence *response selection* and *control*. Once a response is made, feedback is derived from the environment, which is subject to subsequent attentional analysis. This feedback either results in further processing, compensatory responses based on error, or inhibition of the response. This feedback arrangement in conjunction with the other three components is the basis for *sustained attention*. It should be noted that this basic arrangement is similar to that described by Licklider (1960) in his simple model of compensatory tracking.

As the four primary attention factors are composed of a number of components, this simplified model can be expanded to account for a much larger set of determinants. At the very least, attention depends on (1) sensory intake; (2) sensory systems for initial filtering; (3) a system containing sensory comparison processes by which signals are analyzed according to existing neuronal templates; (4) a memory system; (5) an affective weighting system that assigns value or salience to signals and response tendencies; (6) a variable arousal system; (7) a motivational system that creates response pressures based on the drive state; (8) response preparatory and planning systems; (9) feedback arrangements; and (10) a

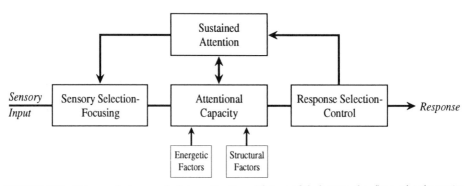

FIGURE 22.1. Primary factors underlying attention. This model depicts the flow of information through the four major components of attention: sensory selection/focusing, response selection/control, capacity, and sustained attention. Attentional capacity is influenced by energetic and structural components. Sustained attention is a product of the information flow through the system and the resulting feedback, which affects each factor.

system for compensatory response adjustments based on errors. As the complexity of the model increases in size very rapidly when these components are inserted, it is easier to consider the sensory selection and response control factors separately.

The models that are described below specify cognitive operations to account for likely processes that underlie the primary attentional factors of sensory selection and focusing and of response selection and control. The models illustrate the sequential flow of information through these cognitive systems, but at certain stages, processing becomes parallel. Attention depends in part on serial operations, which govern the direction and sequence of information flow (represented by arrows in these models). However, with the increasing evidence of parallel attentional processes, it is likely that there is a multitude of reciprocal and transactional relationships across the system's components. Therefore, it is reasonable to assume that, often, the flow of information through the system is not unidirectional. With the exception of several specific pathways, most of the paths within this model are assumed to flow bidirectionally.

Sensory Selection and Focusing

Sensory selection and focusing depend on processes that enable particular features or stimuli to receive more intensive cognitive consideration while other stimuli or processes are ignored. Figure 22.2 presents a more detailed schematic of the processes that may underlie sensory selection and focusing. Again, this model assumes a scenario in which attention is driven by the occurrence of external stimuli. Therefore, response selection and control are minimized, though these components undoubtedly influence sensory selection.

This model has several important features. Attention occurs in a hierarchical and parallel fashion. Such an arrangement enables sensory selection to occur without serial constraints and yet with multiple layers of analysis of each stimulus frame. The model contains several key processes following sensory registration: (1) passive filtering; (2) focusing and enhancement; (3) featural analysis; (4) featural integration; (5) decision bias; and (6) object selection and recognition.

This model accounts for events that occur after perceptual registration. There are, in fact, earlier attentional operations. The orienting response, which has been shown to occur based on changes in stimulus characteristics, may be triggered by preperceptual processes. For instance, early sensory detection based on gross stimulus parameters such as light–dark contrast or movement at the periphery may cause a saccadic eye movements or postural realignment before full sensory registration or perceptual analysis.

Although the attentional shifts associated with the OR are clearly an important aspect of sensory selection, the processes illustrated in Figure 22.2 occur following sensory registration and perceptual analysis. Therefore, this model does not directly address the OR. However, it is easy to envision how the OR could influence sensory focusing, because a sudden automatic shift of attention to a new stimulus (OR) would interfere and compete with ongoing attentional focusing.

Once the stimulus is fully registered in the sensory systems, a number of automatic attentional operations occur. For instance, iconic representations (very-short-term memory), which have been associated with sensory registration, may influence attention. Although the relevance of iconic memory to early attentional processes is not well understood, a number of other automatic processes also occur that are better understood. For instance perceptual analysis involves processes by which stimuli can be discriminated. So that later cognitive operations, such as object recognition and selection, can be performed, the primary featural components of the newly registered stimulus must be differentiated from the background and noise. The differentiation of stimulus features from these extra-

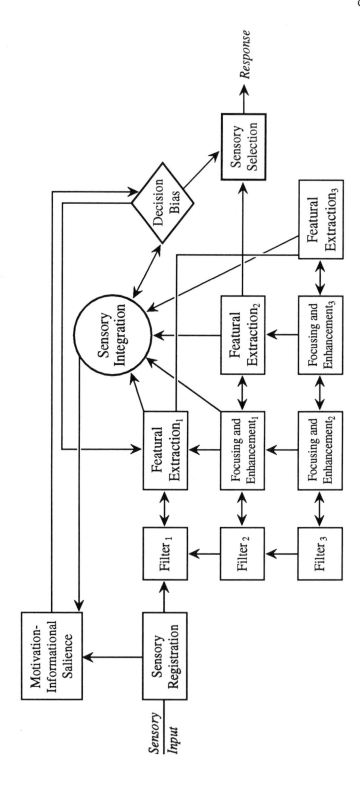

neous variables seems to be highly predetermined based on the tuning of sensory systems. The term *filtering* is used to describe these automatic operations by which stimulus features are sharpened relative to the contrast. This step of stimulus filtering is closely related to visual perception. In fact, some theorists have referred to these operations as preattentional rather than as components of attention. They have been included in the present model, because such processes provide for early featural extraction and selection based on the dominant features of the stimulus. Although while selection of this type is largely automatic and is based on the way the system is tuned to the external environment, it is nonetheless an important initial step in attentional processing.

We propose that, after this early selection stage, information passes through a hierarchically organized processing stage, during which attentional focusing occurs. The stimulus is processed through a multilayer so that it receives different levels of analysis. This processing stage is referred to as *focus enhancement*, as the act of focusing seems to involve selective enhancement of the strength of certain featural components of the stimulus or environment, whereas other components are attenuated. Therefore, the focus enhancement stage probably contains subcomponents that enable excitation to some features and inhibition of other features. How the enhanced and attentuated features compete with each other for ultimate expression is still not clear. It is possible that processes similar to those postulated by neobehavioral theorists (see Chapter 4) result in a *compound stimulus* made up of the interactions of all the inhibitory and excitatory potentials associated with competing stimuli or stimulus features However, it is also possible that an additional mechanism exists to enable the dominant features to be selected once a decision threshold is reached. Such a selection process has been characterized as a winner-take-all mechanism by Feldman and Ballard (1982).

The focus enhancement process results in a parallel set of features that are subject to *feature analysis and then integration*. A set of related features results from this process that are subjected to a final *decision* process, which specifies the focal point of attention by resolving discrepancies arising from the different resolutions of attentional analysis that result from the enhancement processes. The features resulting from this analysis are then subjected to a final operation of object recognition and selection.

Response Selection and Control

A similar model is proposed to account for attentional response selection and control (see Figure 22.3). A parallel multilayered hierarchical system is proposed by which specificity of search is accomplished. This model assumes a scenario in which the direction of attention is driven by internal factors, rather than by the pull of an external stimulus, as

---

FIGURE 22.2. A model of an attentional network that accounts for the primary components of sensory selection and operations before response selection and control. Response selection components are minimized, as the model describes an attentional response driven by visual input. This is a parallel hierarchical network in which stimuli are analyzed by multiple layers of attentional processes, which produce a modulated output. Sensory registration is followed by very early attentional or preattentional operations, including the extraction of figure–ground relations and filtering. The resulting information proceeds through multiple layers of attentional processing, during which operations such as enhancement and focusing occur. The stimulus receives different levels of attentional processing in parallel. Featural extraction and analysis result from this processing. These operations also produce secondary abstracted information that is integrated, which ultimately sets a bias that influences selection decisions. The decision bias, along with the result of actual featural analysis, results in the final operation of sensory attentional selection.

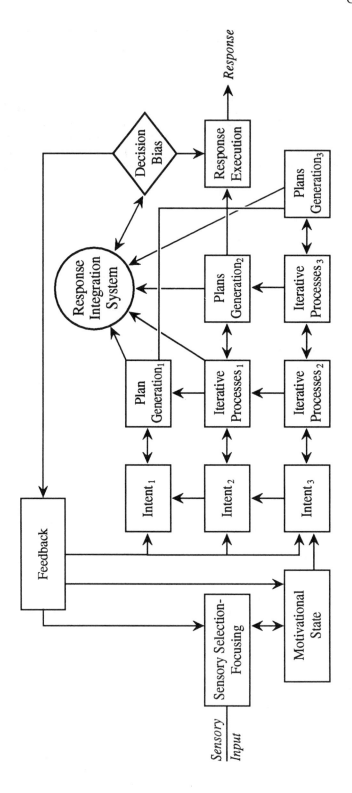

was the case in the previous model. For instance, one might imagine a situation in which a person looks for a lost set of keys in order to operate a car. In such a scenario, attention is a by-product of a motivating pressure to respond.

As the catalyst for the attention search is a motivational state, *motivation* is placed as the catalyst of subsequent selection. The motivational state creates an *intentional* set that establishes a directional character in the motivational state (e.g., "Search the room in order to find the keys"). In response to the intentional set, a set of response *interactions* occur with varying degrees of recursiveness in parallel. These iterations produce likely outcomes based on different levels of analysis of the response alternatives. A set of response *plans* results from this array of iterations, which again are *integrated* and compared. A *decision* process occurs based on system biases created by past experience, level of arousal, motivation, and a number of other factors associated with attentional capacity. The response selection is then processed through an *execution* component, which constructs the actual response.

As responses usually produce outcomes, the system receives *feedback* about the results of the selection. This feedback affects the original motivational state and also modifies the *sensory selection and focusing* system that was discussed previously.

Attentional Capacity

Both the sensory and response selection models described above are subject to influence from the components of attentional capacity. For instance, modifications in the level of arousal or motivational state may affect the decision biases in each model, as well as the intensity or extent of the iterative processes that we have described. Spatial and temporal constraints would also affect both models by limiting the range of the domain subject to attentional search. Of course, memory also has a direct effect on both models by reducing the range of necessary search based on the memory of prior outcomes.

The components of attentional capacity modulate sensory selection and focusing as well as response selection and control. However, complexity becomes excessive if the components of attentional capacity are entered into the models that we have described above. Furthermore, many of the capacity components, particularly energetic factors like arousal and motivation, are organismic by nature and are not easily handled by an information-processing framework. Therefore, these factors are addressed in two subsequent models that consider the neural substrates of attention.

FIGURE 22.3. A model of an attentional network that accounts for the primary components of response selection and control. In contrast to the model in Figure 22.2, this network assumes a case in which attention is being driven by a disposition to respond rather than by an actual stimulus. The result is environmental search. Again, the network contains parallel hierarchical organization, but one driven by a modifiable energetic capacity. As a result of an initial motivational-energetic signal, the system is driven to respond. These impulses are initially analyzed in order to isolate more specific characteristics of the motivational-energetic signal. This process establishes a response intention, as response systems are channeled so as to provide a degree of response specificity. Next, the system engages in series of multilayered intentional operations that generate iterations of possible response outcomes. These iterations are potential response programs or action sequences. Alternative routes of response, or plans, emerge, which are then integrated, and a decision bias is established, which sets the threshold for response selections and execution. The decision bias may result in a tendency toward response initiation, inhibition, shift, or maintenance. Feedback from execution enables the system to redirect responding by influencing future sensory selection and the modulation of motivational state.

NEURAL MECHANISMS OF ATTENTION

Attention is not a unitary process that can be localized to a single neuroanatomical region. This conclusion is confirmed by a vast quantity of clinical and experimental neuropsychological findings, which demonstrate the role of multiple brain systems in the control of attention. Similarly, the term *attention* refers to a class of cognitive and behavioral processes that share one feature; the control and selection of stimuli and responses. As a consequence, the neural mechanisms underlying attention vary as a function of the specific characteristics of the behavioral context and the task demands. Furthermore, attention typically involves sequential operations that control different stages of selection.

In this final section, we consider the flow of information through the neural systems responsible for attentional control. The discussion is limited to visual information, although a similar consideration could be directed at other types of sensory information. Figure 22.4 illustrates the most global level of neural organization necessary to account for the full range of human attentional operations.

Before the cortical registration of sensory information, activation of important subcortical structures occurs. Although this activation may precede cortical registration by only a very short duration, it is nonetheless important as it may cause a shift of attentional bias. For instance, the elicitation of the orienting response seems to be associated with activation along classical sensory pathways that may precede cortical sensory registration. This initial orienting response is often based on gross informational features with very little sensory resolution, that is, the detection of an occurrence of a new stimulus before more detailed processing. The orienting response elicits postural changes and is associated with an automatic shift of attention to some region of space. As discussed elsewhere in this book, there is now abundant evidence that the superior colliculus is involved in the production of saccadic eye movements in response to new stimuli that occur at the periphery. The new incoming stimulus also triggers reticular activation, which is critical in energizing the system for a response and further cognitive operation. The occurrence of these events before cortical registration suggests that the earliest attentional response involves rather automatic activation. The resulting shifts in attentional direction occur as a function of a very gross level of information processing. The resulting shifts in attention are a function of very basic information, such as whether or not a stimulus has occurred.

Once sensory information reaches the sensory cortex, a large number of perceptual processes occur, which provide various levels of perceptual resolution of the critical fea-

---→

FIGURE 22.4. Schematic diagram of the neural systems that enable sensory selective attention to visual information. After retinal registration, visual input flows along the classical visual pathway. (1) The superior colliculus (SC) receives this information, and saccadic movements are facilitated. (2) Projections to the pontine mesencephalic reticular formation and other mesencephalic structures help to produce ascending reticular activation across most cortical systems, either directly or through the nucleus reticularis of the thalamus. (3) The hypothalamus is also activated and directs impulses to other subcortical and cortical systems, where they are modulated. Thalamic systems (THAL) also receive hypothalamic impulses. (4) Visual input from the SC also proceeds to the lateral geniculate nucleus of the THAL, and in interaction with reticular activation, attention is modulated at a second level. (5) Thalamic projections to the primary visual cortex (V1) lead to further visual system evaluation (V2–V4), and (6) eventually to heteromodal areas: the inferior temporal, medial temporal, and inferior parietal areas, where focusing occurs. (7) Motivational and activational signals from the limbic system influences this process through the modulation of the limbic and paralimbic systems. (8) Frontal cortex interaction with these other systems provides for response control over sensory selection. (9) The basal ganglia also seem to facilitate selective attention by coordinating sensorimotor integration.

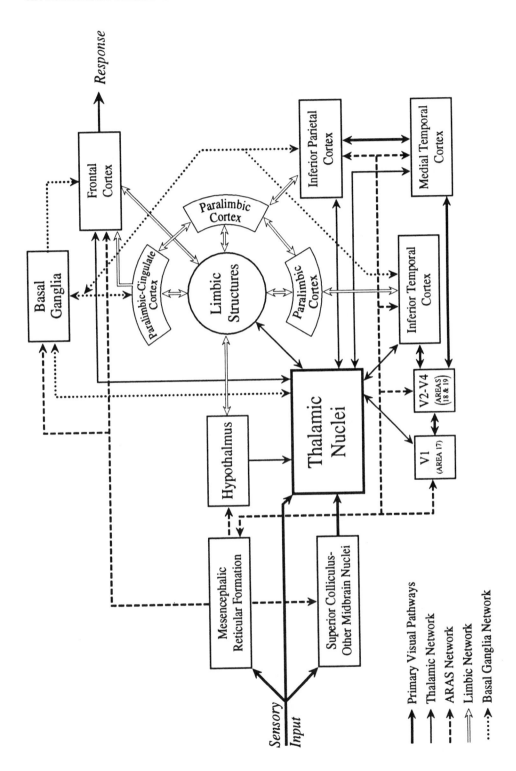

tures of the stimuli. These early perceptual processes probably should not be subsumed under the umbrella of attention, as featural extraction at this point is very automatic, probably not highly modifiable, and somewhat invariant. Sensory systems are "essentially" hardwired at this level. Yet, this stage of perceptual processing is important in subsequent attentional operations, as the fundamental stimulus features are determined.

The extracted stimulus features undergo filtering and analysis during a subsequent stage of processing; the result is a sharpening of important features of the stimulus and the attenuation of other aspects of the information. This processing stage is often considered preattentional, but it actually provides an important attentional operation by which the stimulus develops a strong contrast with its surround (e.g., a figure–ground relationship). At this point, information processing is still relatively automatic and not highly modifiable, though the system has greater degrees of freedom, as this stage depends on the integration of multiple types of featural information. Furthermore, associative information and energetic factors may influence these processes. For visual information, this stage of processing probably occurs in posterior parietal regions consistent with V2, V3, and V4 of primates. It is likely that single neurons and groups of neurons in these areas have filtering capabilities that depend on the complex computations of neural networks (as discussed in Chapter 21). Although some clues to the workings of such systems are beginning to emerge, much more research is necessary before the neurophysiological bases of these computations are understood.

After this preattentional processing, information is integrated within higher cortical (heterotypical) systems. Areas of the inferior parietal and temporal lobes appear to be the location of this level of integration. At this stage, the processing characteristics can be modified, and the biases of the system have a direct impact on attentional selection. As we have discussed previously, the demonstration that the responses of neurons of the inferior parietal lobule vary as a function of the spatial direction of attention suggests that attentional focusing may depend on an enhancement process, which intensifies the response to certain spatial locations, while other locations are minimized.

Thus far, information flow has been traced through sensory analysis to a processing stage that enables the new information to be focused and modified in relation to preexisting biases. Other processes occur concomitantly with this sequence of sensory analysis. As described previously, subcortical activation occurs soon after the initial retinal registration of visual stimuli. Reticular activation elicited at this early stage produces a general energization that affects not only sensory processes, but also the response selection systems of the frontal lobes, as well as limbic and hypothalamic response.

Response selection systems operate somewhat independently of sensory selection. As we live in an environment in which we are constantly bombarded with stimuli, it is often difficult to dissociate these two systems. Yet, in the absence of stimulation, people still experience affective, motivational, and appetitive impulses, which trigger response intention, preparation, planning, initiation, and control. Based on feedback from response selections, new sensory input occurs, which then may affect the bias for sensory selection and may alter the direction of sensory attention.

The frontal lobe has a reciprocal interaction with both the attention systems of the parietal lobe and the limbic system. This interaction is critical in attentional selection, as frontal systems govern the organization of search within the spatial field, as well as the generation of a sequence of attentional responses in complex situations. Although selective attention can be shown to depend largely on the parietal system in certain experimental situations, normally the frontal systems play a critical role. For instance, normal saccadic exploration of space depends on the functioning of the frontal eye fields. The complexity of the frontal systems is minimized in the model shown in Figure 22.4.

The limbic and paralimbic systems also play significant roles in modulating attentional response. As information gains access to the limbic system, it is labeled with affective salience and is integrated according to ongoing pressures from the motivational-drive systems of the hypothalamus. Information also seems to be filtered or gated within the limbic system. The excitatory and inhibitory influences created by the salience of new information in relation to prior patterns of associative connectivity create a bias for certain information. This bias is an important aspect of attention, but an aspect that is frequently overlooked in information-processing models. As a result of limbic processes, information is given different weightings. The salience of information greatly influences the allocation of attention or the intensity of focus. Information weighted as salient receives more elaborated processing and is more likely to gain access to long-term storage (i.e., to be integrated into existing associative networks).

The encoding of new information provides an important rate-limiting factor on attention. Furthermore, the integrity, salience, and representational redundancy of the stimulus item within the associative network influence how that information is handled. Information that is well integrated demands less active (controlled) attentional allocation.

Figure 22.5 details the limbic and subcortical interactions underlying attention control. In this model, the sensory and response selection components are minimized, and the limbic and subcortical interactions are accentuated. The reticular system, which produces ascending activation, catalyzes the overall system and, to a point, increases attentional capacity. However, additional energetic pressures are created by the hypothalamus, which is responsible for many forms of organismic regulation and has often been identified as the site of primitive motivational impulses. Energetic factors from both the reticular system and the hypothalamus create a pressure to act relative to a broad goal (e.g., eating). However, it is only at the level of the limbic system that these pressures are modulated based on interaction with preexisting associative information, and with excitatory or inhibitory signals.

The exact role of the limbic system during attention is undoubtedly very complex, as it depends on the nature of the information being processed. The amygdala and the septal nuclei seem to respond differentially to positive and aversive reinforcement. This differential response probably affects the excitatory and inhibitory valence assigned to input and ultimately affects the direction and intensity of attention. Much still needs to be learned about the exact role of the limbic system relative to different parameters of attention. However, it is safe to say that the limbic system plays a primary role by influencing the weight given to particular information. By assigning different weights or values to information, the limbic system also influences attentional capacity, and attentional bias.

CONCLUSIONS

The neuropsychology of attention is in its infancy. Although attention was a topic of epistemological analysis and introspection among early psychologists, the science of attention has lagged behind many other areas of psychological endeavor. There is a much greater understanding of other neuropsychological functions, such as sensory registration, motor control, and even memory formation. Although the neural representation of language is still a mystery, the basic circuitry for language functions has been known to neuroscientists for many years. Attention has been much more elusive, as it does not have a unitary underlying mechanism. Instead, attention occurs as the by-product of a matrix of interacting processes.

Discomfort is bound to occur in some readers of this book as a result of the extensive array of processes that have been identified as components and/or constraints on attention.

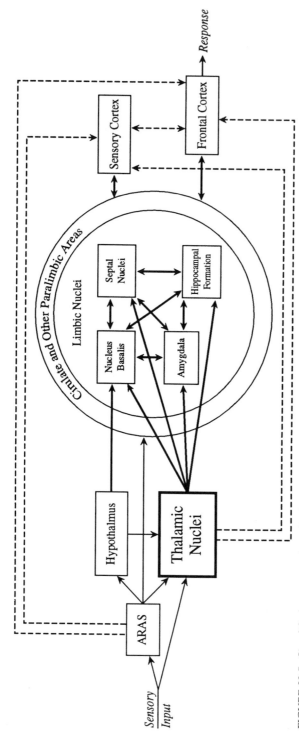

FIGURE 22.5. Simplified representation of subcortical and limbic interactions relative to the sensory and response control systems. (1) The ascending reticular system produces generalized activation, and (2) the hypothalamus generates more specifically directed pressures to respond in accordance with biological state. (3) These impulses create excitation of various structures, including the thalamus and limbic structures such as the hippocampal formation and the septal area. (4) Limbic structures interact with the amygdala, the cingulate cortex, the mammilary bodies, and other limbic nuclei which form a functional circuit with multiple roles for attention. (5) Mesocortical paralimbic areas such as the entorhinal area, the parahippocampal area, and cingulate cortex further modulate salience and integrate motivational signals from the limbic system and (6) interface with the cortical systems, such as the sensory activation cortex and the frontal cortex, that are responsible for sensory selection and response control.

Is attention dependent on so many different component processes that it loses its meaning as a construct? In this book, I have argued that this is not the case. By its nature, attention reflects the interface of stimulus intake, mental experience, and response production. In this capacity, attention is a function of all of its components.

Some theorists may argue that what is being described is a process of sensorimotor integration. Others, stressing a "bottom-up" philosophy, may insist that it is not necessary to maintain a construct that is a composite of smaller component operations. Why not directly address the individual components and avoid the operational complexities of an attentional construct? In the simplest terms, the response is that the construct of attention captures an important aspect of human experience. *Attention* is a label that identifies a complex set of cognitive operations. Just as the term *memory* simplifies the multitude of processes underlying the formation of permanent informational storage, so does the term attention simply refer to the complex array of processes that comprise sensory and response selection. It is a construct that serves as a heuristic to characterize the important interface between the internal and the external.

We can rule out many processes as not being the essence of attention: Attention is not the process of sensory registration, memory formation, symbolic language, emotion, drive state, or motor production. Although all of these processes influence attention, they do not account for the entire process.

Attention is an emergent property of the brain in relationship to the surrounding environment. The actions of individual neurons undoubtedly provide the basic mechanism that makes attention possible. Yet, it seems likely that attention is best seen as a systemic process, one that will eventually be understood as a by-product of the interactions of networks of neurons. Future efforts to understand attention will profit by the integration of the fields of neuropsychology, cognitive and behavioral psychology, and the neurosciences.

References

Adams, J. A. (1956). Vigilance in the detection of low-intensity visual stimuli. *Journal of Experimental Psychology, 52*, 204–208.

Adams, R. D., & Victor, M. (1981). *Principles of neurology* (2nd ed.). New York: McGraw-Hill.

Aggleton, J. P., & Mishkin, M. (1983a). Memory impairments following restricted medial thalamic lesions in monkeys. *Experimental Brain Research, 52*, 199–209.

Aggleton, J. P., & Mishkin, M. (1983b). Visual recognition impairment following medial thalamic lesions in monkeys. *Neuropsychologia, 21*, 189–197.

Aggleton, J. P., & Mishkin, M. (1985). Mammillary-body lesions and visual recognition in the monkey. *Experimental Brain Research, 58*, 190–197.

Aita, J. A., Armitage, S. G., Reitan, R. M., & Rabinovitz, A. (1947). The use of certain psychological tests in the evaluation of brain injury. *Journal of General Psychology, 37*, 25–44.

Albers, H. E., Lydic, R., Gander, P. H., & Moore-Ede, M. C. (1984). Role of the suprachiasmatic nuclei in the circadian timing system of the squirrel monkey: 1. The generation of rhythmicity. *Brain Research, 300*, 275–284.

Albers, H. E., Liou, S. Y., Ferris, C. F., Stopa, E. G., & Zoeller, R. T. (1991). Neurochemistry of circadian timing. In D. C. Klein, R. Y. Moore, & S. M. Reppert (Eds.), *The suprachiasmatic nucleus: The mind's clock.* Oxford: Oxford University Press.

Alkon, D. L. (1982). A biophysical basis for molluscan associative learning. In C. D. Woody (Ed.), *Conditioning: Representation of involved neural function.* New York: Plenum Press.

Allan, L. G. (1977). The time-order error in judgments of duration. *Canadian Journal of Psychology, 31*, 24–31.

Allan, L. G. (1984). Contingent aftereffects in duration judgments. In J. Gibbon & L. Allan (Eds.), *Timing and time perception, Annals of the New York Academy of Sciences* (Vol. 423) (pp. 116–130). New York: New York Academy of Sciences.

Allport, A. (1987). Selection-for-action: Some behavioral and neurophysiological considerations of attention and action. In H. Heuer and A. F. Sanders (Eds.), *Perspectives on perception and acton.* Hillsdale, NJ: Erlbaum.

Alpern, M. (1971). Effector mechanisms in vision. In J. W. Kling & L. A. Riggs (Eds.), *Experimental psychology.* New York: Holt, Rinehart & Winston.

American Psychiatric Association. (1980). *Diagnostic and statistical manual of mental disorders* (3rd ed; DSM-III). Washington, DC: Author.

American Psychiatric Association (1987). *Diagnostic and statistical manual of mental disorders* (3rd ed., rev., DSM-III-R). Washington, DC: Author.

Amsel, A. (1967). Partial reinforcement effects on vigor and persistence: Advances in frustration theory derived from a variety of within-subjects experiments. In K. W. Spence & Janet T. Spence (Eds.), *The psychology of learning and motivation,* Vol. I (pp. 1–65). New York: Academic Press.

Anand, B. K., & Dua, S. (1956). Effect of electrical stimulation of the limbic system ("visceral brain") on gastric secretion and motility. *Indian Journal of Medical Research, 44*, 125–130.

Andersen, P., Sundberg, S. H., Sveen, O., & Wigstrom, H. (1977). Specific long-lasting potentiation of synaptic transmission in hippocampal slices. *Nature, 266*, 736–737.

Anderson, J. A. (1977). Neural models with cognitive implications. In D. LaBerge & S. J. Samuels (Eds.), *Basic processes in reading perception and comprehension* (pp. 27–90). Hillsdale, N.J.: Erlbaum.

Anderson, J. R. (1983). *The architecture of cognition.* Cambridge, MA: Harvard University Press.

Anderson, R. A., & Mountcastle, V. B. (1980). The direction of gaze influences the response of many light sensitive neurons of the inferior parietal lobule (area 7) in waking monkeys. *Neuroscience Abstracts, 6*, 673.

Angell, J. R., & Thompson, H. B. (1899). A study of the relations between certain organic processes and consciousness. *Psychological Review, 6*, 32–53.

Arena, R., Menchetti, G., Tassinari, G., & Tognetti, M. (1979). *Simple and complex reaction time to lateralised visual stimuli in groups of epileptic patients.* 11th Epilepsy International Symposium, Florence, Italy.

Arthur, G. (1947). *A point scale of performance tests* (revised form 2). New York: Psychological Corporation.

Aschoff, J. (Ed.). (1981). *Handbook of behavioral neurobiology: Vol. 4. Biological rhythms.* New York: Plenum Press.

Aschoff, J. (1984). Circadian timing. In J. Gibbon & L. Allan (Eds.), *Timing and time perception, Annals of the New York Academy of Sciences* (Vol. 423, pp. 442–468). New York: New York Academy of Sciences.

Aschoff, J., & Wever, R. (1981). The circadian system of man. In J. Aschoff (Ed.), *Handbook of behavioral neurobiology* (Vol. 4, pp. 311–331). New York: Plenum Press.

Ashcroft, G. W., & Sharman, D. F. (1960). 5-Hydroxyindoles in human cerebral fluid. *Nature, 186*, 1050.

Ashe, J. H., & Libet, B. (1981). Orthodromic production of noncholinergic slow depolarizing response in the superior cervical ganglion of the rabbit. *Journal of Physiology, 320*, 333–346.

Atkinson, R. C., & Estes, W. K. (1963). Stimulus sampling theory. In R. D. Luce, R. R. Bush, & E. Galanter (Eds.), *Handbook of mathematical psychology* (pp. 121–268). New York: Wiley.

Atkinson, R. C., & Shiffrin, R. M. (1967). *Human memory: A proposed system and its control processes.* Technical Report No. 110, Institute for Mathematical Studies in the Social Sciences, Stanford University.

Atkinson, R. C., & Shiffrin, R. M. (1968). Human memory: A proposed system and its control processes. In K. W. Spence & J. T. Spence (Eds.), *The psychology of learning and motivation: Advances in research and theory* (Vol. 2, pp. 89–195). New York: Academic Press.

Atkinson, R. C., & Shiffrin, R. M. (1971). The control of short-term memory. *Scientific American, 224*, 82–90.

Ax, A. F. (1953). The physiological differentiation between fear and anger in humans. *Psychosomatic Medicine, 15*, 433–442.

Bachevalier, J., & Mishkin, M. (1989). Mnemonic and neuropathological effects of occluding the posterior cerebral artery in *macaca mulatta. Neuropsychologia, 27*, 83–105.

Baddeley, A. D. (1966a). The influence of acoustic and semantic similarity on long-term memory for word sequences. *Quarterly Journal of Experimental Psychology, 18*, 302–309.

Baddeley, A. D. (1966b). Short-term memory for word sequences as a function of acoustic, semantic and formal similarity. *Quarterly Journal of Experimental Psychology, 18*, 362–365.

Baddeley, A. D., & Colquhoun, W. P. (1969). Signal probability and vigilance: A reappraisal of the "signal rate" effect. *British Journal of Psychology, 60*, 169–178.

Bagshaw, M. H., & Pribram, J. D. (1968). Effect of amygdalectomy on stimulus threshold of the monkey. *Experimental Neurology, 20*, 197–202.

Bagshaw, M. H., Kimble, D. P., & Pribram, K. H. (1965). The GSR of monkeys during orienting and habituation and after ablation of the amygdala, hippocampus, and inferotemporal cortex. *Neuropsychologia, 3*, 111–119.

Bagshaw, M. H., Mackworth, N. H., & Pribram, K. H. (1970). The effect of inferotemporal cortex ablation on eye movements of monkeys during discrimination training. *International Journal of Neuroscience, 1*, 153–158.

Bagshaw, M. H., Mackworth, N. H., & Pribram, K. H. (1972). The effect of resections of the inferotemporal cortex or the amygdala on visual orienting and habituation. *Neuropsychologia, 10*, 153–162.

Baleydier, C., & Mauguiere, F. (1980). The duality of the cingulate gyrus in monkeys. *Brain, 103*, 525–554.

Ballard, D. H., Hinton, G. E., & Sejnowski, T. J. (1983). Parallel visual computation. *Nature, 306*, 21–26.

Ballenger, J. C., Post, R. M., Gold, P. W., Robertson, G. O., Bunney, W. E., & Goodwin, F. K. (1980). Endocrine correlates of personality and cognition (abstr. 81). Presented at the 133rd Annual

Meeting of the American Psychiatric Association, San Francisco, May. *Scientific Proceedings of the American Psychiatric Association*, *133*, 144.

Ballentine, H. T., Jr., Levey, B. A., Dagi, T. F., & Diriunas, I. B. (1977). Cingulotomy for psychiatric illness: Report of 13 years experience. In W. H. Sweet, S. Obrador, & J. G. Martin-Rodrigues (Eds.), *Neurosurgical treatment in psychiatry, pain and epilepsy* (pp. 333–353). Baltimore: University Park Press.

Baribeau-Braun, J., Picton, T. W., & Gosselin, J. V. (1983). Schizophrenia: A neurophysiological evaluation of abnormal information processing. *Science*, *219*, 874–876.

Barkley, R. A. (1977). The effect of methylphenidate on various measures of activity level and attention in hyperkinetic children. *Journal of Abnormal Child Psychology*, *5*, 351–369.

Barkley, R. A. (1988a). Attention. In M. Tramonthana & S. Hooper (Eds.). *Assessment issues in child neuropsychology* (pp. 115–154). New York: Plenum Press.

Barkley, R. A. (1988b). Attention deficit disorder with hyperactivity. In R. A. Barkley, E. J. Mash, & L. G. Terdal (Eds.), *Behavioral assessment of childhood disorders* (pp. 69–104). New York: Guilford.

Barkley, R. A., DuPaul, G. J., & McMurray, M. B. (1991) Comprehensive evaluation of attention deficit disorder with and without hyperactivity as defined by research criteria. *Journal of Consulting and Clinical Psychology*, *58*, 775–789.

Barkley, R. A., Grodzinsky, G., & DuPaul, G. J. (1992). Frontal lobe funtions in attention deficit disorder with and without hyperactivity: A review and research report. *Journal of Abnormal Child Psychology*, *20*, 163–188.

Barris, R. W., & Schuman, H. R. (1953). Bilateral anterior cingulate gyrus: Syndrome of the anterior cingulate gyri. *Neurology*, *3*, 44–52.

Barry, R. J. (1977). Failure to find evidence of the unitary OR concept with indifferent low-intensity auditory stimuli. *Psychological Psychology*, *5*, 89–96.

Bartlett, F. C. (1932). *Remembering*. Cambridge: Cambridge University Press.

Bartley, S. H. (1981). Fatigue. *Perceptual and Motor Skills*, *53*, 958.

Bartus, R. T., & LeVere, T. E. (1977). Frontal decortication in rhesus monkeys: A test of the interference hypothesis. *Brain Research*, *119*, 233–248.

Basden, B. H. (1969). *A nonselective model of differential cue effectiveness in discrimination learning by rats*. Unpublished doctoral dissertation, University of California, Santa Barbara.

Bashinski, H. S., & Backrach, V. R. (1980). Enhancement of perceptual sensitivity as the result of selectively attending spatial locations. *Perception and Psychophysics*, *28*, 241–248.

Battersby, W. S., Bender, M. B., & Pollack, M. (1956). Unilateral spatial agnosia (inattention) in patients with cerebral lesions. *Brain*, *79*, 68–93.

Baudry, M., & Lynch, G. (1979). Regulation of glutamate receptors by cations. *Nature*, *282*, 748–750.

Baudry, M., & Lynch, G. (1984). Glutamate receptor regulation and the substrates of memory. In G. Lynch, J. L. McGaugh, & N. M. Weinberger (Eds.), *Neurobiology of learning and memory* (pp. 431–450). New York: Guilford Press.

Bauer, R. H. (1974). Brightness discrimination of pretrained and nonpretrained hippocampal rats reinforced for choosing brighter or dimmer alternatives. *Journal of Comparative and Physiological Psychology*, *87*, 987–996.

Bear, D. M., & Fedio, F. (1977). Quantitative analysis of interictal behavior in temporal lobe epilepsy. *Archives of Neurology*, *34*, 454–467.

Beatty, J. (1979). Pupillometric methods of workload evaluation: Present status and future possibilities. In B. O. Harman & R. E. McKenzie (Eds.), *Survey of methods to assess workload*. Neuilly Sur Seine, France: Advisory Group for Aerospace Research and Development, North Atlantic Treaty Organization.

Beatty, T. (1982). Task-evoked pupillary responses, processing load, and the structure of processing resources. *Psychological Bulletin*, *1*(2), 276–292.

Bellack, A. S., & Hersen, M. (1988). *Behavioral assessment* (3rd ed.). New York: Pergamon Press.

Benowitz, L. I., Bear, D. M., Rosenthal, R., Mesulam, M. M., Zaidel, E., & Sperry, R. W. (1983). Hemispheric specialization in nonverbal communication. *Cortex*, *19*, 5–11.

Benson, D. A., Hienz, R. D., & Goldstein, M. H. (1981). Single-unit activity in the auditory cortex of monkeys actively localizing sound sources: Spatial tuning and behavioral dependency. *Brain Research*, *219*, 249–267.

Benson, D. F. (1975). The hydrocephalic dementias. In D. F. Benson & D. Blumer (Eds.), *Psychiatric aspects of neurologic disease*. New York: Grune & Stratton.

Benson, D. F. (1991). The role of frontal dysfunction in attention deficit hyperactivity disorder. *Journal of Child Neurology, 6*, 9–12.

Benton, A. L. (1967). Constructional apraxia and the minor hemisphere. *Confina Neurologica, 29*, 1–16.

Benton, A. L. (1968). Differential behavioral effects in frontal lobe disease. *Neuropsychologia, 6*, 53–60.

Benton, A. L. (1973). Visuoconstructive disability in patients with cerebral disease: Its relationship to side of lesion and aphasic disorder. *Documenta Opthalmologia, 34*, 67–76.

Benton, A. L., & Fogel, M. L. (1962). Three-dimensional constructional praxis. *Archives of Neurology, 7*, 347–354.

Berg, E. A. (1948). A simple objective test for measuring flexibility in thinking. *Journal of General Psychology, 39*, 15–22.

Berlin, C. I., & McNeil, M. R. (1976). Dichotic listening. In N. J. Lass (Ed.), *Contemporary issues in experimental phonetics*. New York: Academic Press.

Berlucchi, G., & Rizzolatti, G. (1987). Selective visual attention. *Neuropsychologia, 25*(1A), 1–3.

Berlyne, D. E. (1960). *Conflict, arousal, and curiosity*. New York: McGraw-Hill.

Berlyne, D. E., & McDonnell, P. (1965). Effects of stimulus complexity and incongruity on duration of EEG desynchronization. *Electroencephalography and Clinical Neurophysiology, 18*, 156–161.

Bernheim, J. W., & Williams, D. R. (1967). Time-dependent contrast effects in a multiple schedule of food reinforcement. *Journal of the Experimental Analysis of Behavior, 10*, 243–249.

Bianchi, L. (1895). The functions of the frontal lobes. *Brain, 18*, 497–522.

Birch, H. G., Belmont, I., & Karp, E. (1967). Delayed information processing and extinction following cerebral damage. *Brain, 90*, 113–130.

Birren, J. E., Woods, A. M., & Williams, M. V. (1980). Behavioral slowing with age: Causes, organization and consequences. In L. W. Poon (Ed.), *Aging in the 1980's*. Washington, DC: American Psychological Association.

Birt, D., & Olds, M. (1981). Associative response changes in lateral midbrain tegmentum and medial geniculate during differential appetitive conditioning. *Journal of Neurophysiology, 46*, 1039–1055.

Bisiach, E., & Luzzatti, C. (1978). Unilateral neglect of representational space. *Cortex, 14*, 29–133.

Bisiach, E., Luzzatti, C., & Perani, D. (1979). Unilateral neglect, representational schema and consciousness. *Brain, 102*, 609–618.

Blakeslee, P. (1979). Attention and vigilance: Performance and skin conductance response changes. *Psychophysiology, 16*, 413–419.

Bleuler, E. (1950). Dementia praecox, or the group of schizophrenias. New York: International University Press.

Block, R. A. (1978). Processing temporal information in single stories: Effects of input sequence. *Journal of Verbal Learning and Verbal Behavior, 17*, 559–572.

Bobrow, D. G., & Norman, D. A. (1975). Some principles of memory schemata. In D. G. Bobrow & A. Collins (Eds.), *Representation and understanding: Studies in cognitive science* (pp. 131–149). New York: Academic Press.

Bonvallet, M., & Bobo, E. G. (1972). Changes in phrenic activity and heart rate elicited by localized stimulation of amygdala and adjacent structures. *Electroencephalography and Clinical Neurophysiology, 32*, 1–16.

Bower, G. H., & Hilgard, E. R. (1981). *Theories of learning* (5th ed.). Englewood Cliffs, NJ: Prentice-Hall.

Bowes, W. A., Brackbill, Y., Conway, E., & Steinschneider, A. (1970). The effects of obstetrical medication on fetus and infant. *Monographs of the Society for Research in Child Development, 35*(4), 3–23.

Bowers, D., & Heilman, K. (1976). Material specific hemispheric arousal. *Neuropsychologia, 14*, 123–127.

Bowers, D., Heilman, K. M., & Van Den Abell, T. (1976). Hemispace-visual half field compatibility. *Neuropsychologia, 19*, 757–765.

Bradshaw, J. L. (1968). Pupil size and problem solving. *Quarterly Journal of Experimental Psychology, 20*, 116–122.

Bradshaw, J. L., Nettleton, N. C., & Geffen, G. (1971). Ear differences and delayed auditory feedback: Effects on a speech and music task. *Journal of Experimental Psychology, 91*, 85–92.

Bradshaw, J. L., Nettleton, N. C., & Geffen, G. (1972). Ear asymmetry and delayed auditory feedback: Effect of task requirements and competitive stimulation. *Journal of Experimental Psychology, 94*, 269–275.

Brand, C. (1981). General intelligence and mental speed: Their relationship and development. In M. P. Friedman, J. P. Das, & N. O'Connor (Eds.), *Intelligence and learning* (pp. 589–593). New York: Plenum Press.

Brecher, M., Porjesz, B., & Begleiter, H. (1987). The N2 component of the event-related potential in schizophrenic patients. *Electroencephalography and Clinical Neurophysiology, 66*, 369–375.

Breitmeyer, B. G. (1975). Simple reaction time as a measure of the temporal response properties of sustained and transient channels. *Vision Research, 15*, 1411–1412.

Breslow, R., Kocsis, J., & Belkin, B. (1980). Memory deficits in depression: Evidence utilizing the Wechsler Memory Scale. *Perceptual and Motor Skills, 51*, 541–542.

Brickner, R. (1934). An interpretation of frontal lobe function based upon the study of a case of partial bilateral frontal lobectomy. *Research Publication of the Association of Research on Nervous and Mental Disorders, 13*, 259–351.

Broadbent, D. E. (1950). *The twenty dials test under quiet conditions.* A. P. Report No. 130.

Broadbent, D. E. (1952). Listening to one of two synchronous messages. *Journal of Experimental Psychology, 44*, 51–55.

Broadbent, D. E. (1957). Effects of noise of high and low frequency on behavior. *Ergonomics, 1*, 21–29.

Broadbent, D. E. (1958). *Perception and communication.* London: Pergamon Press.

Broadbent, D. E. (1963). Some recent research from the Applied Psychological Research Unit, Cambridge. In D. N. Buckner & J. J. McGrath (Eds.), *Vigilance: A symposium.* New York: McGraw-Hill.

Broadbent, D. E. (1970). Stimulus set and response set: Two kinds of selective attention. In D. I. Mostofsky (Ed.), *Attention: Contemporary theory and analysis* (pp. 51–60). New York: Appleton-Century-Crofts.

Broadbent, D. E. (1971). *Decision and stress.* London: Academic Press.

Broadbent, D. E. (1977). The hidden preattentive process. *American Psychologist, 32*(2), 109–118.

Broadbent, D. E. (1979). Is a fatigue test now possible? *Ergonomics, 22*, 1277–1290.

Broadbent, D. E., & Gregory, M. (1963). Vigilance considered as a statistical decision. *British Journal of Psychology, 54*, 309–323.

Broadbent, D. E., & Gregory, M. (1965). Effects of noise and of signal rate upon vigilance analysed by means of decision theory. *Human Factors, 7*, 155–162.

Brodal, A. (1973). Self-observations and neuroanatomical considerations after a stroke. *Brain, 96*, 694.

Brooks, N. (1984). Cognitive deficits after head injury. In N. Brooks (Ed.), *Closed head injury: Psychological, social and family consequences* (pp. 44–73). New York: Oxford University Press.

Bruce, C., Desimone, R., & Gross, C. G. (1981). Visual properties of neurons in a polysensory area in superior temporal sulcus of the macaque. *Journal of Neurophysiology, 46*, 369–384.

Bruhn, P., & Parsons, O. A. (1977). Reaction time variability in epileptic and brain-damaged patients. *Cortex, 13*, 373–384.

Brunton, T. L. (1883). On the nature of inhibition, and the action of drugs upon it. *Nature, 27*, 419–422.

Buchsbaum, M. S., & Sostek, A. J. (1980). An adaptive rate continuous performance test: Vigilance characteristics and reliability for 400 male students. *Perceptual and Motor Skills, 51*, 707–713.

Bullinger, A. (1983). Space, the organism, and objects: Their relationship and development. In A. Hein & M. Jeannerad (Eds.), *Spatially oriented behavior* (pp. 215–222). New York: Springer-Verlag.

Bunney, W. E., Jr., & Davis, J. M. (1965). Norepinephrine in depressive reactions. *Archives of General Psychiatry, 13*, 483–494.

Bush, R. R., & Mosteller, F. (1951). A mathematical model for simple learning. *Psychological Review, 58*, 313–323.

Bushnell, M. C., Goldberg, M. E., & Robinson, D. L. (1981). Behavioral enhancement of visual responses in monkey cerebral cortex: 1. Modulation in posterior parietal cortex related to selective visual attention. *Journal of Neurophysiology, 46*, 755–772.

Butter, C. M. (1964). Habitation of responses to novel stimuli in monkeys with selective frontal lesions. *Science, 144*, 313–315.

Butter, C. M. (1969): Perseveration in extinction and in discrimination reversal tasks following selective frontal ablations in *macaca mulatta. Physiology and Behavior, 4*, 163–171.

Butter, C. M., Mishkin, M., & Rosvold, H. E. (1963). Conditioning and extinction of a food-rewarded response after selective ablations of frontal cortex in rhesus monkeys. *Experimental Neurology, 7*, 65–75.

Butter, C. M., Mishkin, M., & Mirsky, A. F. (1968). Emotional responses toward humans in monkeys with selective frontal lesions. *Physiology and Behavior, 3,* 213–215.

Butter, C. M., Rapcsak, S., Watson, R. T., & Heilman, K. M. (1988). Changes in sensory inattention, directional motor neglect and "release" of the fixation reflex following a unilateral frontal lesion: A case report. *Neuropsychologia, 26,* 533–545.

Butters, N., & Pandya, D. (1969). Retention of delayed-alternation: Effect of selective lesions of sulcus principalis. *Science, 165,* 1271–1273.

Butters, N., Butter, C., Rosen, J., & Stein, D. (1973). Behavioral effects of sequential and one-stage ablations of orbital prefrontal cortex in the monkey. *Experimental Neurology, 39,* 204–214.

Byrne, D. C. (1977). Affect and vigilance performance in depressive illness. *Journal of Psychiatric Research, 13,* 185–191.

Cacioppo, J. T., & Petty, R. E. (1979). Effects of exogenous changes in heart rate on the facilitation of thought and resistance to persuasion. *Journal of Personality and Social Psychology, 378,* 2181–2199.

Cacioppo, J. T., & Petty, R. E. (1981a). Electromyograms as measures of extent and affectivity of information processing. *American Psychologist, 36,* 441–456.

Cacioppo, J. T., & Petty, R. E. (1981b). Electromyographic specificity during covert information processing. *Psychophysiology, 18,* 518–523.

Caine, E. D. (1981). Pseudodementia: Current concepts and future directions. *Archives of General Psychiatry, 38,* 1359–1364.

Caine, E. D. (1986). *The neuropsychology of depression: The pseudodementia syndrome.* In I. Grant & K. M. Adams (Eds.), *Neuropsychological assessment of neuropsychiatric disorders* (pp. 221–243). New York and Oxford: Oxford University Press.

Callaway, E., & Naghdi, S. (1982). An information processing model for schizophrenia. *Archives of General Psychiatry, 39,* 339–347.

Campbell, K. B., Courchesne, E., Picton, T. W., & Squires, K. C. (1979). Evoked potential correlates of human information processing. *Biological Psychology, 8,* 45–68.

Cannon, W. B. (1929). *Bodily changes in pain, horror, fear and rage* (2nd ed.). New York: Appleton.

Cantwell, D., & Carlson, G. (1978). Stimulants. In J. Werry (Ed.), *Pediatric psychopharmacology* (pp. 171–207). New York: Brunner/Mazel.

Carlson, C. L., Lahey, B. B., & Neeper, R. (1986). Direct assessment of the cognitive correlates of attention deficit disorder with and without hyperactivity. *Journal of Psychopathology and Behavioral Assessment, 8,* 69–86.

Carlson, N. R., & Cole, J. R. (1970). Enhanced alternation performance following septal lesions in mice. *Journal of Comparative and Physiological Psychology, 73,* 157–161.

Carlson, N. R., & Norman, R. J. (1971). Enhanced go, no-go single-lever alternation of mice with septal lesions. *Journal of Comparative and Physiological Psychology, 75,* 508–512.

Carlson, N. R., & Vallante, M. A. (1974). Enhanced cue function of olfactory stimulation in mice with septal lesions. *Journal of Comparative and Physiological Psychology, 87,* 237–248.

Carroll, B. J. (1978). Neuroendocrine function in psychiatric disorders. In M. A. Lipton, A. D. Mascio, & K. F. Killan (Eds.), *Psychopharmacology: A generation of progress* (pp. 487–497). New York: Raven Press.

Carroll, B. J., & Davies, B. (1970). Clinical associations of 11-hydroxycorticosteroid suppression and non-suppression in severe depressive illness. *British Medical Journal, 1,* 789–791.

Carroll, B. J., Curtis, G. C., & Mendels, J. (1976). Neuroendocrine regulation in depression. *Archives of General Psychiatry, 33,* 1039–1058.

Castellucci, V., Pinsker, H., Kupfermann, I., & Kandel, E. R. (1970). Neuronal mechanisms of habituation and dishabituation of the gill-withdrawal reflex in *Aplysia. Science, 167,* 1745–1748.

Castellucci, V. F., Carew, T. J., & Kandel, E. R. (1978). Cellular analysis of long-term habituation of the gill-withdrawal reflex in *Aplysia. Science, 202,* 1306–1308.

Cattell, R. B. (1963). Theory of fluid and crystallized intelligence: A critical experiment. *Journal of Educational Psychology, 54,* 1–22.

Cermak, L. S. (1984). The episodic-semantic distinction in amnesia. In L. R. Squire & N. Butters (Eds.), *Neuropsychology of memory* (pp. 55–62) New York: Guilford Press.

Chapman, C. J., & Chapman, J. P. (1973). *Disordered thought in schizophrenia.* New York: Appleton-Century-Crofts.

Chapman, F., & McGhie, A. (1962). A comparative study of disordered attention in schizophrenia. *Journal of Mental Science, 108,* 487–500.

Chapman, L. J., & Chapman, J. P. (1978). The measurement of differential deficit. *Journal of Psychiatric Research, 14,* 303–311.

Chelyne, G. J., Ferguson, W., Koon, R., et al. (1986). Frontal lobe disinhibition in attention deficit disorder. *Child Psychiatry and Human Development, 16,* 221–234.

Cherry, C. T. (1975). Variability and discrimination reversal learning in the open field following septal lesions in rats. *Physiology and Behavior, 15,* 641–646.

Cherry, E. C. (1953). Some experiments on the recognition of speech, with one and with two ears. *Journal of the Acoustical Society of America, 26* 975–979.

Church, R. M. (1984). Properties of the internal clock. In J. Gibbon & L. Allan (Eds.), *Timing and time perception, Annals of the New York Academy of Sciences* (Vol. 423) (pp. 566–582). New York: New York Academy of Sciences.

Churchland, P. M., & Churchland, P. S. (1990). Could a machine think? Classical AI is unlikely to yield conscious machines; Systems that mimic the brain might. *Scientific American, 262,* 32–37.

Clark, C. V. H., & Isaacson, R. L. (1965). Effect of bilateral hippocampal ablation on DRL performance. *Journal of Comparative and Physiological Psychology, 59,* 137–140.

Cohen, R. A. (1991). Autonomic and evoked potential responses associated with intentional dysfunction secondary to bilateral medial cingulotomy. *Journal of Clinical and Experimental Neuropsychology, 13.*

Cohen, R. A., & Albers, H. E. (1991). Disruption of human circadian and cognitive regulation following a discrete hypothalamic lesion: A case study. *Neurology, 41,* 726–729.

Cohen, R. A., & O'Donnell, B. F. (1988). Attention, effort, and fatigue: Neuropsychological perspectives. In R. L. Harris, A. T. Pope, & J. R. Comstock (Eds.), *Proceedings from the First NASA Mental State Estimation Workshop, NASA Publication 2504* (pp. 237–268). Langley, VA: NASA.

Cohen, R. A., & Fisher, M. (1988). Neuropsychological correlates of fatigue associated with multiple sclerosis. *Journal of Clinical and Experimental Neuropsychology, 10*(1), 48.

Cohen, R. A., & Fisher, M. (1989). Amantadine treatment of fatigue associated with multiple sclerosis. *Archives of Neurology, 46,* 676–680.

Cohen, R. A., & Waters, W. (1985). Psychophysiological correlates of levels and states of cognitive processing. *Neuropsychologia, 23*(2), 243–256.

Cohen, R. A., Fennell, E., Bauer, R., & Moscovitch, R. (1983). Neuropsychological concomitants of unipolar and bipolar affective disorders. *International Neuropsychological Society Bulletin,* October, 21.

Cohen, R. A., McCrae, V., Phillips, K., & Wilkinson, H. (1990). Neurobehavioral consequences of bilateral medial cingulotomy, *Neurology, 40*(1), 198.

Cohen, R. A., Smith, T. W., & Fisher, M. (1991). Neglect associated with damage to the anterior basal ganglia: A clinicopathologic study. *Journal of Clinical and Experimental Neuropsychology, 13,* 96.

Cohen, R. M., Weingartner, H., Smallberg, S. A., & Murphy, D. L. (1982). Effort and cognition in depression. *Archives of General Psychiatry, 39,* 593–597.

Coles, M. G. H., & Duncan-Johnson, C. C. (1975). Cardiac activity and information processing: The effects of stimulus significance, and detection and response requirement. *Journal of Experimental Psychology: Human Perception and Performance, 1,* 418–428.

Collard, R. F. A., & Leewenberg, E. L. J. (1981). Temporal order and spatial context. *Canadian Journal of Psychology, 35,* 323–329.

Collins, A. M., & Loftus, E. F. (1975). A spreading-activaton theory of semantic processing. *Psychological Review, 82,* 407–428.

Collins, A. M., & Quillian, M. R. (1969). Retrieval time from semantic memory. *Journal of Verbal Learning and Verbal Behavior, 8,* 240–247.

Colquhoun, W. P. (1961). The effect of unwanted signals on performance on a vigilance task. *Ergonomics, 4,* 41–51.

Colquhoun, W. P. (1966). Training for vigilance: A comparison of different techniques. *Human Factors, 8,* 7–12.

Colquhoun, W. P., & Baddeley, A. D. (1964). Role of retest expectancy in vigilance decrement. *Journal of Experimental Psychology, 68,* 156–160.

Colquhoun, W. P., & Baddeley, A. D. (1967). Influence of signal probability during pretraining on vigilance decrement. *Journal of Experimental Psychology, 73,* 153–155.

Conkey, R. C. (1938). Psychological changes associated with head injuries. *Archives of Psychology, 232,* 1–62.

Connolly, C. J. (1950). *External morphology of the primate brain.* Springfield, IL: Charles C Thomas.

Corcoran, D. W. J., & Houston, T. G. (1977). Is the lemon test an index of arousal level? *British Journal of Psychiatry, 68,* 361–364.

Corcoran, D. W. J., Mullin, J., Rainey, M. T., & Frith, G. (1977). The effects of raised signal and noise amplitude during the course of vigilance tasks. In R. Mackie (Ed.), *Vigilance.* New York: Academic Press.

Corkin, S., Milner, B., & Taylor, L. (1973). Bilateral sensory loss after unilateral cerebral lesion in man. *Transactions of the American Neurological Association, 98,* 25–29.

Corman, D. C., Meyer, P. M., & Meyer, D. R. (1967). Open-field activity and exploration in rats with septal and amygdaloid lesions. *Brain Research, 5,* 469–476.

Cornblatt, B. A., Risch, N. J., Faris, G., Friedman, D., & Erlenmeyer-Kimling, L. (1988). The continuous performance test, identical pairs version (CPT-IP): 1. New findings of sustained attention in families. *Psychiatry Research, 26,* 223–238.

Corvin, S., Milner, B., & Rasmussen, T. (1970). Somatosensory thresholds: Contrasting effects of post-central gyrus and posterior parietal-lobe excisions. *Archives of Neurology, 23,* 41–58.

Coslett, H. B., & Heilman, K. M. (1984). Hemihypokinesia following right hemisphere stroke. *Neurology, 34* (Suppl. 1), 190.

Coslett, H. B., & Heilman, K. M. (1989). Hemihypokinesia after right hemisphere stroke. *Brain and Cognition, 9*(2), 267–278.

Coslett, H. B., Bowers, D., & Heilman, K. M. (1987). Reduction in cerebral activation after right hemisphere stroke. *Neurology, 37*(6), 957–962.

Coslett, H. B., Bowers, D., Fitzpatrick, E., Haws, C., & Heilman, K. M. (1990). Directional hypokinesia and hemispatial inattention in neglect. *Brain, 113,* 475–486.

Courchesne, E., Hillyard, S. A., & Galambos, R. (1975). Stimulus novelty, task relevance and the visual evoked potentials in man. *Electroencephalography and Clinical Neurophysiology, 39,* 131–143.

Cowan, N. (1984). On short and long auditory stores. *Psychological Bulletin, 96,* 341–370.

Cowan, N. (1988). Evolving conceptions of memory storage, selective attention, and their mutual constraints within the human information-processing system. *Psychological Bulletin, 104*(2), 163–191.

Craik, F. I. M., & Blankenstein, K. R. (1975). Psychophysiology and human memory. In P. H. Venables & M. J. Christie (Eds.), *Research in psychophysiology* (pp. 388–417). London: Wiley.

Craik, F. I. M., & Lockhart, R. S. (1972). Levels of processing: A framework for memory research. *Journal of Verbal Learning and Verbal Behavior, 11,* 671–684.

Crick, F. (1984). Memory and molecular turnover. *Nature, 312,* 101.

Crick, F. H. C., & Asanuma, C. (1986). *Certain aspects of the anatomy and physiology of the cerebral cortex in parallel distributed processing: Explorations in the microstructure of cognition* (Vol. 2). Cambridge: MIT Press.

Critchley, M. (1949). Tactile inattention with reference to parietal lesions. *Brain, 72,* 438–561.

Cronholm, B., & Ottosson, J. (1961). Memory functions in endogenous depression. *Archives of General Psychiatry, 5,* 193–197.

Crosson, B. (1985). Subcortical functions of language: A working model. *Brain and Language, 25,* 257–292.

Crow, T. J., & Alkon, D. L. (1980). Associative behavioral modification in *Hermissenda:* Cellular correlates. *Science, 209,* 412–414.

Crowe, D. P., Yeo, C. H., & Russell, I. S. (1981). The effects of unilateral frontal eye field lesions in the monkey: Visual-motor guidance and avoidance behavior. *Behavioral Brain Research, 2,* 165–185.

Curry, S. H. (1981). Event related potentials as indicants of structural and functional damage in closed head injury. *Progress in Brain Research, 54,* 507–515.

Dalland, T. (1970). Response and stimulus perseveration in rats with septal and dorsal hippocampal lesions. *Journal of Comparative and Physiological Psychology, 71,* 114–118.

Dalland, T. (1976). Response perseveration of rats with dorsal hippocampal lesions. *Behavioral Biology, 17,* 473–484.

Damosio, A. R., & Van Hoesen (1983). Emotional disturbances associated with facial lesions of the limbic frontal lobe. In C. M. Heilman & P. Satz (Eds.), *Neuropsychology of Human Emotion*. New York: Guilford Press.

Damasio, A. R., Damasio, H., & Chui, H. C. (1980). Neglect following damage to frontal lobe or basal ganglia. *Neuropsychologia, 18*, 123–132.

Darrow, C. W. (1929). Differences in the physiological reaction to sensory and ideational stimuli. *Psychological Bulletin, 26*, 185–201.

Daugman, J. (1990). Brain Metaphor and Brain Theory. In E. L. Schwartz (Ed.), *Computational neuroscience* (pp. 9–18). Boston: MIT Press.

Davies, D. R., & Parasuraman, R. (1982). *The psychology of vigilance*. New York: Academic Press.

Dawson, M. E., & Nuechterlein, K. H. (1984). Psychophysiological dysfunctions in the developmental course of schizophrenic disorders. *Schizophrenia Bulletin, 10*(2), 204–232.

Delgado, J. M. R., Roberts, W. W., & Miller, N. E. (1954). Learning motivated by electrical stimulation of the brain. *American Journal of Physiology, 179*, 587.

Denny, M. R., (1946). The role of secondary reinforcement in a partial learning situation. *Journal of Experimental Psychology, 36*, 373–389.

Denny, M. R., Wells, R. H., & Maatsch, J. L. (1957). Resistance to extinction as a function of the discrimination habit established during fixed-ratio reinforcement. *Journal of Experimental Psychology, 6*, 451–456.

Denny-Brown, D., & Chambers, R. A. (1958). The parietal lobe and behavior. *Research Publication of the Association for the Research of Nervous and Mental Diseases, 36*, 35–117.

Denny-Brown, D., Meyer, J. S., & Horenstein, S. (1952). The significance of perceptual rivalry. *Brain, 75*, 433–471.

DeRenzi, E., Faglioni, P., & Scotti, G. (1970). Hemispheric contribution to the exploration of space through the visual and tactile modality. *Cortex, 6*, 191–203.

DeRenzi, E., Faglioni, P., & Previdi, P. (1977). Spatial memory and hemispheric locus of lesion. *Cortex, 13*, 424–433.

DeRenzi, E., Colombo, A., Faglioni, P., & Gilbertoni, M. (1982). Conjugate gaze paralysis in stroke patients with unilateral damage. *Archives of Neurology, 39*, 482–486.

Desimone, R., & Gross, C. G. (1979). Visual areas in the temporal cortex of the macaque. *Brain Research, 178*, 363–380.

Desimone, R., & Ungerleider, L. G. (1986). Multiple visual areas in the caudal superior temporal sulcus of the macaque. *Journal of Comparative Neurology, 248*, 164–189.

Desimone, R., Albright, T. D., Gross, C. G., & Bruce, C. J. (1980). Responses of inferior temporal neurons to complex visual stimuli. *Society for Neuroscience Abstracts, 6*, 581.

Desimone, R., Schein, S. J., Moran, J., & Ungerleider, L. G. (1985). Contour, color, and shape analysis beyond the striate cortex. *Vision Research, 25*, 441–452.

Detterman, D. K. (1987). What does reaction time tell us about intelligence? In P. A. Vernon (Ed.), *Speed of information processing and intelligence* (pp. 177–200). Norwood, NJ: Ablex.

Deutsch, C. P. (1953). Differences among epileptics and between epileptics and non-epileptics in terms of some learning and memory variables. *Archives of Neurology and Psychiatry, 70*, 474–482.

Deutsch, J. A., & Deutsch, D. (1963). Attention: Some theoretical considerations. *Psychological Review, 70*, 80–90.

deWied, D. (1974). Pituitary-adrenal system hormones and behavior. In F. O. Schmitt & G. F. Worden (Eds.), *The neurosciences: Third study program* (pp. 653–666). Cambridge: MIT Press.

deWied, D., & Bohus, B. (1979). Modulation of memory processes by neuropeptides of hypothalamic-neurohypophyseal gin. In M. A. B. Brazier (Ed.), *Brain mechanisms in memory and learning: From the single neuron to man*. New York: Raven Press.

Diamond, D. M., & Weinberger, N. M. (1984). Physiological plasticity of single neurons in auditory cortex of cat during acquisition of the pupillary conditioned response: II, secondary field (AII). *Behavioral Neuroscience, 98*, 189–210.

DiCara, L. V. (1966). Effect of amygdaloid lesions on avoidance learning in the rat. *Psychonomic Science, 4*, 279–280.

Dickinson, A. (1972). Septal damage and response output under frustrative nonreward. In R. A. Boakes & M. S. Halliday (Eds.), *Inhibition and learning* (pp. 461–496). London: Academic Press.

Diller, L., & Weinberg, J. (1977). Hemi-attention in rehabilitation: The evolution of a rational remediation program. In E. A. Weinstein & R. P. Friedland (Eds.), *Advances in neurology* (p. 18). New York: Raven Press.

Diller, L., Ben-Yishay, Y., Gerstman, L. J., Goodkin, R., Gordon, W., & Weinberg, J. (1974). *Studies in cognition and rehabilitation in hemiplegia.* (Rehabilitation Monograph No. 50). New York: New York University Medical Center Institute of Rehabilitation Medicine.

Dimken, S. S., Temkin, N., & Armsden, G. (1989). Neuropsychological recovery: Relationship to psychosocial functioning and postconcussional complaints. In H. S. Levin, H. M. Eisenberg, & A. L. Benton (Eds.), *Mild head injury* (pp. 229–241). New York: Oxford University Press.

Dimond, S. J. (1976). Depletion of attentional capacity after total commissurotomy in man. *Brain, 99,* 347–356.

Dodwell, P. C. (1983). Spatial sense of the human infant. In A. Hein & M. Jeannerod (Eds.), *Spatially oriented behavior* (pp. 197–214). New York: Springer-Verlag.

Donahue, J. W., & Palmer, D. A. (1992). *Learning and its Implications for Complex Behavior.* Boston: Allyn & Bacon.

Donchin, E. (1981). Surprise! . . . Surprise? *Psychophysiology, 18,* 493–513.

Donchin, E., Heftley, E., Hillyard, S. A., Loveless, N., Maltzman, I., Ohman, A., Fosler, F., Ruchkin, D., & Siddle, D. (1984). Cognition and event-related potentials: 20. The orienting reflex. In R. Karrer, J. Cohen, & P. Tueting (Eds.), *Brain and information: Event related potentials. Annals of the New York Academy of Sciences, 425,* 39–57.

Donders, F. C. (1969). On the speed of mental processes. In W. G. Koster (Ed. and Trans.), *Attention and performance* (Vol. 2). Amsterdam: North-Holland. (Originally published, 1868.)

Douglas, R. J. (1967). The hippocampus and behavior. *Psychological Bulletin, 67,* 416–422.

Douglas, R. J. (1975). The development of hippocampal function. In R. L. Isaacson & K. H. Pribram (Eds.), *The hippocampus.* New York: Plenum Press.

Douglas, R. J., & Isaacson, R. L. (1964). Hippocampal lesions and activity. *Psychonomic, 1,* 187–188.

Douglas, R. J., & Pribram, K. H. (1969). Distraction and habituation in monkeys with limbic lesions. *Journal of Comparative and Physiological Psychology, 69,* 473–480.

Douglas, V. I. (1983). Attentional and cognitive problems. In M. Rutter (Ed.), *Developmental neuropsychiatry* (pp. 280–329). New York: Guilford Press.

Douglas, V. I., & Peters, K. G. (1979). Toward a clear definition of the attentional deficit of hyperactive children. In A. H. Gordon & M. Lewis (Eds.), *Attention and cognitive development* (pp. 173–246). New York: Plenum Press.

Downer, De, C. J. L. (1962). Interhemispheric integration in the visual system. In V. B. Mountcastle (Ed.), *Interhemispheric relations and cerebral dominance* (pp. 87–100). Baltimore: Johns Hopkins University Press.

Downing, C. J., & Pinker, S. (1985). The spatial structure of visual attention. In M. I. Posner & O. S. Marin (Eds.), *Mechanisms of attention: Attention and performance* (Vol. 11, pp. 171–187). Hillsdale, N.J.: Erlbaum.

Drachman, D. A., & Adams, R. D. (1962). Herpes simplex and acute inclusion body encephalitis. *Archives of Neurology, 7,* 45–63.

Drachman, D. A., & Arbit, J. (1966). Memory and the hippocampal complex. *Archives of Neurology, 15,* 52–61.

Drachman, D. A., & Leavitt, J. L. (1974). Human memory and the cholinergic system: A relationship to aging? *Archives of Neurology, 30,* 113–121.

Duffy, E. (1962). *Activation and behavior.* New York: Wiley.

Duffy, E. (1972). Activation. In N. S. Greenfield & R. A. Sternbach (Eds.), *Handbook of psychophysiology.* New York: Holt, Rinehart & Winston.

Duncan, C. C. (1988). Event related brain potentials: A window on information processing in schizophrenia. *Schizophrenia Bulletin, 14,* 199–203.

Duncan, C. C., Morihisa, J. M., Fawcett, R. W., & Kirch, D. G. (1987). P300 in schizophrenia: State or trait marker? *Psychopharmacology Bulletin, 23,* 497–501.

Duncan-Johnson, C., & Donchin, E. (1977). On quantifying surprise: The variation of event-related potentials with subjective probability. *Psychophysiology, 14,* 456–467.

Duncan-Johnson, C. C., Roth, W., & Koppell, B. S. (1984). Effects of stimulus sequence on P300 and reaction time in schizophrenics. In R. Karrer, J. Cohen, & P. Tueting (Eds.), *Brain and information: Event-related potentials. Annals of the New York Academy of Sciences, 425,* 570–577.

Dykman, R. A., Holcomb, P. J., Ackerman, P. T., & McCray, D. S. (1983). Auditory ERP augmentation-reduction and methylphenidate dosage needs in attention and reading disordered children. *Psychiatry Research, 9,* 255–269.

Easterbrook, J. A. (1959). The effects of emotion on cur utilization and the organization of behavior. *Psychological Review, 66,* 183–201.

Ebbinghaus, H. (1973). *Psychology: An elementary text-book.* New York: Arno.

Eccles, J. C. (1964). *The physiology of the synapses.* Berlin: Springer.

Edelbrock, C., Costello, A., & Kessler, M. D. (1984). Empirical corroboration of attention deficit disorder. *Journal of the American Academy of Child Psychiatry, 23,* 285–290.

Eidelberg, E., & Schwartz, A. J. (1971). Experimental analysis of the extinction phenomenon in monkeys. *Brain, 94,* 91–108.

Eisler, H. (1984). Subjective duration in rats: The psychophysical function. In J. Gibbon & L. Allan (Eds.), *Timing and time perception, Annals of the New York Academy of Sciences* (Vol. 423, pp. 43–51). New York: New York Academy of Sciences.

Eslinger, P. J., & Damasio, A. R. (1985). Severe disturbance of higher cognition after bilateral frontal lobe ablation: Patient EVR. *Neurology, 35*(12), 1731–1741.

Estes, W. K. (1950). Toward a statistical theory of learning. *Psychological Review, 57,* 94–107.

Estes, W. K. (1959). The statistical approach to learning theory. In S. Koch (Ed.), *Psychology: A study of a science* (Vol. 2, pp. 380–491). New York: McGraw-Hill.

Estes, W. K., & Burke, C. J. (1953). A theory of stimulus variability in learning. *Psychological Review, 60,* 276–286.

Estes, W. K., & Burke, C. J. (1955). Application of a statistical model to simple discrimination learning in human subjects. *Journal of Experimental Psychology, 50,* 81–88.

Fairbanks, G., Guttman, N., & Miron, M. S. (1957). Effects of time compression upon the comprehension of connected speech. *Journal of Speech and Hearing Disorders, 22,* 10–19.

Fantz, R. L. (1958a). Pattern vision in young infants. *Psychological Record, 8,* 43–48.

Fantz, R. L. (1958b). Visual discrimination in a neonate chimpanzee. *Perceptual and Motor Skills, 8,* 59–66.

Fantz, R. L. (1965). Visual perception from birth as shown by pattern selectivity. *Annals of the New York Academy of Sciences, 118,* 793–814.

Fantz, R. L. (1967). Visual perception in infancy. In H. Stevenson, E. Hess, & H. Rheingold (Eds.), *Early behavior: Comparative and developmental approaches.* New York: Wiley.

Farkas, T., Wolf, A. P., Jaeger, J., Cancro, R., Christman, D., & Fowler, J. (1981). *Regional cerebral glucose utilization in chronic schizophrenia.* Third World Congress Biological Psychiatry. Symposium on Cerebral Circulation and Metabolism Related to Psychopathology, Stockholm, Sweden.

Faux, S. F. Shenton, M. E., McCarley, R. W., Nestor, P. G., Marcy, B., & Ludwig, A. (1990). Preservation of P300 event-related potential topographic asymmetries in schizophrenia with use of either linked-ear or nose reference sites. *Electroencephalography and Clinical Neurophysiology, 75,* 378–391.

Fedio, P., & Mirsky, A. F. (1969). Selective intellectual deficits in children with temporal lobe or centrecephalic epilepsy. *Neuropsychologia, 7,* 287–300.

Feldman, J. A. (1982). Dynamic connections in neural networks. *Biological Cybernetics, 46,* 27–39.

Feldman, J. A., & Ballard, D. H. (1982). Connectionist models and their properties. *Cognitive Sciences, 6,* 205–254.

Ferris, C. F., & Albers, H. E. (1984). Effect of peptides on flank gland grooming following microinjection into the medial preoptic area of golden hamsters. *Neuroscience Abstracts, 10,* 170.

Ferris, C. F., Singer, E. A., Meenan, D. M. J., & Albers, H. E. (1988). Inhibition of vasopressin-stimulated flank marking behavior by V_2-receptor antagonists. *European Journal of Pharmacology, 154,* 153–159.

Ferro, J. M., Kertesz, A., & Black, S. E. (1987). Subcortical neglect: Quantitation, anatomy, and recovery. *Neurology, 37,* 1487–1492.

Filby, R. A., & Gazzaniga, M. S. (1969). Splitting the normal brain with reaction time. *Psychonomic Science, 17,* 335–336.

Findlay, J. M. (1983). Visual information processing for saccadic eye movements. In A. Hein & M. Jeannerod (Eds.), *Spatially oriented behavior* (pp. 281–304). New York: Springer-Verlag.

Finger, S., & Stein, D. G. (1982). *Brain damage and recovery: Research and clinical perspectives*. New York and London: Academic Press.

Fischer, B., & Breitmeyer, B. (1987). Mechanisms of visual attention revealed by saccadic eye movements. *Neuropsychologia, 25*, 73–83.

Fisk, A. D., & Schneider, W. (1984). Memory as a function of attention, level of processing, and automization. *Journal of Experimental Psychology: Learning, Memory and Cognition, 10*(2), 181–197.

Flicker, C., Dean, R. L., Watkins, D. L., Fisher, S. K., & Bartus, R. T. (1983). Behavioral and neuro-chemical effects following neurotoxic lesions of a major cholinergic input to the cerebral cortex in the rat. *Pharmacology, Biochemistry, and Behavior, 18*, 973–981.

Flor-Henry, P. (1983). *Cerebral basis of psychopathology*. Boston: John Wright.

Flor-Henry, P., & Yeudall, L. T. (1979). Neuropsychological investigation of schizophrenia and manic-depressive psychoses. In J. Gruzelier & P. Flor-Henry (Eds.), *Hemisphere asymmetries of function in psychopathology*. Amsterdam: Elsevier/North-Holland.

Folkard, S. (1979a). Changes in immediate memory strategy under induced muscle tension and with time of day. *Quarterly Journal of Experimental Psychology, 31*, 621–633.

Folkard, S. (1979b). Time of day and level of processing. *Memory and Cognition, 7*, 247–252.

Folkard, S., & Greeman, A. L. (1974). Salience induced muscle tension, and the ability to ignore irrelevant information. *Quarterly Journal of Experimental Psychology, 26*, 360–367.

Folkard, S., & Monk, T. H. (1980). Circadian rhythms in human memory. *British Journal of Psychology, 71*, 295–307.

Fonberg, E. (1973). The normalizing effect of lateral amygdalar lesions upon the dorsomedial amygdalar syndrome in dogs. *Acta Neurobiologiae Experimentalis, 33*, 449.

Franz, S. I. (1907). On the function of the cerebrum: The frontal lobes. *Archives of Psychology, 2*, 1–64.

Freal, J. E., Kraft, G. H., & Coryell J. K. (1984). Symptomatic fatigue in multiple sclerosis. *Archives of Physical Medicine and Rehabilitation, 65*, 135–138.

Freedman, B. J., & Chapman, L. J. (1973). Early subjective experience in schizophrenic episodes. *Journal of Abnormal Psychology, 82*, 46–54.

Freeman, G. L. (1948). *The energetics of human behavior*. Ithaca, NY: Cornell University Press.

Friedman, D. B., Hakerem, G., Sutton, S., & Fleiss, J. L. (1973). Effect of stimulus uncertainty on the pupillary dilatation response and the vertex evoked potential. *Electroencephalography and Clinical Neurophysiology, 34*, 475–484.

Frith, C. D., Stevens, M., Johnstone, E. C., Deakin, J. F., Lancer, P., & Crow, T. J. (1983). Effects of ECT and depression on various aspects of memory *British Journal of Psychiatry, 142*, 610–617.

Furedy, J. J. (1968). Novelty and the measurement of the GSR. *Journal of Experimental Psychology, 76*, 501–503.

Fuster, J. M. (1989). *The prefrontal cortex: Anatomy, physiology, and neuropsychology of the frontal lobe*. New York: Raven Press.

Fuster, J., Bauer, R. H., & Jervey, J. P. (1982). Cellular discharge in the dorsolateral prefrontal cortex of the monkey in cognitive tasks. *Experimental Neurology, 77*, 679–694.

Gabriel, M., Miller, J. D., & Saltwick, S. E. (1976). Multiple unit activity of the rabbit medial geniculate nucleus in conditioning, extinction and reversal. *Psychological Psychology, 4*, 124–134.

Gale, A., Dunkin, N., & Coles, M. (1969). Variation in visual input and the occipital EEG. *Psychonomic Science, 14*, 262–263.

Gaska, J. P., Jacobson, L. D., & Pollen, D. A. (1988). Spatial and temporal frequency selectivity of neurons in the visual cortical area. V3A of the macaque monkey. *Vision Research, 28*(11), 1179–1191.

Gatchel, R. J., & Lang, P. J. (1974). Effects of interstimulus interval length and variability on habituation of autonomic components of the orienting response. *Journal of Experimental Psychology, 103*, 802–804.

Gawryszewski, L. D. G., Riggio, L., Rizzolatti, G., & Umilta, C. (1987). Movements of attention in the three spatial dimensions and the meaning of "neutral" cues. *Neuropsychologia, 25*(1A), 19–29.

Gazzaniga, M. S. (1970). *The bisected brain*. New York: Appleton-Century-Crofts.

Gazzaniga, M. S., & Ladavas, E. (1987). Disturbances of spatial attention following lesion or disconnection of the right parietal lobe. In M. Jeannerod (Ed.), *Neurophysiological and neuropsychological aspects of spatial neglect*. New York: Elsevier.

Geer, J. H. (1966). Effect of interstimulus intervals and rest-period length upon habituation of the orienting response. *Journal of Experimental Psychology, 72*, 617–619.

Gentilini, M., Nichelli, P., & Schoenhuber, R. (1989). Neuropsychological recovery: Relationship to psychosocial functioning and postconcussional complaints. In H. S. Levin, H. M. Eisenberg, & A. L. Benton (Eds.), *Mild head injury* (pp. 163–175). New York: Oxford University Press.

Geschwind, N. (1979). Specializations of the human brain. *Scientific American, 241,* 180.

Gesell, A., & Ilg, F. L. (1949). *Child development: An introduction to the study of human growth.* New York: Harper & Row.

Gibbon, J. (1981). Two kinds of ambiguity in the study of psychological time. In M. L. Commons & J. A. Nevins (Eds.), *Quantitative analysis of behavior: Discriminative properties of reinforcement schedules* (pp. 157–189). Cambridge, MA: Ballinger.

Gibbon, J., Church, R. M., & Meck, W. H. (1984). Scalar timing in memory. In J. Gibbon & L. Allan (Eds.), *Timing and time perception, Annals of the New York Academy of Sciences* (Vol. 423, pp. 52–77). New York: New York Academy of Sciences.

Gibson, E., & Rader, N. (1979). Attention: The perceiver as performer. In A. H. Gordon & M. Lewis (Eds.), *Attention and cognitive development* (pp. 1–21). New York: Plenum Press.

Gibson, J. J. (1950). *The perception of visual world.* Boston: Houghton Mifflin.

Gibson, J. J. (1979). *Ecological approach to visual perception.* Boston: Houghton Mifflin.

Gittelman, R., Abikoff, H., Pollack, E., Klein, D. F., Katz, S., & Mattes, J. (1980). A controlled trial of behavior modification and methylphenidate in hyperactive children. In C. K. Whalen & B. Henker (Eds.), *Hyperactive children: The social ecology of identification and treatment* (pp. 107–138). New York: Academic Press.

Gjerde, P. F. (1983). Attentional capacity dysfunction and arousal in schizophrenia. *Psychological Bulletin, 93,* 57–72.

Glassman, W. E. (1972). Subvocal activity and acoustic confusions in short term memory. *Journal of Experimental Psychology, 96,* 164–169.

Glick, S. D., Goldfarb, T. L., & Jarvik, M. E. (1969). Recovery of delayed matching performance following lateral frontal lesions in monkeys. *Communications in Behavior and Biology, 3,* 299–303.

Glowinsky, H. (1973). Cognitive deficits in temporal lobe epilepsy: An investigation of memory functioning. *Journal of Nervous and Mental Diseases, 157,* 129–137.

Gold, R. M., & Proulx, D. M. (1972). Bait-shyness acquisition is impaired by VMH lesions that produce obesity. *Journal of Comparative and Physiological Psychology, 79,* 201–209.

Goldberg, M. E., & Bruce, C. J. (1986). The role of arcuate frontal eye fields in the generation of saccadic eye movements. *Progress in Brain Research, 64,* 143–154.

Goldberg, M. E., & Bushnell M. D. (1981). Behavioral enhancement of visual response in monkey cerebral cortex: 2. Modulation in frontal eye fields specifically related to saccades. *Journal of Neurophysiology, 46,* 773–787.

Goldberg, M. E., & Robinson, D. L. (1977). Visual responses of neurons in inferior parietal lobule: The physiological substrate of attention and neglect. *Neurology, 27,* 350–362.

Goldberg, M. E., & Robinson, D. L. (1980). The significance of enhanced visual responses in posterior parietal cortex. *Behavior and Brain Science, 3,* 503–505.

Goldberg, M. E., & Segraves, M. A. (1987). Visuospatial and motor attention in the monkey. *Neuropsychologia, 25*(1A), 107–118.

Goldberg, M. E., & Wurtz, R. H. (1972). Activity of superior colliculus in behaving monkey: 1. Visual receptive fields of single neurons. *Journal of Neurophysiology, 35,* 542–559.

Goldberg, R. B., & Fuster, J. M. (1974). Neuronal responses to environmental stimuli of behavior significance in the thalamus and frontal cortex of the squirrel monkey (*Saimiri sciureus*). In *Program and abstracts, 4th annual meeting* (p. 231). Rockville, MD: Society for Neuroscience.

Goldstein, K. (1944). The mental changes due to frontal lobe damage. *Journal of Psychology, 17,* 187–208.

Goldstein, K. H., & Sheerer, M. (1941). Abstract and concrete behavior: An experimental study with special tests. *Psychological Monographs, 53,*(2) (Whole No. 239).

Goodglass, H., & Kaplan, E. (1979). Assessment of cognitive deficit in the brain-injured patient. In M. S. Gazzaniga (Ed.), *Handbook of behavioral neurobiology: Vol. 2. Neuropsychology.* New York: Plenum Press.

Goodin, D. S., & Aminoff, M. J. (1984). The relationship between the evoked potential and brain events in sensory discrimination and motor response. *Brain, 107,* 241–251.

Goodin, D. S., Squires, K. C., & Starr, A. (1978). Long latency event-related components of the auditory evoked potential in dementia. *Brain, 101,* 635–648.

Goodin, D. S., Squires, K. C., Henderson, B. H., & Starr, A. (1978). Age-related variations in evoked potentials to auditory stimuli in normal subjects. *Electroencephalography and Clinical Neurophysiology, 44*, 447–458.

Goodin, D. S., Squires, K. C., & Starr, A. (1983). Variations in early and late event-related components of the auditory evoked potential with task difficulty. *Electroencephalography and Clinical Neurophysiology, 55*, 680–686.

Goodman, S. J. (1968). Visuo-motor reaction times and brain stem multiple-unit activity. *Experimental Neurology, 22*, 367–378.

Gordon, M. (1983). *The Gordon Diagnostic System.* Boulder, CO: Clinical Diagnostic Systems.

Gottesman, I. I., & Shields, J. (1982). *Schizophrenia: The epigenetic puzzle.* Cambridge: Cambridge University Press.

Gottschalk, Ch., Grusser, O-J., & Lindau, M. (1978). Tracking movement of the eyes elicited by auditory stimuli at a constant angular velocity. *Pflugers Archiv, 377*, 46.

Graham, F. K. (1973). Habituation and dishabituation of responses innervated by the autonomic nervous system. In H. V. S. Peke & M. J. Herz (Eds.), *Habituation: Vol. 1. Behavioral Studies* (pp. 163–218). New York: Academic Press.

Graham, F. K. (1979). Distinguishing among orienting, defense, and startle reflexes. In H. D. Kimmel, E. H. van Olst, & J. F. Orlebeke (Eds.), *The orienting reflex in humans* (pp. 137–167). Hillsdale, N.J.: Erlbaum.

Graham, F. K., & Clifton, R. K. (1966). Heart-rate change as a component of the orienting response. *Psychological Bulletin, 65*, 305–320.

Grant, D. A., & Norris, E. B. (1947). Eyelid conditioning as influenced by the presence of sensitized beta-responses. *Journal of Experimental Psychology, 37*, 423-433.

Grant, I., McDonald, W. I., Trimble, M. R., Smith, E., & Reed, R. (1984). Deficient learning and memory in early and middle phases of multiple sclerosis. *Journal of Neurology, Neurosurgery, and Psychiatry, 47*, 250–255.

Grastyan, E., Szabo, I., Molnar, P., & Kolta, P. (1968). Rebound, reinforcement and self-stimulation. *Communications in Behavior and Biology, Part A, 2*, 235–266.

Gray, J. A. (1970). Sodium amobarbital, the hippocampal theta rhythm, and the partial reinforcement extinction effect. *Psychological Reviews, 77*, 465–480.

Green, D. M. (1958). Detection of multiple component signals in noise. *Journal of the Acoustical Society of America, 30*, 904–911.

Green, D. M., & Swets, J. A. (1966). *Signal detection theory and psychophysics.* New York: Wiley.

Green, M. F., Neuchterlein, K. H., & Satz, P. (1989). The relationship of symptomatology and medication to electrodermal activity in schizophrenia. *Psychophysiology, 26*, 148–165.

Grice, G. R. (1971). A threshold model for drive. In H. H. Kendler & J. T. Spence (Eds.), *Tenets of neurobehaviorism* (pp. 285–312). New York: Appleton-Century-Crofts.

Gronwall, D. (1987). Advances in the assessment of attention and information processing after head injury. In H. S. Levin, J. Grafman, & H. M. Eisenberg (Eds.), *Neurobehavioral recovery from head injury* (pp. 355–371). New York: Oxford University Press.

Gronwall, D. M. A., & Sampson, H. (1974). *The psychological effects of concussion.* Auckland, New Zealand: Auckland University Press/Oxford University Press.

Gronwall, D. M. A., & Wrightson, P. (1974). Delayed recovery of intellectual function after minor head injury. *Lancet, 2*(7874), 1452.

Grossberg, S. (1976a). Adaptive pattern classification and universal recoding: Parallel development and coding of neural feature detectors. *Biological Cybernetics, 23*, 121–134.

Grossberg, S. (1976b). Adaptive pattern classification and universal recoding: 2. Feedback, expectation, olfaction, and illusions. *Biological Cybernetics, 23*, 187–202.

Grossberg, S. (1980). How does the brain build a cognitive code? *Psychological Review, 87*, 1–51.

Grossberg, S. (1988). *Neural networks and natural intelligence* Cambridge: MIT Press.

Grossman, S. P. (1976). Behavioral functions of the septum: A re-analysis. In J. F. DeFrance (Ed.), *The septal nuclei* (pp. 361–422). New York: Plenum Press.

Grossman, S. P., Dacey, D., Halaris, A. E., Collier, T., & Routtenberg, A. (1978). Aphasia and adipsia after preferential destruction of nerve cell bodies in hypothalamus. *Science, 202*, 537–539.

Groves, P. M., & Lynch, G. S. (1972). Mechanisms of habituation in the brain stem. *Psychological Review*, *79*(3), 237–244.

Groves, P. M., & Thompson, R. F. (1970). Habituation: A dual-process theory. *Psychological Review*, *77*, 419–450.

Grueninger, W. E., & Pribram, K. H. (1969). Effects of spatial and nonspatial distractors on performance latency of monkeys with frontal lesions. *Journal of Comparative and Physiological Psychology*, *68*, 203–209.

Grusser, O-J. (1983). Multimodal structure of the extrapersonal space. In A. Hein & M. Jeannerod (Eds.), *Spatially oriented behavior* (pp. 327–352). New York: Springer-Verlag.

Gruzelier, J. H., & Venables, P. H. (1972). Skin conductance orienting activity in a heterogeneous sample of schizophrenics. *Journal of Nervous and Mental Disease*, *155*, 277–287.

Guitton, D., Buchtel, H. A., & Douglas, R. M. (1985). Frontal lobe lesions in man cause difficulties in suppressing reflexive glances and in generating goal-directed saccades. *Experimental Brain Research*, *58*, 455–472.

Hackley, S. A., & Graham, F. K. (1987). Effects of attending selectively to the spatial position of reflex-eliciting and reflex-modulating stimuli. *Journal of Experimental Psychology: Human Perception and Performance*, *13*, 411–424.

Haier, R. J., Siegel, B. J., Nuechterlein, K. H., & Hazlett, E. (1988). Cortical glucose metabolic rate correlates of abstract reasoning and attention studied with positron emission tomography. *Intelligence*, *12*(2), 199–217.

Hale, G. A. (1979). Development of children's attention to stimulus components. In A. H. Gordon & M. Lewis (Eds.), *Attention and cognitive development* (pp. 43–64). New York: Plenum Press.

Halgren, E., Squires, N. K., Rohrbaugh, J. W., Babb, T. L., & Crandall, P. H. (1980). Endogenous potentials generated in the human hippocampal formation and amygdala by infrequent events. *Science*, *210*, 803–805.

Halgren, E., Stapleton, J. M., Smith, M., & Altafullah, I. (1986). Generators of the human scalp P3(s). In R. Q. Cracco & I. Bodis-Wollner (Eds.), *Evoked potentials* (pp. 269–284). New York: Alan Liss.

Hallett, P. E., & Lightstone, A. D. (1976). Saccadic eye movement towards stimuli triggered by prior saccades. *Vision Research*, *16*, 99–106.

Hansch, E. C., Syndulko, K., Cohen, S. N., Goldberg, Z. I., Potvin, A. R., & Tourtellotte, W. W. (1982). Cognition in Parkinson disease: An event-related potential perspective. *Annals of Neurology*, *11*, 599–607.

Harlow, J. M. (1868). Recovery from the passage of an iron bar through the head. *Publications of the Massachusetts Medical Society*, *2*, 237–246.

Harter, M. R., Aine, C., & Schroeder, C. (1982). Hemispheric differences in the neural processing of stimulus location and type: Effects of selective attention on visual evoked potentials. *Neuropsychologia*, *20*, 42–438.

Harter, M. R., Diering, S., & Wood, F. B. (1988). Separate brain potential characteristics in children with reading disability and attention deficit disorder: Relevance-independent effects. *Brain and Cognition*, *7*, 54–86.

Harting, J. K., Huerta, M. F., Frankfurter, A. J., Strominger, N. L., & Royce, G. J. (1980). Ascending pathways from the monkey superior colliculus: An autoradiographic analysis. *Journal of Comparative Neurology*, *192*, 853–882.

Hasher, L., & Zacks, R. T. (1979). Automatic and effortful processes in memory. *Journal of Experimental Psychology: General*, *108*, 356–388.

Hasher, L., & Zacks, R. T. (1984). Automatic processing of fundamental information: The case of frequency of occurrence. *American Psychologist*, *39*, 1372–1388.

Hassler, R., Mundinger, F., & Reichert, T. (1979). *Stereotaxis in Parkinson syndrome*. New York: Springer-Verlag.

Hastings, J. E., & Barkley, R. A. (1978). A review of psychophysiological research with hyperkinetic children. *Journal of Abnoraml Child Psychology*, *6*, 413–447.

Hatton, H. M., Berg, W. K., & Graham, F. K. (1970). Effects of acoustic rise time on heart rate response. *Psychnomic Science*, *19*, 101–103.

Hawkins, R. D., & Kandel, E. R. (1984). Steps toward a cell-biological alphabet for elementary forms of learning. In G. Lynch, J. L. McGaugh, & N. M. Weinberger (Eds.), *Neurobiology of learning and memory* (pp. 385–404. New York: Guilford Press.

Hawkins, R. D., Abrams, T. W., Carew, T. J., & Kandel, E. R. (1983). A cellular mechanism of classical conditioning in Aplysia: Activity dependent amplification of presynaptic facilitation. *Science, 219,* 400–404.

Heath, R. G., & Mickle, W. A. (1960). Evaluation of seven years' experience with depth electrode studies in human patients. In E. R. Ramsey & D. S. O'Doherty (Eds.), *Electrical studies of the unanesthetized brain* (pp. 214–242). New York: Hoever.

Heaton, R. K., & Crowley, T. J. (1981). Effects of psychiatric disorders and their somatic treatments on neuropsychological test results. In S. B. Filskov & T. J. Boss (Eds.), *Handbook of clinical neuropsychology.* New York: Wiley.

Heaton, R. K., Baade, L. E., & Johnson, K. L. (1978). Neuropsychological test results associated with psychiatric disorders in adults. *Psychological Bulletin, 85,* 141–162.

Heaton, R. K., Nelson, L. M., Thompson, D. S., Burks, J. S., & Franklin, G. M. (1985). Neuropsychological findings in relapsing/remitting and chronic/progressive multiple sclerosis. *Journal of Consulting and Clinical Psychology, 53,* 103–110.

Hebb, D. O. (1945). Man's frontal lobes: A critical review. *Archives of Neurology and Psychiatry, 54,* 10–24.

Hebb, D. O. (1949). *The organization of behavior.* New York: Wiley.

Hebb, D. O., & Penfield, W. (1940). Human behavior after extensive bilateral removal from the frontal lobes. *Archives of Neurology and Psychiatry, 44,* 421–430.

Hecaen, H., & Ajuriaguerra, J. (1954). Balint's syndrome (psychic paralysis of visual fixation) and its minor forms. *Brain, 77,* 373–400.

Hecaen, H., & Ajuriaguerra, J. (1956). *Troubles mentaux au cours des tumeurs intracranniennes.* Paris: Masson.

Hecaen, H., & Albert, M. L. (1975a). Disorders of mental functioning related to frontal lobe pathology. In D. F. Benson & D. Blumer (Eds.), *Psychiatric aspects of neurologic disease* (pp. 137–149). New York: Grune & Stratton.

Hecaen, H., & Albert, M. L. (1975b). Mental symptoms associated with tumors of the frontal lobe. In J. M. Warren & K. Akert (Eds.), *The frontal granular cortex and behavior* (pp. 335–352). New York: McGraw-Hill.

Hecaen, H., Penfield, W., Bertrand, C., & Malmo, R. (1956). The syndrome of apractognosia due to lesions of the minor hemisphere. *Archives of Neurology and Psychiatry, 75,* 400–434.

Heilman, K. M. (1979). Neglect and related disorders. In K. M. Heilman & E. Valenstein (Eds.), *Clinical neuropsychology* (pp. 268–307). New York: Oxford University Press.

Heilman, K. M. (1991). Anosognosia: Possible neuropsychological mechanisms. In G. P. Prigatano & D. L. Schachter (Eds.). *Awareness of deficit after brain injury: Clinical and theoretical issues* (pp. 53–62). New York: Oxford University Press.

Heilman, K. M., & Satz, P. (1983). Advances in Neuropsychology and behavioral neurology. In K. M. Heilman & P. Satz, (Eds.), *Neuropsychology of human emotion,* (Vol. 1). New York and London: Guilford Press.

Heilman, K. M., & Valenstein, E. (1972). Frontal lobe neglect in man. *Neurology, 22,* 660–664.

Heilman, K. M., & Valenstein, E. (1979). Mechanisms underlying hemispatial neglect. *Annals of Neurology, 5,* 166–170.

Heilman, K. M., & Van Den Abell, T. (1979). Right hemispheric dominance for mediating cerebral activation. *Neuropsychologia, 17,* 315–321.

Heilman, K. M., & Van Den Abell, T. (1980). Right hemispheric dominance for attention: The mechanisms underlying hemispheric asymmetries of inattention (neglect). *Neurology, 30,* 327–330.

Heilman, K. M., & Watson, R. T. (1976). The neglect syndrome—A unilateral defect of the orienting response. In S. Harnad, R. Doty, L. Goldstein, J. Jaynes, & E. Krauthamer (Eds.), *Lateralization in the nervous system* (pp. 285–302). New York: Academic Press.

Heilman, K. M., Pandya, D. N., Karol, E. A., & Geschwind, N. (1971). Auditory inattention. *Archives of Neurology, 24,* 323–325.

Heilman, K. M., Schwartz, H., & Watson, R. T. (1978). Hypoarousal in patients with the neglect syndrome and emotional indifference. *Neurology (Minneapolis), 28,* 229–232.

Heilman, K. M., Bowers, D., Coslett, H. B., & Watson, R. T. (1983). Directional hypokinesia in neglect. *Neurology, 2,* 104.

Heilman, K. M., Valenstein, E., & Watson, R. T. (1983). Localization of neglect. In A. Kertesz (Ed.), Localization in neuropsychology (pp. 471–492). New York: Academic Press.

Heilman, K.M., Watson, R. T., & Valenstein, E. (1985). Neglect and related disorders. In K. M. Heilman & E. Valenstein (Eds.), Clinical neuropsychology (2nd ed., pp. 243–293). New York and Oxford: Oxford University Press.

Heilman, K. M., Watson, R. T., Valenstein, E., & Goldberg, M. E. (1988). Attention: Behavior and neural mechanisms. Attention, 11, 461–481.

Heilman, K. M., Kytja, K. S., Voeller, K. K. S., & Nadeau, S. E. (1991). A possible pathophysiologic substrate of attention deficit hyperactivity disorder. Journal of Child Neurology, 6:S76–S81.

Hein, A., & Diamond, R. M. (1972). Locomotory space as a prerequisite for acquiring visually guided reaching in kittens. Journal of Comparative and Physiological Psychology, 81, 394–398.

Hein, A., & Diamond, R. (1983). Contribution of eye movement to the representation of space. In A. Hein & M. Jeannerod (Eds.), Spatially oriented behavior (pp. 119–134). New York: Springer-Verlag.

Hein, A., & Held, R. (1967). Dissociation of the visual placing response into elicited and guided components. Science, 158, 390–392.

Heinemann, E. G. (1984). A model for temporal generalization and discrimination. In J. Gibbon & L. Allan (Eds.), Timing and time perception, Annals of the New York Academy of Sciences (Vol. 423), pp. 361–371). New York: New York Academy of Sciences.

Held, R., & Hein, A. (1963). Movement-produced stimulation in the development of visually guided behavior. Journal of Comparative and Physiological Psychology, 56, 872–876.

Henke, P. G., Allen, J. D., & Davidson, C. (1972). Effect of lesions in the amygdala on behavioral contrast. Psychology and Behavior, 8, 173–176.

Hersen, M., & Barlow, D. H. (1976). Single-case experimental designs: Strategies for studying behavior change. New York: Pergamon Press.

Hess, W. R. (1957). The functional organization of the diencephalon. New York: Grune & Stratton.

Hess, W. R. (1969). Hypothalamus and thalamus: Experimental documentation. Stuttgart: Georg Thieme Verlag.

Heston, L. L. (1966). Psychiatric disorders in foster home reared children of schizophrenic mothers. British Journal of Psychiatry, 112, 819–825.

Hetherington, A. W., & Ranson, S. W. (1942). The spontaneous activity and food intake of rats with hypothalamic lesions. American Journal of Physiology, 136, 609–617.

Hick, W. E. (1952a). On the rate of gain of information. Quarterly Journal of Experimental Psychology, 4, 11–26.

Hick, W. E. (1952b). Why the human operator? Transactions of the Society of Instrument Technology, 4, 67–77.

Hicks, R. E. (1975). Intrahemispheric response competition between vocal and unimanual performance in normal adult human males. Journal of Comparative and Physiological Psychology, 89, 50–60.

Hier, D. B., Mondlock, J., & Caplan, L. R. (1983). Behavioral abnormalities after right hemisphere stroke. Neurology, 33, 337–344.

Hillyard, S. A. (1985). Electrophysiology of human selective attention. Trends in Neurosciences, 8, 401.

Hillyard, S. A., & Hansen, J. C. (1986). Attention: Electrophysiological approaches. In M. G. H. Coles, E. Donchin, & S. W. Porges (Eds.), Psychophysiology: Systems, processes, and applications (pp. 227–243). New York: Guilford Press.

Hillyard, S. A., & Kutas, M. (1983). Electrophysiology of cognitive processing. Annual Review of Psychology, 34, 1983.

Hillyard, S. A., & Munte, T. F. (1984). Selective attention to color and location: An analysis with event-related potentials. Perception and Psychophysics, 36, 185–198.

Hillyard, S. A., Hink, R. F., Schwent, V. L., & Picton, T. W. (1973). Electrical signs of selective attention in the human brain. Science, 182, 177–180.

Hinshaw, S. (1987). On the distinction between attentional deficits/hyperactivity and conduct problems/aggression in child psychopathology. Psychological Bulletin, 101, 250–265.

Hinton, G. E. (1981). Implementing semantic networks in parallel hardware. In G. E. Hinton & J. A. Anderson (Eds.), Parallel models of associative memory (pp. 161–188). Hillsdale, NJ: Erlbaum.

Hinton, G. E., & Sejnowski, T. J. (1983). Analyzing cooperative computation. Proceedings of the Fifth Annual Conference of the Cognitive Science Society.

Hinton, G. E., & Sejnowski, T. J. (1986). *Learning and relearning in Boltzmann machines in parallel distributed processing: Explorations in the microstructure of cognition* (Vol. 1). Cambridge: MIT Press.

Hinton, G. E., Sejnowski, T. J., & Ackley, D. H. (1984). Boltzmann machines: Constraint satisfaction networks that learn. (Tech. Rep. CMU-CS-84-119). Pittsburgh, Carnegie-Mellon University, Department of Computer Science.

Hirst, W. (1986). The psychology of attention. In J. E. Ledoux & W. Hirst (Eds.), *Mind and brain: Dialogues in cognitive neuroscience* (pp. 105–141). New York: Cambridge University.

Hirst, W., Spelke, E. S., Reaves, C. C., Caharack, G., & Neisser, U. (1980). Dividing attention without alternation or automaticity. *Journal of Experimental Psychology: General, 109,* 98–117.

Hochberg, J. E. (1970). Attention, organization, and consciousness. In D. I. Mostofsky (Ed.), *Attention, contemporary theory and analysis* (pp. 99–124). New York: Appleton-Century-Crofts.

Hockey, G. R. J. (1970a). Effect of loud noise on attentional selectivity. *Quarterly Journal of Experimental Psychology, 22,* 28–36.

Hockey, G. R. J. (1970b). Signal probability and spatial location as possible bases for increased selectivity in noise. *Quarterly Journal of Experimental Psychology, 22,* 37–42.

Hockey, G. R. J. (1978). Attentional selectivity and the problems of replication: A reply to Forster and Grierson. *British Journal of Psychiatry, 69,* 499–503.

Hockey, G. R. J. (1979). Stress and the cognitive components of skilled performance. In V. Hamilton & D. M. Warburton (Eds.), *Human stress and cognition.* Chichester, England: Wiley.

Hockey, G. R. J., & Colquhoun, W. P. (1972). Diurnal variation in human performance: A review. In W. P. Colquhoun (Ed.), *Aspects of human efficiency: Diurnal rhythm and loss of sleep.* London: English Universities Press.

Hoebel, B. G., & Teitelbaum, P. (1966). Weight regulation in normal and hypothalamic hyperphagic rats. *Journal of Comparative and Physiological Psychology, 61,* 189–193.

Hoffman, J. E., Simons, R. F., & Houck, M. R. (1983). Event-related potentials during controlled and automatic target detection. *Psychophysiology, 20,* 625–632.

Hoffmann, K. P., & Schoppmann, A. (1975). Retinal input to direction selective cells in the nucleus tractus opticus of the cat. *Brain Research, 99,* 359–366.

Hoffmann, K. P., & Schoppmann, A. (1981). A quantitative analysis of the direction-specific response of neurons in the cat's nucleus of the optic tract. *Experimental Brain Research, 42,* 1–12.

Holcomb, P. J., Ackerman, P. T., & Dykman, R. A. (1985). Cognitive event-related brain potentials in children with attention and reading deficits. *Psychophysiology, 22,* 656–667.

Holloway, F. A., & Parsons, O. A.. (1978). Psychophysiology: Brain damaged patients. *Handbook of biological psychiatry (vol. 3): Brain mechanisms and abnormal behavior.* New York: Dekker.

Homberg, V., Hefter, H., Granseyer, G., Strauss, J., Lange, P., & Hennerici, R. (1986). Event-related potentials in patients with Huntington's disease and relative at-risk in relation to detailed psychometry. *Electroencephalography and Clinical Neurophysiology, 63,* 552–569.

Honig, W. K. (1969). Attention factors governing the slope of the generalization gradient. In R. M. Gilbert & N. S. Sutherland (Eds.), *Animal discrimination learning.* New York: Academic Press.

Honig, W. K. (1970). Attention and the modulation of stimulus control. In D. I. Mostofsky (Ed.), *Attention: Contemporary theory and analysis.* New York: Appleton-Century-Crofts.

Hopkins, G. W. (1984). Ultrastable stimulus-response latencies: Towards a model of response-stimulus synchronization. In J. Gibbon & L. Allan (Eds.), *Timing and time perception, Annals of the New York Academy of Sciences, 423,* 16–29.

Hopkins, G. W., & Kristofferson, A. B. (1980). Ultrastable stimulus-response latencies: Acquisition and stimulus control. *Perceptual Psychophysiology, 27(3),* 241–250.

Hopkins, W. F., & Johnston, D. (1984). Frequency-dependent noradrenergic modulation of long-term potentiation in the hippocampus. *Science, 226,* 350–352.

Horn, J. L., & Cattell, R. B. (1967). Age differences in fluid and crystallized intelligence. *Acta Psychologica, 25,* 107–129.

Houck, R. L., & Mefferd, R. B., Jr. (1969). Generalization of GSR habituation to mild intramodal stimuli. *Psychophysiology, 6,* 202–206.

Hovland, C. I., & Riesen, A. H. (1940). Magnitude of galvanic and vasomotor response as a function of stimulus intensity. *Journal of General Psychology, 23,* 103–121.

Howes, D., & Boller, F. (1975). Evidence of focal impairments from lesions of the right hemisphere. *Brain, 98,* 317–332.

Hubel, D. M., & Wiesel, T. N. (1963). Receptive fields of cells in the striate cortex of very young, visually inexperienced kittens. *Journal of Neurophysiology, 106,* 994–1002.

Hubel, D. H., & Wiesel, T. N. (1968). Receptive fields and functional architecture of monkey striate cortex. *Journal of Physiology (London), 195,* 215–243.

Hubel, D. H., & Wiesel, T. N. (1977). Functional architecture of macaque monkey visual cortex. *Proceedings of the Royal Society of London, Series B, 198,* 1–59.

Huber, S. J., Shuttleworth, E. C., Freidenberg, D. O. (1989). Neuropsychological differences between dementias of Alzheimer's and Parkinson's diseases *Archives of Neurology, 46,* 1287–1291.

Hughes, H. C., & Zimba, L. D. (1987). Natural boundaries for the spatial spread of directed visual attention. *Neuropsychologia, 25*(1A), 5–18.

Hull, C. L. (1943). *Principles of behavior.* New York: Appleton-Century.

Humphreys, M. S., Revelle, W., Simon, L., & Gilliland, K. (1980). Individual differences in diurnal rhythms and multiple activation states: A reply to M. W. Eysenck and Simon Folkard. *Journal of Experimental Psychology, 109,* 42–48.

Hyman, R. (1953). Stimulus information as a determinant of reaction times. *Journal of Experimental Psychology, 45,* 188–196.

Hynd, G. W., Semrud-Clikeman, M., Lorys, A. R., Novey, E. S., & Eliopulos, D. (1990). Brain morphology in developmental dyslexia and attention deficit disorder/hyperactivity. *Archives of Neurology, 47,* 919–926.

Hynd, G. W., Semrud-Clikeman, M., Lorys, A. R., Novey, E. S., Eliopulos, D., & Lyytinen, H. (1991a). Corpus callosum morphology in attention deficit-hyperactivity disorder: Morphometric analysis of MRI. *Journal of Learning Disabilities, 24,* 141–146.

Hynd, G. W., Lorys, A. R., Semrud-Clikeman, M., Nieves, N., Heuttner, M. I. S., & Lahey, B. B. (1991b). Attention deficit disorder without hyperactivity: A distinct behavioral and neurocognitive syndrome. *Journal of Child Neurology, 6,* 37–43.

Hyvarinen, J., Poranen, A., & Jokinen, Y. (1980). Influence of attentive behavior on neuronal responses to vibration in primary somatosensory cortex of the monkey. *Journal of Neurophysiology, 43,* 870–882.

Isaacson, R. L. (1972). Neural systems of the limbic brain and behavioral inhibition. In R. Boakes & J. Halliday (Eds.), *Inhibition and learning.* New York: Academic Press.

Isaacson, R. L. (1980). Limbic system contributions to goal-directed behavior. In R. F. Thompson, L. H. Hicks, & V. B. Schvyrkov (Eds.), *Neuronal mechanisms of goal-directed behavior and learning* (pp. 409–423). New York: Academic Press.

Isaacson, R. L. (1982a). The hippocampal formation and its regulation of attention and behavior. In E. Grastyan & P. Molnar (Eds.), *Sensory functions: Advances in physiological sciences* (Vol. 16). New York: Pergamon Press.

Isaacson, R. L. (1982b). *The limbic system* (2nd ed). New York and London: Plenum Press.

Isaacson, R. L., & Kimble, D. P. (1972). Lesions of the limbic system: Their effects upon hypotheses and frustration. *Behavioral Biology, 7,* 767–793.

Isaacson, R. L., & Wickelgren, W. O. (1962). Hippocampal ablation and passive avoidance. *Science, 138,* 1104–1106.

Isaacson, R. L., Douglas, R. J., & Moore, R. Y. (1961). The effect of radical hippocampal ablation on acquisition of avoidance response. *Journal of Comparative and Physiological Psychology, 54,* 625–628.

Israel, J. B., Chesney, G. L., Wickens, C. D., & Donchin, E. (1980). P300 and tracking difficulty: Evidence for multiple resources in dual-task performance. *Psychophysiology, 17,* 259–273.

Israel, J. B., Wickens, C. D., Chesney, G. L., & Donchin, E. (1980). The event-related brain potential as an index of display-monitoring workload. *Human Factors, 22,* 211–224.

Isseroff, A., Rosvold, H. E., Galkin, T. W., & Goldman-Rakic, P. S. (1982). Spatial memory impairment following damage to the mediodorsal nucleus in the thalamus of rhesus monkeys. *Brain Research, 232,* 97–113.

Ivry, R. B., Keele, S. B., & Diener, H. C. (1988). Dissociation of the lateral and medial cerebellum in movement timing and movement execution. *Experimental Brain Research, 73*(1), 167–180.

Izawa, C. (1971). Massed and spaced practice in paired-associate learning: List versus item distributions. *Journal of Experimental Psychology, 89,* 10–21.

Jackson, J. C. (1974). Amplitude and habituation of the orienting reflex as a function of stimulus intensity. *Psychophysiology, 11,* 647–659.

Jackson, J. H. (1932). *Selected writings of John Hughlings Jackson* (J. Taylor, ed.). London: Hodder and Stoughton.

Jackson, J. H. (1958). *Selected writings.* New York: Basic Books.

Jackson, J. L., Michon, J. A., & Vermeeren, A. (1984). The processing of temporal information. In J. Gibbon & L. Allan (Eds.), *Timing and time perception* (pp. 603–604). New York: New York Academy of Sciences.

Jacobsen, C. F. (1931). A study of cerebral function in learning: The frontal lobes. *Journal of Comparative Neurology, 52,* 271–340.

Jacobsen, C. F. (1936). Studies of cerebral functions in primates: 1. The functions of the frontal association areas in monkeys. *Comparative Psychology, 13,* 3–60.

Jacobsen, C. F., & Nissen, H. W. (1937). Studies of cerebral function in primates: 4. The effects of frontal lobe lesions on the delayed alternation habit in monkeys. *Journal of Comparative and Physiological Psychology, 23,* 101–112.

Jacobsen, E. (1938). *Progressive relaxation* (rev. ed.). Chicago: University of Chicago Press.

James, W. (1884). What is an emotion? *Mind, 9,* 188–204.

James, W. (1890). *Principles of psychology.* New York: Holt.

James, W. (1922). What is emotion? In Dunlap (Ed.), *The emotions.* Baltimore: Williams & Wilkins.

Jamieson, D. G. (1977). Two presentation order effects. *Canadian Journal of Psychology, 31,* 184–194.

Jamieson, D. G., & Petrusic, W. M. (1976). On a bias induced by the provision of feedback in psychophysical experiments. *Acta Psychologica, 40,* 127–152.

Jamieson, D. G., Slawinska, E., Cheesman, M. F., & Espinoza-Varas, B. (1984). Timing perturbations with complex auditory stimuli. In J. Gibbon & L. Allan (Eds.), *Timing and time perception, Annals of the New York Academy of Sciences* (Vol. 423, pp. 96–102). New York: New York Academy of Sciences.

Janer, K. W., & Pardo, J. V. (1991). Deficits in selective attention following bilateral anterior cingulotomy. *Journal of Comparative Neuroscience, 3*(3), 231–241.

Jasper, H., Ricci, G., & Doane, B. (1962). Microelectrode analysis of discharges of cortical cells during the elaboration of conditioned defensive reflexes in monkeys. *Electroencephalographic investigation of higher nervous activity* M., Izd-vo AN SSSR.

Jeannerod, M. (1983). How do we direct our actions in space? In A. Hein & M. Jeannerod (Eds.), *Spatially oriented behavior* (pp. 1–14). New York: Springer-Verlag.

Jenkins, H. M. (1984). Time and conditioning in classical conditioning. In J. Gibbon & L. Allan (Eds.), *Timing and time perception, Annals of the New York Academy of Sciences* (Vol. 423) (pp. 242–253). New York: New York Academy of Sciences.

Jennett, B., & Teasdale, G. (1981). *Management of head injuries.* Philadelphia: F. A. Davis.

Jennings, J. R. (1971). Cardiac reactions and different developmental levels of cognitive functioning. *Psychophysiology, 8,* 433–450.

Jennings, J. R. (1986a). Bodily changes during attending. In M. G. H. Coles, E. Donchin, & S. W. Porges (Eds.), *Psychophysiology: Systems, processes, and applications* (pp. 268–289). New York: Guilford Press.

Jennings, J. R. (1986b). Memory, thought, and bodily response. In M. G. H. Coles, E. Donchin, & S. W. Porges (Eds.), *Psychophysiology: Systems, processes, and applications* (pp. 290–308). New York: Guilford Press.

Jennings, J. R., & Hall, S. W., Jr. (1980). Recall, recognition, and rate: Memory and the heart. *Psychophysiology, 17,* 37–46.

Jennings, J. R., Lawrence, B. E., & Kasper, P. (1978). Changes in alertness and processing capacity in a serial learning task. *Memory and Cognition, 6,* 45–63.

Jennings, J. R., Averill, R. J., Opton, M. E., & Lazarus, R. S. (1980). Some parameters of heart rate change: Perceptual versus motor task requirements, noxiousness, and uncertainty. *Psychophysiology, 7,* 194–212.

Jensen, A. R. (1978). The current status of the IQ controversy. *Australian Psychologist, 13,* 7–27.

Jensen, A. R. (1982). Reaction time and psychometric g. In H. J. Eysenk (Ed.), *A model for intelligence*. New York: Springer-Verlag.

Jensen, A. R., & Vernon, P. A. (1986). Jensen's reaction time studies: A reply to Longstreth. *Intelligence, 10*, 153–179.

Jerison, H. J. (1957). Performance on a simple vigilance task in noise and quiet. *Journal of the Acoustical Society of America, 29*, 1163–1165.

Jerison, H. J. (1959). Effects of noise on human performance. *Journal of Applied Psychology, 43*, 96–101.

Jimerson, D., Gordon, E. K., Post, R. M., & Goodwin, F. K. (1975). Central norepinephrine function in man: VMA in the CSF. *Brain Res, 99*, 434–439.

John, E. R. (1967). *Mechanisms of memory*. New York: Academic Press.

John, E. R. (1972). Switchboard versus statistical theories of learning and memory. *Science, 11*, 850–864.

Johnson, W. A., & Dark, V. A. (1986). Selective attention. *Annual Review of Psychology, 37*, 43–75.

Johnson, W. A., & Dark, V. J. (1982). In defense of intraperceptual theories of attention. *Journal of Experimental Psychology: Human Perception and Performance, 8*(3), 407–421.

Jones, M. R. (1984). The patterning of time and its effects of perceiving. In J. Gibbon & L. Allan (Eds.), *Timing and time perception, Annals of the New York Academy of Sciences* (Vol. 423, pp. 158–16?). New York: New York Academy of Sciences.

Jones, M. R., & Boltz, M. (1989). Dynamic attending and responses to time. *Psychological Review, 96*(3), 459–491.

Jonides, J. (1981). Voluntary versus automatic control over the mind's eye movements. In J. Long & A. Baddeley (Eds.), *Attention and performance* Vol. 9. Hillsdale, N.J.: Erlbaum.

Joynt, R. J. (1977). Inattention syndromes in split-brain man. In E. A. Weinstein & R. P. Friedland (Eds.), *Advances in neurology: Vol. 18. Hemi-inattention and hemisphere specialization* (pp. 33–39). New York: Raven Press.

Kagan, J. (1966). Reflection-impulsivity: The generality and dynamics of conceptual tempo. *Journal of Abnormal Psychology, 71*, 17–24.

Kahneman, D. (1973). *Attention and effort*. Englewood Cliffs, NJ: Prentice-Hall.

Kahneman, D., & Beatty, J. (1966). Pupil diameter and load on memory. *Science, 154*, 1583–1585

Kahneman, D., & Treisman, A. (1984). Changing views of attention and automaticity. In R. Parasuraman & D. R. Davies (Eds.), *Varieties of attention*. New York: Academic Press.

Kahneman, D., Beatty, J., & Pollack, I. (1967). Perceptual deficit during a mental task. *Science, 157*, 218–219.

Kahneman, D., Tursky, B., Shapiro, D., & Crider, A. (1969). Pupillary, heart rate and skin resistance changes during a mental task. *Journal of Experimental Psychology, 79*, 164–167.

Kamikawa, K., McIlwain, J. T., & Adey, W. R. (1964). Response pattern of thalamic neurons during classical conditioning. *Electroencephalography and Clinical Neurophysiology, 17*, 485–496.

Kamin, L. J. (1968). "Attention-like" processes in classical conditioning. In M. R. Jones (Ed.), *Miami symposium on the prediction of behavior: Aversive stimulation*. Miami: University of Miami Press.

Kamin, L. J. (1969). Predictability, surprise, attention, and conditioning. In R. Church & B. Campbell (Eds.), *Punishment and aversive behavior* (pp. 279–296). New York: Appleton-Century-Crofts.

Kandel, E. R. (1978). *A cell-biological approach to learning*. Bethesda, MD: Society for Neuroscience.

Kandel, E. R., & Schwartz, J. H. (1982). Molecular biology of memory: Modulation of transmitter release. *Science, 218*, 433–443.

Kandel, E. R., & Schwartz, J. H. (1983). *Principles of neural science*. New York: Elsevier/North Holland.

Kandel, E.R., & Spencer, V. A. (1968). Cellular neurophysiological approaches in the study of learning. *Physiology Review, 48*, 65–134.

Kant, I. (1931). *Critique of pure reason* (N. Kemp Smith, Trans.). London: Macmillan.

Kaplan, J. (1968). Approach and inhibitory reactions in rats after bilateral hippocampal damage. *Journal of Comparative and Physiological Psychology, 65*, 274–281.

Kaplan, R. F., Verfaellie, M., DeWitt, L. D., & Caplan, L. R. (1990). Effects of changes in stimulus contingency on visual extinction. *Neurology, 40*, 1299–1301.

Kasamatsu, T. (1983). Neuronal plasticity maintained by the central norepinephrine system in the cat visual cortex. In J. M. Sprague & A. N. Epstein (Eds.), *Progress in psychobiology and physiological psychology* (pp. 1–83). New York: Academic Press.

Kasamatsu, T., Pettigrew, J., & Ary, M. (1979). Restoration of visual cortical plasticity by local microperfusion of norepinephrine. *Journal of Comparative Neurology, 185*, 163–182.

Katkin, E. S. (1985). Blood, sweat, and tears: Individual differences in autonomic self-perception. *Psychophysiology, 22*(2), 125–137.

Kaufman, A. S. (1979). *Intelligence testing with the WISC-R*. New York: John Wiley.

Keele, S. W. (1968). Movement control in skilled motor performance. *Psychological Bulletin, 70*, 387–403.

Keele, S. W. (1973). *Attention and human performance*. Pacific Palisades, CA: Goodyear.

Keele, S. W. (1981). Behavioral analysis of movement. In V. B. Brooks (Eds.), *Handbook of physiology (Vol. 2): Motor control, part 2*. Baltimore, MD: American Physiological Society.

Kemble, E. D., & Beckman, G. J. (1970). Vicarious trial and error following amygdaloid lesions in rats. *Neuropsychologia, 8*, 161–169.

Kemper, T. (1986). Neuroanatomical and neuropathological changes in normal aging and in dementia. In M. L. Albert (Ed.), *Clinical neurology of aging* (pp. 9–52). New York: Oxford Press.

Kendler, T. S. (1971). Continuity theory and cue-dominance. In H. H. Kendler & J. T. Spence (Eds.), *Tenets of neurobehaviorism* (pp. 237–264). New York: Appleton-Century-Crofts.

Kendler, H.H., & Kendler, T. S. (1962). Vertical and horizontal processes in problem solving. *Psychological Review, 69*, 1–16.

Kennard, M. A. (1939). Alterations in response to visual stimuli following lesions of frontal lobe in monkeys. *Archives of Neurology and Psychiatry, 41*, 1153–1165.

Kennard, M. A., & Ectors, L. (1938). Forced circling movements in monkeys following lesions of the frontal lobe. *Journal of Neurophysiology, 1*, 45–54.

Kennard, M. A., Spencer, S., & Fountain, G. (1941). Hyperactivity in monkeys following lesions of the frontal lobes. *Journal of Neurophysiology, 4*, 512–524.

Kety, S. (1970). The biogenic amines in the central nervous system: Their possible role in arousal, emotion and learning. In F. O. Schmitt (Ed.), *The neurosciences: Second study program*. Cambridge: MIT Press.

Kety, S. S. (1980). The syndrome of schizophrenia: Unresolved questions and opportunities for research. *British Journal of Psychiatry, 136*, 421–436.

Khachaturian, Z. S. (1985). Diagnosis of Alzheimer's disease. *Archives of Neurology, 42*, 1097–1105.

Khomskaya, E. D., & Luria, A. R. (Eds.). (1977). *Problems in neuropsychology: Psychophysiological investigations*. Moscow: Nauka.

Kievit, J., & Kuypers, H. G. J. M. (1975). Basal forebrain and hypothalamic connections to frontal and parietal cortex in the rhesus monkey. *Science, 187*, 660–662.

Killeen, P. R. (1984). Incentive theory: 3. Adaptive clocks. In J. Gibbon & L. Allan (Eds.), *Timing and time perception, Annals of the New York Academy of Sciences* (Vol. 423, pp. 515–527). New York: New York Academy of Sciences.

Killeen, P. R., & Fetterman, J. G. (1988). A behavioral theory of timing. *Psychological Review, 92*(2), 274–295.

Kimble, D. P. (1968). Hippocampus and internal inhibition. *Psychological Bulletin, 70*, 285–295.

Kimble, D. P., & Greene, E. G. (1968). Absence of latent learning in rats with hippocampal lesions. *Psychonomic Science, 11*, 99–100.

Kimble, D. P., & Kimble, R. J. (1970). The effect of hippocampal lesions on extinction and "hypothesis" behavior in rats. *Physiology and Behavior, 5*, 735–738.

Kimble, G. A., & Ost, J. W. P. (1961). A conditioned inhibitory process in eyelid conditioning. *Journal of Experimental Psychology, 61*, 150–156.

Kimble, D. P., Bagshaw, M. H., & Pribram, K. H. (1965). The GSR of monkeys during orienting and attention after selective ablation of the cingulate and frontal cortex. *Neuropsychologia, 3*, 121–128.

Kimble, D. P., Kirkby, R. J., & Stein, D. G. (1966). Response perseveration interpretation of passive avoidance deficits in hippocampectomized rats. *Journal of Comparative and Physiological Psychology, 61*, 141–143.

Kimmel, H., Van Olst, E. H., & Orlebeke, J. F. (Eds.), (1979). *The orienting reflex in humans*. Hillsdale, NJ: Erlbaum.

Kimura, D. (1967). Functional asymmetry of the brain in dichotic listening. *Cortex, 3*, 163–178.

Kinchla, R. A. (1980). The measurement of attention. In R. S. Nickerson (Ed.), *Attention and performance* (Vol. 8, pp. 213–238). Hillsdale, N.J.: Erlbaum.

King, C., & Young, R. (1982). Attentional deficits with and without hyperactivity: teacher and peer perceptions. *Journal of Abnormal Child Psychology, 10*, 483–496.

Kinsbourne, M. (1970). A model for the mechanism of unilateral neglect of space. *Transactions of the American Neurological Association, 95*, 143.

Kinsbourne, M. (1974). Direction of gaze and distribution of cerebral thought processes. *Neuropsychologia, 12,* 270–281.

Kinsbourne, M. (1982). Hemispheric specialization and the growth of human understanding. *American Psychologist, 37,* 411–420.

Kirsner, K., & Smith, M. C. (1974). Modality effects in word recognition. *Memory and Cognition, 2,* 637–640.

Klein, D., Moscovitch, M., & Vigna, C. (1976). Attentional mechanisms and perceptual asymmetries in tachistoscopic recognition of words and faces. *Neuropsychologia, 14,* 55–66.

Kleinman, J. E., Casanova, M. F., & Jaskiw, G. E. (1988). The neuropathology of schizophrenia. *Schizophrenia Bulletin, 14,* 209–216.

Kleinsmith, L. J., & Kaplan, S. (1963). Paired-associate learning as a function of arousal and interpolated interval. *Journal of Experimental Psychology, 65,* 190–193.

Kleist, K. (1907). Corticale (innervatorische) Apraxie. *Journal of Psychiatry, 28,* 65–72.

Kleitman, N. (1963). *Sleep and wakefulness.* Chicago: University of Chicago Press.

Kleitman, N., & Jackson, D. P. (1951). *Journal of Abnormal Physiology, 3,* 309–328.

Klorman, R., Brumaghim, J. T., Salzman, L. F., et al. (1990). Effects of methylphenidate on processing negativities in patients with attention-deficit hyperactivity disorder. *Psychophysiology, 27,* 328–337.

Klove, H. (1963). Clinical neuropsychology. In F. M. Forster (Ed.), *The medical clinics of North America.* New York: Saunders.

Kluver, H., & Bucy, P. C. (1939). Preliminary analysis of the temporal lobe functions in monkeys. *Archives of Neurology and Psychiatry, 47,* 979–1000.

Koch, C., & Ullman, S. (1985). Shifts in selective visual attention: Toward the underlying neural circuitry. *Human Neurobiology,* 291–227.

Kohler, W. (1947). *Gestalt psychology.* New York: Liveright.

Kojima, S., & Goldman-Rakic, P. S. (1982). Delay-related activity of prefrontal neurons in rhesus monkeys performing delayed response. *Brain Research, 248,* 43–49.

Kojima, S., & Goldman-Rakic, P. S. (1984). Functional analysis of spatially discriminative neurons in prefrontal cortex of rhesus monkeys. *Brain Research, 291,* 229–240.

Kojima, S., Matsumara, M., & Kubota, K. (1981). Prefrontal neuron activity during delayed-response performance without imperative GO signals in the monkey. *Experimental Neurology, 74,* 369–407.

Kojima, S., Kojima, M., & Goldman-Rakic, P. S. (1982). Operant behavioral analysis of memory loss in monkeys with prefrontal lesions. *Brain Research, 248,* 51–59.

Konorski, J. (1948). *Conditioned reflexes and neuron organization.* Cambridge, England: Cambridge University Press.

Konorski, J. (1957). On the hyperactivity in animals following lesions of the frontal lobes. In *Problems of physiology of the central nervous system* (pp. 285–293). Moscow: USSR Academy of Sciences.

Konorski, J. (1970). *Integrative activity of the brain.* Chicago and London: University of Chicago Press.

Konorski, J. (1971). The role of prefrontal control in programming of motor behaviour. In J. D. Maser (Ed.), *Efferent organization and integrative behaviour.* London: University of Chicago Press.

Konorski, J. (1972). Physiological mechanisms of internal inhibition. In R. A. Boakes & M. S. Halliday (Eds.), *Inhibition and learning.* London: Academic Press.

Kornblith, C., & Olds, J. (1973). Unit activity in brain stem reticular formation of the rat during learning. *Journal of Neurophysiology, 36,* 1211–1344.

Korner, P. L. (1971). Integrative neural cardiovascular control. *Physiological Review, 51,* 312–367.

Kotliar, B. I. (1969). Activity of the nervous cells at the time of the formation of a temporary connection. *Nauchn. dokl. vyssh. shkoly,* ser. biol. nauki, *12.*

Kotliar, B. I. (1971). Electrophysiological investigation of the formation of a temporary connection at the systemic and neuronal levels. *Avtoref. dokt. diss. M.*

Kotliar, B. E. (1983). *Neural mechanism of conditioning.* (N. M. Weinberger, Ed. and Trans.). New York: Pergamon Press.

Kotliar, B. I., & Yeroshenko, T. (1971). Hypothalamic glucoreceptors: The phenomenon of plasticity. *Physiology and Behavior, 7,* 609–615.

Kraepelin, E. (1931). *Dementia praecox and paraphrenia.* Edinburgh: Livingstone.

Kraiuhin, C., Gordon, E., Meares, R., & Howson, A. (1986). Psychometrics and event-related potentials in the diagnosis of dementia. *Journal of Gerontology, 41,* 154–162.

Kramer, A., Schneider, W., Fisk, A., & Donchin, E. (1986). The effects of practice and task structure on the components of the event-related brain potential. *Psychophysiology, 23,* 33–47.

Krane, R. V., & Ison, J. R. (1971). Positive induction in differential instrumental conditioning. *Journal of Comparative and Physiological Psychology, 75*, 129–135.

Krasne, F. B. (1976). Invertebrate systems as a means of gaining insight into the nature of learning and memory. In M. R. Rosenzweig & E. L. Bennett (Eds.), *Neural mechanisms of learning and memory* (pp. 401–429). Cambridge, MA: MIT Press.

Kristofferson, A. B. (1977). A real-time criterion theory of duration discrimination. *Perceptual Psychophysiology, 21*(2), 105–117.

Kristofferson, A. B. (1980). A quantal step function in duration discrimination. *Perceptual Psychophysiology, 27*(4), 300–306.

Kristofferson, A. B. (1984). Quantal and deterministic timing in human duration discrimination. In J. Gibbon & L. Allan (Eds.), *Timing and time perception, Annals of the New York Academy of Sciences* (Vol. 423, pp. 3–15). New York: New York Academy of Sciences.

Krupp, L. B., Alvarez, L. A., LaRocca, N. G., & Scheinberg, L. C. (1988). Fatigue in multiple sclerosis. *Archives of Neurology, 45*, 435–437.

Kuffler, S. W. (1953). Discharge patterns and functional organization of the mammalian retina. *Journal of Neurophysiology, 16*, 37–68.

Kutas, M., McCarthy, G., & Donchin, E. (1977). Augmenting mental chronometry: The P300 as a measure of stimulus evaluation time. *Science, 197*, 792–795.

LaBerge, D. (1990). Thalamic and cortical mechanisms of attention suggested by recent positron emission tomographic experiments. *Journal of Comparative Neuroscience, 2*(4), 358–373.

LaBerge, D., & Brown, V. (1989). Theory of attentional operations in shape identification. *Psychological Review, 96*, 101–124.

LaBerge, D., Van Gilder, P., & Yellott, S. (1971). A cueing technique in choice reaction time. *Journal of Experimental Psychology, 87*, 225–228.

LaBerge, D., Petersen, R.J., & Norden, M. J. (1977). Exploring the limits of cueing. In S. Dornic (Ed.), *Attention and performance VI*. London: Academic Press.

Lacey, B. C., & Lacey, J. I. (1978). Two way communications between the heart and the brain. *American Psychologist, 33*, 99–113.

Lacey, J. I. (1959). Psychophysiological approaches to the evaluation of psychotherapeutic process and outcome. In E. A. Rubenstein & M. B. Parloff (Eds.), *Research in psychotherapy* (pp. 160–208). Washington, DC: American Psychological Association.

Lacey, J. I. (1967). Somatic response patterning and stress: Some revisions of activation theory. In M. H. Appley & R. Trumbull (Eds.), *Psychological stress: Issues in research*. New York: Appleton-Century-Crofts.

Lacey, J. I., Kagan, J., Lacey, B., & Moss, H. A. (1963). The visceral level: Situational determinants and behavioral correlates of autonomic response patterns. In P. H. Knapp (Ed.), *Expression of the emotions in man*. New York: International Universities Press.

Lahey, B. B., Shaughency, E., Strauss, C., & Frame, C. (1984). Are attention deficit disorders with and without hyperactivity similar or dissimilar disorders? *Journal of the American Academy of Child Psychiatry, 23*, 302–309.

Lamb, M. R., Robertson, L. C., & Knight, R. T. (1989). Attention and interference in the processing of global and local information: Effects of unilateral temporal-parietal lobe lesions. *Neuropsychologia, 27*(4), 471–483.

Lane, D. M. (1980). Incidental learning and the development of selective attention. *Psychological Review, 87*, 316–319.

Langfitt, T. W., Obrist, W. D., Alavi, A., Grossman, R., Zimmerman, R., Jaggi, J., Uzzell, B., Reivich, M., & Patton, D. (1987). Regional structure and function in head injured patients: Correlation of CT, MRI, PET, CBF, and neuropsychological assessment. In H. S. Levin, J. Grafman, & H. M. Eisenberg (Eds.), *Neurobehavioral recovery from head injury*. New York: Oxford University Press.

Laplane, D., Degos, J. D., Baulac, M., & Gray, F. (1981). Bilateral infarction of the anterior cingulate gyri and of the fornices. *Journal of the Neurological Sciences, 51*, 289–300.

Lashley, K. S. (1929). *Brain mechanisms and intelligence: A quantitative study of injuries to the brain*. Chicago: University of Chicago Press.

Lawrence, D. H. (1949). Acquired distinctiveness of cues: 1. Transfer between discriminations on the basis of familiarity with the stimulus. *Journal of Experimental Psychology, 39*, 770–784.

LeDoux, J. E., Thompson, M. E., Iadecola, C., Tucker, L. W., & Reis, D. J. (1983). Local cerebral blood flow increases during auditory and emotional processing in the conscious rat. *Science, 221*, 576–578.

Lestienne, F., Whittington, D., & Bizzi, E. (1983). Coordination of eye-head movements in alert monkeys: Behavior of eye-related neurons in the brain stem. In A. Hein & M. Jeannerod (Eds.), *Spatially oriented behavior* (pp. 105–118). New York: Springer-Verlag.

Leuba, C., Birch, L., & Appleton, J. (1968). Human problem solving during complete paralysis of the voluntary musculature. *Psychological Reports, 22*, 849–855.

Levin, H. S., Benton, A. L., & Grossman, R. G. (1982). *Neurobehavioral consequences of closed head injury.* New York: Oxford University Press.

Levit, R. A., Sutton, S., & Zubin, J. (1973). Evoked potential correlates of information processing in psychiatric patients. *Psychological Medicine, 3*, 487–494.

Levy, J. (1974). Cerebral asymmetries as manifested in split-brain man. In M. Kinsbourne & W. L. Smith (Eds.), *Hemispheric disconnection and cerebral function.* Springfield, IL: C. C. Thomas.

Levy, J., & Trevarthen, C. (1976). Meta-control of hemispheric function in human split-brain patients. *Journal of Experimental Psychology: Human Perception, 2*, 299–312.

Levy, J., Trevarthen, C., & Sperry, R. W. (1972). Perception of bilateral chimeric figures following hemispheric deconnection. *Brain, 95*, 61–78.

Lewis, M., & Baldini, N. (1979). Attentional processes and individual differences. In A. H. Gordon & M. Lewis (Eds.), *Attention and cognitive development* (pp. 135–172). New York: Plenum Press.

Lezak, M. D. (1978). Subtle sequelae of brain damage: Perplexity, distractibility and fatigue. *American Journal of Physical Medicine, 57*, 9–15.

Lezak, M. D. (1979). *Behavioral concomitants of configurational disorganization.* Paper presented at the seventh annual meeting of the International Neuropsychological Society, New York City.

Lezak, M. D. (1983). *Neuropsychological assessment* (2nd ed.). New York: Oxford University Press.

Libet, B. (1970). Generation of slow inhibitory and excitatory postsynaptic potentials. *Federation Proceedings, 29*, 1945–1956.

Libet, B. (1984). Heterosynaptic interaction at a sympathetic neuron as a model for induction and storage of a postsynaptic memory trace. In G. Lynch, J. L. McGaugh, & N. M. Weinberger (Eds.), *Neurobiology of learning and memory* (pp. 405–430). New York: Guilford Press.

Libet, B., & Owman, C. (1974). Concomitant changes in formaldehyde-induced fluorescence of dopamine interneurones and in slow inhibitory postsynaptic potentials of rabbit superior cervical ganglion, induced by stimulation of preganglionic nerve by a muscarinic agent. *Journal of Physiology (London), 237*, 635–662.

Libet, B., & Tosaka, T. (1970). Dopamine as a synaptic transmitter and modulator on sympathetic ganglia: A different mode of synaptic action. *Proceedings of the National Academy of Sciences, 67*, 667–673.

Licklider, J. C. R. (1960). *Quasi-linear operator models in the study of manual tracking.* Glencoe, IL: Free Press.

Lindsley, D. B. (1952). Psychological phenomena and the electroencephalogram. *Electroencephalography and Clinical Neurophysiology, 4*, 443–456.

Lindsley, D. B. (1960). Attention, consciousness, sleep and wakefulness. In J. Field, H. W. Magoun, & V. E. Hall (Eds.), *Handbook of physiology* (Vol. 3, pp. 1553–1593). Washington, DC: American Physiological Society.

Lindsley, D. B. (1970). The role of nonspecific reticulo-thalamo-cortical systems in emotion. In P. Black (Ed.), *Physiological correlates of emotion.* New York: Academic Press.

Lindsley, D. B., Bowden, J. W., & Magoun, H. W. (1949). Effect upon the EEG of acute injury to the brain stem activating system. *Electroencephalography and Clinical Neurophysiology, 1*, 475–486.

Lloyd, D. P. C. (1941). A direct central inhibitory action of dromically conducted impulses. *Journal of Neurophysiology, 4*, 184–190.

Lloyd, D. P. C. (1946). Facilitation and inhibition of spinal motoneurons. *Journal of Neurophysiology, 9*, 421–438.

Locke, L. J., & Fehr, F. S. (1970). Young children's use of the speech code in a recall task. *Journal of Experimental Child Psychology, 10*, 367–373.

Loeb, M., & Alluisis, E. (1984). Theories of vigilance. In J. S. Warm (Ed.), *Sustained attention in human performance* (pp. 179–205). London: Wiley.

Logan, F. A. (1972). Essentials of a theory of discrimination learning. In H. H. Kendler & J. T. Spence (Eds.), *Tenets of neurobehaviorism* (pp. 265–284). New York: Appleton-Century-Crofts.

Loiselle, D., Stamm, J. S., Maintinsky, S., & Whipple, S. C. (1980). Evoked potential and behavioral signs of attentive dysfunctions in hyperactive boys. *Psychophysiology, 17*, 193–201.

Loiseau, P., Stube, E., Broustet, D., Batteleochi, S., Gomeni, C., & Morselli, P. D. (1980). Evaluation of memory function in a population of epileptic patients and matched controls. *Acta Neurologica Scandinavica, 62*, 58–61.

Loney, J., Langhorne, J., & Paternite, C. (1978). An empirical basis for subgrouping the hyperkinetic/minimal brain dysfunction syndrome. *Journal of Abnormal Psychology, 87*, 431–441.

Lou, H. C., Henriksen, L., & Bruhn, P. (1984). Focal cerebral hypoperfusion in children with dysphasia and/or attention deficit disorder. *Archives of Neurology, 41*, 825–829.

Lou, H. C., Henriksen, L., Bruhn, P., Borner, H., & Neilson, J. B. (1989). Striatal dysfunction in attention deficit and hyperkinetic disorder. *Archives of Neurology, 46*, 48–52.

Lovejoy, E. P. (1965). An attention theory of discrimination learning. *Journal of Mathematical Psychology, 2*, 342–362.

Lovibond, S. H. (1969). Habituation of the orienting response to multiple stimulus sequences. *Psychophysiology, 5*, 435–439.

Luce, R. D. (1960). The theory of selective information and some of its behavioral applications. In R. D. Luce (Ed.), *Developments in mathematical psychology* (pp. 5–119). Glencoe, IL: Free Press.

Luria, A. R. (1966). *Higher cortical functions in man* (B. Haigh, trans.). New York: Basic Books.

Luria, A. R., & Khomskaya, E. D. (1962). An objective study of ocular movements and their control. *Psychol. Beitr., 6*.

Luria, A. R., & Khomskaya, E. D. (Eds.). (1966). *The frontal lobes and regulation of psychological processes.* Moscow: Moscow University Press.

Luria, A. R., & Vinogradova, O. S. (1959). An objective investigation of the dynamics of semantic systems. *British Journal of Psychology, 50*, 89–105.

Luria, A. R., Karpov, B. A., & Yarbus, A. L. (1966). Disturbances of active visual perception with lesions of the frontal lobes. *Cortex, 2*, 202–212.

Lydic, R., Albers, H. E., Tepper, B., & Moore-Ede, M. C. (1982). Three-dimensional structure of the mammalian suprachiasmatic nuclei: a comparative study of five species. *Journal of Comparative Neurology, 204*, 225–237.

Lynch, G. (1986). *Synapses, circuits, and the beginnings of memory.* Cambridge: MIT Press.

Lynch, G., & Baudry, M. (1984). The biochemistry of memory: A new and specific hypothesis. *Science, 224*, 1057–1063.

Lynch, J. C. (1980). The functional organization of the posterior parietal association cortex. *Behavior and Brain Science, 3*, 485–534.

Lynch, J. C., Mountcastle, V. B., Talbot, W. H., & Yin, T. C. T. (1977). Directed visual attention. *Journal of Neurophysiology, 40*, 362–389.

Lynn, R. (1966). *Attention, arousal and the orientation reaction.* Oxford, England: Pergamon Press.

MacDougall J. M., Van Hoesen, G. W., & Mitchell J. C. (1969). Anatomical organisation of septal projections in maintenance of DRL behavior. *Journal of Comparative and Physiological Psychology, 68*, 568–575.

MacKay, D. (1951). In search of basic symbols. In Heinz Von Foerster (Ed.), *Cybernetics* (pp. 181–221). New York: Josiah Macy Jr. Foundation.

Mackintosh, N. J. (1965). Selective attention in animal discrimination learning. *Psychological Bulletin, 64*, 124–150.

Mackworth, J. F. (1965). Deterioration of signal detectability during a vigilance teak as a function of background event rate. *Psychnomic Science, 3*, 421–422.

Mackworth, J. F. (1969). *Vigilance and habituation.* Baltimore: Penguin.

Mackworth, J. F., & Taylor, M. M. (1963). The d' measure of signal detectability in vigilance-like situations. *Canadian Journal of Psychology, 17*, 302–325.

Mackworth, N. H. (1950). Researches in the measurement of human performance. *MRC Special Report Series*, No. 268. London: H.M. Stationery Office.

Magnun, G. R., & Hillyard, S. A. (1987). The spatial allocation of visual attention as indexed by event-related brain potentials. *Human Factors, 29*, 195–212.

Magnun, G. R., & Hillyard, S. A. (1988). Spatial gradients of visual attention: Behavioral and electro-physiological evidence. *Electroencephalography and Clinical Neurophysiology, 70,* 417–428.

Mahut, H., Moss, M., & Zola-Morgan, S. (1981). Retention deficits after combined amygdalo-hippocampal and selective hippocampal resections in the monkey. *Neuropsychologia, 19,* 201–225.

Malmo, R. B. (1942). Interference factors in delayed response in monkeys after removal of frontal lobes. *Journal of Neurophysiology, 5,* 295–308.

Malmo, R. B., & Surwillo, W. W. (1960). Sleep deprivation: Changes in performance and physiological indicants of activation. *Psychological Monographs, 74* (Whole No. 502).

Malone, J. R. L., & Hemsley, D. R. (1977). Lowered responsiveness and auditory signal detectability during depression. *Psychosomatic Medicine, 7,* 717–722.

Maltzman, I. (1955). Thinking: From a behavioristic point of view. *Psychological Review, 62,* 275–286.

Maltzman, I. (1968). Theoretical conceptions of semantic conditioning and generalization. In T. R. Dixon & D. L. Horton (Eds.), *Verbal behavior and general behavior theory* (pp. 291–339). Englewood Cliffs, NJ: Prentice-Hall.

Maltzman, I. (1979). Orienting reflexes and classical conditioning in humans. In H. D. Kimmel, E. H. van Olst, & J. F. Orlebeke (Eds.), *The orienting reflex in humans* (pp. 323–352). Hillsdale, NJ: Erlbaum.

Maltzman, I., Langdon, B., & Feeney, D. (1970). Semantic generalization without prior conditioning. *Journal of Experimental Psychology, 83,* 73–75.

Mandel, I. J., & Bridger, W. H. (1973). Is there classical conditioning without cognitive expectancy? *Psychophysiology, 10,* 87–90.

Mandell, M. P. (1968). Instructions, attitudinal factors and anxiety in "semantic conditioning" situations involving physiological and performance measures. *Dissertation Abstracts, 29,* 4403–B. (University Microfilms No. 69-7255.)

Mangun, S. R., & Hillyard, S. A. (1988). Spatial gradients of visual attention: Behavioral and electro-physiological evidence. *Electroencephalography and Clinical Neurophysiology, 70,* 417–428.

Marsh, G. G., Markham, C. M., & Ansel, R. (1971). Levodopa's awakening effect on patients with Parkinsonism. *Journal of Neurology, Neurosurgery, and Psychiatry, 34,* 209–218.

Marshall, J. F., Turner, B. H., & Teitelbaum, P. (1971). Sensory neglect produced by lateral hypothalamic damage. *Science, 174,* 523–525.

Mason, S. T. (1981). Noradrenaline in the brain: Progress in theories of behavioral function. *Progress in Neurobiology, 16,* 263–303.

Massaro, D. W. (1972). Preperceptual images, processing time, and perceptual units in auditory perception. *Psychological Review, 79,* 124–145.

Massaro, D. W. (1975). *Experimental psychology and information processing.* Chicago: Rand McNally.

May, J. R., & Johnson, H. J. (1973). Physiological activity to internally elicited arousal and inhibitory thoughts. *Journal of Abnormal Psychology, 82,* 239–245.

Mayeux, R. (1983). Emotional changes associated with basal ganglia disorders. In K. M. Heilman & P. Satz (Eds.), *Neuropsychology of human emotion.* New York: Guilford Press.

Mayeux, R., Stern, Y., Rosen, J., & Leventhal, J. (1981). Depression, intellectual impairment, and Parkinson disease. *Neurology, 31,* 645–650.

Maylor, E. A., & Hockey, R. (1987). Effects of repetition on the facilitatory and inhibitory components of orienting in visual space. *Neuropsychologia, 25,* 41–54.

Mays, L. E., & Sparks, D. L. (1980). Saccades are spatially, not retinocentrically, coded. *Science, 208,* 1163–1165.

McCarley, R. W., Faux, S. F., Shenton, M. E., Nestor, P. G., & Adams, J. (1991). Event-related potentials in schizophrenia: Their biological and clinical correlates and a new model of schizophrenic patho-physiology. *Schizophrenia Research, 4,* 209–231.

McCarley, R. W., Shenton, M. E., O'Donnell, B. F., Faux, S. F., Kikinis, R., Nestor, P. G., & Jolesz, F. A. (1992). Auditory P300 abnormalities and left posterior temporal gyrus volume reduction in schizophrenia. *Archives of General Psychiatry,* in press.

McCarthy, G., & Donchin, E. (1981). A comparison of P300 latency and reaction time. *Science, 211,* 77–80.

McCleary, R. A. (1966). Response-modulating functions of the limbic system: Initiation and suppression. In E. Stellar & J. M. Sprague (Eds.), *Progress in physiological psychology* (Vol. 1). New York: Academic Press.

McClelland, J. L. (1979). On the time relations of mental processes: An examination of systems of processes in cascade. *Psychological Review, 86*, 287–330.

McClelland, J. L., & Rumelhart, D. E. (1986). A distributed model of human learning and memory. In J. L. McClelland & D. E. Rumelhart (Eds.), *Parallel distributed processing: Explorations in the microstructure of cognition. Volume 2: Psychological and biological models.* Cambridge, MA: MIT Press.

McClelland, J. L., & Rumelhart, D. E. (1986). *Parallel distributed processing: Explorations in the microstructure of cognition* (Vols. 1, 2). Cambridge: MIT Press.

McGaugh, J. L. (1966). Time-dependent processes in memory storage. *Science, 153*, 1351–1358.

McGhie, A., & Chapman, J. (1961). Disorders of attention and perception in early schizophrenia. *British Journal of Medical Psychology, 34*, 103–116.

McGrath, J. J. (1963). Irrelevant stimulation and vigilance performance. In J. Buckner & F. F. McGrath (Eds.), *Vigilance: A symposium.* New York: McGraw-Hill.

McGrath, J. J. (1965). Performance sharing in an audio-visual vigilance task. *Human Factors, 7*, 141–153.

McGuigan, F. J. (1978). Imagery and thinking: Covert functioning of the motor system. In G. E. Schwartz & D. Shapiro (Eds.), *Consciousness and self-regulation: Advances in research and theory* (Vol. 2). New York: Plenum Press.

McGuigan, F. J., & Rodier, W. I., III. (1968). Effects of auditory stimulation on covert oral behavior during silent reading. *Journal of Experimental Psychology, 76*, 649–655.

McIntyre, D. C. (1979). Effects of focal vs. generalized kindled convulsions from anterior neocortex or amygdala on CER acquisition in rats. *Physiology and Behavior, 23*, 855–859.

McLean, O. (1959). The limbic system with respect to two life principles. In *2nd Macy Conference: The Central Nervous System and Behavior.* Bethesda, MD: National Institutes of Health.

McLeod, P., & Posner, M. I. (1984). Privileged loops from perception to act. In H. Bouma & D. Bowhius (Eds.), *Attention and performance* (Vol. 10). Hillsdale, NJ: Erlbaum.

McNaughton, B. L., Barnes, C. A., & O'Keefe, J. (1983). The contributions of position, direction, and velocity to single unit activity in the hippocampus of freely moving rats. *Experimental Brain Research, 52*, 41–49.

Meadows, M. E. (1992). Emotional responsivity following right hemisphere damage: A psychophysiological and behavioral analysis. Ph.D. diss, Boston University, Boston, MA.

Meadows, M. E., & Kaplan, R. F. (1992). Dissociation of autonomic and subjective responses to emotional slides in right hemisphere damaged patients. *Journal of Clinical and Experimental Neuropsychology, 14*, 404.

Meck, W. H. (1984). Attentional bias between modalities: Effect on the internal clock, memory, and decision stages used in animal time discrimination. In J. Gibbon & L. Allan (Eds.), *Timing and time perception, Annals of the New York Academy of Sciences* (pp. 528–541). New York: New York Academy of Sciences.

Meck, W. H., Komeily-Zadeh, F., & Church, R. M. (1981). *Interference of signal timing by response timing.* Paper presented at meeting of the Psychonomic Society, Philadelphia.

Melzac, R. (1973). The puzzle of pain. New York: Basic Books.

Melzac, R., & Wall, P. D. (1965). Pain mechanisms: A new theory. *Science, 150*, 971.

Merzenich, M. M., Kaas, J. H., Wall, J. T., Sur, M., Nelson, R. J., & Feldman, D. J. (1983). Progression of change following median nerve section in the cortical representation of the hand in areas 3b and 1 in adult owl and squirrel monkeys. *Neuroscience, 10*, 639–665.

Mesulam, M. A. (1981). A cortical network for directed attention and unilateral neglect. *Archives of Neurology, 10*, 304–325.

Mesulam, M-M. (1985). *Principles of behavioral neurology.* Philadelphia: F. A. Davis.

Mesulam, M. M., Van Hoesen, G. W., Pandya, D. N., & Geschwind, N. (1977). Limbic and sensory connections of the inferior parietal lobule (area PG) in the rhesus monkey: A study with a new method for horseradish peroxidase histochemistry. *Brain Research, 136*, 393–414.

Meyer, D. R., & Harlow, H. F. (1952). Effects of multiple variables on delayed response performance by monkeys. *Journal of Genetic Psychology, 81*, 53–61.

Michon, J. A., & Jackson, J. L. (1984). Attentional effort and cognitive strategies in the processing of temporal information. In J. Gibbon & L. Allan (Eds.), *Timing and time perception, Annals of the New York Academy of Sciences* (Vol. 423, pp. 298–321). New York: New York Academy of Sciences.

Miles, F. A., & Evarts, E. V. (1979). Concepts of motor organization. *Annual Review of Psychology, 43*, 327–362.

Miller, G. A. (1956). The magical number seven, plus or minus two: Some limits on our capacity for processing information. *Psychological Review, 63,* 81–97.

Miller, G. A., & Frick, F. C. (1949). Statistical behavioristics and sequences of responses. *Psychological Review, 56,* 311–324.

Miller, M. H., & Orbach, J. (1972). Retention of spatial alternation following frontal lobe resections in stump-tailed macaques. *Neuropsychologia, 10,* 291–298.

Milner, B. (1959). The memory defect in bilateral hippocampal lesions. *Psychiatric Research, 11,* 43–58.

Milner, B. (1962). Laterality effects in audition. In V. B. Mountcastle (Ed.), *Interhemispheric relations and cerebral dominance.* Baltimore: Johns Hopkins University Press.

Milner, B. (1963). Effects of different brain lesions on card sorting. *Archives of Neurology, 9,* 90–100.

Milner, B. (1964). Some effects of frontal lobotomy in man. In J. M. Warren & K. Akert (Eds.), *The frontal granular cortex and behavior* (pp. 313–334). New York: McGraw-Hill.

Milner, B. (1965). Visually-guided maze learning in man: Effects of bilateral hippocampal, bilateral frontal and unilateral cerebral lesions. *Neuropsychologia, 3,* 317–338.

Milner, B. (1967). Brain mechanisms suggested by studies of temporal lobes. In F. L. Darley (Ed.). *Brain mechanisms underlying speech and language* (pp. 122–145). New York: Grune & Stratton.

Milner, B. (1968). Visual recognition and recall after right temporal lobe excision in man. *Neuropsychologia, 6,* 191–209.

Milner, B. (1971). Interhemispheric differences in the localization of psychological processes in man. *British Medical Bulletin, 27,* 272.

Milner, B. (1975). Psychological aspects of focal epilepsy and its neurosurgical management. *Advances in Neurology, 8,* 299–321.

Milner, B. (1982). Some cognitive effects of frontal-lobe lesions in man. *Philosophical Transactions of the Royal Society of London, [Biol. J.], 298,* 211–226.

Mindham, H. S. (1970). Psychiatric syndromes in Parkinsonism. *Journal of Neurology, Neurosurgery, and Psychiatry, 30,* 188–191.

Minsky, M., & Papert, S. (1969). *Perceptrons.* Cambridge: MIT Press.

Mirsky, A. F. (1978). Attention: A neuropsychological perspective. In *Education and the brain.* Chicago: National Society for the Study of Education.

Mirsky, A. F. (1989). The neuropsychology of attention: Elements of a complex behavior. In E. Perelman (Ed.), *Integrating theory and practice in clinical neuropsychology.* Hillsdale, NJ: Erlbaum Associates.

Mirsky, A. F., & Duncan, C. C. (1986). Etiology and expression of schizophrenia: neurobiological and psychosocial factors. *Annual Review of Psychology, 37,* 291–319.

Mirsky, A. F., Primac, D. W., Marsan, C. A., Rosvold, H. E., & Stevens, J. R. (1960). A comparison of the psychological test performance of patients with focal and non-focal epilepsy. *Experimental Neurology, 2,* 75–89.

Mirsky, A. F., Silberman, E. K., Latz, A., & Nagler, S. (1985). Adult outcomes of high-risk children: Differential effects of town and kibbutz rearing. *Schizophrenia Bulletin, 11,* 150–154.

Mischel, W. Shoda, Y., & Rodriguez, M. L. (1989). Delay of gratification in children. *Science, 244,* 933–938.

Mishkin, M. (1957). Effects of small frontal lesions on delayed alternation in monkeys. *Journal of Neurophysiology, 20,* 615–622.

Mishkin, M. (1964). Perseveration of central sets after frontal lesions in monkeys. In J. M. Warren & K. Akert (Eds.), *The frontal granular cortex and behavior* (pp. 219–241). New York: McGraw-Hill.

Mishkin, M. (1978). Memory in monkeys severely impaired by combined but not by separate removal of amygdala and hippocampus. *Nature, 273,* 297–298.

Mishkin, M. (1982). A memory system in the monkey. *Philosophical Transactions of the Royal Society of London, B298,* 85–95.

Mishkin, M., & Bachevalier, J. (1983). Object recognition impaired by ventromedial but not dorsolateral prefrontal cortical lesions in monkeys. *Society for Neurosciences Abstracts, 9,* 29.

Mishkin, M., Rosvold, H. E., & Pribram, K. H. (1953). Effects of Nembutal in baboons with frontal lesions. *Journal of Neurophysiology, 16,* 155–159.

Mishkin, M., Ungerleider, L.G., & Macko, K. A. (1983). Object vision and spatial vision: Two cortical pathways. *Trends in Neuroscience, 6,* 414–417.

Mishkin, M., Malamut, B., & Bachevalier, J. (1984). Memories and habits: Two neural systems. In G.

Lynch, J. L. McGaugh, & N. M. Weinberger (Eds.), *Neurobiology of learning and memory* (pp. 65–77). New York: Guilford Press.

Molnar, P., & Grastyan, E. (1972). Inhibition in motivation and reinforcement. In R. A. Boakes & M. S. Halliday (Eds.), *Inhibition and learning*. London: Academic Press.

Moore, R.Y. (1964). Effects of some rhinencephalic lesions on retention of conditioned avoidance behavior in cats. *Journal of Comparative and Physiological Psychology, 53,* 540–548.

Moray, N. (1959). Attention in dichotic listening: Affective cues and the influence of instructions. *Quarterly Journal of Experimental Psychology, 11,* 56–60.

Moray, N. (1970). *Attention: Selective processes in vision and learning.* New York: Academic Press.

Morrell, F. (1967). *Electrical signs of sensory coding.* New York: Rockefeller University Press.

Mortimer, J. A., Christensen, K. J., & Webster, D. D. (1984). Parkinson dementia. In G. W. Bruyn & H. L. Klawans (Eds.), *Handbook of clinical neurology: Vol. 46. Neurobehavioral disorders.* Amsterdam: Elsevier.

Moruzzi, G., & Magoun, H. W. (1949). Brain stem reticular formation and activation of the EEG. *Electroencephalography and Clinical Neurophysiology, 1,* 455–473.

Moscovitch, M. (1982). Multiple dissociations of function in amnesia. In L. Cermak (Ed.), *Human memory and amnesia* (pp. 337–370). Hillsdale, NJ: Erlbaum.

Moscovitch, M., & Klein, D. (1977). *Material specific interference effects and their relation to functional hemispheric asymmetrics.* Paper presented at the International Neuropsychological Society Meeting, Santa Fe, New Mexico.

Moscovitch, M., Scullian, D., & Christie, D. (1976). Early versus late stages of processing and their relation to functional hemispheric asymmetries in face recognition. *Journal of Experimental Psychology: Human Perception and Performance, 2,* 401–416.

Motter, B. C., & Mountcastle, V. B. (1981). The functional properties of the light-sensitive neurons of the posterior parietal cortex studied in waking monkeys: Foveal sparing and opponent vector organization. *Journal of Neuroscience, 1,* 3–26.

Mountcastle, V. (1978). Brain mechanisms for directed attention. *Journal of the Royal Society of Medicine, 71,* 14–27.

Mountcastle, V. B. (1979). An organizing principle for cerebral function: The unit module and the distributed system. In F. O. Schmitt & F. G. Worden (Eds.), *The neurosciences* (pp. 21–42). Cambridge: MIT Press.

Mountcastle, V. B., Lynch, J. C., Georgopoulos, A., Sakata, H., & Acuna, C. (1975). Posterior parietal association cortex of the monkey: Command function from operations within extrapersonal space. *Journal of Neurophysiology, 38,* 871–908.

Mountcastle, V. B., Anderson, R. A., & Motter, B. C. (1981). The influence of attentive fixation upon the excitability of the light sensitive neurons of the posterior parietal cortex. *Journal of Neuroscience, 1,* 1218–1235.

Mountcastle, V. B., Motter, B. C., Steinmetz, M. A., & Duffy, C. J. (1984). In G. M. Edelman, W. E. Gall, & W. M. Cowan (Eds.), *Dynamic aspects of neocortical functions* (pp. 159–193). New York: Wiley.

Mozer, M. C. (1988). A connectionist model of selective attention in visual perception. In *Proceedings of the 10th Conference of the Cognitive Science Society* (pp. 195–201). Montreal: Cognitive Science Society.

Murray, E. A., & Mishkin, M. A. (1983). A further examination of the medial temporal lobe structures involved in recognition memory in the monkey. *Society for Neurosciences, Abstracts, 9,* 27.

Murray, E. A., & Mishkin, M. (1985). Amygdalectomy impairs crossmodel association in monkeys. *Science, 228,* 601–605.

Murray, E. A., & Mishkin, M. (1986). Visual recognition in monkeys following rhinal cortical ablations combined with either amygdalectomy or hippocampectomy. *Journal of Neuroscience, 6,* 1991–2003.

Näätänen, R. (1982). Processing negativity: An evoked potential reflection of selective attention. *Psychological Bulletin, 92,* 605–640.

Nadeau, S. E., & Heilman, K. M. (1991). Gaze-dependent hemianopia without hemispatial neglect. *Neurology, 41,* 1244–1250.

Nakamura, Y., Goldberg, L. J., & Clemente, C. D. (1967). Nature of suppression of the masseteric monosynaptic reflex induced by stimulation of the orbital gyrus of the cat. *Brain Research, 6,* 184–198.

Nauta, W. J. H. (1946). Hypothalamic regulation of sleep in rats: Experimental study. *Journal of Neurophysiology, 9,* 285–316.

Nauta, W. J. H. (1961). Fiber degeneration following lesions of the amygdaloid complex in the monkey. *Journal of Anatomy, 95*, 515–531.

Nauta, W. J. H. (1964). Some efferent connections of the prefrontal cortex in the monkey. In J. Warren & K. Akert (Eds.), *The frontal granular cortex and behavior* (pp. 397–407). New York: McGraw-Hill.

Nauta, W. J. H. (1972). Neural associations of the frontal cortex. *Acta Neurobiological Experimentalis, 32*, 125–140.

Nauta, W. H. J., & Haymaker, W. (1969). Hypothalamic nuclei and fiber connections. In W. Haymaker, E. Anderson, & W. J. H. Nauta (Eds.), *The hypothalamus* (pp. 136–210). Springfield, IL: Thomas.

Naveh-Benjamin, M. (1987). Coding of spatial location information: An automatic process? *Journal of Experimental Psychology: Learning, Memory, and Cognition, 13*, 595–605.

Navon, D. (1985). Attention division or attention sharing? In M. I. Posner, & O. S. M. Marin (Eds.), *Attention and performance* (Vol. 11, pp. 133–146). Hillsdale, NJ: Erlbaum.

Navon, D., & Gopher, D. (1979). On the economy of the human-processing system. *Psychological Review, 86*, 214–255.

Navon, D., & Gopher, D. (1980). Task difficulty, resources, and dual-task performance. In R. S. Nickerson (Ed.), *Attention and performance* (Vol. 8, pp 297–315). Hillsdale, NJ: Erlbaum.

Neale, J. M., & Oltmanns, T. F. (1980). *Schizophrenia*. New York: Wiley.

Nehemkis, A. M., & Lewinsohn, P. M. (1972). Effects of left and right cerebral lesions in the naming process. *Perceptual and Motor Skills, 35*, 787–798.

Neisser, U. (1967). *Cognitive psychology*. New York: Appleton-Century-Crofts.

Neisser, U. (1969). *Selective reading: A method for the study of visual attention*. Presented at the 19th International Congress of Psychology, London.

Neisser, U. (1976). *Cognition and reality*. San Francisco: Freeman.

Neisser, U., & Becklen, R. (1975). Selective looking: Attending to visually-specified events. *Cognitive Psychology, 7*, 480–494.

Nelson, H. E. A. (1976). A modified card sorting test sensitive to frontal lobe defects. *Cortex, 12*, 318–324.

Neumann, O. (1987). Beyond capacity: A functional view of attention. In H. Heuer and A. F. Sanders (eds.), *Perspectives on Perception and Action*. Hillsdale, NJ: Erlbaum.

Newcombe, F., Ratcliff, G., & Damasio, H. (1987). Dissociable visual and spatial impairments following right posterior cerebral lesions. Clinical, neuropsychological, and anatomical evidence. *Neuropsychologia, 25*, 149–161.

Newell, A., & Simon, H. (1972). *Human problem solving*. Englewood Cliffs, NJ: Prentice-Hall.

Norman, D. A. (1968). Toward a theory of memory and attention. *Psychological Review, 75*(6), 522–536.

Norman, D. A., & Bobrow, D. A. (1975). On data-limited and resource-limited processes. *Cognitive Psychology, 7*, 44–64.

Norman, D. A., & Rumelhart, D. E. (1975). *Explorations in cognition*. San Francisco: Freeman.

Norman, D. A., & Shallice, T. (1984). Attention to action: Willed and automatic control of behavior. In R. J. Davidson, G. E. Schwartz, and D. Shapiro (Eds.), *Consciousness and self-regulation* (Vol. 4, pp. 3–16). New York: Plenum Press.

Norman, R. J., Buchwald, J. S., & Villablanca, J. R. (1977). Classical conditioning with auditory discrimination of the eyeblink in decerebrate cats. *Science, 196*, 551–553.

Nuechterlein, K. H. (1977). Reaction time and attention in schizophrenia: A critical evaluation of the data and theories. *Schizophrenia Bulletin, 3*, 373–428.

Nuechterlein, K. H., & Dawson, M. E. (1984). Information processing and attentional functioning in the developmental course of schizophrenic disorders. *Schizophrenia Bulletin, 10*, 160–203.

Oakley, D. A., & Russell, I. S. (1972). Neocortical lesions and classical conditioning. *Physiology and Behavior, 8*, 915–926.

O'Brien, J. H., & Fox, S. S. (1969). Single-cell activity in cat motor cortex: 2. Functional characteristic of the cell related to conditioning changes. *Journal of Neurophysiology, 32*, 267–284.

Obrist, P. A. (1981). *Cardiovascular psychophysiology: A perspective*. New York: Plenum Press.

Obrist, P. A., Webb, R. A., & Sutterer, J. R. (1969). Heart rate and somatic changes during aversive conditioning and a simple reaction time task. *Psychophysiology, 5*, 696–712.

O'Donnell, B. F., & Cohen, R. A. (1988). The N2-P3 complex of evoked potential and human performance. In R. L. Harris, A. T. Pope, & J. R. Comstock (Eds.), *Proceedings from the First NASA Mental-State Estimation Workshop* (pp. 269–286). Langley, VA: NASA.

O'Donnell, B. F., Squires, N. K., Martz, M. J., Chen, J. R., & Phay, A. J. (1987). Evoked potential changes and neuropsychological performance in Parkinson's disease. *Biological Psychology, 24*, 23–37.

O'Donnell, B. F., Drachman, D. A., Lew, R. A., & Swearer, J. M. (1988). Measuring dementia: Assessment of multiple deficit domains. *Clinical Psychology, 44*, 916–923.

O'Donnell, B. F., Friedman, S., Squires, N. K., Maloon, A., Drachman, D. A., & Swearer, J. M. (1990). Active and passive P3 latency in dementia: Relationship to psychometric, EEG, and CT measures. *Neuropsychiatry, Neuropsychology and Behavioral Neurology, 3*, 164–179.

Ohman, A. (1979). The orienting response, attention, and learning: An information-processing perspective. In H. D. Kimmel, E. H. van Olst, & J. F. Orlebeke (Eds.), *The orienting reflex in humans* (pp. 443–471). The Hague: Mouton.

Ohman, A. (1983). The orienting response during Pavlovian conditioning. In D. Siddle (Ed.), *Orienting and habituation: Perspectives in human research* (pp. 315–370). New York: Wiley.

O'Keefe, J., & Nadel, L. (1978). *The hippocampus as a cognitive map.* Oxford: Clarendon Press.

Olds, J. (1955). Physiological mechanisms of reward. In *Nebraska Symposium on Motivation.* Lincoln: University of Nebraska Press.

Olds, J. (1958a). Effects of hunger and male sex hormone on self-stimulation of the brain. *Journal of Comparative and Physiological Psychology, 51*, 320–324.

Olds, J. (1958b). Self-stimulation of the brain. *Science, 127*, 315–324.

Olds, J. (1962). Hypothalamic substrates of reward. *Physiological Review, 42*, 554–604.

Olds, J., & Hirano, T. (1969). Conditioned responses of hippocampal and other neurons. *EEG Clinical Neurophysiology, 26*, 159–166.

Olds, J., & Milner, P. (1954). Positive reinforcement produced by electrical stimulation of septal area and other regions of rat brain. *Journal of Comparative and Physiological Psychology, 47*, 419–427.

Olds, J., Mink, W. D., & Best, Ph. J. (1969). Single unit patterns during anticipatory behavior. *Electroencephalography and Clinical Neurophysiology, 26*, 144–158.

Olds, J., & Olds, M. E. (1958). Positive reinforcement produced by stimulating the hypothalamus. *Science, 127*, 325–334.

Olds, J., & Olds, M. (1965). Drives, rewards, and the brain. In *New directions in physiology* (pp. 329–410). New York: Holt, Rinehart & Winston.

Olds, M. E. (1973). Short-term changes in the firing pattern of hypothalamic neurons during Pavlovian conditioning. *Brain Research, 58*, 95–116.

Olds, M. E., & Frey, J. (1971). Effects of hypothalamic lesions on escape behavior produced by midbrain electrical stimulation. *American Journal of Physiology, 221*, 8–18.

Olds, M. E., & Olds, J. (1962). Approach-escape interactions in the rat brain. *American Journal of Physiology, 203*, 803–810.

Olds, M. E., & Olds, J. (1963). Approach-avoidance analysis of rat diencephalon. *Journal of Comparative Neurology, 120*, 259–295.

Oleson, T., Ashe, J., & Weinberger, N. M. (1975). Modification of auditory and somatosensory activity during pupillary conditioning in the paralyzed cat. *Journal of Neurophysiology, 38*, 1114–1139.

Oltmanns, T. F., Ohayon, J., & Neale, J. M. (1978). The effect of anti-psychotic medication and diagnostic criteria on distractability in schizophrenia. *Journal of Psychiatric Research, 14*, 81–91.

Ornstein, R. E. (1969). *On the experience of time.* Harmondsworth, England: Penguin Books.

Oscar-Berman, M. (1975). The effects of dorsolateral-frontal and ventrolateral-orbitofrontal lesions on spatial discrimination learning and delayed response in two modalities. *Neuropsychologia, 13*, 237–246.

Oscar-Berman, M., & Gade, A. (1979). Electrodermal measures of arousal in humans with cortical or subcortical brain damage. In H. D. Kimmel, E. H. Van Olst, & J. F. Orlebeke (Eds.), *The orienting reflex in humans* (pp. 665–676). Hillsdale, NJ: Lawrence Erlbaum Associates.

Paller, K. A., Zola-Morgan, S., Squire, L. R., & Hillyard, S. A. (1988). P3-like brain waves in normal monkeys and in monkeys with medial temporal lesions. *Behavioral Neuroscience, 102*, 714–725.

Papanicolaou, A. C. (1987). Electrophysiological methods for the study of attentional deficits in head injury. In H. S. Levin, J. Grafman, & H. M. Eisenberg (Eds.), *Neurobehavioral recovery from head injury* (pp. 379–397). New York: Oxford University Press.

Papanicolaou, A. C., Loring, D. W., Raz, N., & Eisenberg, H. M. (1985). Relationship between stimulus intensity and the P300. *Psychophysiology, 22*, 326–329.

Papez, J. W. (1937). A proposed mechanism of emotion. *Archives of Neurology and Psychiatry, 38,* 725–743.

Parasuraman, R. (1984). Sustained attention in detection and discrimination. In R. Parasuraman & D. R. Davies (Eds.), *Varieties of attention* (pp. 243–289). New York: Academic Press.

Parasuraman, R., & Davies, D. R. (Eds.). (1984). *Varieties of attention.* New York: Academic Press, Series in Cognition and Perception.

Paterson, A., & Zangwill, O. L. (1944). Disorders of visual space perception associated with lesions of the right cerebral hemisphere. *Brain, 67,* 331.

Pavlov, I. P. (1927). *Conditioned reflexes* (G. V. Anrep, Trans.). London: Oxford University Press.

Payne, R. W., Mattussek, P., & George, E. I. (1959). An experimental study of schizophrenic thought disorder. *Journal of Mental Science, 105,* 627–652.

Pendergrass, V. E., & Kimmel, H. D. (1968). UCR diminution in temporal conditioning and habituation. *Journal of Experimental Psychology, 77,* 1–6.

Penfield, W. (1958). *The excitable cortex in conscious man.* Liverpool, England: Liverpool University Press.

Penfield, W., & Milner, B. (1958). Memory deficit produced by bilateral lesions in the hippocampal zone. *Archives of Neurology and Psychiatry, 79,* 475–497.

Penfield, W., & Rasmussen, T. (1950). *The cerebral cortex of man.* New York: Macmillan.

Penfield, W., & Roberts, L. (1959). Speech and brain mechanisms. Princeton: Princeton University Press.

Pepper, G. M., & Krieger, D. T. (1984). Hypothalamic-pituitary-adrenal abnormalities in depression: Their possible relation to central mechanisms regulating ACTH release. In R. M. Post & J. C. Ballenger (Eds.), *Neurobiology of mood disorders* (pp. 245–270). J. H. Wood & B. R. Brooks (Series Eds.), *Frontiers of Clinical Neuroscience* (Vol. 1). Baltimore: Williams & Wilkins.

Perenin, M. T., & Jeannerod, M. (1979). Subcortical vision in man. *Trends in Neuroscience, 2,* 204–207.

Perenin, M. T., & Jeannerod, M. (1989). Subcortical vision in man. *Trends in Neuroscience, 2,* 204–207.

Petersen, S. E., Robinson, D. L., & Keys, W. (1985). Pulvinar nuclei of the behaving rhesus monkey: Visual responses and their modulation. *Journal of Neurophysiology, 54,* 207–226.

Petersen, S. E., Robinson, D. L., & Morris, J. D. (1987). Contributions of the pulvinar to visual spatial attention. *Neuropsychologia, 25,* 97–105.

Petersen, S. E., Fox, P. T., Posner, M. I., Mintun, M., & Raichle, M. E. (1989). Positron emission tomographic studies of the processing of single words. *Journal of Cognitive Neuroscience, 1(2),* 153–170.

Peterson, L. R., & Peterson, M. J. (1959). Short-term retention of individual verbal items. *Journal of Experimental Psychology, 58,* 193–198.

Pfeffer, R. I., & Van der Noort, S. (1978). Parkinson's disease: Correlation of clinical and chemical features. In A. A. Buerger & J. S. Tobis (Eds.), *Neurophysiologic aspects of rehabilitation medicine* (pp. 299–316). Springfield, IL: Thomas.

Pfefferbaum, A., Ford, J. M., Roth, W. T., & Kopell, B. S. (1980). Age differences in P3-reaction time associations. *Electroencephalography and Clinical Neurophysiology, 49,* 257–265.

Pfefferbaum, A., Wenegrat, B. G., Ford, J. M., Roth, W. T., & Kopell, B. S. (1984). Clinical application of the P3 component of the event-related potentials: 2. Dementia, depression and schizophrenia. *Electroencephalography and Clinical Neurophysiology, 59,* 104–124.

Phillips, M. I., & Olds, J. (1969). Unit activity: Motivation-dependent response from midbrain neurons. *Science, 165,* 1269–1271.

Phillips, R. R., Malamut, B. L., Bachevalier, J., & Mishkin, M. (1988). Dissociation of the effects of inferior temporal and limbic lesions on object discrimination learning with 24-h intertrial intervals. *Behavioural Brain Research, 27,* 99–107.

Phillips, W. A. (1974). On the distinction between sensory storage and short-term visual memory. *Perception and Psychophysics, 16,* 283–290.

Pillsbury, W. B. (1908). *Attention.* New York: Macmillan.

Pirozzolo, F. J., & Rayner, K. (1977). Hemispheric specialization in reading and word recognition. *Brain and Language, 4,* 248–261.

Pirozzolo, F. J., Hansch, E. C., & Mortimer, J. A. (1982). Dementia in Parkinson disease: A neuropsychological analysis. *Brain and Cognition, 1,* 71–83.

Pittendrigh, C. (1981). Circadian systems: Entrainment. In J. Aschoff (Ed.), *Handbook of behavioral neurobiology: Vol. 4. Biological rhythms* (pp. 95–124). New York: Plenum Press.

Platt, J. R. (1984). Motivational and response factors in temporal differentiation. In J. Gibbon & L. Allan

(Eds.), *Timing and time perception, Annals of the New York Academy of Sciences* (Vol. 423, pp. 646–648). New York: New York Academy of Sciences.

Plum, F. (1972). Organic disturbances of consciousness. In M. Critchley & J. L. O'Leary (Eds.), *Scientific foundations of neurology*. Philadelphia: F. A. Davis.

Polich, J. (1987). Comparison of P300 from a passive tone sequence paradigm and an active discrimination task. *Psychophysiology, 24,* 41–46.

Polich, J. (1989). P300 from a passive auditory paradigm. *Electroencephalography and Clinical Neurophysiology, 74,* 312–320.

Polich, J., Howard, L., & Starr, A. (1983). P300 latency correlates with digit span. *Psychophysiology, 20,* 665–669.

Polich, J., Ehlers, C. L., Otis, S., Mandell, A. J., & Bloom, F. E. (1986). P300 latency reflects the degree of cognitive decline in dementing illness. *Electroencephalography and Clinical Neurophysiology, 63,* 138–144.

Pollen, D. A., & Ronner, S. F. (1975) Periodic excitability changes across the receptive field of complex cells in the striate and parastriate cortex of the cat. *Journal of Physiology, 245,* 667–697.

Pollen, D. A., Jacobson, L. D., & Gaska, J. P. (1988). Responses of simple and complex cells to sine-wave gratings. *Vision Research, 28*(1), 25–39.

Pollen, D. A., Gaska, J. P., & Jacobson, L. D. (1990). Physiological constraints on models of visual cortical function. In R. M. J. Cotterill (Ed.), *Models of brain function*. New York: Cambridge University Press.

Ponsford, J. L., & Kinsella, G. (1988). The evaluation of a remedial program for attentional deficits following closed head injury. *Journal of Clinical and Experimental Neuropsychology, 10,* 693–708.

Poppelreuter, W. L. (1917). *Die psychischen Schadigungen durch Kopfschuss Krieg im 1914–1916: Die Storungen der niederen und hoheren Leistungen durch Verletzungen des Oksipitalhirns* (Vol. 1). Leipzig: Leopold Voss.

Porrino, L. J., & Goldman-Rakic, P. (1982). Brainstem innervation of prefrontal and anterior cingulate cortex in the rhesus monkey revealed by retrograde transport of HRP. *Journal of Comparative Neurology, 205,* 63–76.

Posner, M. I. (1975). Psychobiology of attention. In M. S. Gazzaniga & C. Blakemore (Eds.), *Handbook of psychobiology*. New York: Academic Press.

Posner, M. I. (1978). *Chronometric explorations of mind*. Hillsdale, NJ: Erlbaum.

Posner, M. I. (1980). Orienting of attention: The VIIth Sir Frederic Bartlett Lecture. *Quarterly Journal of Experimental Psychology, 32,* 3–25.

Posner, M. I. (1986). *Chronometric explorations of the mind*. New York: Oxford University Press.

Posner, M. I., & Cohen, Y. (1984). Facilitation and inhibition in shifts of visual attention. In H. Bouma & D. Bowhuis (Eds.), *Attention and performance* (Vol. 10). Hillsdale, NJ: Erlbaum.

Posner, M. I., & Snyder, C. R. R. (1975). Attention and cognitive control. In R. L. Solso (Ed.), *Information processing and cognition: The Loyola Symposium* (pp. 55–84). Hillsdale, NJ: Erlbaum.

Posner, M. I., Snyder, C. R., and Davidson, B. J. (1980). Attention and the detection of signals. *Journal of Experimental Psychology: General, 109,* 160–174.

Posner, M. I., Cohen, Y., & Rafal, R. D. (1982). Neural systems control of spatial orienting. *Philosophical Transactions of the Royal Society of London, B298,* 187–198.

Posner, M. I., Walker, J. A., Friedrich, F. J., & Rafal, R. D. (1984). Effects of parietal lobe injury on covert orienting of visual attention. *Journal of Neuroscience, 4*(7), 1863–1874.

Posner, M. I., Walker, J. A., Friedrich, F. A., & Rafal, R. D. (1987). How do the parietal lobes direct covert attention? *Neuropsychologia, 25*(1A), 135–145.

Posner, M. I., Peterson, S. E., Fox, P. T., & Raichle, M. E. (1988). Localization of cognitive operations in the human brain. *Science, 240,* 1627–1631.

Post, R. M., & Ballenger, J. C. (Eds.). (1984). Neurobiology of mood disorders. In J. H. Wood & B. R. Brooks (Eds.), *Frontiers of clinical neuroscience* (Vol. 1). Baltimore: Williams & Wilkins.

Poulton, E. C. (1979). Composite model for human performance in continuous noise. *Psychological Review, 86,* 361–375.

Precht, W., & Strata, P. (1980). On the pathway mediating optkinetic responses in vestibular nuclear neurons. *Neuroscience, 5,* 777–787.

Pribram, K. H. (1955). Lesions of "frontal eye fields" and delayed response of baboons. *Journal of Neurophysiology, 18,* 105–112.

Pribram, K. H. (1961). A further experimental analysis of the behavioral deficit that follows injury to the primate frontal cortex. *Experimental Neurology, 3*, 432–466.

Pribram, K. H. (1967). Neurophysiology and learning: 1. Memory and the organization of attention. In D. B. Lindsley & A. A. Lumsdaine (Eds.), *Brain function: Vol. 4. Brain function and learning* (pp. 79–93). Berkeley: University of California Press.

Pribram, K. H. (1969). The neurobehavioral analysis of limbic forebrain mechanisms: Revision and progress report. In *Advances in the study of behavior* (Vol. 2). New York: Academic Press.

Pribram, K. H. (1971). *Languages of the brain: Experimental paradoxes and principles in neuropsychology.* Englewood Cliffs, NJ: Prentice-Hall.

Pribram, K. H. (1976). Problems concerning the structure of consciousness. In G. Globus, G. Maxell, & I. Savodnik (Eds.), *Science and the mind-brain puzzle.* New York: Plenum Press.

Pribram, K. H. (1980). Mind, brain, and consciousness: The organization of competence and conduct. In J. M. Davidson & R. J. Davidson (Eds.), *The psychobiology of consciousness* (pp. 47–63). New York and London: Plenum Press.

Pribram, K. H., & Bagshaw, M. (1953). Further analysis of the temporal lobe syndrome utilize frontotemporal ablations. *Journal of Comparative Neurology, 99*, 347–375.

Pribram, K. H., & McGuiness, D. (1975). Arousal, activation and effort in the control of attention. *Psychological Review, 82*, 116–149.

Pribram, K. H., Mishkin, M., Rosvold, H. E., & Kaplan, S. J. (1952). Effects of delayed-response performance of lesions of dorsolateral and ventromedial frontal cortex of baboons. *Journal of Comparative Physiological and Psychology, 45*, 565–575.

Pribram, K. H., Douglas, R. J., & Pribram, B. J. (1969). The nature of nonlimbic learning. *Journal of Comparative and Physiological Psychology, 69*, 765–772.

Prigatano, G. P. (1978). Wechsler memory scale: A selective review of the literature. *Journal of Clinical Psychology, 34*, 816–832.

Pritchard, W. S., Brandt, M. E., Shappell, S. A., O'Dell, T., & Barratt, E. S. (1986). No decrement in visual P300 amplitude during extended performance of the oddball task. *International Journal of Neuroscience, 29*, 199–204.

Pylyshyn, Z. W. (1973). What the mind's eye tells the mind's brain: A critique of mental imagery. *Psychological Bulletin, 80*, 1–24.

Ramos, A., Schwartz, E. L., & John, E. R. (1976). Stable and plastic unit discharge patterns during behavioral generalization. *Science, 192*, 393–396.

Rao, S. M. (1986). Neuropsychology of multiple sclerosis: A critical review. *Journal of Clinical and Experimental Neuropsychology, 8*(5), 503–542.

Rapcsak, S. Z., Verfaellie, M., Fleet, W. S., & Heilman, K. M. (1989). Selective attention in hemispatial neglect. *Archives of Neurology, 46*, 178–182.

Raphaelson, A. C., Isaacson, R. L., & Douglas, R. J. (1966). The effect of limbic damage on the retention and performance of a runway response. *Neuropsychologia, 4*, 253–264.

Rapoport, J. L., Buchsbaum, M. S., Zahn, T. P., Weingartner, H., Ludlow, C., & Mikkelsen, E. J. (1978). Dextroamphetamine: Cognitive and behavioral effects in normal prepubertal boys. *Science, 199*, 560–563.

Raskin, A., Friedman, A. S., & DiMascio, A. (1982). Cognitive and performance deficits in depression. *Psychopharmacology Bulletin, 18*, 196–202.

Raskin, D. C. Kotses, H., & Bever, J. (1969). Autonomic indicators of orienting and defensive reflexes. *Journal of Experimental Psychology, 80*, 423–433.

Ratcliff, G. (1982). Disturbances of spatial orientation associated with cerebral lesions. In M. Pategal (Ed.), *Spatial abilities: Development and physiological foundations.* New York: Academic Press.

Ratcliff, G., & Newcombe, F. (1973). Spatial orientation in man: Effects of left, right, and bilateral posterior lesions. *Journal of Neurology, Neurosurgery, and Psychiatry, 36*, 448–454.

Rausch, R., Lieb, J. P., & Crandall, P. H. (1978). Neuropsychologic correlates of depth spike activity in epileptic patients. *Archives of Neurology, 35*, 699–705.

Ray, C. L., Mirsky, A. F., & Pragay, E. B. (1982). Functional analysis of attention-related unit activity in the reticular formation of the monkey. *Experimental Neurology, 77*, 544–562.

Ray, R. L. (1979). The effect of stimulus intensity and intertrial interval on long-term retention of the OR. In H. D. Kimmel, E. H. van Olst, & J. F. Orlebeke (Eds.), *The orienting reflex in humans* (pp. 373–380). Hillsdale, NJ: Erlbaum.

Recht, L. D., McCarthy, K., O'Donnell, B. F., Cohen, R. A., & Drachman, D. A. (1989). Tumor associated aphasia in left hemisphere primary brain tumors: The importance of age and tumor grade. *Neurology, 38,* 48–50.

Reichlan, S., Baldessarini, R. J., & Martin, J. B. (1978). *The hypothalamus.* New York: Raven Press.

Reis, D. J., & McHugh, P. R. (1968). Hypoxia as a cause of bradycardia during amygdala stimulation in monkey. *American Journal of Physiology, 214,* 601–610.

Reitan, R. M. (1958). Validity of the Trail Making Test as an indication of organic brain damage. *Perceptual and Motor Skills, 8,* 271–276.

Rescorla, R. A. (1967). Pavlovian conditioning and its proper control procedures. *Psychological Review, 74,* 71–90.

Rescorla, R. A. (1969). Conditioned inhibition of fear. In N. J. Mackintosh & W. K. Honig (Eds.), *Fundamental issues in associative learning* (pp. 65–89). Halifax, Canada: Dalhousie University Press.

Rescorla, R. A., & Wagner, A. R. (1972). A theory of Pavlovian conditioning: Variation in the effectiveness of reinforcement and nonreinforcement. In A. H. Black and W. F. Prakasy (Eds.), *Classical conditioning II: Current research and theory* (pp. 64–99). New York: Appleton-Century-Crofts.

Restle, F. (1955). A theory of discrimination learning. *Psychology Review, 62,* 11–19.

Reuter-Lorenz, P. A., & Fendrich, R. (1990). Orienting attention across the vertical meridian: Evidence form callosotomy patients. *Journal of Cognitive Neuroscience, 2*(3), 232–239.

Revelle, W., Humphreys, M. S., Simon, L., & Gilliland, K. (1980). The interactive effect of personality, time of day, and caffeine: A test of the arousal model. *Journal of Experimental Psychology, 108,* 1–31.

Riddoch, J. M., & Humphreys, G. W. (1983). The effects of cueing on unilateral neglect. *Neuropsychologia, 21,* 589–599.

Rimel, R. W., Giordani, B., Barth, J. T., Boll, T. J., & Jane, J. A. (1981). Disability caused by minor head injury. *Neurosurgery, 9,* 221–228.

Risberg, J. (1980). Regional cerebral blood flow measurements by 133Xe-inhalation: Methodology and applications in neuropsychology and psychiatry. *Brain and Language, 9,* 9–34.

Ritter, W., Vaughn, H. G., & Costa, L. D. (1968). Orienting and habituation to auditory stimuli: A study of short term changes in averaged evoked responses. *Electroencephalography and Clinical Neurophysiology, 25,* 550–556.

Ritter, W., Simson, R., & Vaughan, H. G. (1972). Association cortex potentials and reaction time in auditory discrimination. *Electroencephalography and Clinical Neurophysiology, 33,* 547–555.

Ritter, W., Vaughn, H. G., & Friedman, D. (1979). A brain event related to the making of a sensory discrimination. *Science, 203,* 1358–1361.

Rizzo, M., & Robin, D. A. (1990). Simultanagosia: A defect of sustained attention yields insights on visual information processing. *Neurology, 40,* 447–455.

Rizzolatti, G. (1983). Mechanisms of selective attention in mammals. In J. P. Ewert, R. R. Capranica, & D. J. Ingle (Eds.), *Advances in vertebrate neuroethology.* New York: Plenum.

Rizzolatti, G., Scandolara, C., Matelli, M., & Gentilucci, M. (1981a). Afferent properties of periarcuate neurons in macaque monkeys: 1. Somatosensory responses. *Behavior and Brain Research, 2,* 125–146.

Rizzolatti, G., Scandolara, C., Matelli, M., & Gentilucci, M. (1981b). Afferent properties of periarcuate neurons in macaque monkeys: 2. Visual responses. *Behavior and Brain Research, 2,* 147–163.

Rizzolatti, G., Riggio, L., Dascola, I., & Umilta, C. (1987). Reorienting attention across the horizontal and vertical meridians: Evidence in favor of a pre-motor theory of attention. *Neuropsychologia, 25*(1A), 31–40.

Roberts, S. (1982). Cross-modal use of an internal clock. *Journal of Experimental Psychology of Animal Behavioral Processes, 8,* 2–22.

Roberts, W., A., & Kraemer, P. J. (1982). Some observations of the effects of intertrial interval and delay on delayed matching to sample in pigeons. *Journal of Experimental Psychology, 8,* 342–353.

Robertson, L. C. (1989). Anomalies in the laterality of omissions in unilateral left visual neglect: Implications for attentional theory. *Neuropsychologia, 27,* 157–165.

Robertson, L. C., Lamb, M. R., & Knight, R. T. (1988). Effects of lesions of temporal-parietal junction on perceptual and attentional processing in humans. *Journal of Neuroscience, 8*(10), 3757–3769.

Robinson, D. A. (1974). Occulomotor control signals. In G. Lennerstrand & P. Bach-y-Rita (Eds.), *Basic mechanisms of ocular motility and their clinical implications* (pp. 337–374). Oxford: Pergamon Press.

Robinson, D. E., & Peterson, S. E. (1986). The neurobiology of attention. In J. E. Ledoux & W. Hirst

(Eds.), *Mind and brain: Dialogues in cognitive neuroscience* (pp. 143–186). New York: Cambridge University Press.

Rohrbaugh, J. W. (1984). The orienting reflex: Performance and CNS manifestations. In R. Parasuraman (Ed.), *Varieties of Attention*. New York: Academic Press.

Rosenbaum, D. A. (1991). Human motor control. New York: Academic Press.

Rosenblatt, F. (1962). *Principles of neurodynamics*. New York: Spartan.

Rosenthal, D., Wender, Ph. H., Kety, S. S., Welner, J., & Schulsinger, F. (1971). The adopted away offspring of schizophrenics. *American Journal of Psychiatry, 128*, 307–311.

Rosenthal, N. E., & Blehar, M. (Eds.). (1989). *Seasonal affective disorders and phototherapy*. New York: Guilford Press.

Rosenthal, R. H., & Allen, T. W. (1978). An examination of attention arousal and learning dysfunctions of hyperkinetic children. *Psychological Bulletin, 85*, 689–715.

Rosvold, H. E., Mirsky, A. F., Sarandon, I., Bransome, E. D., & Beck, L. H. (1956). A continuous performance test of brain damage. *Journal of Consulting Psychology, 20*, 343–350.

Roth, W. T., Horvath, T. B., Pfefferbaum, A., & Kopell B. S. (1980). Event-related potentials in schizophrenics. *Electroencephalography and Clinical Neurophysiology, 48*, 127–139.

Roth, W. T., Pfefferbaum, A., Horvath, T. B., Berger, P. A., & Kopell, B. S. (1980). P3 reduction in auditory evoked potentials of schizophrenics. *Electroencephalography and Clinical Neurophysiology, 49*, 497–505.

Ruchkin, D. S., & Sutton, S. (1978). Equivocation and P300 amplitude. In D. Otto (Ed.), *Multidisciplinary perspectives in event-related brain potential research* (pp. 175–177). EPA-600/9-77-043. Washington, DC: Government Printing Office.

Rumelhart, D. E., & Norman, D. A. (1982). Simulating a skilled typist: A study of skilled cognitive-motor performance. *Cognitive Sciences, 6*, 1–36.

Rumelhart, D. E., & Zipser, D. (1985). Feature discovery by competitive learning. *Cognitive Science, 9*, 75–112.

Rumelhart, D. E., & Zipser, D. (1986). *Feature discovery by competitive learning in parallel distributed processing: Explorations in the microstructure of cognition* (Vol. 1). Cambridge: MIT Press.

Rumelhart, D. E., Hinton, G. E., & McClelland, J. L. (1986). A general framework for parallel distributed processing. In J. L. McClelland & D. E. Rumelhart (Eds.), *Parallel distributed processing: Explorations in the microstructure of cognition* (Vol. 1, pp. 45–77). Cambridge: MIT Press.

Rutter, M. (1983a). Behavioral studies: Questions and findings on the concept of a distinctive syndrome. In M. Rutter (Ed.), *Developmental neuropsychiatry* (pp. 259–279). New York: Guilford Press.

Rutter, M. (1983b). Issues and prospects in developmental neuropsychiatry. In M. Rutter (Ed.), *Developmental neuropsychiatry* (pp. 577–598). New York: Guilford Press.

Rylander, G. (1939). *Personality changes after operations on the frontal lobes*. London: Oxford University Press.

Ryugo, D. K., & Weinberger, N. M. (1976). Differential plasticity of morphologically distinct neuron populations in the medial geniculate body of the cat during classical conditioning. *Behavioral Biology, 22*, 275–301.

Salthouse, T. A. (1982). *Adult cognition*. New York: Springer-Verlag.

Sanders, R. E., Gonzalez, E. G., Murphy, M. D., Liddle, C. L., & Vitina, J. R. (1987). Frequency of occurrence and the criteria for automatic processing. *Journal of Experimental Psychology: Learning, Memory and Cognition, 13*, 241–250.

Sandon, P. A. (1990). Simulating visual attention. *Journal of Cognitive Neuroscience, 2*, 213–231.

Sanides, F. (1970). Functional architecture of motor and sensory cortices in primates in the light of a new concept of neocortex evolution. In C. R. Noback & Montagna (Eds.), *The primate brain* (pp. 137–208). New York: Appleton-Century-Crofts.

Satterfield, J. H., Schell, A. M., Nicholas, T., & Backs, R. W. (1988). Topographic study of auditory event-related potentials in normal boys and boys with attention deficit disorder with hyperactivity. *Psychophysiology, 25*, 591–606.

Satterfield, J. H., Schell, A. M., Nicholas, T. W., Satterfield, B. T., & Freese, T. E. (1990). Ontogeny of selective attention effects on event-related potentials in attention-deficit hyperactivity disorder and normal boys. *Biological Psychiatry, 28*, 879–903.

Schachar, R., Rutter, M., & Smith, A. (1981). The characteristics of situationally and pervasively hyperactive children: Implications for syndrome definition. *Journal of Child Psychology and Psychiatry, 22,* 375–392.

Schacter, D. L. (1985). Multiple forms of memory in humans and animals. In N. M. Weinberger, G. Lynch, & J. McGaugh (Eds.), *Memory systems of the brain: Animal and human cognitive processes* (pp. 351–379). New York: Guilford Press.

Schacter, D. L., & Prigatano, G. P.(1991). Forms of unawareness. In G. P. Prigatano & D. L. Schacter (Eds.), *Awareness of deficit after brain injury: Clinical and theoretical issues* (pp. 258–262). New York: Oxford University Press.

Schachter, S., & Singer, J. E. (1962). Cognitive, social and physiological determinants of emotional state. *Psychological Review, 69,* 379–399.

Schaub, R. E. (1965). The effect of interstimulus interval of GSR adaptation. *Psychonomic Science, 2,* 361–362.

Schildkraut, J. J. (1965). The catecholamine hypothesis of affective disorders: A review of supporting evidence. *American Journal of Psychiatry, 122,* 509–522.

Schildkraut, J. J. (1977). Biochemical research in affective disorders. In G. Usdin (Ed.), *Depression: Clinical, biological and psychological perspectives* (pp. 166–197). New York: Brunner/Mazel.

Schiller, P. H., True, S. D., & Conway, J. L. (1979). Paired stimulation of the frontal eye fields and the superior colliculus of the rhesus monkey. *Experimental Brain Research, 179,* 162–164.

Schlag, J., & Schlag-Rey, M. (1983). Interface of visual input and oculomotor command for directing the gaze on target. In A. Hein & M. Jeannerod (Eds.), *Spatially oriented behavior* (pp.87–104). New York: Springer-Verlag.

Schlag-Rey, M., & Schlag, J. (1981). Eye movement-related neuronal activity in the central thalamus of monkeys. In A. Fuchs & W. Becker (Eds.), *Progress in oculomotor research.* New York: Elsevier/North-Holland.

Schmaltz, L. W., & Isaacson, R. L. (1966). The effects of preliminary training conditions upon DRL 20 performance in the hippocampectomized rat. *Physiology and Behavior, 1,* 175–182.

Schneider, W., & Fisk, A. D. (1984). Automatic category search and its transfer. *Journal of Experimental Psychology: Learning, Memory, and Cognition, 10,* 1–15.

Schneider, W., & Shiffrin, R. M. (1977). Controlled and automatic human information processing: 1. Detection, search, and attention. *Psychological Review, 84,* 1–66.

Schneider, W., Dumais, S. T., & Shiffrin, R. M. (1984). Automatic and control processing and attention. In R. Parasuraman & D. R. Davies (Eds.), *Varieties of attention* (pp. 1–27). New York: Academic Press.

Schvaneveldt, R., & Meyer, D. E. (1973). Retrieval and comparison processes in semantic memory. In S. Kornblum (Ed.), *Attentional and performance* (Vol. 4). New York: Academic Press.

Schwartz, F., Carr, A. C., Munich, R. L., Glauber, S., Lesser, B., & Murray J. (1989). Reaction time impairment in schizophrenia and affective illness: The role of attention. *Biological Psychiatry, 25,* 540–548.

Schwartz, G. E. (1986). Emotion and psychophysiological organization: A systems approach. In M. G. H. Coles, E. Donchin, & S. W. Porges (Eds.), *Psychophysiology: Systems, processes, and applications* (pp. 354–377). New York: Guilford Press.

Schwartz, G. E., & Higgins, J. D. (1971). Cardiac activity preparatory to overt and covert behavior. *Science, 173,* 1144–1145.

Schwartz, W. J., Davidsen, L. C., & Smith, C. B. (1980). In vivo metabolic activity of a putative circadian oscillator, the rat suprachiasmatic nucleus. *Journal of Comparative Neurology, 189,* 157–167.

Schwartzbaum, J. S., Kellicut, M. H., Spieth, T. M., & Thompson, J. B. (1964). Effects of septal lesions in rats on response inhibition associated with food reinforced behavior. *Journal of Comparative and Physiological Psychology, 58,* 217–224.

Schweickert, R. J. (1984). The representation of mental activities in critical path networks. In J. Gibbon & L. Allan (Eds.), *Timing and time perception, Annals of the New York Academy of Sciences* (Vol. 423, pp. 82–95). New York: New York Academy of Sciences.

Scoville, W. B. (1949). Selective cortical undercutting as a means of modifying and studying frontal lobe function in man. *Journal of Neurosurgery, 6,* 65–73.

Scoville, W. B. (1973). Surgical locations for psychiatric surgery with special reference to orbital and cingulate operations. In L. V. Laitinen & K. E. Livingston (Eds.), *Surgical approaches in psychiatry* (pp. 29–36). Baltimore: University Park Press.

Scoville, W. B., & Milner, B. (1957). Loss of recent memory after bilateral hippocampal lesions. *Journal of Neurology, Neurosurgery, and Psychiatry, 20,* 11–21.

Searle, J. (1990). Is the brain's mind a computer program? No. A program merely manipulates symbols, whereas a brain attaches meaning to them. *Scientific American, 262,* 26–31.

Sechenov, L. M. (1956). *Selected physiological and psychological works.* Moscow: Foreign Languages Publishing House.

Segal, M. (1973). Flow of conditioned responses in limbic telecephalic system of the rat. *Journal of Neurophysiology, 36,* 840–854.

Segal, M. (1977). Excitability changes in rat's hippocampus during conditioning. *Experimental Neurology, 55,* 67–73.

Segraves, M. A., Goldberg, M. E., Deng, S. Y., Bruce, C. J., Ungerleider, L. G., & Mishkin, M. (1987). The role of striate cortex in the guidance of eye movements in the monkey. *Journal of Neuroscience, 7,* 3040–3058.

Sejnowski, T. J. (1981). Skeleton filters in the brain. In G. E. Hinton & J. A. Anderson (Eds.), *Parallel models of associative memory* (pp. 49–82). Hillsdale, NJ: Erlbaum.

Sejnowski, T. J. (1986). *Open questions about computation in cerebral cortex in parallel distributed processing: Explorations in the microstructure of cognition* (Vol. 2). Cambridge: MIT Press.

Semjen, A. G., Garcia-Colera, A., & Requin, J. (1984). On controlling force and time in rhythmic movement sequences: The effect of stress location. In J. Gibbon & L. Allan (Eds.), *Timing and time perception* (pp. 168–182). New York: New York Academy of Sciences.

Senf, G. M., & Miller, N. E. (1967). Evidence for Pavlovian induction in discrimination learning. *Journal of Comparative and Physiological Psychology, 64,* 121–127.

Shaffer, L. H. (1975). Multiple attention in continuous verbal tasks. In P. M. Babbitt & S. Dornic (Eds.), *Attention and performance* (Vol. 5, pp. 157–167). New York: Academic Press.

Shallice, T. (1972). Dual functions of consciousness. *Psychological Review, 79*(5), 383–393.

Shannon, C. E. (1948). A mathematical theory of communication. *Bell System Technical Journal, 27,* 379–423, 623–656.

Shannon, C. E. (1951). Prediction and entropy in the English language. *Bell System Technical Journal, 30,* 50–64.

Shannon, C. E., & Weaver, W. (1949). *The mathematical theory of communication.* Urbana: University of Illinois Press.

Shaywitz, S. E., & Shaywitz, B. A. (1987). Attention deficit disorder: Current perspectives. *Pediatric Neurology, 3,* 129–135.

Shaywitz, B. A., & Shaywitz, S. E. (1991). Comorbidity: A critical issue in attention deficit disorder. *Journal of Child Neurology, 6,* S13–S21.

Shelton, R. C., & Weinberger, D. R. (1986). X-Ray computerized tomography studies in schizophrenia: A review and synthesis. in H. A. Nasrallah & D. R. Weinberger (Eds.), *The neurology of schizophrenia* (Vol. 1, pp. 207–250). Amsterdam: Elsevier.

Shenton, M. E., Kikinis, R., Jolesz, F. A., Pollak, S. D., LeMay, M., Martin, J., Metcalf, D., Coleman, M., & McCarley, R. W. (1992). Left temporal lobe abnormalities in schizophrenia. *New England Journal of Medicine, 327,* 604–612.

Sheperd, G. M. (1979). *The synaptic organization of the brain.* New York: Oxford University Press.

Sherrington, C. S. (1947). *The integrative action of the nervous system* (7th ed). London: Cambridge University Press.

Shiffrin, R. M., & Schneider, W. (1977). Controlled and automatic human information processing: 2. Perceptual learning, automatic attending and a general theory. *Psychological Review, 84,* 127–190.

Siddle, D. A. T., & Spinks, J. A. (1979). Orienting response and information processing: Some theoretical and empirical problems. In H. D. Kimmel, E. H. Van Olst, & J. F. Orlebeke (Eds.), *The orienting reflex in humans.* Hillsdale, NJ: Erlbaum.

Siddle, D., Stephenson, D., & Spinks, J. A. (1983). Elicitation and habituation of the orienting response. In D. Siddle (Ed.), *Orienting and habituation: Perspectives in human research* (pp. 109–182). New York: Wiley.

Sifneos, P. E. (1973). The prevalence of alexythymic characteristics in psychosomatic patients. *Psychotherapy & Psychosomatics, 22,* 255–262.

Silverstein, L. D., & Berg, W. K. (1977, October). *Repetition and distribution effects on memory: A psychophysiological analysis*. Presented at the annual meeting of the Society for Psychophysiological Research.

Simson, R., Vaughan, H. G., & Ritter, W. (1976). The scalp topography of potentials associated with missing visual or auditory stimuli. *Electroencephalography and Clinical Neurophysiology, 40*, 33–42.

Simson, R., Vaughan, H. G., & Ritter, W. (1977). The scalp topography of potentials in auditory and visual discrimination tasks. *Electroencephalography and Clinical Neurophysiology, 42*, 528–535.

Singer, M. T., & Wynne, L. C. (1966). Principles for scoring communication defects and deviances in parents of schizophrenics: Rorschach and TAT scoring manuals. *Psychiatry, 29*, 260–288.

Singer, W. (1979). Central-core control of visual cortex functions. In F. O. Schmitt & F. G. Worden (Eds.), *The neurosciences* (pp. 1093–1109). Cambridge: MIT Press.

Singer, W. (1982). Central core control of developmental plasticity in the kitten visual cortex: 1. Diencephalic lesions. *Experimental Brain Research, 47*, 209–222.

Skelly, J. J., Rizzuto, A., & Wilson, G. (1984). Temporal patterning and selective attention effects on the human evoked response. In J. Gibbon & L. Allan (Eds.), *Timing and time perception, Annals of the New York Academy of Sciences* (Vol. 423, pp. 646–648). New York: New York Academy of Sciences.

Skinner, B. F. (1938). *The behavior of organisms*. New York: Appleton-Century-Crofts.

Small, I. F., Heimburger, R. F., Small, J. G., Milstein, V., & Moore, D. F. (1977). Follow-up of stereotaxic amygdalotomy for seizure and behavior disorders. *Biological Psychiatry, 12*, 401–411.

Smith, A. (1967). The serial sevens subtraction test. *Archives of Neurology, 17*, 78–80.

Smith, A. (1968). The Symbol Digit Modalities Test: A neuropsychologic test for economic screening of learning and other cerebral disorders. *Learning Disorders, 3*, 83–91.

Smith, A. (1973). *Symbol Digit Modalities test manual*. Los Angeles: Western Psychological Services.

Smith, A. P., Jones, D. M., & Broadbent, D. E. (1981). The effects of noise on recall of categorized lists. *British Journal of Psychiatry, 72*, 299–316.

Smith, E. E., Shoben, E. J., & Rips, L. J. (1974). Structure and process in semantic memory: A featural model for semantic decisions. *Psychological Review, 81*, 214–241.

Smolensky, P. (1984). The mathematical role of self-consistency in parallel computation. In *Proceedings of the 6th Annual Conference of the Cognitive Science Society*.

Smolensky, P. (1986). Information processing in dynamical systems: Foundations of harmony theory. In D. E. Rumelhart & J. L. McLelland (Eds.), *Parallel distributed processing: Explorations in the microstructure of cognition* (Vol. 1). Cambridge: MIT Press.

So, N., Gloor, P., Quesney, L. F., Jones-Gotman, M., Olivier, A., & Andermann, F. (1989). Depth electrode investigations in patients with bitemporal epileptiform abnormalities. *Annals of Neurology, 25*, 423–431.

Sokolov, E. N. (1960). Neuronal models and the orienting reflex. In M. A. B. Brazier (Ed.), *The central nervous system and behavior* (3rd conference, pp. 187–286). New York: Josiah Macy, Jr. Foundation.

Sokolov, E. N. (1963). *Perception and the conditioned reflex*. Oxford: Pergamon Press.

Sokolov, E. N. (1969). The modeling properties of the nervous system. In M. Cole & I. Maltzman (Eds.), *A handbook of contemporary Soviet psychology* (pp. 671–704). New York: Basic Books.

Sokolov, E. N. (1976). Learning and memory: Habituation as negative learning. In M. R. Rosenzweig & E. L. Bennett (Eds.), *Neural mechanisms of learning and memory* (pp. 475–482). Cambridge MA: MIT Press.

Sparks, D. L., & Mays, L. E. (1980). Movement of saccade-related burst neurons in the monkey superior colliculus. *Brain Research, 190*, 39–50.

Spearman, C. (1927). *The abilities of man*. London: Macmillan.

Spelke, E. S., Hirst, W. C., & Neisser, U. (1976). Skills of divided attention. *Cognition, 4*, 215–230.

Spence, K. W. (1936). The nature of discrimination learning in animals. *Psychological Review, 57*, 427–449.

Spence, K. W. (1951). Theoretical interpretations of learning. In S. S. Stevens (Ed.), *Handbook of experimental psychology*. New York: Wiley.

Spence, K. W. (1956). *Behavior theory and conditioning*. New Haven: Yale University Press.

Spencer, W. A., Thompson, R. F., & Nielson, D. R., Jr. (1966). Decrement of ventral root electronus and intracellularly recorded PSPs produced by iterated cutaneous afferent volleys. *Journal of Neurophysiology, 29*, 253–273.

Sperling, G. (1960). The information available in brief visual presentations. *Psychological Monographs, 74*, 498.

Sperling, G. (1984). A unified theory of attention and signal detection. In *Varieties of attention* (pp. 103–182). New York: Academic Press, Series in Cognition and Perception.

Sperling, G., & Melchner, M. J. (1978). Visual search, visual attention, and the attention operating characteristic. In J. Requin (Ed.), *Attention and performance* (Vol. 7, pp. 675–686). Hillsdale, NJ: Erlbaum.

Sperry, R. W. (1952). Neurology and the mind-brain problem. *American Scientist, 40,* 291–312.

Sperry, R. W. (1969). A modified concept of consciousness. *Psychological Review, 76,* 532–536.

Spiegler, B. J., & Mishkin, M. (1981). Evidence for the sequential participation of inferior temporal cortex and amygdala in the acquisition of stimulus-reward associations. *Behavioral Brain Research, 3*(3), 303–317.

Spinks, J. A., & Siddle, D. A. T. (1976). Effects of stimulus information and stimulus duration on amplitude and habituation of the electrodermal orienting response. *Biological Psychology, 4,* 29–39.

Spinks, J. A., & Siddle, D. (1983). The functional significance of the orienting response. In D. Siddle (Ed.), *Orienting and habituation: Perspectives in human research* (pp. 237–314). New York: Wiley.

Spinnler, H., Sterzi, R., & Vallar, G. (1984). Selective visual interference with right hemisphere performance in verbal recall: A divided field study. *Neuropsychologia, 22,* 353–361.

Spitzer, H., Desimone, R., & Moran, J. (1988). Improved orientation tuning is also found in V4, but not V1, when repetition of a visual pattern triggers a behavioral response. *Science, 240,* 388.

Sprague, J. M., Chambers, W. W., & Stellar, E. (1961). Attentive, affective, and adaptive behavior in the cat. *Science, 133,* 165–173.

Sprague, R. L. (1983). Behavior modification and educational techniques. In M. Rutter (Ed.), *Developmental neuropsychiatry* (pp. 404–421). New York: Guilford Press.

Spreen, O., & Benton, A. L. (1965). Comparative studies of some psychological tests for cerebral damage. *Journal of Nervous and Mental Disease, 140,* 323–333.

Spreen, O., & Benton, A. L. (1969). *Neurosensory Center Comprehensive Examination for Aphasia.* Victoria, BC: Neuropsychological Laboratory Department of Psychology, University of Victoria.

Springer, S. P. (1986). Dichotic listening. In H. J. Hannay (Ed.), *Experimental techniques in human neuropsychology.* New York: Oxford University Press.

Squire, L. R. (1981). Two forms of human amnesia: An analysis of forgetting. *Journal of Neuroscience, 1,* 635–640.

Squire, L. R. (1984). The neuropsychology of memory. In P. Marler & H. S. Terrace (Eds.), *The biology of learning* (pp. 667–685). Berlin: Springer-Verlag.

Squire, L. R. (1987). *Memory and brain.* New York: Oxford University Press.

Squire, L. R., & Zola-Morgan, S. (1985). Neuropsychology of memory: New links between humans and experimental animals. In D. Olton, S. Corkin, & E. Gamzu (Eds.), *Memory dysfunctions: An integration of animal and human research from preclinical and clinical perspectives.* New York: New York Academy of Sciences.

Squires, K. C., Wickens, C., Squires, N. K., & Donchin, E. (1976). The effect of stimulus sequence on the waveform of the cortical event-related potential. *Science, 193,* 1142–1146.

Squires, N. K., & Ollo, C. (1986). Human evoked potential techniques: Possible applications to neuropsychology. In J. H. Hannay (Ed.), *Experimental techniques in human neuropsychology* (pp. 386–418). New York: Oxford University Press.

Squires, N. K., Squires, K. C., & Hillyard, S. A. (1975). Two varieties of long-latency positive waves evoked by unpredictable auditory stimuli in man. *Electroencephalography and Clinical Neurophysiology, 38,* 387–401.

Squires, N. K., Donchin, E., & Squires, K. C. (1977). Bisensory stimulation: Inferring decision-related processes from the P300 component. *Journal of Experimental Psychology: Human Perception and Performance, 3,* 299–315.

Squires, N. K., Halgren, E., Wilson, C., & Crandall, P. (1983). Human endogenous limbic potentials: Cross-modality and depth/surface comparisons in epileptic subjects. In A. W. K. Gaillard & W. Ritter (Eds.), *Tutorials in event related potential research: Endogenous components* (pp. 217–232). New York: North-Holland.

Squires, N. K., Sanders, D., & Wanser, R. (1986). Comparison of attend and non-attend paradigms for the evaluation of ERP changes in normal aging and neurologic dysfunction. In J. W. Rohrbaugh, R.

Johnson, & R. Parasuraman (Eds.), *Eighth International Conference on Event-Related Potentials of the Brain: Research Reports* (pp. 137–139). Palo Alto, CA: Stanford.

Staddon, J. E. R. (1984). Time and memory. In J. Gibbon & L. Allan (Eds.), *Timing and time perception, Annals of the New York Academy of Sciences* (Vol. 423, pp. 322–334). New York: New York Academy of Sciences.

Stankov, L. (1988). Aging, attention, and intelligence. *Psychology and Aging, 3,* 59–74.

Stapleton, J. M., Halgren, E., & Moreno, K. A. (1987). Endogenous potentials after anterior temporal lobectomy. *Neuropsychologia, 25,* 549–557.

Stelmach, G. E., Mullins, D. A., & Teuling, H. L. (1984). Motor programming and temporal patterns in handwriting. In J. Gibbon & L. Allan (Eds.), *Timing and time perception* (pp. 144–157). New York: New York Academy of Sciences.

Stephenson, D. (1982). *Habituation and systemic desensitization.* Unpublished doctoral dissertation, University of Southampton.

Stephenson, D., & Siddle, D. (1983). Theories of habituation. In D. Siddle (Ed.), *Orienting and habituation: Perspectives in human research* (pp. 183–236). New York: Wiley.

Stepien, I. (1972). The magnet reaction, a symptom of prefrontal ablation. *Acta Biologia Experimentia, 34,* 145–160.

Sternberg, S. (1966). High-speed scanning in human memory. *Science, 153,* 652–654.

Sternberg, S. (1969). The discovery of processing stages: Extensions of Donder's method. In W. G. Koster (Ed.), *Attention and performance: II.* Amsterdam: North-Holland.

Storandt, M., Botwinick, J., Danzinger, W. L., Berg, L., & Hughes, C. P. (1984). Psychometric differentiation of mild senile dementia of the Alzheimer type. *Archives of Neurology, 41,* 497–499.

Stromgren, L. S. (1977). The influence of depression on memory. *Acta Psychiatria Scandinavica, 56,* 109–128.

Stroop, J. R. (1935). Studies of interference in serial verbal reactions. *Journal of Experimental Psychology, 18,* 643–662.

Stubbs, A. (1968). The discrimination of stimulus duration by pigeons. *Journal of Experimental Analysis of Behavior, 11,* 223–258.

Stubbs, D. A. (1979). Temporal discrimination and psychophysics. In M. D. Zeiler & P. Harzem (Eds.), *Advances in the analysis of behavior: Reinforcement and the organization of behavior* (Vol. 1, pp. 341–369). Chichester, England: Wiley.

Stuss, D. T. (1987). Contribution of frontal lobe injury to cognitive impairment after closed head injury: Methods of assessment and recent findings. In H. S. Levin, J. Grafman, & H. M. Eisenberg (Eds.), *Neurobehavioral recovery from head injury* (pp. 166–177). New York: Oxford University Press.

Stuss, D. T. (1991). Disturbances of self-awareness after frontal system damage. In G. P. Prigatano & D. L. Schacter (Eds.), *Awareness of deficit after brain injury: Clinical and theoretical issues* (pp. 63–83). New York: Oxford University Press.

Stuss, D. T., Eli, P., Hugenholtz, H., Richard, M. T., LaRochelle, S., Poirier, C. A., & Bell, I. (1985). Subtle neurological deficits in patients with good recovery after closed head injury. *Neurosurgery, 17,* 41–47.

Stuss, D. T., Stethem, L. L., Hugenholtz, H., Picton, T., Pivik, J., & Richard, M. T. (1989). Reaction time after head injury: Fatigue, divided and focused attention, and consistency of performance. *Journal of Neurology, Neurosurgery, and Psychiatry, 52,* 742–748.

Suess, W. M., & Berlyne, D. E. (1978). Exploratory behavior as a function of hippocampal damage, stimulus complexity, and stimulus novelty in the hooded rat. *Behavioral Biology, 23,* 487–499.

Sutton, S., & Ruchkin, D. S. (1984). The late positive complex: Advances and new problems. In R. Karrer, J. Cohen, & P. Tueting (Eds.), *Brain and information: Event-related potentials. Annals of the New York Academy of Sciences, 425,* 1–23.

Sutton, S., Braren, R., Zubin, J., & John, E. R. (1965). Evoked-potential correlates of stimulus uncertainty. *Science, 150,* 1187–1188.

Swets, J. A. (Ed.). (1964). *Signal detection and recognition by human observers.* New York: Wiley.

Swets, J. A. (1973). The relative operating characteristic in psychology. *Science, 182,* 990–1000.

Swets, J. A. (1984). Mathematical models of attention. In R. Parasuraman & D. R. Davies (Eds.), *Varieties of attention* (pp. 183–242). New York: Academic Press.

Sykes, D. H., Douglas, V. I., & Morgenstern, G. (1973). Sustained attention in hyperactive children. *Journal of Child Psychology and Psychiatry, 14,* 213–220.

Syndulko, K., Hansch, E. C., Cohen, S. N., Pearce, J. W., Goldberg, Z., Montan, B., Tourtellotte, W. W., & Potvin, A. R. (1982). Long-latency event-related potentials in normal aging and dementia. In J. Courjon, F. Mauguire, & M. Revol (Eds.), *Clinical applications of evoked potentials in neurology* (pp. 278–285). New York: Raven Press.

Talland, G. A., & Schwab, R. S. (1964). Performance with multiple sets in Parkinson's disease. *Neuropsychologia, 2*, 45–53.

Tanner, W. P., Jr., & Norman, R. Z. (1954). The human use of information: 2. Signal detection for the case of an unknown signal parameter. In *Transactions of the Institute of Radio Engineers, Professional Group on Information Theory, PGIT-R* (pp. 222–227).

Tartaglione, A., Bino, G., Manzino, M., Spadevecchia, L., & Favale, E. (1986). Simple reaction-time changes in patients with unilateral brain damage. *Neuropsychologia, 24*(5), 649–658.

Tassinari, G., Aglioti, S., Chelazzi, L., Marzi, C. A., & Berlucchi, G. (1987). Distribution in the visual field of the costs of voluntarily allocated attention and of the inhibitory aftereffects of covert orienting. *Neuropsychologia, 25*(1A), 55–71.

Taub, E., Williams, M., Barro, G., & Steiner, S. S. (1978). Comparison of the performance of differential and intact monkeys on continuous and fixed rate schedules of reinforcement. *Experimental Neurology, 58*, 1–13.

Taylor, J. A. (1951). The relationship of anxiety to the conditioned eyelid response. *Journal of Experimental Psychology, 41*, 81–92.

Taylor, M. A., Abrams, R., & Gaztanaga, P. (1975). Manic-depressive illness and schizophrenia: A partial validation of research diagnostic criteria utilizing neuropsychological testing. *Comprehensive Psychiatry, 16*, 91–96.

Taylor, M. A., Greenspan, B., & Abrams, R. (1979). Lateralized neuropsychological dysfunction in affective disorder and schizophrenia. *American Journal of Psychiatry, 136*, 1031–1034.

Taylor, M. A., Redfield, J., & Abrams, R. (1981). Neuropsychological dysfunction in schizophrenia and affective disease. *Biological Psychiatry, 16*, 467–478.

Teasdale, G., & Jeannett, B. (1974). Assessment of coma and impaired consciousness. *Lancet, 2*, 81–84.

Teasdale, G., & Mendelow, D. (1984). Pathophysiology of head injuries. In N. Brooks (Ed.), *Closed head injury: Psychological, social and family consequences* (pp. 4–36). New York: Oxford University Press.

Terman, L. M. (1916). *The measurement of intelligence.* Boston: Houghton Mifflin.

Terman, M. (1983). Behavioral analysis and circadian rhythms. In M. D. Zeiler & P. Harzem (Eds.), *Advances in Analysis of Behaviour* (Vol. 3, pp. 103–141). Chichester, England: Wiley.

Terrace, H. S. (1963). Discrimination learning with and without errors. *Journal of the Experimental Analysis of Behavior, 6*, 1–27.

Terrace, H. S. (1968). Discrimination learning, the peak shift, and behavioral contrast. *Journal of the Experimental Analysis of Behavior, 11*, 727–741.

Terrace, H. S. (1971a). Byproducts of discrimination learning. In G. Bower & J. Spence (Eds.), *The psychology of learning and motivation* (Vol. 5). New York: Academic Press.

Terrace, H. S. (1971b). Escape from S⁻. *Learning and Motivation, 2*, 148–163.

Teuber, H. L. (1960). *Visual field defects after penetrating missile wounds of the brain.* Cambridge: Harvard University Press.

Thomas, E. (1972). Excitatory and inhibitory processes. In R. A. Boakes & M. S. Halliday (Eds.), *Inhibition and learning.* London: Academic Press.

Thompson, R. F., & Spencer, W. A. (1966). Habituation: A model phenomenon for the study of neuronal substrates of behavior. *Psychological Review, 73*, 16–43.

Thompson, R. F., Berger, T. W., Berry, S. D., Clark, G. A., Kettner, R. E., Lavond, D. G., Mauk, M. D., McCormick, D. A., Solomon, P. R., & Weisz, D. J. (1982). Neuronal substrates of learning and memory: Hippocampus and other structures. In C. D. Woody (Ed.), *Conditioning: Representation of involved neural functions.* New York: Plenum Press.

Thompson, R.F., Clark, G. A., Donegan, N. H., Lavond, D. G., Madden, J., IV, Mamounas, L. A., Mauk, M. D., & McCormick, D. A. (1984). Neuronal substrates of basic associative learning. In N. Butters & L. Squires (Eds.), *Neuropsychology of memory.* New York: Guilford Press.

Thorndike, E. L. (1911). *Animal intelligence.* New York: Macmillan.

Thorndike, E. L. (1931). *Human learning.* New York: Appleton-Century-Crofts.

Thurstone, L. L. (1938). *Primary mental abilities.* Chicago: University of Chicago Press.

Tikhomirov, O. K., & Vinogradov, Y. E. (1970). Emotions in the function of heuristics. *Soviet Psychology, 8,* 198–223.

Titchener, E. B. (1908). *Lectures on the elementary psychology of feeling and attention.* New York: Macmillan.

Trabasso, T., & Bower, G. H. (1968). *Attention in learning theory and research.* New York: Wiley.

Tranel, D., & Damasio, H. (1989). Intact electrodermal skin conductance responses after bilateral amygdala damage. *Neuropsychologia, 27*(4), 381–390.

Treisman, A. M. (1960). Contextual cues in selective listening. *Quarterly Review of Experimental Psychology, 12,* 242–248.

Treisman, A. M. (1964). Selective attention in man. *British Medical Bulletin, 20,* 12–16.

Treisman, A. M. (1967). Verbal cues, language and meaning in selective attention. *American Journal of Psychology, 77,* 206–219.

Treisman, A. M. (1969). Strategies and models of selective attention. *Psychological Review, 76,* 282–299.

Treisman, A. M., & Davies, A. (1973). Divided attention to ear and eye. In S. Kornblum (Ed.), *Attention and performance IV.* New York: Academic Press.

Treisman, A. M., & Geffen, G. (1967). Selective attention: Perception or response? *Quarterly Journal of Experimental Psychology, 19,* 1–18.

Treisman, A., & Gelade, G. (1980). A feature integration theory of attention. *Cognitive Psychology, 12,* 97–136.

Treisman, M. (1963). Temporal discrimination and the indifference interval: Implications for a model of the "internal clock." *Psychology Monographs, 77,* 1–31.

Treisman, M. (1984). Temporal rhythms and cerebral rhythms. In J. Gibbon & L. Allan (Eds.), *Timing and time perception, Annals of the New York Academy of Sciences* (Vol. 423, pp. 542–565). New York: New York Academy of Sciences.

Trimble, M. R., & Thompson, P. J. (1986). Neuropsychological aspects of epilepsy. In I. Grant & K. Adams (Eds.), *Neuropsychological assessment of neuropsychiatric disorders* (pp. 321–346). New York and Oxford: Oxford University Press.

Trommer, B. L., Hoeppner, J. B., Lorber, R., & Armstrong, K. J. (1988). The go/no-go paradigm in attention deficit disorder. *Annals of Neurology, 24,* 610–614.

Tsukahara, N. (1981). Synaptic plasticity in the mammalian central nervous system. *Annual Review of Neuroscience, 4,* 351–379.

Tsukahara, N. (1984). Classical conditioning mediated by the red nucleus: An approach beginning at the cellular level. In G. Lynch, J. L. McGaugh, & N. M. Weinberger (Eds.), *Handbook of learning and memory* (pp. 165–180). New York: Guilford Press.

Tsukahara, N., Oda, Y., & Notsu, T. (1981). Classical conditioning mediated by the red nucleus in the cat. *Journal of Neuroscience, 1,* 72–79.

Tulving, E. (1983). *Elements of episodic memory.* Oxford, England: Clarendon Press.

Tulving, E., & Thomson, D. M. (1973). Encoding specificity and retrieval processes in episodic memory. *Psychological Review, 80,* 352–373.

Turner, B. H., Mishkin, M., & Knapp, M. (1980). Organization of the amygdalopetal projections from modality-specific cortical association areas in the monkey. *Journal of Comparative Neurology, 191,* 515–543.

Turpin, G., & Siddle, D. A. T. (1979). Effects of stimulus intensity on electrodermal activity. *Psychophysiology, 16,* 582–591.

Tursky, B., Schwartz, G. E., & Crider, A. (1970). Differential patterns of heart rate and skin resistance during a digit-transformation task. *Journal of Experimental Psychology, 83,* 451–457.

Turvey, M. T. (1977). Preliminaries to a theory of action with reference to vision. In R. Shaw & J. Bransford (Eds.), *Perceiving, acting, and knowing: Toward an ecological psychology.* Hillsdale, NJ: Erlbaum.

Tzeng, D. L. J., Lee, A. T., & Wetzel, C. D. (1979). Temporal coding in verbal information processing. *Journal of Experimental Psychology: Human Learning and Memory, 5,* 52–64.

Underwood, G. (1976). *Attention and memory.* New York: Pergamon Press.

Ungerleider, L. G. (1985). The cortical pathways for object recognition and spatial perception. In C. Chagas, R. Grattass, & C. Gross (Eds.), *Pattern recognition mechanisms.* Berlin: Springer.

Ungerleider, L. G., & Desimone, R. (1986). Cortical connections of visual area MT in the macaque. *Journal of Comparative Neurology, 248,* 190–222.

Ungerleider, L. G., & Mishkin, M. (1982). Two cortical visual systems. In D. J. Ingle, M. A. Goodale, & R. J. W. Mansfield (Eds.), *The analysis of visual behavior* (pp. 549–586). Cambridge: MIT Press.

Ursin, H., Wester, K., & Ursin, R. (1979). Habituation to electrical stimulation of the brain in unanesthetized cats. *EEG Clinical Neurophysiology, 23*, 41–49.

Valenstein, E., & Heilman, K. M. (1981). Unilateral hypokinesia and motor extinction. *Neurology, 31*, 445–448.

Valenstein, E., Van Den Abell, T., Watson, R. T., & Heilman, K. M. (1982). Nonsensory neglect from parietotemporal lesions in monkeys. *Neurology, 32*, 1198–1201.

Van Hoesen, G. W. (1982). The parahippocampal gurus. *Trends in Neuroscience, 5*, 345–350.

Van Hoesen, G. W., & Pandya, D. N. (1975). Some connections of the entirhinal (area 28) and perirhinal (area 35) cortices of the rhesus monkey: 3. Efferent connections. *Brain Research, 95*, 39–59.

Van Hoesen, G. W., MacDouglass, J. M., & Mitchell, J. C. (1969). Anatomical specificity of septal projections in active and passive avoidance behavior in the rat. *Journal of Comparative and Physiological Psychology, 68*, 80–89.

Van Hoesen, G. W., Pandya, D. N., & Butters, N. (1972). Cortical afferents to the entorhinal cortex of the rhesus monkey. *Science, 175*, 1471–1473.

Van Zomeren, A. H., & Van Den Burg, W. (1985). Residual complaints of patients 2 years after severe head injury. *Journal of Neurology, Neurosurgery, and Psychiatry, 48*, 21–28.

Van Zomeren, A. H., Brouwer, W. H., & Deelman, B. G. (1984). Attentional deficits: The riddles of selectivity, speed and alertness. In N. Brooks (Ed.), *Closed head injury: Psychological, social and family consequences* (pp. 74–107). New York: Oxford University Press.

Vasko, T., & Kulberg, G. (1979). Results of psychological testing of cognitive functioning in patients undergoing stereotactic psychiatric surgery. In E. R. Hitchcock, H. T. Ballentine, & B. A. Meyerson (Eds.), *Modern concepts in psychiatric surgery*. Amsterdam: Elsevier.

Verbaten, M. N., Woestenburg, J. C., & Sjouw, W. (1979). The influence of visual information on habituation of the electrodermal and the visual orienting reaction. *Biological Psychology, 8*, 189–201.

Verfaellie, M., & Heilman, K. M. (1987). Response preparation and response inhibition after lesions of the medial frontal lobe. *Archives of Neurology, 44*(12). 1265–1271.

Verfaellie, M., Bowers, D., & Heilman, K. M. (1988a). Hemispheric asymmetries in mediating intention, but not selective attention. *Neuropsychologia, 26*(4), 521–531.

Verfaellie, M., Bowers, D., & Heilman, K. M. (1988b). Attentional factors in the occurrence of stimulus-response compatibility effects. *Neuropsychologia, 26*, 435–444.

Verfaellie, M., Rapcsak, S., & Heilman, K. M. (1990). Impaired shifting of attention in Balint's syndrome. *Brain and Cognition, 12*, 195–204.

Verleger, R., & Cohen, R. (1978). Effects of certainty, modality shift, and guess outcome on evoked potentials and reaction times in chronic schizophrenics. *Psychological Medicine, 8*, 81–93.

Vernon, P. A. (1987). *Speed of information processing and intelligence*. Norwood, NJ: Ablex.

Vilkki, J. (1984). Visual hemi-inattention after ventrolateral thalamotomy. *Neuropsychologia, 22*(4), 399–408.

Vinogradova, O. S. (1970). The hippocampus and the orienting reflex. In *Neuronal mechanisms of the orienting reflex* IZD-VO MGU.

Viviani, P., & Terzulo, V. (1980). Space-time invariance in learned motor skills. In G. E. Stelmach & J. Requin (Eds.), *Tutorials in motor behavior* (pp. 525–539). Amsterdam: North Holland.

Von Economo, C. (1931). *Encephalitis lethargica: Its sequelae and treatment*. (K. D. Newman, Trans.). London: Oxford University Press.

Voorhis, S. V., & Hillyard, S. A. (1977). Visual evoked potentials and selective attention to points in space. *Perception and Psychophysics, 22*, 54–62.

Vygotsky, L. S. (1962). *Thought and language* (E. Hanfmann & G. Vakar, Eds. and Trans.). Cambridge: MIT Press.

Wada, J. A. (1986). *Kindling* (3rd ed.). New York: Raven Press.

Wagner, A. R. (1976). Priming in STM: An information-processing mechanism for self-generated or retrieval-generated depression in performance. In T. J. Tighe & A. N. Leaton (Eds.), *Habituation: Perspectives from child development, animal behavior and neurophysiology* (pp. 95–128). Hillsdale, NJ: Erlbaum.

Wagner, A. R. (1979). Habituation and memory. In A. Dickenson & R. A. Boakes (Eds.), *Mechanisms of learning and motivation: A memorial volume to Jerzy Konorski* (pp. 53–82). Hillsdale, NJ: Erlbaum.

Wagner, A. R. (1981). SDP: A model of automatic memory processing in animal behavior. In N. E. Spear

& R. R. Miller (Eds.), *Information processing in animals: Memory mechanisms* (pp. 5–48). Hillsdale, NJ: Erlbaum.

Walker, P. (1978). Short-term visual memory: The importance of the spatial and temporal separation of successive stimuli. *Quarterly Journal of Experimental Psychology, 30,* 665–679.

Walton, P., Halliday, R., Naylor, H., & Callaway, E. (1986). Stimulus intensity, contrast and complexity have additive effects on P3 latency. In J. W. Rohrbaugh, R. Johnson, & R. Parasuraman (Eds.), *Eighth International Conference on Event-Related Potentials of the Brain* (pp. 409–411). Stanford.

Warren, L. R., & Marsh, G. R. (1979). Changes in event related potentials during processing of stroop stimuli. *International Journal of Neurosciences, 9,* 217–223.

Warrington, E. K., & James, M. (1967). An experimental investigation of facial recognition in patients with unilateral cerebral lesions. *Cortex, 3,* 317–326.

Wasserman, E. A., DeLong, R. E., & Larew, M. B. (1984). Temporal order and duration: Their discrimination and retention by pigeons. In J. Gibbon & L. Allan (Eds.), *Timing and time perception, Annals of the New York Academy of Sciences* (Vol. 423, pp. 103–115). New York: New York Academy of Sciences.

Watanbe, M. (1986a). Prefrontal unit activity during delayed conditional go-nogo discrimination in the monkey: 1. Relation to the stimulus. *Brain Research, 382,* 1–14.

Watanbe, M. (1986b). Prefrontal unit activity during delayed conditional go-nogo discrimination in the monkey: 2. Relation to go and no-go responses. *Brain Research, 382,* 15–27.

Waters, W. F., & McDonald, D. G. (1974). Effects of "below-zero" habituation on spontaneous recovery and dishabituation of the orienting response. *Psychophysiology, 11,* 548–558.

Waters, W. F., & McDonald, D. G. (1975). Stimulus and temporal variables in the "below-zero" habituation of the orienting response. *Psychophysiology, 12,* 461–464.

Waters, W. F., & McDonald, D. G. (1976). Repeated habituation and overhabituation of the orienting response. *Psychophysiology, 13,* 231–235.

Waters, W. F., McDonald, D. G., & Koresko, R. L. (1977). Habituation of the orienting response: A gating mechanism subserving selective attention. *Psychophysiology, 14*(3), 228–236.

Waters, W. F., & Wright, D. C. (1979). Maintenance and habituation of the phasic orienting response to competing stimuli in selective attention. In H. D. Kimmel, E. H. Van Olst, & J. F. Orlebeke (Eds.), *The orienting response in humans* (pp. 101–121). Hillsdale, NJ: Erlbaum.

Watson, J. B. (1913). Psychology as the behaviorists view it. *Psychological Review, 20,* 158–177.

Watson, J. B. (1958). *Behaviorism*. Chicago: University of Chicago Press.

Watson, R. T., Heilman, K. M., Cauthen, J. C., & King, F. A. (1973). Neglect after cingulectomy. *Neurology, 23,* 1003–1007.

Watson, R. T., Heilman, K. M., Miller, B. D., & King, F. A. (1974). Neglect after mesencephalic reticular formation lesions. *Neurology, 24,* 294–298.

Watson, R. T., Andriola, M., & Heilman, K. M. (1977). The electroencephalogram in neglect. *Journal of the Neurological Sciences, 34,* 343–348.

Watson, R. T., Miller, B. D., & Heilman, K. M. (1978). Nonsensory neglect. *Annals of Neurology, 3,* 505–508.

Watson, R. T., Valenstein, M., & Heilman, K. M. (1981). Thalamic neglect: The possible role of the medial thalamus and nucleus reticularis thalami in behavior. *Archives of Neurology, 38,* 501–507.

Wechsler, D. (1945). A standardized memory scale for clinical use. *Journal of Psychology, 19,* 87–95.

Wechsler, D. (1981). *The Wechsler Adult Intelligence Scale—Revised Manual*. New York: Psychological Corporation.

Weerts, T. C., & Roberts, R. (1976). The physiological effects of imagining anger provoking and fear provoking scenes. *Psychophysiology, 13,* 174.

Weinberger, D. A., Schwartz, G. E., & Davidson, R. J. (1979). Low anxious, high anxious, and repressive coping styles: Psychometric patterns and behavioral and physiological responses to stress. *Journal of Abnormal Psychology, 88,* 369–380.

Weinberger, N. M., Hopkins, W., & Diamond, D. M. (1984). Physiological plasticity of single neurons in auditory cortex of cat during acquisition of the pupillary conditioned response: 1. Primary fields (AI). *Behavioral Neuroscience, 98,* 171–188.

Weingartner, H., Gold, P., Ballenger, J. D., Smallberg, S. A., Summers, R., Rubinon, D. R., Post, R. M., & Goodwin, F. K. (1981). Effects of vasopressin on human memory functions. *Science, 211,* 601–603.

Weinstein, E. A., & Friedland, R. P. (1977). Hemi-inattention and hemispheric specialization. In E. A. Weinstein & R. P. Friedland (Eds.), *Advances in neurology: Vol. 18, Hemi-inattention and hemispheric specialization*. New York: Raven Press.

Weintraub, S., & Mesulam, M. M. (1985). Mental state assessment of young and elderly adults in behavioral neurology. In M. M. Mesulam (Ed.), *Principles of behavioral neurology* (pp. 71–115). Philadelphia: F. A. Davis.

Weiss, G. (1983). Long term outcome: Findings, concepts and practical implications. In M. Rutter (Ed.), *Developmental neuropsychiatry* (pp. 422–426). New York: Guilford Press.

Welch, K., & Stuteville, P. (1958). Experimental production of neglect in monkeys. *Brain, 81,* 341–347.

Wever, R. A. (1979). *The circadian system of man: Results of experiments under temporal isolation*. New York, Berlin and Heidelberg: Springer-Verlag.

Whitaker, L. A. (1982). Stimulus-response compatibility for left-right discriminations as a function of stimulus position. *Journal of Experimental Psychology: Human Perception and Performance, 8*(6), 865–874.

White, N. (1971). Perseveration by rats with amygdaloid lesions. *Journal of Comparative and Physiological Psychology, 77,* 416–426.

Whitehead, W. E., Drescher, V. M., & Blackwell, B. (1976). Lack of relationship between Autonomic Perception Questionnaire scores and actual sensitivity for perceiving one's heart beat (Abstract). *Psychophysiology, 13,* 177.

Whitehead, W. E., Drescher, V. M., Heiman, P., & Blackwell, B. (1977). Relation of heart rate control to heart beat perception. *Biofeedback and Self-Regulation, 2,* 371–392.

Whitehouse, P. J., Price, D. L., Clark, A. W., Coyle, J. T., & DeLong, M. R. (1981). Alzheimer disease: Evidence for selective loss of cholinergic neurons in the nucleus basalis. *Annals of Neurology, 10,* 122–126.

Wickelgren, W. A. (1975). The long and the short of memory. In D. Deutsch & J. A. Deutsch (Eds.), *Short-term memory*. New York: Academic Press.

Wickelgren, W. A. (1979). Chunking and consolidation: A theoretical synthesis of semantic networks, configuring in conditioning, S-R versus cognitive learning, normal forgetting, the amnesic syndrome, and the hippocampal arousal system. *Psychological Review, 86,* 44–60.

Wickelgren, W. O., & Isaacson, R. L. (1963). Effect of the introduction of an irrelevant stimulus in runway performance of the hippocampectomized rat. *Nature, 200,* 48–50.

Wickens, C. D. (1984). Processing resources in attention. In R. Parasuraman & D. R. Davies (Eds.), *Varieties of attention* (pp. 63–102). New York: Academic Press.

Wickens, C., Kramer, A., Vanasse, L., & Donchin, E. (1983). Performance of concurrent tasks: A psychophysiological analysis of the reciprocity of information-processing resources. *Science, 226,* 1080–1082.

Wielgus, M. S., & Harvey, P. D. (1988). Dichotic listening and recall in schizophrenia and mania. *Schizophrenia Bulletin, 14,* 689–700.

Wiener, N. (1948). *Cybernetics*. New York: Wiley.

Wieser, H. G. (1983). Depth recorded limbic seizures and psychopathology. *Neuroscience and Biobehavioral Review, 7,* 427–440.

Wigal, T., Goodlett, C., Eisenberg, S., Spear, N., Hannigan, J. H., Jr., Donovick, P., Burright, R., & Isaacson, R. (1981). The effects of home contextual cues on spontaneous alternation and conditional place aversion in rats with septal or hippocampal lesions. *Neuroscience Abstracts, 7,* 649.

Wilkinson, R. T. (1962). Muscle tension during mental work under sleep deprivation. *Journal of Experimental Psychology, 64,* 565–571.

Williamson, D. A., & Blanchard, E. B. (1979). Heart rate and blood pressure biofeedback: 2. A review and integration of recent theoretical models. *Biofeedback and Self-Regulation, 4,* 35–50.

Wing, A. M., Keele, S., & Margolin, D. I. (1984). Motor disorder and the timing of repetitive movements. In J. Gibbon & L. Allan (Eds.), *Timing and time perception* (pp. 183–192). New York: New York Academy of Sciences.

Wing, A. M., & Kristofferson, A. B. (1973). Response delays and the timing of discrete motor responses. *Perception and Psychophysics, 14*(1), 5–12.

Winokur, G., Stewart, M., Stern, J., & Pfeiffer, J. (1962). A dynamic equilibrium in GSR habituation: The effect of interstimulus interval. *Journal of Psychosomatic Research, 6,* 117–122.

Wise, S. P., & Desimone, R. (1988). Behavioral neurophysiology: Insights into seeing and grasping. *Science, 242*, 736–741.

Witkin, H. A. (1959). The perception of the upright. *Scientific American, 200*, 50–70.

Wood, R. L. (1987). *Brain injury rehabilitation: A neurobehavioral approach*. Rockville, MD: Aspen.

Woodworth, R. S. (1938). *Experimental psychology*. New York: Holt, Rinehart & Winston.

Woody, C. D. (1967). Characterization of an adaptive filter for the analysis of variable latency neuroelectric signals. *Medical and Biological Engineering, 5*, 539–553.

Woody, C. D. (1970). Conditioned eye blink: Gross potential activity at coronal-pericruciate cortex of the cat. *Journal of Neurophysiology, 33*, 838–850.

Wundt, W. M. (1973). *An introduction to psychology*. New York: Arno.

Wurtz, R. H., Goldberg, M. E., & Robinson, E. L. (1980). Behavioral modulation of visual responses in the monkey: Stimulus selection for attention and movement. *Progress in Psychobiology and Physiological Psychology, 9*, 43–83.

Wurtz, R. H., Goldberg, M. E., & Robinson, D. L. (1982). Brain mechanisms of visual attention. *Scientific American, 246*, 124–135.

Wurtz, R. H., Richmond, B. J., & Newsome, W. T. (1984). Modulation of cortical visual processing by attention, perception, and movement. In G. M. Edelman, W. E. Gall, & W. M. Cowan (Eds.), *Dynamic aspects of neocortical functions* (pp. 195–217). New York: Wiley.

Yarbus, A. L. (1965). *The role of eye movements in the perception of pictures*. Moscow: Nauka.

Yaremko, R. M., & Keleman, K. (1972). The orienting reflex and amount and direction of conceptual novelty. *Psychonomic Science, 27*, 195–196.

Yaremko, R. M., Blair, M. W., & Leckhart, B. T. (1970). The orienting reflex to changes in a conceptual stimulus dimension. *Psychnomic Science, 21*, 115–116.

Yaremko, R. M., Glanville, B. B., & Leckart, B. T. (1972). Imagery-mediated habituation of the orienting reflex. *Psychonomic Science, 27*, 204–206.

Yerkes, R. M., & Dodson, J. D. (1908). The relation of strength of stimulus to rapidity of habit formation. *Journal of Comparative Neurology and Psychology, 18*, 459–482.

Zahn, T. P. (1988). Studies of the autonomic psychophysiology and attention in schizophrenia. *Schizophrenia Bulletin, 14*, 205–208.

Zahn, T. P., Rapoport, J. L., & Thompson, C. L. (1981). Autonomic effects of dextroamphetamine in normal men: Implications for hyperactivity and schizophrenia. *Psychiatry Research, 4*, 39–47.

Zahn, T. P., Van Kammen, D. P., Schooler, C., & Mann, L. S. (1982). Autonomic activity in schizophrenia: Relationships to cortical atrophy and symptomatology. *Psychophysiology, 19*, 593.

Zaidel, D., & Sperry, R. W. (1973). Performance on the Raven's colored progressive matrices test by subjects with cerebral commissurotomy. *Cortex, 9*, 34–39.

Zametkin, A. J., Nordahl, T. E., Gross, M., *et al.* (1990). Cerebral glucose metabolism in adults with hyperactivity of childhood onset. *New England Journal of Medicine, 323*, 1361–1366.

Zaret, B., & Cohen, R. A. (1986). Reversible valproic acid dementia: A case report. *Epilepsia, 27*(3), 234–240.

Zeaman, D., & House, B. J. (1963). The role of attention in retardate discrimination learning. In N. R. Ellis (Ed.), *Handbook of mental deficiency* (pp. 159–223). New York: McGraw-Hill.

Zeki, S., & Shipp, S. (1988). The functional logic of cortical connections. *Nature, 335*, 311–317.

Zola-Morgan, S., & Squire, L. R. (1985a). Amnesia in monkeys following lesions of the mediodorsal nucleus of the thalamus. *Annals of Neurology, 17*, 558–564.

Zola-Morgan, S., & Squire, L. R. (1985b). Complementary approaches to the study of memory: Human amnesia and animal models. In N. Weinberger, J. McGaugh, & G. Lynch (Eds.), *Memory systems of the brain: Animal and human cognitive processes* (pp. 463–477). New York: Guilford Press.

Zola-Morgan, S., & Squire, L. R. (1986). Memory impairment in monkeys following lesions of the hippocampus. *Behavioral Neuroscience, 100*, 155–160.

Zola-Morgan, S., Squire, L. R., & Mishkin, M. (1982). The neuroanatomy of amnesia: Amygdala-hippocampus vs. temporal stem. *Science, 218*, 1337–1339.

Zolovick, A. J. (1972). Effects of lesions and electrical stimulation of the amygdala on hypothalamic-hypophyseal regulation. In B. E. Eleftheriou (Ed.), *The neurobiology of the amygdala* (pp. 643–683). New York: Plenum Press.

Index